Nursing Now!

Nursing Now!
Today's Issues, Tomorrow's Trends

Seventh edition

Joseph T. Catalano, PhD, RN
Program Consultant, Author
President, Oklahoma Nurses Association
Ada, Oklahoma

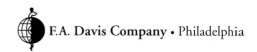 F.A. Davis Company • Philadelphia

F. A. Davis Company
1915 Arch Street
Philadelphia, PA 19103
www.fadavis.com

Printed in the United States of America

Last digit indicates print number: 10 9 8 7 6 5 4 3 2 1

Acquisitions Editor: Megan Klim
Publisher: Joanne P. DaCunha, RN, MSN
Director of Content Development: Darlene D. Pedersen, MSN, APRN, BC
Content Project Manager: Christina L. Snyder
Illustration and Design Manager: Carolyn O'Brien

As new scientific information becomes available through basic and clinical research, recommended treatments and drug therapies undergo changes. The author(s) and publisher have done everything possible to make this book accurate, up to date, and in accord with accepted standards at the time of publication. The author(s), editors, and publisher are not responsible for errors or omissions or for consequences from application of the book, and make no warranty, expressed or implied, in regard to the contents of the book. Any practice described in this book should be applied by the reader in accordance with professional standards of care used in regard to the unique circumstances that may apply in each situation. The reader is advised always to check product information (package inserts) for changes and new information regarding dose and contraindications before administering any drug. Caution is especially urged when using new or infrequently ordered drugs.

Library of Congress Cataloging-in-Publication Data

Catalano, Joseph T., author.
  Nursing now! : today's issues, tomorrow's trends / Joseph T. Catalano. — Seventh edition.
    p. ; cm.
  Includes bibliographical references and index.
  ISBN 978-0-8036-3972-0
  I. Title.
  [DNLM: 1. Nursing—trends. 2. Nursing Care—trends. WY 16.1]

RT82
610.7306'9—dc23

2014027951

Dedication

To all the present and future leaders of the nursing profession who have and will dedicate their time, efforts, and talents to empower nurses across all specialties and practice settings to promote the profession of nursing and improve health care.

Major revisions was the name of the game for the seventh edition of *Nursing Now: Today's Issues, Tomorrow's Trends,* with tons of new information and topics! We believe you will be very pleased with how it turned out. It remains truly unique among issues and trends books. The seventh edition retains the eye-appealing and user-friendly format that made previous editions so popular.

The changes keep coming in health care since the last publication of this text. Major demographic shifts are occurring as baby boomers reach retirement age and the population of new immigrants rapidly expands. As the health-care reform bill continues to be implemented, large groups of individuals now have health-care insurance who didn't in the recent past. Nurses, as always, are at the forefront of these changes, providing care for the elderly and those who speak English as a second language. They have to implement reforms that look more to quality of care rather than the number of services provided.

Thanks to our readers' suggestions, we have added several new chapters. Chapter 13, "Understanding and Dealing Successfully With Difficult Behavior," is an outgrowth of Chapter 12 on communication. It organizes difficult behavior around the five elements of the grieving process. It also provides examples of both what clients might say or do when being difficult and the appropriate responses by the nurse. Because of the emphasis placed on quality of care and outcomes of care in the health-care reform bill, Chapter 15, "Ensuring Quality Care," was added to clearly define what quality is and means and the efforts to achieve it. Chapter 19, "The Politically Active Nurse," discusses the pros and cons of health-care reform in a balanced manner. It is very timely, as the health-care reform bill will be fully implemented over the next few years. Every nurse has noticed the increase of the elderly in the health-care system, so Chapter 23, "Impact of

the Aging Population on Health-Care Delivery," was added and discusses how the large influx of the elderly have added additional stress to an already stressed system of care.

It is also impossible to deny that there has been an increase in natural and man-made disasters over the past few years. Disaster preparedness is something all nurses need to be familiar with, and new Chapter 26, "Preparing for Functioning Effectively in a Disaster," discusses both the role of the public in preparing for disasters and the special preparation nurses need to have to function after a disaster in providing care for the victims.

The chapter on the NCLEX exam was updated to reflect the recent changes by the National Council of State Boards of Nursing, including samples of the new alternative-format questions. All other chapters were revised with the addition of new content and resources. There is new material on bioethics and leadership and management; expanded discussion of SBAR, QSEN, and Six Sigma; discussion of the LACE model and future plans for advanced practice nurses; expanded information on writing and submitting online résumés; and many other new developments in health care.

Graduates from today's nursing programs have opportunities for professional practice and advancement that could only be dreamed of a few years ago. Yes, the demands are many, but the rewards are great. Today's nursing students must learn more, do more, and be more. Students entering nursing schools today come from diverse cultural, personal, and educational backgrounds. They must master a tremendous amount of information and learn a wide variety of skills so that they can pass the licensure exam and become highly skilled registered nurses.

The seventh edition of *Nursing Now! Today's Issues, Tomorrow's Trends* offers students a starting point to influence the future of health care in the

United States. We are very excited about the revised text and believe its quality and content meet the high standards demanded by our readers.

As in past editions, we have retained the interactive format of the text, in addition to the journal layout, current issues boxes, and integrated questions throughout. There are many new graphic illustrations and case studies. We also added a number of new illustrations to increase the visual appeal of the book. The available website with interactive learning activities for students has been updated and expanded.

The book's primary purpose remains the same as in past editions. It presents an overview and synthesis of the important issues and trends that are basic to the development of professional nursing and that affect nursing both today and into the future. Our readers tell us that the book can be used both at the beginning of the student's educational process as an "Introduction to Nursing" course, and also toward the end of the process as an "Issues and Trends" course. Some instructors even use it throughout their programs, incorporating chapters as the content is reflected in their course presentations. Nursing students remain the primary intended audience for *Nursing Now!* However, practicing nurses have reported there is a sufficiently wide range of current issues and topics covered in enough depth to be useful for their practice.

Another dichotomy that nurses face on a daily basis is the ability to hold on to key unchanging principles while working in a constantly changing environment. Simply stated, a nurse's ability to adapt to changes in the health-care system while remaining focused on providing high-quality care is the basis for a successful professional practice. The only way that nurses will be able to effectively practice their profession in a demanding health-care system is to remain firmly rooted in those values and beliefs that have always served as their source of strength. Even more so than in the past, nurses need to look to each other for the inspiration and the strength that allow them to succeed. Professional organizations still serve as the single most powerful force for nurses, and membership in professional organizations is becoming increasingly important.

It is our belief that this book will help future nurses become familiar with the important issues and trends that affect the profession and health care. The nursing profession needs highly skilled nurses who can be civil, teach, do research, solve complicated client problems, provide highly skilled care, obtain advanced degrees, and influence the political realm that so affects all aspects of health care. The leaders of the profession will come from those students who have a clear understanding of what it means to be a professional nurse and are willing to invest effort in attaining their goals.

Joseph T. Catalano, PhD, RN

Acknowledgments

I would like to express my sincere thanks to my students and colleagues who have given their time, knowledge, creativity, and understanding of what is required to promote the profession of nursing both in the present and for the future. I would also like to thank Pam, Sarah, Amanda, Dandy, and Pepper for their tolerance and encouragement as I ignore them while I'm on the computer. And a special thank you to Sharon Bator, whose tireless work and outstanding organizational skills contributed to the editing and revision of several chapters.

Contributors

Mary Abadie, RN, MSN, CPNP
Assistant Professor
Southern University and A&M College
School of Nursing
Baton Rouge, Louisiana

Tonia Aiken, RN, BSN, JD
President and CEO
Aiken Development Group
New Orleans, Louisiana

Sharon M. Bator, RN, MSN, CPE
Assistant Professor
Southern University and A&M College
School of Nursing
Baton Rouge, Louisiana

Barbara Bellfield, MS, RNP-C, RN
Family Nurse Practitioner
Ventura County Public Health
Loma Vista Road
Ventura, California

Cynthia Bienemy, RN, PhD
Director, Louisiana Center for Nursing
Louisiana State Board of Nursing
Baton Rouge, Louisiana

Doris Brown, Med, MS, RN, CNS
Public Health Executive Director
Robert Wood Johnson Nurse Fellow 2006–2009
Baton Rouge, Louisiana

Sandra Brown, RN, DNS, APRN, FNP-BC
Professor
Southern University and A&M College
School of Nursing
Baton Rouge, Louisiana

Joseph T. Catalano, PhD, RN
Program Consultant, Author
Ada, Oklahoma

Sarah T. Catalano
Public Relations Coordinator
Cothran Development Strategies
Ada, Oklahoma

Captain Dr. Leah S. Cullins, MSN, APRN, FNP-BC
NIH-NINR SGI Fellow
Louisiana Commission on HIV, AIDS,
and Hepatitis C
Assistant Professor
Southern University School of Nursing
Undergraduate & Graduate Programs
Southern University and A&M College
Baton Rouge, Louisiana

Lydia DeSantis, RN, PhD, FAAN
University of Miami
School of Nursing
Miami, Florida

Joan Anny Ellis, RN, PhD
Director, Educational Services
Woman's Hospital
Baton Rouge, Louisiana
Associate Professor
Southern University and A&M College
School of Nursing
Baton Rouge, Louisiana

Mary Evans, JD, RN
316 N. Tejon
Colorado Springs, Colorado

Betty L. Fomby-White, RN, PhD
Southern University and A&M College
School of Nursing
Baton Rouge, Louisiana
Associate Faculty
University of Phoenix Online

Donna Gentile O'Donnell, RN, MSN
Deputy Health Commissioner (Retired)
Philadelphia, Pennsylvania

Anita H. Hansberry, RN, MS
Assistant Professor
Southern University and A&M College
School of Nursing
Baton Rouge, Louisiana

Nicole Harder, RN, BN, MPA
Coordinator, Learning Laboratories
Helen Glass Centre for Nursing
Faculty of Nursing
University of Manitoba
Winnipeg, Manitoba, Canada

Jacqueline J. Hill, RN, PhD
Associate Professor & Chair
Undergraduate Nursing Program
Southern University A&M College
Baton Rouge, Louisiana

Edna Hull, PhD, RN, CNE
Associate Professor & Program Director
Our Lady of the Lake College
Metropolitan New Orleans Center
New Orleans, Louisiana

Sharon W. Hutchinson, PhD, MN, RN, CNE
Associate Professor and Chair
Graduate Nursing Programs
Southern University School of Nursing
Southern University and A&M College
Baton Rouge, Louisiana

Joyce Miller, BSN, CPE, CCM
Clarity Hospice of Baton Rouge
Baton Rouge, Louisiana

Karen Mills, MSN, RN
Nurse Family Partnership State Nurse Consultant
Louisiana Office of Public Health
Baton Rouge, Louisiana

Roberta Mowdy, MS, RN
Instructor
Department of Nursing
East Central University
Ada, Oklahoma

Joseph Mulinari, PhD, RN
College of Mt. St. Vincent
Department of Nursing
Riverdale, New York

Linda Newcomer, RN, MSN
Instructor
Department of Nursing
East Central University
Ada, Oklahoma

Robert Newcomer, PhD
Assistant Professor
East Central University
Ada, Oklahoma

Anyadie Onu, RN, MS
Assistant Professor
Southern University and A&M College
School of Nursing
Baton Rouge, Louisiana

Janet S. Rami, RN, PhD
Southern University and A&M College
School of Nursing
Baton Rouge, Louisiana

Mary Ann Remshardt, EdD, RN
Assistant Professor
Department of Nursing
East Central University
Ada, Oklahoma

Viki Saidleman, MS, RN
Instructor
Department of Nursing
East Central University
Ada, Oklahoma

Nancy C. Sharts-Hopko, RN, PhD, FAAN
Professor
Villanova University
Villanova, Pennsylvania

Enrica K. Singleton, RN, PhD
Professor
Southern University and A&M College
School of Nursing
Baton Rouge, Louisiana

Wanda Raby Spurlock, DNS, RN, BC, CNS, FNGNA
Associate Professor
Southern University and A&M College
School of Nursing
Baton Rouge, Louisiana

Melissa Stewart DNS, RN, CPE
Assistant Professor
Our Lady of the Lake College
School of Nursing
Baton Rouge, Louisiana

Cheryl Taylor, PhD, RN
Associate Professor of Nursing
Director Office of Nursing Research
NLN Consultant to National Student Nurses
Association
Southern University and A&M College
School of Nursing
Baton Rouge, Louisiana

Karen Tomajan, MS, RN, NEA-BC
Clinical/Regulatory Consultant
INTEGRIS Baptist Medical Center
Oklahoma City, Oklahoma

Esperanza Villanueva-Joyce, EdD, CNS, RN
National Dean for Academics
Education Affiliates

Kathleen Mary Young, RN, C, MA
Instructor
Western Michigan University
Kalamazoo, Michigan

Contents

Unit 1 **The Growth of Nursing** 1

1   The Development of a Profession   3
2   Historical Perspectives   20
3   Theories and Models of Nursing   38
4   The Process of Educating Nurses   72
5   The Evolution of Licensure, Certification, and Nursing Organizations   99

Unit 2 **Making the Transition to Professional** 119

6   Ethics in Nursing   121
7   Bioethical Issues   145
8   Nursing Law and Liability   178
9   NCLEX: What You Need to Know   205
10   Reality Shock in the Workplace   226

Unit 3 **Leading and Managing** 255

11   Leadership, Followership and Management   257
12   Communication, Negotiation, and Conflict Resoloution   285
13   Understanding and Dealing Successfully With Difficult Behavior   310
14   Health-Care Delivery Systems   353
15   Ensuring Quality Care   376
16   Delegation in Nursing   396
17   Incivility: The Antithesis of Caring   411
18   Nursing Informatics   429
19   The Politically Active Nurse   452

Unit 4 **Issues in Delivering Care** 483

20   The Healt-Care Debate: Best Allocation of Resources for the Best Outcomes   485
21   Spirituality and Health Care   519
22   Cultural Diversity   540
23   Impact of the Aging Population on Health-Care Delivery   565

24   Nursing Research and Evidence-Based Practice   581
25   Integrative Health Practices   611
26   Preparing for Functioning Effectively in a Disaster   646
27   Developments in Current Nursing Practice   674

Glossary   688
Index   705

1

The Growth of Nursing

The Development of a Profession

1

Joseph T. Catalano

Learning Objectives

After completing this chapter, the reader will be able to:

- Define the terms **position, job, occupation,** and **profession**
- Compare the three approaches to defining a profession
- Analyze those traits defining a profession that nursing has attained
- Evaluate why nursing has failed to attain some of the traits that define a profession
- Correlate the concept of power with its important characteristics

WHAT IS A PROFESSION?

Since the time of Florence Nightingale, each generation of nurses, in its own way, has fostered the movement to professionalize the image of nurses and nursing. The struggle to change the status of nurses—from that of female domestic servants to one of high-level health-care providers who base their protocols on scientific principles—has been a primary goal of nursing's leaders for many years. Yet some people, both inside and outside the profession of nursing, question whether the search for and attainment of professional status is worth the effort and price that must ultimately be paid.

At some levels in nursing, the question of **professionalism** takes on immense significance. However, to the busy **staff nurse**—who is trying to allocate client assignments for a shift, distribute the medications at 9 a.m. to 24 clients, and supervise two aides, a licensed practical nurse (LPN) or licensed vocational nurse (LVN) and a nursing student—the issue may not seem very significant at all.

Indeed, when nurses were first developing their identity separately from that of physicians, there was no thought about their being part of a **profession.** Over the years, as the scope of practice and responsibilities have expanded, nurses have increasingly begun to consider what they do to be professional activities.

This chapter presents some of the current thoughts concerning professions and where nursing stands in relation to these viewpoints.

APPROACHES TO DEFINING A PROFESSION

In common use, terms such as *position, job, occupation, profession, professional,* and *professionalism* often are used interchangeably and incorrectly. The following definitions will clarify what is meant by these terms within this text:

Position: A group of tasks assigned to one individual

Job: A group of positions similar in nature and level of skill that can be carried out by one or more individuals

Occupation: A group of jobs similar in type of work that are usually found throughout an industry or work environment

Profession: A type of occupation that requires prolonged preparation and formal qualifications and meets certain higher level criteria (discussed later in this chapter) that raise it to a level above that of an occupation[1]

Professional: A person who belongs to and practices a profession (The term *professional* is probably the most misused of all these terms when describing people who are clearly involved in jobs or occupations, such as a "professional truck driver," "professional football player," or even "professional thief.")

Professionalism: The demonstration of high-level personal, ethical, and skill characteristics of a member of a profession[2]

For almost 100 years, experts in social science have been attempting to develop a "foolproof" approach to determining what constitutes a profession but with only minimal success. Three common models are the process approach, the power approach, and, most widely accepted, the trait approach.

Process Approach

The process approach views all occupations as points of development into a profession situated along a continuum ranging from position to profession:

Continuum of Professional Development:

Position $\longleftrightarrow$ Profession

Using this approach, the question becomes not whether nursing and truck driving are professions but where they are located along the continuum. Occupations such as medicine, law, and the ministry are widely accepted by the public as being closest to the professional end of the continuum.[3] Other occupations may be less clearly defined.

What Do You Think?

Do you really care if nursing is a profession? How will it affect the way you practice nursing?

The major difficulty with this approach is that it lacks criteria on which to base judgments. Final determination of the status of an occupation or profession depends almost completely on public perception of the activities of that occupation. Nursing has always had a rather negative public image when it comes to being viewed as a profession.

> *Over the years, as the scope of practice and responsibilities have expanded, nurses have increasingly begun to consider what they do to be professional activities.*

Power Approach

The power approach uses two criteria to define a profession:

1. How much independence of practice does this occupation have?
2. How much power does this occupation control?

The concept of power is discussed later in this chapter, but in this context, it refers to political power and the amount of money that the person in that occupation earns.[4]

Using this determinant, occupations such as medicine, law, and **politics** clearly would be considered professions. The members of these occupations earn high incomes, practice their skills with a great deal of independence; and exercise significant power over individuals, the public, and the political community, both individually and in organized groups. The ministry is generally perceived as having power and influence. However, most people in this group, except for a few individuals such as television evangelists, have relatively low income levels. Nursing, of course, with its comparatively lower salaries, low membership in professional organizations, and perceived lack of political power, would clearly not meet the power criteria for a profession.

The question that comes to mind is whether power, independence of practice, and high income are the only elements that determine professional status. Although those three factors confer status in our culture, other elements can be considered significant in how a profession is viewed. For example, to many people, members of the clergy have a great deal of power when they act as counselors, speakers of the truth, and community leaders.

Trait Approach

Of the many researchers and theorists who have attempted to identify the traits that define a profession, Abraham Flexner, Elizabeth Bixler, and Eliza Pavalko are most widely accepted as the leaders in the field. These three social scientists have determined that the following common characteristics are important:

- High intellectual level
- High level of individual responsibility and **accountability**
- Specialized body of knowledge
- Knowledge that can be learned in institutions of higher education
- Public service and altruistic activities
- Public service valued over financial gain
- Relatively high degree of **autonomy** and independence of practice
- Need for a well-organized and strong organization representing the members of the profession and controlling the quality of practice
- A **code of ethics** that guides the members of the profession in their practice
- Strong professional identity and commitment to the development of the profession
- Demonstration of professional competency and possession of a legally recognized license[4]

NURSING AS A PROFESSION

How does nursing compare with other professions when measured against these widely accepted professional traits? The profession of nursing meets most of the criteria but falls short in a few areas.

High Intellectual Level

In the early stages of the development of nursing practice, this criterion did not apply. Florence Nightingale raised the bar for education, and graduates of her school were considered to be highly educated compared with other women of that time.

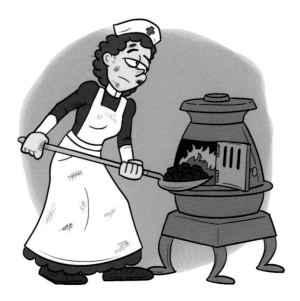

However, by today's standards, most of the tasks performed by these early nurses are generally considered to be menial and routine.

On the other hand, as health care has advanced and made great strides in technology, pharmacology, and all branches of the physical sciences, a high level of intellectual functioning is required for even relatively simple nursing tasks, such as taking a client's temperature or blood pressure using automated equipment. On a daily basis, nurses use **assessment** skills and knowledge, have the ability to reason, and make routine judgments based on clients' conditions. Without a doubt, professional nurses must function at a high intellectual level.

High Level of Individual Responsibility and Accountability

Not too long ago, a nurse was rarely, if ever, named as a **defendant** in a malpractice suit. In general, the public did not view nurses as having enough knowledge to be held accountable for errors that were made in client care. This is not the case in the health-care system today. Nurses are often the primary, and frequently the only, defendants named when errors are made that result in injury to the client. Nurses must be accountable and demonstrate a high level of individual responsibility for the care and services they provide.[5]

The concept of accountability has legal, ethical, and professional implications that include accepting responsibility for actions taken to provide **client** care and for the consequences of actions that are not performed. Nurses can no longer state that "the physician told me to do it" as a method of avoiding responsibility for their actions.

Specialized Body of Knowledge

Most early nursing skills were based either on traditional ways of doing things or on the intuitive knowledge of the individual nurse. As nursing developed into an identifiable, separate discipline, a specialized body of knowledge called *nursing science* was compiled through the research efforts of nurses with advanced educational degrees.[6] As the body of specialized nursing knowledge continues to grow, it forms a theoretical basis for the best practices movement in nursing today. As more nurses obtain advanced degrees, conduct research, and develop philosophies and theories about nursing, this body of knowledge will increase in scope and quantity.

Evidence-Based Practice

In professional nursing today, there is an increasing emphasis on evidence-based practice. Almost all of the currently used nursing theories address this issue in some way. Simply stated, evidence-based practice is the practice of nursing in which interventions are based on data from research that demonstrates that they are appropriate and successful. It involves a systematic process of uncovering, evaluating, and using information from research as the basis for making decisions about and providing client care.[7] Many nursing practices and interventions of the past were performed merely because they had always been done that way (accustomed practice) or because of deductions from physiological or pathophysiological information. Clients are now more sophisticated and knowledgeable about health-care issues and demand a higher level of knowledge and skill from their health-care providers.

The development of information technology has made evidence-based practice in nursing a reality. In the past, nurses relied primarily on units within their own facilities for information about the success of treatments, decisions about health care, and outcomes for clients. Nursing education now requires nursing students to perform Web-based research for papers and projects so that by the time of graduation, they feel comfortable accessing a

> " *Evidence-based practice is the practice of nursing in which interventions are based on data from research that demonstrates that they are appropriate and successful.* "

wide range of the best and most current information through electronic sources. Of course, one of the key limiting factors of evidence-based practice is the quality of the information on which the practice is based. Evaluating the quality of information on the Web can be difficult at times.

The first step in developing an evidence-based practice is to identify exactly what the intervention is supposed to accomplish. Once the goal or client outcome is identified, the nurse needs to evaluate current practices to determine whether they are delivering the desired client outcomes. If the current practices are unsuccessful or if the nurse feels they can be more efficient with fewer complications, research sources need to be collected. These can be from published journal articles (either electronic or hard copy) and from presentations at research or practice conferences, which often present the most current information. Then a plan should be developed to implement the new findings. This process can be applied to changing policy and procedures or developing training programs for facility staff. Research data should always be used when initiating new practices or modifying old ones.

Public Service and Altruistic Activities

When defining nursing, almost all major nursing theorists include a statement that refers to a goal of helping clients adapt to illness and achieve their highest level of functioning. The public (variously referred to as *consumers, patients, clients, individuals,* or *humans*) is the focal point of all nursing models and nursing practice. The public service function of nursing has always been recognized and acknowledged by society's willingness to continue to educate nurses in public, tax-supported institutions and in private schools. In addition, nursing has been viewed universally as an altruistic profession composed of selfless individuals who place the lives and well-being of their clients above their personal safety. In the earliest days, dedicated nurses provided care for victims of deadly plagues with little regard for their own welfare. Today, nurses are found in remote and often hostile areas, providing care for the sick and dying, working 12-hour shifts, being on call, and working rotating shifts.

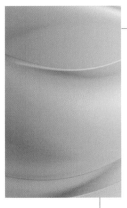

Issues Now

Websites: Friends or Foes?

Have a paper or report to do for class? Need information on pheochromocytoma, Smith-Strang disease, Kawasaki disease? No problem, look it up on the Web, right? Well, yes and no. Without question, there is a tremendous amount of information about almost any subject available just a few mouse clicks away. But the bigger question is, How good is that information? Anyone can post almost anything online these days, and there are no organizations or agencies that oversee or review the information for quality, accuracy, or objectivity. So how are you supposed to know what is good and what is not? Although there is no foolproof method for determining the quality of any given website, some telltale markers can point you in the right direction when you are rating the quality of the information you seek.

Marker 1: Peer Review

All major professional journals have a peer-review process that requires any manuscripts submitted to be reviewed by two or three professionals who are considered experts, or at least knowledgeable, in the subject matter. Peer review is one of the key elements in ensuring the accuracy of the information in the manuscript. When considering a Web source, look for a clear statement of the source of the information and how that information is reviewed. If the information is from an established source, such as a recognized professional journal, it has been peer reviewed and has a higher degree of accuracy. Examine the format and writing style of the document. If it seems to be very choppy, or if the style, tone, or point of view changes throughout the article, it is an indication that it was not well edited and probably not peer reviewed. Use the information with caution.

Marker 2: Author Credentials

The name of the author and his or her titles and credentials should be listed. Be cautious if no author or publisher is listed. Of course, anyone can use another person's name as the author, but it is relatively easy to cross-check authors' names through other databases, such as those found in libraries. Before accepting the information as gospel, it is probably worth looking up the author and seeing what other articles or books he or she has written. Another key to determining author credentials is to establish who owns the website. In general, personal website pages are less likely to contain authoritative information. You can also look at the last three letters in the website address. The ones that end in *.gov, .org,* or *.edu* tend to have higher-quality information. Also, see whether the information has a copyright. If the information is copyrighted, the person felt strongly enough about what he or she was posting to go to the effort of making sure that no one else could use it as their original information.

Marker 3: Prejudice and Bias

Although there is almost always a small degree of prejudice and bias in all written material, most legitimate authors strive to be as objective as possible. Many times, if you read a document with a critical eye, you can discern obvious prejudicial

(continued)

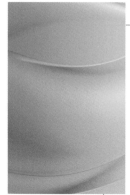

Issues Now continued

viewpoints. See if the author has a vested interest in the content of the document. For example, an article about the effects of tobacco use on the respiratory system written by a scientist who was hired by the R. J. Reynolds Company would probably have a decidedly different viewpoint than an article written by a scientist who was employed by the National Health Information Center. See if contact information is provided by the author and who the sponsor or publisher of the document is. If these are not provided, be suspicious about the information.

Marker 4: Timeliness

Of course, all of us want the most recent information we can find and sometimes mistakenly assume that because it is on the Web, it is new. Some forms of the Web have been around since Tim Berners-Lee invented the World Wide Web in 1989, so some of the material can be very outdated. See if you can determine when the site was last updated and how extensively the information was revised. It is also a good practice to look to other sources (e.g., Web, journals, books) to compare the material for currency. Many websites have links where you can access other related information. If those links have messages such as "Page not found" or "Link no longer available," be extremely cautious with the information. Good links should connect you to other reliable sites.

Marker 5: Presentation

Although the old saying is that "you can't tell a book by its cover," experienced Web surfers can often tell a lot about a website by its presentation. Some look well developed and professional, and others look very amateurish. There is no guarantee that the slick-looking websites are better, but it is one factor to consider in the overall evaluation of the information you are seeking. Take a look at the graphics. They should be balanced with the text and help explain or demonstrate information in the text. If the graphics seem to be just decorative, it should raise a red flag about the content of the site. Some sites use a compressed format that requires special programs such as Adobe Acrobat to view them. If you do not have access to these programs, the information in the site is unusable. Move on to the next site.

In summary, the Internet can be a valuable source of information about a wide variety of subjects. However, each source needs to be evaluated carefully. Following the five markers discussed here will place you on the path to deciding the quality of the information presented in any website.

Sources: Carlson EA. What to look for when evaluating Web sites. *Orthopaedic Nursing*, 28(4): 199–202, 2009; Golterman L, Banasiak NC. Primary care approaches. Evaluating web sites. Reliable child health resources for parents. *Pediatric Nursing*, 37(2):81–83, 2011; Spector ND, Matz PS, Levine LJ, Gargiulo KA, McDonald MB 3rd, McGregor RS. e-Professionalism: Challenges in the age of information. *Journal of Pediatrics*, 156(3):345–346, 2010.

Few individuals enter nursing to become rich and famous. It is likely that those who do so for these reasons quickly become disappointed and move on to other career fields. Although the pay scale has increased tremendously since the 1990s, nursing is, at best, a middle-income occupation. Surveys among students entering nursing programs continue to indicate that the primary reason for wishing to become a nurse is to "help others" or "make a difference" in someone's life and to have "job security." Rarely do these beginning students include "to make a lot of money" as their motivation.[7]

Well-Organized and Strong Representation

Professional organizations represent the members of the profession and control the quality of professional practice. The National League for Nursing (NLN) and the American Nurses Association (ANA) are the two major national organizations that represent nursing in today's health-care system. The NLN is primarily responsible for regulating the quality of the educational programs that prepare nurses for the practice of nursing, whereas the ANA is more concerned with the quality of nursing practice in the daily health-care setting. These and other organizations are discussed in more detail in Chapter 5.

Both these groups are well organized, but neither can be considered powerful when compared with other professional organizations, such as the American Hospital Association, the American Medical Association (AMA), or the American Bar Association (ABA). One reason for their lack of strength is that fewer than 10 percent of all nurses in the United States are members of any professional organization at the national level.[3] Many nurses do belong to specialty organizations that represent a specific area of practice, but these lack sufficient political power to produce changes in health-care laws and policies at the national level.

Nurses' Code of Ethics

Nursing has several codes of ethics that are used to guide nursing practice. The ANA Code of Ethics for Nurses, the most widely used in the United States, was first published in 1971 and updated in 1985 and 2001. In 2013, the ANA began surveying its members for input into possible changes in the Code. The current 2014 ANA Code of Ethics, while maintaining the integrity found in earlier versions, is now more relevant to current health-care and nursing practices.

This code of ethics is recognized by other professions as a standard with which others are compared. The nurses' code of ethics and its implications are discussed in greater detail in Chapter 6.

Competency and Professional License

Nurses must pass a national licensure examination to demonstrate that they are qualified to practice nursing. Nurses are allowed to practice only after passing this examination. The granting of a nursing **license** is a legal activity conducted by the individual state under the **regulations** contained in that state's nurse practice act.

WHEN NURSING FALLS SHORT OF THE CRITERIA

Before Florence Nightingale practiced nursing, people considered it to be unnecessary, if not outright dangerous, to educate nurses through independent nursing programs in publicly supported educational institutions. As nursing has developed, particularly in the United States, the recognition of the intellectual nature of the practice, as well as the vast amount of knowledge required for the job, has led to a belief by some nursing leaders that college education for nurses is now a necessity.[8-10]

Autonomy and Independence of Practice

Historically, the handmaiden or servant relationship of the nurse to the physician was widely accepted.[11] It was based on several factors, including social norms. For example, women became nurses, whereas men became physicians; women were subservient to men, the nature of the work being such that nurses cleaned and physicians cured. In terms of the relative levels of education of the two groups, the average nursing program lasted for 1 year, whereas physician education lasted for 6 to 8 years.

Unfortunately, despite efforts to expand nursing practice into more independent areas through updated nurse practice legislation, nursing retains much of its subservient image. In reality, nursing is both an independent and interdependent discipline. Nurses in all health-care settings must work closely with physicians, hospital administrators, pharmacists, and other groups in the provision of care. In some cases, nurses in **advanced practice** roles, such as **nurse practitioners,** can and do establish their own independent practices. Most state

nurse practice acts allow nurses more independence in their practice than they realize. To be considered a true profession, nursing will need to be recognized by other disciplines as having practitioners who practice nursing independently.

Professional Identity and Development

The issue of job versus career is in question here. A job is a group of positions, similar in nature and level of skill, that can be carried out by one or more individuals. There is relatively little commitment to a job, and many individuals move from one job to another with little regard to the long-term outcomes. A career, in contrast, is usually viewed as a person's major lifework, which progresses and develops as the person grows older. Careers and professions have many of the same characteristics, including a formal education, full-time employment, requirement for lifelong learning, and a dedication to what is being achieved. Although an increasing number of nurses view nursing as their life's work, many still treat nursing more as a job.

The problem becomes circular. The reason nurses lack a strong professional identity and do not consider nursing as a lifelong career is that nursing does not have full status as a profession.[11] Until nurses are fully committed to the profession of nursing, identify with it as a profession, and are dedicated to its future development, nursing will probably not achieve professional status.

MEMBERS OF THE HEALTH-CARE TEAM

The health-care delivery system employs large numbers of diagnosticians, technicians, direct care providers, administrators, and support staff (Table 1.1). It is estimated that more than 300 job titles are used to describe health-care workers. Among these are nurses, physicians, physician assistants, social workers, physical therapists, occupational therapists, respiratory therapists, clinical psychologists, and pharmacists. All these individuals provide services that are essential to daily operation of the health-care delivery system in this country.

Of particular importance among this array of health-care workers are various types of nurses: Registered nurses, licensed practical (vocational) nurses, nurse practitioners, case managers, and clinical nurse specialists. Each of these requires a different type of educational background, clinical expertise, and, sometimes, professional credentialing. In general, all nurses make valuable contributions within the health-care delivery system. There has been an increased demand for nurses who are educated to deliver care in the community setting and in long-term health-care settings rather than in the hospital. There has also been a need for nurse case managers who are prepared to coordinate care for vulnerable populations requiring costly services over extended periods. Nursing education programs are attempting to meet these needs by preparing individuals who can practice independently and autonomously, network, collaborate, and coordinate services. These programs also offer more clinical experiences in rehabilitation, nursing home, and community settings.

What Do You Think?

List and rate several of your recent experiences with the health-care system. In what roles did you observe registered nurses functioning?

Registered Nurses, Licensed Practical Nurses, and Unlicensed Assistive Personnel

Registered nurses (RNs) who have been educated at the associate, diploma, or baccalaureate level have traditionally been considered the cornerstone of the current health-care delivery system. In the past, most RNs worked within hospital settings and provided direct client care and nursing administration functions within these facilities. Owing to past trends in health-care funding, there were fewer hospital admissions, which temporarily decreased the demand for RNs in acute care facilities and increased the need for well-prepared nurses who could function autonomously within the community. However, current trends in population and health care have demonstrated a need for RNs in both acute care and community settings. The need still remains within institutional settings for licensed practical nurses (LPNs) and unlicensed assistive personnel (UAPs) who work under the supervision of an RN. This pattern of care is particularly evident in nursing homes and other long-term care facilities.[12]

Advanced Practice Nurses

For individuals who are unfamiliar with the health-care delivery system, it is sometimes difficult to

Table 1.1 **Other Key Health-Care Team Members**

Title	Credential	Practice
Physician (MD)	License—Medical	Medical—limited only by specialization; some serve as primary care providers.
Physician (DO)	License—Osteopath	Medical, with focus on body movement and holistic health—similar to MD. Can serve as primary care providers.
Physician (DC)	License—Chiropractor	Limited—focus on spinal column and nervous system. Unable to prescribe medications.
Physician (DPM)	License—Podiatry	Limited—foot problems. Can prescribe medications, perform foot surgery.
Physician assistant	Certification—no individual license	Practices on physician's license. Practice limited by medical practice act and wishes of supervising physician.
Social worker	License	Increasingly important as health care becomes more complex. Resolves financial, housing, psychosocial, and employment problems; does discharge planning and assists clients in transfer between facilities. May serve in case management roles to coordinate services.
Physical therapist	License	Focuses on helping clients maintain or regain the highest level of function possible after strokes, spinal cord injury, arthritis, or residual effects of traumatic accidents. Helps prevent physical decline and regain the ability to groom, eat, and walk through individualized range of motion and exercise programs. Therapy occurs in hospitals, clinics, or the community.
Respiratory therapist	License	Strives to restore normal or as near to normal pulmonary functioning as possible by conducting diagnostic tests and administering treatments that have been prescribed by a physician.
Clinical psychologist	License	Helps clients to manage mental health problems. Private practice, clinics.
Pharmacist	License	Distributes prescribed and over-the-counter medications, educates clients, monitors appropriate medication selections, detects interactions and untoward responses in community pharmacies and institutional settings. Valuable resource for nurses.

understand the similarities and differences between nursing titles and roles. This confusion is particularly evident in the case of clinical nurse specialists (CNSs) and nurse practitioners (NPs), who are sometimes collectively referred to as advanced practice registered nurses (APRNs).[13]

The Nurse Practitioner

In general, NPs are prepared to provide direct client care in primary care settings, focusing on health promotion, illness prevention, early diagnosis, and treatment of common health problems. Their educational preparation varies, but in most cases individuals successfully complete a graduate nurse practitioner program and are certified by the American Nurses Credentialing Center (ANCC) or an appropriate professional nursing organization. Depending on the individual state nurse practice act, NPs have a range of responsibilities for diagnosing diseases and prescribing both treatments and medications. A growing number of states now grant

NPs direct third-party reimbursement for their services without a physician.

The Clinical Nurse Specialist

Clinical nurse specialists usually practice in secondary- or tertiary-care settings and focus on care of individuals who are experiencing an acute illness or an exacerbation of a chronic condition. In general, they are prepared at the graduate level and are ANCC certified.[14] These highly skilled practitioners are comfortable working in high-tech environments with seriously ill individuals and their families. Because of the nature of their work, they are excellent health-care educators and physician collaborators.

Attempts have been made to combine the roles of the CNS and NP so that the best qualities of both roles are preserved. The goal of this combination is to provide high-quality care to individuals in a wide array of health-care settings who have a wide range of health problems. Advocates of this movement include the NLN, the American Association of Colleges of Nursing (AACN), and the ANA. Titling for this new blended role is unconfirmed, and state legislatures may make the final decisions through their licensing laws.[14] As such, titling, educational preparation, and practice privileges will probably vary from one state to another.

Case Managers

One argument for the blended NP–CNS role is the need for case managers who possess the expertise of both levels of preparation. Case managers coordinate services for clients with high-risk or long-term health problems who have access to the full continuum of health-care services. Case managers provide services in various settings, such as acute care facilities, rehabilitation centers, and community agencies. They also work for managed care companies, insurance companies, and private case management agencies. Their roles vary according to the circumstances of their employment; however, their overall goal is to coordinate the use of health-care services in the most efficient and cost-effective manner possible.[15]

Case management is the glue that holds health-care services together across practitioners, agencies, funding sources, locations, and time. Titling, educational preparation, and certification of nurse case managers are now available. The ANCC has developed certification eligibility criteria for nurse case managers, and an examination is available. At this time, case managers can be physicians, social workers, RNs, and even well-intentioned laypersons with little health-care education.

EMPOWERMENT IN NURSING

One concern that has plagued nursing, almost from its development as a separate health-care specialty, is the relatively large amount of personal responsibility shouldered by nurses combined with a relatively small amount of control over their practice. Even in the more enlightened atmosphere of today's society, with its concerns about equal opportunity, equal pay, and collegial relationships, many nurses still seem uncomfortable with the concepts of power and control in their practice. Their discomfort may arise from the belief that nursing is a helping and caring profession whose goals are separate from issues of power.

Historically, nurses have been mostly powerless, and previous attempts at gaining power and control over their practice have been met with much resistance from groups who benefit from making sure that nurses remain without authority. Nevertheless, all nurses use an authoritative voice in their daily practice, even if they do not realize it. Until nurses understand the sources of their influence, how to increase it, and how to use it in providing client care, they will be relegated to a subservient position in the health-care system.

The Nature of Power

The term *power* has many meanings. From the standpoint of nursing, power is probably best defined as the ability or capacity to exert influence over another person or group of persons.[16] In other words, power is the ability to get other people to do things even when they do not want to do them. Although power in itself is neither good nor bad, it can be used to produce either good or bad results.

> *Depending on the individual state nurse practice act, NPs have a range of responsibilities for diagnosing diseases and prescribing both treatments and medications.*

Power is always a two-way street. By its very definition, when power is exerted by one person, another person is affected; that is, the use of power by one person requires that another person give up some of his or her power. Individuals are always in a state of change, either increasing their power or losing some; the balance of power rarely remains static. **Empowerment** refers to the increased amount of power that an individual or group is either given or gains.

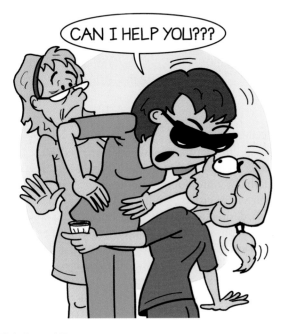

CAN I HELP YOU???

Origins of Power

If power is such an important part of nursing and the practice of nurses, where does it come from? Although there are many sources, some of them would be inappropriate or unacceptable for those in a helping and caring profession. The following list includes some of the more accessible and acceptable sources of power that nurses should consider using in their practice:[16]

- Referent
- Expert
- Reward
- Coercive
- Legitimate
- Collective

Referent Power

The referent source of power depends on establishing and maintaining a close personal relationship

with someone. In any close personal relationship, one individual often will do something he or she would really rather not do because of the relationship. This ability to change the actions of another is an exercise of power.

Nurses often obtain power from this source when they establish and maintain good therapeutic relationships with their clients. Clients take medications, tolerate uncomfortable treatments, and participate in demanding activities that they would likely prefer to avoid because the nurse has good relationships with them. Likewise, nurses who have good collegial relationships with other nurses, departments, and physicians are often able to obtain what they want from these individuals or groups in providing care to clients.

Expert Power

The expert source of power derives from the amount of knowledge, skill, or expertise that an individual or group has. This power source is exercised by the individual or group when knowledge, skills, or expertise is either used or withheld in order to influence the behavior of others. Nurses should have at least a minimal amount of this type of power because of their education and experience. It follows logically that increasing the level of nurses' education will, or should, increase this expert power. As nurses attain and remain in positions of power longer, the increased experience will also aid the use of expert power. Nurses in advanced practice roles are good examples of those who have expert power. Their additional education and experience provide these nurses with the ability to practice skills at a higher level than nurses prepared at the basic education level.

By demonstrating their knowledge of the client's condition, recent laboratory tests, and other elements that are vital to the client's recovery, nurses demonstrate their expert power. This knowledge may increase the amount of respect they are given by physicians. Nurses access this expert source of power when they use their knowledge to teach, counsel, or motivate clients to follow a plan of care. Nurses can also use expert power when dealing with physicians.

Power of Rewards

The reward source of power depends on the ability of one person to grant another some type of reward for specific behaviors or changes in behavior. The rewards can take on many different forms, including personal favors, promotions, money, expanded privileges, and eradication of punishments. Nurses, in their daily provision of care, can use this source of power to influence client behavior. For example, a nurse can give a client extra praise for completing the prescribed range-of-motion exercises. There are many aspects of the daily care of clients over which nurses have a substantial amount of reward power. This reward source of power is also the underlying principle in the process of behavior modification.

Coercive Power

The coercive source of power is the flip side of the reward source. The ability to reprimand, withhold rewards, and threaten punishment is the key element underlying the coercive source of power. Although nurses do have access to this source of power, it is probably one that they use minimally, if at all. Not only does the use of coercive power destroy therapeutic and personal relationships, but it can also be considered unethical and even illegal in certain situations. Threatening clients with an injection if they do not take their oral medications may motivate them to take those medications, but it is generally not considered to be a good example of a therapeutic communication technique.

Legitimate Power

The legitimate source of power depends on a legislative or legal act that gives the individual or organization a right to make decisions that they might not otherwise have the authority to make. Most obviously, political figures and **legislators** have this source of power. This power can also be disseminated and delegated to others through legislative acts. In nursing, the state board of nursing has access to the legitimate source of power because of its establishment under the nurse practice act of that state. Similarly, nurses have access to the legitimate source of power when they are licensed by the state under the provisions in the nurse practice act or when they are appointed to positions within a health-care agency. Nursing decisions made about client care can come only from individuals who have a legitimate source of power to make those decisions—that is, licensed nurses.

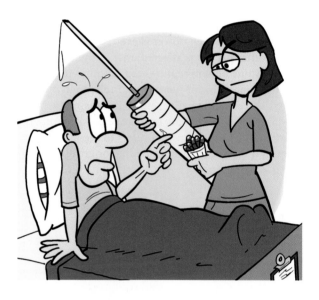

Collective Power

The collective source of power is often used in a broader context than individual client care and is the underlying source for many other sources of power. When a large group of individuals who have similar beliefs, desires, or needs become organized, a collective source of power exists.[17] For individuals who belong to professions, the professional organization is the focal point for this source of power. The main goal of any organization is to influence policies that affect the members of the organization. This influence is usually in the form of political activities carried out by politicians and **lobbyists.**

Professional organizations that can deliver large numbers of votes have a powerful means of influencing politicians. The use of the collective source of power contains elements of reward, coercive, expert, and even referent sources. Each source may come into play at one time or another.

How to Increase Power in Nursing

Despite some feelings of powerlessness, nurses really do have access to some important, and rather substantial, sources of power. What can nurses, either as individuals or as a group, do to increase their power?

Issues in Practice

Kasey is an RN who has worked on the busy surgical unit of a large city hospital for the past 6 years. As one of three RNs on the unit's day shift, she often serves as the charge nurse when the assigned charge nurse has a day off. She is hard working, caring, and well organized and provides high-quality care for the often very unstable postoperative clients they receive on a daily basis.

About 2 weeks ago, Kasey's mother was admitted for a high-risk surgical removal of a brain tumor that was not responding to chemotherapy or radiation therapy. The surgery did not go well, and Kasey's mother was admitted to the surgical unit after the procedure. During the past 2 weeks, she has shown a gradual but steady decline in condition and is no longer able to recognize her family, speak, or do any self-care. It is believed she will probably not live more than another week.

Per hospital policy, Kasey is not assigned to care for her mother; however, during her shifts, Kasey is spending more and more time with her mother, sometimes to the detriment of her assigned clients. She is also beginning to make more demands on the unit nursing staff, often overseeing their care and requesting that only certain nurses care for her mother. One of the other nurses on the unit suggested that Kasey's mother be moved to a less specialized unit. When Kasey heard about the suggestion, she became livid and loudly scolded the nurse for her insensitivity in the middle of the nurses' station.

Questions for Thought

1. Is the practice of not allowing nurses to provide care for their relatives evidence-based or accustomed practice?
2. Identify the steps in making this policy evidence based.
3. Do you think nurses should be allowed to care for relatives? Why? Why not?

Professional Unity

Probably the first, and certainly the most important, way in which nurses can gain power in all areas is through professional unity. The most powerful groups are those that are best organized and most united. The power that a professional organization has is directly related to the size of its membership. According to the ANA, there are approximately 2.7 million nurses in the United States. It is not difficult to imagine the power that the ANA could have to influence legislators and legislation if all of those nurses were members of the organization rather than the 250,000 who actually do belong. This point—that nurses need to belong to their national nursing organization—cannot be emphasized enough.

Political Activity

A second way in which nurses can gain power is by becoming involved in **political action.** Although this produces discomfort in many, nurses must realize that they are affected by politics and political decisions in every phase of their daily nursing activities.

> *By demonstrating their knowledge of the client's condition, recent laboratory tests, and other elements that are vital to the client's recovery, nurses demonstrate their expert power. This knowledge may increase the amount of respect they are given by physicians.*

The simple truth is that if nurses do not become involved in politics and participate in important legislation that influences their practice, someone other than nurses will be making those decisions for them. Nurses need to become involved in political activities from local to national levels. The average legislator knows little about issues such as clients' rights, national health insurance, quality of nursing care, third-party reimbursement for nurses, and expanded practice roles for nurses, yet they make decisions about these issues almost daily. It would seem logical that more informed and better decisions could be made if nurses took an active part in the legislative process.

Accountability and Professionalism

A third method of increasing power is by demonstrating the characteristics of accountability and professionalism. Nursing has made great strides in these two areas in recent years. Nurses, through professional organizations, have been working hard to establish standards for high-quality client care. More important, nurses are now concerned with demonstrating competence and delivering high-quality client care through processes such as peer review and evaluation. By accepting responsibility for the care that they provide and by setting the standards to guide that care, nurses are taking the power to govern nursing away from non-nursing groups.

Networking

Finally, nurses can gain power through establishing a nurse support network. It is common knowledge that the "old boy" system remains alive and well in many segments of our seemingly enlightened 21st-century society. The old boy system, which is found in most large organizations, ranging from universities to businesses and governmental agencies, provides individuals, usually men, with the encouragement, support, and nurturing that allow them to move up quickly through the ranks in the organization to achieve high administrative positions. An important element in making this system work involves never criticizing another "old boy" in public, even though there may be major differences of opinion in private. Presentation of a united front is extremely important in maintaining power within this system. Nursing and nursing organizations have never had this type of system for the advancement of nurses.

Part of the difficulty in establishing a nurse support network is that nurses have not been in high-level positions for very long. The framework for a support system for nurses is now in place; with some commitment to the concept and some activity, it can grow into a well-developed network to allow the brightest, best, and most ambitious people in the profession to achieve high-level positions.[16]

Future Trends in the Nursing Profession

Clearly, it would be difficult to make an airtight case for nursing as a profession. Yet nursing does meet many of the criteria proposed for a profession. Although it would probably be most accurate to call nursing a developing or aspiring profession, for the purposes of this book, nursing will be referred to as a profession. Only when nurses begin to think of nursing as a profession, work toward raising the educational standards for entry level, and begin practicing independently as professionals will the status of profession become a reality for nursing. The movement of any discipline from the status of occupation to one of profession is a dynamic and ongoing process with many considerations.

Experts now predict a severe shortage of professional nurses, ranging from 200,000 to 800,000, by the year 2025. In the past, the way that nursing shortages were handled was to use a quick-fix method of producing more nurses in a shorter period of time by reducing the educational requirements. The current nursing education system is producing approximately 40,000 graduates from diploma and associate degree programs every year.[10] Although this number may help alleviate the nursing shortage, the more critical question to ask is whether this level of education is going to prepare nurses to meet the challenges of a rapidly changing and demanding health-care system.

As the national employment picture continues to evolve for registered nurses, from bedside caregivers to coordinators of care, and as financial resources become stressed, perhaps more nurses will begin to look on what they do as a lifelong commitment. Professional commitment is a complicated issue, but little doubt exists that nurses will not have increased independence of practice until they begin to demonstrate that they are professionals committed to the field of nursing.

> " *Probably the first, and certainly the most important, way in which nurses can gain power in all areas is through professional unity. The most powerful groups are those that are best organized and most united.* "

Conclusion

Ongoing changes in the health-care system will have a major impact on how and where nursing is practiced, and even on who practices it. If nurses utilize their tremendous potential power by banding together as a profession, they will be able to influence decisions about the direction in which health-care is going. Subsequently, nurses, rather than politicians, physicians, hospital administrators, and insurance companies, will be shaping the future of the nursing profession. The move toward mandated staffing ratios is one way that nurses are demonstrating their power to achieve a goal when they band together and exert power as a group.

Nursing has taken great strides forward in achieving professional status in the health-care system. Currently, many nurses accept the premise that nursing is a profession and therefore are not very concerned about furthering the process. Even as nursing has matured and evolved into a field of study with an identifiable body of knowledge, the questions and problems that have plagued this profession persist. In addition, advances in technology, management, and society have raised new questions about the nature and role of nursing in the health-care system. Only by understanding and exploring the issues of professionalism will nurses be prepared to practice effectively in the present and meet the complex challenges of the future.

Critical Thinking Exercises

- Distinguish between an occupation and a profession.
- Is nursing a profession? Defend your position.
- Discuss four ways in which nursing can improve its professional status.
- Name the three sources of power to which nurses have the most access. Discuss how nurses can best use these sources of power to improve nursing, nursing care, and the health-care system.

References

1. Gokenbach V. Professionalism in nursing: What does it really mean? *Nurse Together*, 2012. Retrieved March 2013 from http://www.nursetogether.com/Career/ Career-Article/itemid/ 2245.aspx

2. Russell KA, Beaver LK. Professionalism extends beyond the workplace. *Journal of Nursing Regulation*, 3(4):15–18, 2013.

3. Stagen M. The five C's of professionalism. *Healthcare Traveler* 17(12):16, 2010.

4. Hahn J. Integrating professionalism and political awareness into the curriculum. *Nurse Educator* 35(3):110–113, 2010.

5. Cox C. Legal responsibility and accountability. *Nursing Management* (UK), 17(3):18–20, 2010.

6. Nairn S. A critical realist approach to knowledge: implications for evidence-based practice in and beyond nursing. *Nursing Inquiry*, 19(1):6–17, 2012.

7. Eley D, Eley R, Bertello M, Rogers-Clark C. Why did I become a nurse? Personality traits and reasons for entering nursing. *Journal of Advanced Nursing*, 68(7):1546–1555, 2012.

8. Elcock K. What is nursing? Exploring theory and practice. *Nursing Standard*, 24(25):30, 2010.

9. Lane SH, Kohlenberg E. The future of baccalaureate degrees for nurses. *Nursing Forum*, 45(4):218–227, 2010.

10. Smith TG. A policy perspective on the entry into practice issue. *Online Journal of Issues in Nursing*, 15(1):2, 2010.

11. Cabaniss R. Educating nurses to impact change in nursing's image. *Teaching and Learning in Nursing*, 6(3):112–118, 2011.

12. Martin K, Wilson CB. Newly registered nurses' experience in the first year of practice: A phenomenological study. *International Journal for Human Caring*, 5(2):21–27, 2011.

13. Hartigan C. APRN regulation: The licensure-certification interface. *Advanced Critical Care*, 22(1):50–67, 2011.

14. Cahill M, Hysong A. Moving forward with role recognition for clinical nurse specialists. *Journal of Nursing Regulation*, 3(3): 47–50, 2012.

15. Stachowiak ME, Bugel MJ. The clinical nurse leader and the case manager: Are both roles needed? *American Journal of Nursing*, 113(1):59–63, 2013.

16. Rudge T, Holmes D, Perron AE. The rise of practice development within reformed bureaucracy: Discourse, power and the government of nursing. *Journal of Nursing Management*, 19(7):837–844, 2011.

17. Bogue RJ, Joseph ML, Sieloff CL. Shared governance as vertical alignment of nursing group power and nurse practice council effectiveness. *Journal of Nursing Management*, 17(1):4–14, 2009.

Historical Perspectives

Joseph T. Catalano

UNDERSTANDING OUR HISTORY

Knowledge about the profession's past can help us understand how nursing developed and even suggest solutions to problems that face the profession today. Several threads run throughout the history of nursing, including society's beliefs about the causes of illness, the value placed on individual life, and the role of women in society. The wars of modern history have also had a significant impact on nursing, particularly in influencing the development of technology and guiding the direction of health care. This chapter is not a treatise on the history of health care and nursing but presents some key historical milestones and individuals that helped to form the foundations of health and nursing care.

ORIGINS OF NURSING

According to the American Nurses Association (ANA), the modern definition of nursing is the protection, promotion, and optimization of clients' health and abilities, the prevention of disease and illness, and the alleviation of suffering through the diagnosis and treatment of human response to disease and injury. This comprehensive and modern definition of nursing was only arrived at after centuries of development. However, one of the common elements seen throughout the history of nursing is the belief that by providing care to the ill and injured, including individuals, families, and communities, optimal health and quality of life could be restored or maintained.

Before Nursing

Current nursing practice is a relatively recent development. The major concern of most early civilizations was the survival of the group, and because illness and injury threatened this survival, many primitive health-care practices grew from processes of trial and error. In prehistoric times, women tended to care for the ill and injured. Evil spirits were thought to be the cause of illness, and the medicine men and women who practiced witchcraft were considered religious figures.

Driving Out Demons

In ancient Eastern civilizations, starting from about 3500 BC, health care was intertwined with religion. Taoism emphasized balance and the driving of demons out of the ailing body. Acupuncture developed over the next several thousands of years, and medicinal herbs were used in preventive health care.

In Southeast Asia, Hinduism emphasized the need for good hygiene, and written records would soon chronicle a number of surgical procedures. This was also the first culture to document medical treatment outside the home, although women were prohibited from working. The rise of Buddhism around 530 BC caused a surge in interest in health care, with the development of public hospitals, the requirement of high standards for doctors and other hospital workers, and an emphasis on hygiene and prevention of disease. The development of medical knowledge was somewhat hindered by the refusal of physicians to come in contact with blood and infectious body secretions and the prohibition against dissection of the human body.

Ancient Sciences

During the same period, the ancient Egyptians' belief that all disease was caused by evil spirits and punishing gods was changing. Health-care providers from that time showed a well-developed understanding of the basis of disease. Writings from 1500 BC refer to surgical procedures, the role of the midwife, bandaging, preventive care,

" The major concern of most early civilizations was the survival of the group, and because illness and injury threatened this survival, many primitive health-care practices grew from processes of trial and error. "

and even birth control. Women enjoyed a higher status in Egyptian society and even worked in hospitals.[1] Physicians, however, were still men, who served in multiple roles as surgeons, priests, architects, and politicians.

The Babylonian Empire, united in 2100 BC, was a civilization that focused on astrology. Its health-care practices included special diets, massage therapy, and rest to drive evil spirits from a body. People would go to the marketplace to seek advice on how to treat their ailments. During the height of the empire, strict guidelines governed doctors' fees and responsibilities in medical practice. There is also evidence from this period of child care and treatment of some diseases, but most care still took place in the home.

By 1900 BC, the Hebrews had formed a nation along the Mediterranean and adopted many of the health practices of their neighbors. They integrated elements of the Egyptian sanitary laws to form the Mosaic Code of Laws which, as in many other cultures, mixed religion and medicine. Caring for widows, orphans, and other strangers in need was part of daily life. Hebrews had good knowledge of anatomy and physiology, especially the circulatory system. Physician-priests routinely performed operations such as cesarean deliveries (named later by the Romans), amputations, and circumcisions. They also enforced rules of purification, performed sacrifices, and conducted rituals related to food preparation.

What Do You Think?

Is the study of history really necessary for nursing students? Why or why not?

The Father of Medicine

Ancient Greek culture focused on appeasing the gods, and its medical practice was no exception. The god Apollo was devoted to medicine and good health. The Greeks performed sacrifices to appease the gods and practiced abortion and infanticide in an attempt to control the population. People took hot baths at spas to improve health, but the sick and injured were cared for at clinics. Although women were held in high esteem, they were not permitted to provide any health care outside the home.

Around 400 BC, the writings of Hippocrates began to change medical practice in Greece. One of a roving group of physician-priests, Hippocrates was called "the father of medicine." His beliefs focused on harmony with the natural law instead of on appeasing the gods. He emphasized treating the whole client—mind, body, spirit, and environment—and making diagnoses on the basis of symptoms rather than on an isolated idea of a disease. He was also concerned with ethical standards for physicians, expressed in the now-famous Hippocratic Oath. (See http://www.medterms.com/script/main/art.asp?articlekey=20909 for a copy of the oath.)

Health Care in the Roman Empire

Ancient Romans clung to superstitions and polytheism as the foundations for medical and religious practices. The dominant Roman Empire ruled from around 290 BC and absorbed useful elements of whatever culture it conquered—including the Greeks and Hebrews. The Romans developed quite an advanced system of medicine and a pharmacology that included more than 600 medications derived from herbs and plants. Roman physicians were eventually able to distinguish among various conditions and performed many surgeries. They also did physical therapy for athletes; diagnosed symptoms of infections; identified job-related dangers of lead, mercury, and asbestos; and published medical textbooks.

The Romans' advances in creating an unlimited supply of clean water through aqueducts were critical in maintaining the good health of the citizens, as were central heating, spas and baths, and more advanced systems for sewage disposal. Because the great Roman armies were so crucial to the empire, they developed early hospitals to care for sick and injured soldiers. These were mobile and were staffed by female and male attendants who performed duties that would today be thought of as nursing care: Cleaning and bandaging wounds, feeding and cleaning clients, and providing comfort to the wounded and dying. In many ways, women enjoyed an equal place in society, and they provided home health care and midwifery.

Early Efforts at Nursing

Although caring for the ill and injured had become an established element in most early societies, the concept of a special group to provide this care evolved some time later. The concept of "nurse" grew primarily from the care provided by Christian orders of nuns who were solely dedicated to the care of the sick and dying. Even today, these early roots are reflected in Great Britain, where nurses are still referred to as "sisters."

The Sanctity of Life

The rise of Christianity, starting from AD 30, brought with it a strong belief in the sanctity of all human life. Christians considered practices such as human sacrifice, infanticide, and abortion—which had been common in Roman society—to be murder. Following the teachings of Jesus meant that caring for the sick, poor, and disadvantaged was of primary importance, and groups of believers soon organized to offer care for those in need.

Early writings of the Christian period record women's important role in ministering to the sick and providing food and care for the poor and homeless. Wealthy Roman women who had converted to Christianity established hospital-like institutions and residences for these caregivers in their homes. The term *nurse* is thought to have originated in this period, from the Latin word *nutrire*, meaning to nourish, nurture, or suckle a child. The majority of care was still provided by a family member in the home. Most early Christian hospitals were roadside houses for the sick, poor, or destitute who were cared for by male and female attendants alike. The attendants learned from a process of trial and error and from observing others.

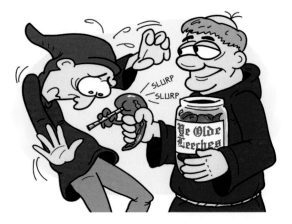

A Time of Disease

The Dark Ages, from roughly AD 500 to 1000, were marked by widespread poverty, illness, and death. Plagues and other diseases such as smallpox, leprosy, and diphtheria ravaged the known world and killed large segments of populations. Health care at this time was almost nonexistent.

However, the strong beliefs of the Catholic Church, which was based in Rome, produced monasteries and convents that became centers for the care of the poor and the sick. By AD 500, there were several religious nursing orders in what is today England, France, and Italy. Men and women worked there and also traveled to rural areas where they were needed, combining religious rituals with home remedies and providing treatments such as bandaging, cautery, bloodletting, enemas, and leeching. The biggest contribution to health care in this period may have been the insistence on cleanliness and hygiene, which lessened the spread of infections. Medieval nurses did not have any formal schooling but learned through apprenticeships with older monks or nuns. Eventually hospitals came to be built outside of monastery grounds. Secular orders were also established, which could provide a wider range of services to the sick because they were not limited by religious restrictions and obligations.

The term nurse is thought to have originated in this period, from the Latin word nutrire, meaning to nourish, nurture, or suckle a child.

Early Military Hospitals

At the end of the Dark Ages, there was a series of holy wars and invasions, including the Crusades, which produced many sick and injured who were far from home. Military nursing orders developed to care for the soldiers, but these were made up exclusively of men who wore suits of armor to protect themselves and their hospitals against attacks. These orders, with the emblem of the Red Cross, were extremely well organized and dedicated, and they existed well into the Renaissance.

Development of the Modern Nurse

It is hard to argue with the fact that technology and scientific advancements have changed the way nurses practice in today's society. However, technological advancements both solve and create problems. Nurses have proven themselves to be highly resourceful in dealing with issues related to technology. Current society readily accepts technology and scientific breakthroughs; however, earlier religion-based societies had more difficulty moving forward with these developments, which were sometimes seen as works of Satan. The Renaissance developed into a battle between progressive thinkers and a very conservative governance structure that resisted change.

Health Care in the Renaissance

In the intellectual reawakening of the Renaissance in Europe, starting in about 1350, nursing emerged in a recognizable form, although it did not grow steadily as a profession during this period. Inventions from this time include the microscope and thermometer, but the use of more modern diagnoses and treatments was viewed with skepticism. Monastic hospitals still regarded the restoration of health as secondary to the salvation of the soul. Major political changes initiated by the Protestant Reformation in 1517 had the greatest effect on the health care of the period. In Catholic nation-states, including Italy, France, and Spain, health care remained generally unchanged from that of the Middle Ages, although the number of male nursing orders gradually decreased. By 1500, the majority of health care was provided by female religious orders.

What Do You Think?

Imagine yourself living in one of the historical periods discussed in this chapter. Given your or your family's health-care problems, how would your lives be different?

A Nursing Hierarchy

In the nation-states that broke away from the Catholic Church, such as England, Germany, and the Netherlands, health care soon degenerated to a condition even worse than that of the Middle Ages. The role of women was reduced under Protestant leadership, and the male nurse all but disappeared. Secular nursing orders gradually took over the duties of the many substandard hospitals that had been established in metropolitan areas. The most famous of these was the Sisters of Charity, established in 1600.

These orders were the first to establish a nursing hierarchy. Primary nurses were called *sisters,* and those assisting them were called *helpers* and *watchers.* At this time, people began to recognize the benefit of skilled nursing care. The first nursing textbooks appeared, and the use of midwives became widespread. Although hospitals were gaining importance, most clients still received health care at home.

The Industrial Revolution (1760–1840) caused a flood of people throughout Europe to move from rural areas into cities, and cramped living situations caused very bad health conditions and the spread of disease and plagues. Factory owners supported some forms of health care to keep their workers on the job, and this led to an early form of community health nursing. The Sisters of Charity expanded their care to include home care. Only a few male nursing orders survived the Protestant Reformation and Industrial Revolution. Several non-Catholic nursing orders were founded, including the one by the famous Quaker, Elizabeth Fry, who established the Society of Protestant Sisters of Charity in London in 1840, which provided training to nurses who cared for the sick and poor, including prisoners and children.

NURSING IN THE UNITED STATES

Five hospitals existed in America before the Revolutionary War that housed the homeless and the poor and included rudimentary infirmaries. However, there were no identifiable groups of nurses for these infirmaries.[2] Health care in America at this time reflected that of the European countries from which the settlers had come. Infant mortality rates were very high, ranging between 50 and 75 percent. One of the first schools of nursing was established in 1640 by the Sisters of St. Ursula in Quebec, and Spanish and French religious orders would establish hospital-based training schools in the New World over the next 100 years.

In Colonial Times

During the Revolutionary War, there was no organized medical or nursing corps, but small groups of untrained volunteers cared for the wounded and sick in their homes or in churches or barns. In 1751, Benjamin Franklin founded Pennsylvania Hospital, the first U.S. hospital dedicated to treating the sick.

Between the Revolutionary and Civil Wars, health care in the United States increased markedly with the influx of religious nursing orders from Europe. More early schools of nursing developed at this time. Despite the rapid increase in the number of hospitals, most nursing care was still given at home by family members. Hospitals were considered a last resort and still had very high mortality rates.

When the States Went to War

The Civil War caused more death and injury than any war in the history of the United States, and the demand for nurses increased dramatically. Women volunteers (as many as 6000 for the North and 1000 for the South) began to follow the armies to the battlefields to provide basic nursing care, although many of them were untrained. Navy Nurses, the American Red Cross, and the Army Nurse Corps all date from this period. Large numbers of women came out of their homes to work in the hospitals, and a number of African American volunteers in the North paved the way for others to enter the health-care field in the future.

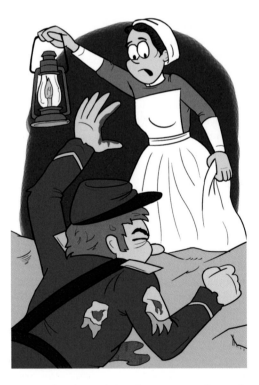

Technological developments in the 19th century included medications such as morphine and codeine for pain and quinine to treat malaria. The arrival of 30 million immigrants in this century meant that the need for health care increased accordingly.

Hospitals sprang up, and many instituted their own schools of nursing. Still, home care was the preferred type of nursing.

After 1914

Nursing and nurses still had a very negative image prior to the beginning of World War I. Their primary duties were to carry out the orders of physicians, clean, cook, and empty bedpans. Most of the duties carried out by physicians would fall well within the current-day scope of practice for nurses. However, in the face of the large numbers of injured produced in World War I, nurses' roles rapidly expanded and they began to be recognized for their skills in providing care and saving lives.

Untrained Nurses

At the beginning of World War I, there were only about 400 nurses in the Army Nurse Corps, but by 1917, that number had swelled to 21,000. Because many hospitals were recruiting untrained women to provide basic care, a committee on nursing was formed to establish standards, and eventually the Red Cross began a training program for nurse's aides. This was supported by physicians but opposed by many nursing leaders who were concerned that it relegated nursing to "women's work," which would be seen as something anyone could do with minimal training. Because nurse's aides were a cheap source of labor, they began to replace more trained nurses in hospitals. Unfortunately, this also resulted in a lower quality of care.

Between Wars

After the war, a segment of the nursing profession began to focus on improving the educational standards of nursing care. At the time, 90 percent of nursing care was still given at home, but nurses began to practice in industry and in branches of government outside of the military. The standards of nursing care were low, and external quality controls were nonexistent.

The Great Depression took its toll on health care and nursing, as jobs became scarce and many nursing schools closed. At this time, the federal government became one of the largest employers of nurses. The newly organized Joint Committee on Nursing recommended that jobs go to more qualified nurses and that the workday be reduced from 12 to 8 hours, although these measures were not widely implemented. During this period, hospitals became the primary source of health care, supported by hospital insurance programs. As the size of hospitals increased, more nursing jobs became available.

Establishing Standards

World War II produced another nursing shortage, and in response, Congress passed the Bolton Act, which shortened hospital-based training programs from 36 to 30 months. The new Cadet Nurse Corps established minimum educational standards for nursing programs and forbade discrimination on the basis of race, creed, or sex.[2] Many schools revised and improved their curricula to meet these new standards.

To encourage more nurses to enter the military, the U.S. government granted women full commissioned status and gave them the same pay as men with the same rank. By the end of the war, African American and male nurses were also admitted to the armed services.

> *Medieval nurses did not have any formal schooling but learned through apprenticeships with older monks or nuns.*

Modern Times: Emerging Specialties

The single largest transformation of the practice of nursing occurred during World War II. Navy and army nurses had such a positive image that it attracted more volunteers than any other occupation at the time. Nurses were revered as selfless heroes under fire in several movies produced during the war. Even nurses captured by the Japanese were allowed to keep practicing because their role was so highly respected. On the battlefields and at rear area hospitals, they often worked together with untrained care providers and physicians, thus initiating the concept of a health-care team.

A Team of Nurses

The advancements in health care made during World War II required that nurses receive more highly specialized education to meet clients' unique needs. After the war, many nurses left the profession to raise families, and the spaces were filled by graduates of new programs that trained licensed practical nurses (LPNs) and licensed vocational nurses (LVNs) in just 1 year. At this time, the concept of team nursing came to be widely accepted, although it removed the registered nurses (RNs) from direct client care, requiring them to serve as team leaders.

A Growing Need

Technical nursing programs, which granted associate degrees (associate degree nurse [ADN]) at 2-year community colleges, were developed to help with the nursing shortage. With the baby boom, the need for nurses continued to grow, and what had been a quick-fix solution began to take a stronger hold. By the mid-1960s, ADNs outnumbered the nurses with baccalaureate degrees (BSN) and the technical LPNs. Also, ADNs won the right to take the same licensing examinations as RN graduates from diploma and BSN programs.

Still, as the health-care system became increasingly complicated, some nursing leaders questioned whether 1- or 2-year LPN and ADN programs were adequate to meet the needs of the profession. Slowly, the number of BSN programs and graduate-level programs began to increase.

Vietnam: Traveling Hospitals

The mobile army surgical hospital (MASH) units that had been developed during the Korean War were replaced during the Vietnam War with medical unit, self-contained transportable (MUST) hospitals, which were staffed by nurses and physicians. Some 5000 nurses served in this war, and for the first time, graduates of 2-year ADN programs were commissioned into the armed services. Several navy nurses were injured in the line of duty, and one army nurse was killed. The efforts of these and other women who served are recognized at the Vietnam Women's Memorial in Washington, dedicated in 1993.

> *Large numbers of women came out of their homes to work in the hospitals, and a number of African American volunteers in the North paved the way for others to enter the health-care field in the future.*

THE EVOLUTION OF SYMBOLS IN NURSING

All professions have symbols that are easily identified and connected with the work and services they provide. In the past, when most of the population was illiterate, these were helpful in distinguishing one professional from another. In modern society, the symbols connect the professions to their historical roots and provide the philosophical basis for the work they do.

The Lamp

The simple definition of a lamp is a device that provides a continuous source of light for an extended period of time. The first evidence of lamp use can be traced back to 10,000 BC, when a hollowed out stone with oil residue was found in a cave. Early variations on the oil lamp included seashell lamps and coconut lamps. Since then, technology has advanced lamps to clay bowls, pottery, and various types of metals.

Pushing Back Darkness

The significance of the lamp is really the significance of light. Its origins can be traced back to the first attempts of human beings to control fire and use it as a tool of survival. These early humans soon found that fire was a source of warmth on cold nights, kept wild animals from attacking, and was useful for cooking.

Light, first in the form of torches and candles and later in the form of the oil lamp, has been used by human beings for thousands of years to push back the darkness of night. It dispelled fear and allowed people to pursue learning long after the sun went down.

The lamp has long been used as a religious symbol. It often represents the eternal flame that dispels darkness and evil. Commonly found in Christian symbolism is the "Lady of Light," often depicted as radiant and glowing brightly and filled with goodness, purity, and wisdom. The lamp can also represent the flame of life, eventually extinguished by death.

As schools and universities developed during the Middle Ages, many adopted the lamp as a symbol of learning. The burning of the lamp signified the continual seeking of knowledge. It also symbolizes the enlightenment that accompanies knowledge. The coats of arms or logos used by many universities contain the image of a lamp.

A Sign of Caring

The lamp was first introduced as a symbol for the nursing profession at the time of Florence Nightingale. In addition to her fame as an early health-care reformer and pioneer, she became well known for her role in caring for injured soldiers during the Crimean War. She made history when she took her 38 nurses to Turkey to try to improve the squalid, filthy conditions she found in the primitive British field hospitals. As Nightingale and her nurses made their night rounds, caring for the wounded in unlit wards, they carried oil lamps to light the way. For the wounded and suffering, these lamps became signs of caring, comfort, and often the difference between life and death.

Nightingale's lamp was not the often-depicted "genie" or "Aladdin's" lamp. Rather, Nightingale would have used one of the many lamps in circulation around the wards, picking up whichever was closest at hand—an ordinary camp lamp or a Turkish candle lantern. She later became immortalized as the "lady with a lamp" in a poem written by Longfellow ("Santa Filomena"). In our modern society, oil lamps are sometimes used for atmosphere or nostalgic reminders of the past, although when the power goes out, they can be very handy. However, for graduate nurses, the lamp, or its close cousin the candle, retains its significance as a symbol of the ideals and selfless devotion of Florence Nightingale. It also signifies the knowledge and learning that the graduates have attained during their years in the nursing program. Even though the nursing graduates may not physically carry an oil lamp during pinning ceremonies, they symbolically carry the brightly burning lamp of their care and devotion as they minister to the sick and injured in their nursing practice.

> " *The Civil War caused more death and injury than any war in the history of the United States, and the demand for nurses increased dramatically.* "

The Nursing Pin

Unlikely as it may seem, the modern nursing pin can trace its origins to the heavy protective war shields used by soldiers as far back as the Greek and Roman Empires. The primary purpose of these shields was to protect the warriors from the spears, swords, and arrows of the opposing army. Adorned with the emblems of the soldier's country and his particular unit in the army, these ancient war shields also served as a quick way to distinguish friend from foe.

During the Crusades, the Knights Hospitallers were formed to provide medical care for the wounded and sick. The Knights wore black tunics over their armor, carried no weapons, and wore a white Maltese cross on chains around their necks. Those wearing this cross became known for their skills in treating the injured and healing the wounded. Since that time, the Maltese cross has been recognized as a symbol of those who care for the sick. Although large by today's standards, the Maltese cross is often considered the first true nursing pin.

The shields of some medieval knights were painted with the coats of arms of the kings they were defending. Only the best knights, recognized for their skills in battle, strength, honesty, and dedication to the service of the king, were permitted to use the king's coat of arms on their shields. The coat of arms displayed to the world the characteristics by which the king wished to be known. A classic example is the symbol of the lion, found on the shields of the knights who served King Richard the Lionheart, which indicated the king's fearlessness and power.

Similarly, during the Middle Ages when most of the population was illiterate, tradesmen and craft guilds began adopting symbols as pictorial representations of their services, skills, and crafts. Modern companies use trademarks and brand names in the same way today. Medieval schools and universities also began using symbols to represent their values and goals. The modern practice of "branding the university," or adopting an official symbol or logo for the school, can be traced back to these early practices. These symbols were embossed on clothing, buttons, badges, and pins that were worn by members of the group. Also traceable to this time in history are the "shields" and badges worn by firefighters and law enforcement officers. Although these shields offer little in the way of protection from arrows and spears, they symbolize official authority and identify the wearer as belonging to a unique, specially trained group.

The first modern nursing pin is attributed to Florence Nightingale. After receiving the medal of the Red Cross of St. George from Queen Victoria for her selfless service to the injured and dying in the Crimean War, Nightingale chose to extend the honor she had received to her most outstanding graduate nurses by awarding each of them a "badge of excellence." The badge or pin she designed for her school is a deep-blue Maltese cross (Fig. 2.1). In the center of the cross is a relief image of Nightingale's head. As the number of nursing schools increased, each program designed a unique pin to represent its own particular values, philosophies, beliefs, and goals.

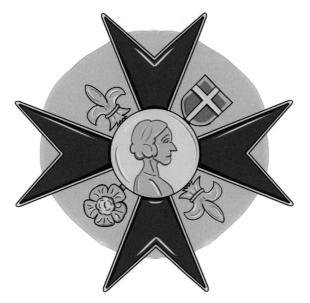

Figure 2.1 Florence Nightingale's nursing excellence pin

The pinning ceremony is part of a long tradition that acknowledges nursing graduates as belonging to a unique group and identifies them as new members of the health-care community. The historical origins of the pin remind nursing professionals of what it symbolizes. Like the badge worn by law enforcement officers, it is also a sign of their legal authority as licensed professionals. Nursing graduates wear their pins proudly in the work setting as evidence of their successful completion of the nursing program.

Question for Thought

Obtain a picture of your nursing school's pin. What do the various symbols on the pin signify?

The Cap

It is rare to see a nurse wearing the traditional "nursing cap" in today's modern hospitals. However, the cap has a long, rich history. Although it may seem sexist by today's standards, throughout much of history, women were required to keep their heads covered with some type of garment. This practice was prevalent in the early Hebrew, Greek, and Roman cultures that served as the roots for modern Western society and the current profession of nursing.

A Symbol of Service

The origins of what we identify as modern nursing can be traced back to an early Christian era group of women called *deaconesses*. Deaconesses were set apart from other women of the period by their white head coverings, which indicated that their primary service was to care for the sick. Originally this head covering was more like a veil that nuns wear, but after the Victorian era, it evolved into a cap. During the early centuries of Christianity, groups of deaconesses banded together and formed what later became the religious orders that were so prevalent in the Holy Roman Empire. The former deaconesses, now recognized as religious order nuns, remained the primary providers of care for the sick throughout the Middle Ages. The traditional garb of nuns, the long-robed habit with the wimple or veil, can be considered the first official nurse's uniform. Each religious order had its own unique style of habit and wimple. The order the nun belonged to could be easily identified from the habit or veil she was wearing.

Religious orders continued to be the primary source of care for the sick well into the 19th century. However, as the Industrial Revolution progressed and the concept of the modern hospital developed, the care of the sick moved away from religious orders to care by laypeople who did not wear the nun's robe and veil.

By the time Florence Nightingale trained at the Institute of Protestant Deaconesses in Germany, the veil had evolved into a white cap that signified "service to others." However, Florence Nightingale lived and practiced nursing during the Victorian era, which required "proper" women to keep their heads covered. The nursing cap Florence Nightingale wore was similar to the head garb worn by cleaning ladies of the day. It was hood shaped with a ruffle around the face and tied under the chin (Fig. 2.2). This early cap served multiple purposes. It met the requirements of the times for women to keep their heads covered; it kept the nurse's long hair, which was fashionable during the Victorian era, up and off her face; and it kept the hair from becoming soiled.

A Cap for Every School

In the United States, the first standardized nursing cap is generally attributed to Bellevue Training School in New York City around 1874. The cap's primary purpose was to keep the nurse's long hair from getting in the way, but it also identified nurses who had graduated from Bellevue. The Bellevue cap

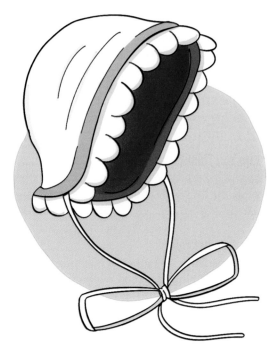

Figure 2.2   Florence Nightingale's nursing cap

covered the whole head to just above the ears and resembled a modern knitted ski hat, except for being white linen with a rolled fringe at the bottom.

As the number of nursing schools increased, there was a corresponding increase in the need for unique caps. Each nursing school designed its own cap. Nursing caps became very frilly, elaborate, and sometimes large and unwieldy. Some caps adopted the upside-down ice cream cone shape, similar to the cloth cone through which ether was given as an anesthetic. By looking at the cap, a person could still determine the school from which the nurse had graduated.

Traditionally, in the 3-year hospital-based schools of nursing, there were two separate ceremonies—one for capping and one for pinning. The capping ceremony usually took place after the student completed the initial 6 months of classroom education, which was considered the probationary period of the program. Capping indicated that the student was now off probation and that she had earned the right to wear the cap during clinical rotations in the hospital.

During nursing school, the cap was also used as a sign of rank and status. In the 3-year hospital-based nursing schools, first-year students wore plain white caps. Second-year students had a vertical black

band added to the edge of the cap, and third-year students were given a second vertical black band. When the student graduated, the vertical black bands were removed, and a horizontal black band was placed across the front of the cap.

Unchanging Values

As shorter hair became an acceptable style for women in the 20th century, the nursing cap lost its function of controlling long hair. However, it continued as a status symbol and a source of pride and identity for the graduates of nursing schools into the 1970s. As technology increased in the health-care work environment, the traditional nursing cap became more of an obstacle for nurses in the practice setting. Also, research demonstrated that the cap, rather than protecting clients from infection by organisms from the nurse's hair, actually helped to colonize organisms. By the 1980s, health-care facilities no longer required nurses to wear caps as part of the uniform, and nursing schools eliminated the cap as a mandatory item of students' uniforms.

Most nursing programs have eliminated the capping ceremony as a throwback to an era that was repressive to women. However, the nursing cap connects graduates to a rich and long history. It retains its significance, from the time of Florence Nightingale, as a sign that the primary goal of nursing is "service to those in need." The nursing cap is a reminder of the unchanging values of wisdom, faith, honesty, trust, and dedication. These values are as important in today's modern, technology-filled hospitals as they were in the era when washing floors was a required basic nursing skill.

What Do You Think?

Does your nursing school have a unique nursing cap that was used in the past? What is the symbolism of the cap's design?

NURSING LEADERS

The nursing profession as it is practiced today owes a great deal to several outstanding nurses who had a vision for the future. The few discussed here are representative of the great drive and dedication of the many individuals who created change and influenced the development of the nursing profession.

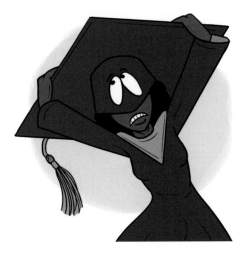

Florence Nightingale (1820–1910)

Universally regarded as the founder of modern nursing, Florence Nightingale dedicated her long life to improving health care and nursing standards. Raised in England, Nightingale was considered highly educated for her time. Through travels with her family, she became aware of the substandard health care in many countries in Europe. In 1851, she attended a 3-month nurses' training program at the church-run hospital in Kaiserswerth, Germany. She was impressed with the program but believed this brief training was insufficient. She later ran a private nursing home and realized that the only way to improve health care was to educate women to be reliable, high-quality nurses.[3]

Volunteering Under Fire

Plans to develop a school of nursing in England were interrupted in 1854 by a cholera epidemic. Nightingale volunteered her services and learned a great deal about how to prevent the spread of disease. When the Crimean War broke out that same year, she obtained permission to take a group of 37 volunteer nurses into the battlefield area. British medical officers initially refused their assistance, but as conditions worsened, the nurses were admitted to the hospital.

After just 6 months of the nurses cleaning and bandaging wounds, cooking, and cleaning the wards, the mortality rate dropped from 42 percent to 2 percent.[3] Nightingale expanded her reform to include supplies, a military post office, convalescent camps for long-term recovery, and residences for soldiers' families. She also began to help with the care given at the front lines. At the height of her work in the war, Nightingale supervised 125 nurses in several large hospitals, and her accomplishments were recognized by the Queen of England with an Order of Merit, the highest award given to English civilians.

What Do You Think?

What would current nursing practice and nursing education be like without the influences of Florence Nightingale?

A Health-Care Reformer

The war experience strengthened Nightingale's convictions that nursing education required major reform. Believing that nursing schools should be run by nurses and be independent of hospitals and physicians, she advocated a program of at least 1 year that included basic biological science, techniques to improve nursing care, and supervised practice. She regarded nursing as a lifelong endeavor and felt that nurses should be in direct contact with clients rather than doing menial jobs such as cooking and cleaning. She worked tirelessly for the reform of health care and nursing and was appointed to many related committees and commissions. A prolific writer, she wrote extensively about improving hospital conditions, sanitation, nursing education, and health care in general.

Her famous Florence Nightingale School of Nursing and Midwifery opened in 1860 and began to train nurses, who were in great demand throughout Europe and the United States. At this school, Nightingale advocated health maintenance and the concept that nursing was both an art and a science. She taught that each person should be treated as an individual and that nurses should meet the needs of clients, not the demands of physicians.

The school flourished, although it faced strong opposition from physicians who felt that nurses were already overtrained. Many early graduates went on to become important nursing leaders. Nightingale's ideas were somewhat diluted during the first half of the 20th century, but they have since resurfaced and are now evaluated in the light of a rapidly changing health-care system.[3]

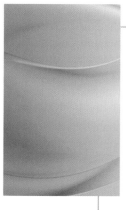

Issues Now

Travel Nursing as a Career

As a nursing student, you may have heard of *travel nursing* or *traveling nurses* but not really know what they are or if it might be something you would be interested in as a career. Much like the recruitment posters for the armed services, "See the World" seems to be an attractive slogan for those looking for new experiences and adventure. However, there may be some drawbacks to travel nursing.

In general, travel nurse staffing companies require a BSN or higher degree. This standard allows the nurses to meet any staffing requirements of individual facilities, and research has demonstrated good client outcomes. Travel nurses differ from agency nurses in several ways. Travel nurses are usually committed to working for a facility for a predetermined length of time, usually about 3 months. To allow preparation for travel to the facility, they are scheduled for their time about 2 months before their start date. Agency nurses generally work on a per diem (by the day) basis and live near the facility. They work a few days at a time to meet a short-term staffing need. Travel nurses provide more continuity of care and fill in for long-term needs, such as extended illness, maternity leave, or even sabbatical leave.

Travel nurses can select where they want to work and the time period of the work schedule. They usually follow the schedule required by the facility but have scheduled days off like other nurses. Their salaries tend to be higher, and, depending on the company, the benefits may range from "bare bones" to what regular staffers would receive at a large health-care facility. The staffing agency also pays for the nurse's license and housing costs. Staffing agencies have a group of employees who support the nurse and act as liaisons with the facilities to resolve any problems that may arise.

A nurse must be careful when selecting a travel nurse staffing company. The nurse should investigate the company carefully, talk to other nurses it employs, and examine the benefits closely. Generally, the larger the firm, the more locations it serves and the better the benefits and support services. Some nurses use travel nurse employment to research locations in which they may be interned and then permanently relocate when they find the ideal location.

So, if you want to be a travel nurse, the opportunities are out there. Travel nursing certainly provides a high degree of autonomy and control of your schedule and career. One of the key elements reported by nurses for career satisfaction is quality of life. The freedom of choice provided by travel nursing would certainly fulfill that need.

Sources: Nurses RX. AMN Health Care Company. Retrieved April 2013 from http://www.nursesrx. com/; Travel Nursing: The Authority in Travel Nursing. Retrieved April 2013 from http://www. travelnursing.com/

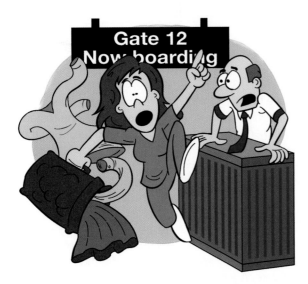

TRAVELING NURSES SEE THE WORLD

Isabel Adams Hampton Robb (1860–1910)

Isabel Adams Hampton Robb started out as a teacher in her home province of Ontario, Canada, but in 1881 she went to New York City to train to be a nurse. After graduation, she moved to Rome and became a superintendent of a hospital there. She had always focused on the academic rather than the clinical side of nursing, but in Italy, her conviction grew that nurses needed a solid theoretical education—a belief that was not well accepted by the medical community of the time. From that point on, she dedicated her life to raising the standards of nursing education in the United States, first as director of the Illinois Training School for Nurses, a school that was unique for its time in that it was university based and emphasized academic learning. Some of her unique ideas for the time were to develop and implement a grading policy for nursing students that required nurses to prove their abilities in order to be awarded a diploma. She also advocated for the reduction of the long hours involved in training nurses. She later headed the new Johns Hopkins Training School for Nurses and would implement her ideas there as well.[4]

Hampton Robb brought together leaders from key nursing schools to form the American Society of Superintendents of Training Schools for Nurses, and she served as its chairwoman. The group was the precursor to the National League for Nursing, which was dedicated to improving the standards for nursing education. In 1896, Hampton

Robb became the first president of a group for staff nurses in active practice called the Nurses Associated Alumnae of the United States and Canada, which would later become the American Nurses Association (ANA), dedicated to the improvement of clinical practice.[4] She later helped develop the *American Journal of Nursing*, the first professional journal dedicated to the improvement of nursing, which is still the official journal of the ANA.

Lillian Wald (1867–1940)

Lillian Wald was raised in Ohio and graduated from the New York Hospital Training School for Nurses in 1901. After working as a hospital nurse, she entered medical school, but encounters with New York's poor and sick caused her to change direction. She instead opened the Henry Street Settlement, a storefront health clinic in one of the poorest sections of the city, which organized nurses to make home visits, focusing on sanitary conditions and children's health.[5] Wald became a dedicated social reformer, an efficient fundraiser, and an eloquent speaker. Although women still did not have the right to vote, her political influence was felt worldwide.

Under Wald's auspices, Columbia University developed courses to prepare nurses for careers in public health. Wald also advocated wellness education, which the medical community did not value at the time. However, the Metropolitan Life Insurance Company saw the value in her beliefs and asked her to organize its nursing branch. She is also credited with founding the American Red Cross's Town and Country Nursing Service and with initiating the concept of school nursing. In 1912, she founded and became the first president of the National Organization for Public Health Nursing. She was the first to place nurses in public schools.[5] Many child health and wellness programs in use today are based on her efforts. Current proposals for health-care reform often include her ideas about public health nursing, independent clinics, and health maintenance.

What Do You Think?

Who is your favorite historical nursing leader? What are some of that person's characteristics that appeal to you? Is there a current nurse or nurse educator who is a role model for you? What are some of that person's characteristics that appeal to you?

Lavinia Lloyd Dock (1858–1956)

Lavinia Lloyd Dock left her home in Pennsylvania in 1885 to attend New York's Hunter-Bellevue School of Nursing. Her contributions as a reformer focused on the professionalization of nursing and the equality of women.[6] She noticed that many of her fellow students struggled to learn about all the medications that were becoming available, and she would later write the first medication textbook for nurses. She worked alongside Lillian Wald at the Henry Street Settlement and Isabel Hampton Robb at Johns Hopkins Hospital.

Like Wald, Dock believed that poverty and squalor contributed to poor health, and she dedicated herself to social reform to address these problems.[6] However, she soon learned that she was limited in her influence because she was a woman, and she spent most of her career dedicated to the pursuit of equal rights. For 20 years, she lobbied legislators at all levels about women's right to vote, believing that this was the only way to influence social reform and health care. An excellent example of the diverse ways that nurses can help achieve higher-quality health care, she is considered one of the most influential leaders in the early 20th century.

Annie W. Goodrich (1866–1954)

Annie Goodrich provided nursing care at Lillian Wald's Henry Street Settlement in New York after receiving her nursing degree. She was known as an outstanding nursing educator and ran a number of nursing schools in New York. In 1910, she was appointed as state inspector of nursing schools, a position that up to that time had been held only by physicians. After the U.S. Army asked her to survey its hospital nursing departments, Goodrich proposed that it organize its own nursing school. The school opened later that year, with her as its dean, and this school would serve as the model for others established at army hospitals during World War I.

To respond to the need for nurses in the war, Goodrich also established a nursing training program at Vassar College. After the war, other colleges and universities slowly began to develop their own nursing programs. Goodrich had demonstrated that teaching theoretical information in a classroom was just as important in training highly skilled nurses as clinical practice. When the war was over, Goodrich returned to the Henry Street Settlement and then became a nursing educator, eventually serving as dean at the Yale School of Nursing. Her many writings about nursing education and her experiences with military nursing have been a great contribution to the nursing profession.[7]

Loretta C. Ford (1920–)

Credited with founding nurse practitioner (NP) practice, Loretta C. Ford was born in New York City. She received her diploma in nursing from the Robert Wood Johnson University Hospital in New Brunswick, New Jersey. She held a staff nurse position there until she accepted a commission as an officer in the U.S. Army Air Force in 1943. After the war, she was accepted into the Bachelor of Science (BS) program at the University of Colorado College of Nursing. She earned her BS in 1949 and her Master of Science in nursing in 1951. Subsequently, she worked as a public health nurse in Boulder, Colorado, and then for the Boulder County Health Department, where she served as director from 1956 to 1958.[8]

Ford began her career in education in 1955, when she was appointed assistant professor at the University of Colorado College of Nursing in Denver. She received her doctorate in education from the University of Colorado in 1961 and became a professor in 1965.

During her time at University of Colorado, she began working with a pediatrician, Dr. Henry K. Silver. Together, they noted that there was a severe regional shortage of family care physicians and pediatricians, particularly in the rural and underserved areas of Colorado. In response, they came up with an innovative approach to the health-care provider shortage. They applied for and received a small grant from the university in 1965, which led to the creation of a demonstration project that focused on extending

> *" The war experience strengthened Nightingale's convictions that nursing education required major reform. Believing that nursing schools should be run by nurses and be independent of hospitals and physicians, she advocated a program of at least 1 year that included basic biological science, techniques to improve nursing care, and supervised practice. "*

the role of the nurse in the health-care community.[9] It was so effective that they published their findings, which later became the blueprint for an educational curriculum for NPs.

Soon after the pilot project was completed, the University of Colorado started the first formal NP program in the country. Initially, it was a certificate program for nurses with a baccalaureate in nursing degree. Ford believed that the nurse practitioner philosophy should be to provide a holistic approach to the client's health. Nurse practitioners should focus on health, functionality, and daily living, as well as give the client feedback on how they are progressing.[8]

At first, the NP program prepared nurses in child and family care, educating clients in preventive health. The program became extremely popular and moved up to a master's degree program. It also expanded its focus to a broader population as it grew, including caring for adults. Ford's program educated NPs to integrate the traditional role of the nurse with advanced medical training and community health, thereby providing clients with high-quality care and education not found in the traditional health-care setting.

NPs are found in every corner of the health-care system today. There are over 150,000 NPs working within the United States, and the number grows daily. In many states, NPs can function independently and provide services such as ordering, performing, and interpreting diagnostic tests. They can diagnose and treat acute and chronic conditions such as diabetes, high blood pressure, infections, and injuries. In some states they are legally permitted to prescribe medications independently. Although still receiving some resistance from physicians' groups, NPs have transformed both the health-care system and the profession of nursing.[8]

Ford became the founding dean of the University of Rochester School of Nursing and director of the Nursing Service at the University Hospital in 1972. The school now has nine specialty NP programs, including child psychiatry, which helps fill a need for mental health services in rural upstate New York.[9] In 2003, she was awarded the Blackwell Award (named for the first female doctor in America) from Hobart and William Smith Colleges, which is given to a woman whose life exemplifies outstanding service to humanity. Among many other accolades, she was inducted into the National Women's Hall of Fame in 2011 for being recognized as an internationally renowned nursing leader who has transformed the profession of nursing and made health care more accessible to the general public. Ford is now retired and living in Florida; however, she has remained involved with the University of Rochester School of Nursing. She still consults and lectures on the historical development of the nurse practitioner along with issues in advanced nursing practice and health-care policy.

Conclusion

Many of the problems and difficulties with today's health-care system, and those of nursing in particular, are based in the historical development of the profession. Knowledge of these historical roots can help us understand why the profession of nursing is the way it is and even suggest solutions to problems that may seem unsolvable. For example, nursing today appears to be a profession with a high level of responsibility but a low level of power.

How did this situation develop? What can be done about it? A great deal of confusion exists about the education of nurses, unlike the situation in other health-care professions. Why does nursing have this problem, and how can this confusion be addressed? Those who belong to the nursing profession have a responsibility not only to learn how these and other conditions developed but also to relate that knowledge to nursing's possibility for growth in the future.

Issues in Practice: Case Study

Mrs. Lee, a 56-year-old high school teacher, had been "feeling something in her eye" for 3 days. She visited the retail optometry store where she had purchased her last pair of glasses. The optometrist at the store examined her and did not find any foreign objects in her eye or scratches on her cornea. However, he felt that the symptoms were serious enough to have Mrs. Lee visit the emergency department (ED) at a local hospital.

At the hospital, the ED triage nurse assessed Mrs. Lee's vital signs, which were normal, and also gave her a basic eye examination for visual acuity. The exam revealed 20/200 vision in the right eye and 20/30 vision in the left eye (20/20 is normal).

The triage nurse had a second-year ophthalmology resident from the hospital's outpatient vision clinic examine Mrs. Lee. The resident examined both eyes but extensively examined the right eye, which had the worse vision. He could find no irregularities and sent Mrs. Lee home with eyedrops and an appointment to see an ophthalmologist the next day. The ophthalmologist ordered a computed tomography (CT) scan, which was taken the same day. He also sent Mrs. Lee home with an appointment to see a neurologist the next day.

Mrs. Lee went home after the CT scan. She collapsed and died from a ruptured cerebral aneurysm before the scan was read by the hospital radiology department and before she could see the neurologist. The family filed a malpractice law suit against the triage nurse, the physicians, and the hospital.

After a lengthy trial, the jury in the Supreme Court of Kings County, New York, concluded that ED personnel committed negligence by failing to have the client examined by a neurologist at admission to the ED. Expert witness testimony convinced the jury that the great disparity in the vision between the two eyes was a primary indicator of some type of brain problem. This should have been recognized immediately by the nurse and ED staff, and a neurologist should have been part of the team from the beginning. The jury awarded $2.15 million to the family.

Questions for Thought

1. Do you think there was any malpractice involved in this case? If yes, what is its nature?
2. Should the triage nurse have noticed any abnormalities that might suggest the condition was worse than an eye problem?
3. What would you have done differently in this case if you were the triage nurse?

Source: Collazo v. NY Eye and Ear Infirmary, 2009 WL 1199357. Superior County Kings Court, New York, March 18, 2009.

Critical Thinking Exercises

1. Trace the history of your nursing school. Who were the leaders in the foundation of the school? Write a short biography for each one, listing their accomplishments.
2. If you know any elderly nurses, contact them and ask them if they would be willing to talk to you about their practice. Develop an oral history of what they experienced and compare it to nursing practice today.
3. Start a journal of your own experiences as a nursing student. Maintain this journal throughout your career. Make sure to include interesting instructors and clients with whom you are in contact.

References

1. Griffin GJ, King J. *History and Trends in Professional Nursing.* St. Louis: CV Mosby, 2003.
2. Judd D. *History of American Nursing: Trends and Eras* (10th ed.). Burlington, MA: Jones & Bartlett Publishers, 2009.
3. Florence Nightingale: A Biography. Retrieved April 2013 from http://www.biography.com/people/florence-nightingale-9423539
4. Isabel Hampton Robb—Nursing Theorist. Retrieved April 2013 from http://nursing-theory.org/nursing-theorists/Isabel-Hampton-Robb.php
5. Lilian Wald: The Henry Street Settlement. Retrieved April 2013 from http://www.henrystreet.org/about/history/lillian-wald.html
6. Burtram MAB. Lavinia Lloyd Dock: An activist in nursing and social reform. Retrieved April 2013 from http://etd.ohiolink.edu/view.cgi?acc_num=osu1269373366
7. Annie Warburton Goodrich (1866–1954) 1976 Inductee, American Nurses Association. Retrieved April 2013 from http://www.nursingworld.org/AnnieWarburtonGoodrich
8. Ridgway S. Loretta Ford, Founded Nurse Practitioner Movement. Profiles in Nursing. Retrieved April 2013 from http://www.workingnurse.com/articles/Loretta-Ford-Founded-Nurse-Practitioner-Movement
9. Loretta Ford, 91, Started Nurse Practitioner Movement. Senior Spirit. 2012. Retrieved April 2013 from http://www.csa.us/email/spirit/ssarticles/1012SeniorSpotlight.html

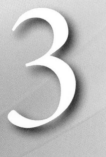

3

Theories and Models of Nursing

Joseph T. Catalano

Joseph T. Catalano

Learning Objectives

After completing this chapter, the reader will be able to:

- Explain why theories and models are important to the profession of nursing
- Analyze the four key concepts found in nursing theories and models
- Interrelate systems theory as an important element in understanding nursing theories and models
- Evaluate how the four parts of all systems interact
- Synthesize three nursing theories, identifying how the different nursing theorists define the key concepts in their theories
- Compare and contrast a middle-range theory with a major nursing theory

CARING FOR REAL PEOPLE

For many nurses, and for most nursing students, the terms *theory* and *model* evoke images of textbooks filled with abstract, obscure words and convoluted sentences. The visceral response is often, "Why is this important? I want to take care of real people!" The simple answer is that understanding and using nursing theories or models will help you be a better nurse and provide better care to real people.

DIFFERENCES BETWEEN THEORIES AND MODELS

What Is a Theory?

Although the terms *theory* and *model* are not synonymous, in nursing practice they are often used interchangeably. Strictly speaking, a theory refers to a speculative statement involving some element of reality that has not been proved. For example, the theory of relativity has never been proved, although the results have often been observed.

The nursing profession tends to use the term *theory* when attempting to explain apparent relationships between observed behaviors and their effects on a client's health. In this nursing context, the goal of a theory is to describe and explain a particular nursing action to make a **hypothesis,** which predicts the effect on a client's outcome, such as improved health or recovery from illness. For example, the action of turning an unresponsive client from side to side every 2 hours should help to prevent skin breakdown and improve respiratory function.

In recent years, nursing has been moving toward using research findings to guide nursing practice. This approach, called *evidence-based practice,* is an important element in improving nursing care and proving many of the long-standing theories that the nursing profession has developed over the years.[1]

What Is a Model?

A model is a hypothetical representation of something that exists in reality. The purpose of a model is to explain a complex reality in a systematic and organized manner. For example, a hospital organizational chart is a model that attempts to demonstrate the interrelationships of the various levels of the hospital's administration.

What Do You Think?

Do you consider yourself to be healthy? What factors make you healthy? What factors are indicators of illness?

What Do Nurses Do?

Although a model tends to be more concrete than a theory, they both help explain and direct nursing actions. This ability, using a systematic and structured approach, is one of the key elements that raises nursing from a task-oriented job to the level of a profession that uses judgment and knowledge to make informed decisions about client care. With the use of a **conceptual model,** nurses can provide intelligent and thoughtful answers to the question, "What do nurses do?" Consider the quoted scenario above.

> *Mr. X had surgery for intestinal cancer 4 days ago. He has a colostomy and needs to learn how to take care of it at home because he is going to be discharged from the hospital in 2 days. When the nurses attempt to teach him colostomy care, he looks away, makes sarcastic personal comments about the nurses, and generally displays a belligerent and hostile attitude.*

Without an understanding of the underlying dynamics involved, the nurses might themselves become sarcastic and scold the client about his behavior or simply minimize their contact with him. This type of response will not improve Mr. X's health status. If, however, the nurses knew about and understood the dynamics of grief theory, they would realize that Mr. X was probably in the anger stage of the grief process. This understanding would direct the nurses to allow, or even to encourage, Mr. X to express his anger and **aggressiveness** without condemnation and to help him deal with his feelings in a constructive manner. Once Mr. X gets past the anger stage, he can move on to taking a more active part in his care and

thus improve his health status. The **client goals** would then be achieved.

If a researcher were to stop 10 people at random on the street and ask the question, "What do nurses do," he or she would likely get 10 different answers, but the confusion about nurses' activities extends far beyond the public at large. What if the researcher asked 10 hospital administrators, 10 physicians, or even 10 nurses the same question? The answers would probably vary almost as much as the answers from laypersons.

The Iowa Project

In an attempt to identify what exactly it is that nurses do, J. C. McCloskey and G. M. Bulechek, two nurse researchers at the University of Iowa, have been conducting a research project since 1990 to develop a **taxonomy** of the **interventions** that nurses use in their practice (Box 3.1). This research has been called Nursing Interventions Classification (NIC), the Iowa Interventions Project, or simply the Iowa Project.[2–5]

A Classification System

The Iowa Project addresses an ongoing need for nurses to be able to identify and quantify what they do. In the current era of concern for high-quality health care, this need has become even more acute. The first results, published in 1994, categorized and ranked 336 interventions that nurses use when they provide care to clients. A follow-up study was conducted about 2 years after the original study categorized and ranked 433 interventions used by nurses. McCloskey and Bulechek[6] also investigated which nursing interventions were commonly used by nurses in specialty settings. Forty specialty areas responded, and the researchers were able to develop a table that lists what core skills are used by each organization. In 2008, the list was again updated. It now contains 542 interventions within a taxonomy of seven domains (i.e., physiological: basic; physiological: complex; behavioral; safety; family; health systems; and community) and 30 classes of interventions.

Research into nursing intervention classification systems is ongoing and has served as the

Box 3.1

What Constitutes Care?

At first glance, it would seem that everybody knows that nurses take care of clients. But what constitutes care? A study conducted by the faculty of the University of Iowa, called the Nursing Interventions Classification (NIC) or simply the Iowa Project, has identified 336 tasks or interventions for which nurses are responsible in their care of patients. Not all nurses carry out all 336 of these tasks all the time, but during an average career, a nurse would likely be involved in the majority of these tasks. Although this project was undertaken in the mid-1990s, it remains the benchmark study. Since the original study, several additional studies have been conducted that reaffirm the findings of the Iowa Project, and several researchers have undertaken projects to use the data generated by the Iowa Project in actual client-care situations.

This project is an excellent example of how a nursing theory led to a research project that developed information that can be used by nurses in their daily practice. On the principle that nursing interventions are specific actions that a nurse can perform to bring about the resolution of a potential or actual health-care problem, the NIC attempted to identify and classify nursing interventions. It also attempted to rank those interventions according to the number of times a nurse was likely to perform one during a working day. The goal of the project was to develop a nursing information system that could be incorporated into the current information systems of all clinical facilities. By using the NIC system, hospital administrators, physicians, nurses, and even the public should be better able to recognize and evaluate the multiple interventions that nurses are responsible for in their daily work.

It is a generally acknowledged fact that nurses, as the largest single group of health-care providers, are essential to the welfare and care of most clients. Yet, in an age of health-care reform, nurses are finding it increasingly difficult to delineate the specific contributions they make to health care. If nurses are unable to define the care they provide, how are the reformers, politicians, and public going to be able to identify the unique contribution made by nursing?

Unfortunately, many of the contributions that nurses make to health care are currently invisible because there is no method of classification for them in the computerized database systems now in use. Commonly used nursing interventions such as active listening, emotional support, touch, skin surveillance, and even family support cannot be measured and quantified by most current information systems.

The large number of interventions used daily by nurses demonstrates the complex and demanding nature of the profession. The breadth and depth of knowledge and skills demanded of nurses on a daily basis are much greater than are found in many other health-care professions. One study found that nurses working in general medical-surgical units during a 6-month period were likely to care for 500 clients with more than 600 individual diagnoses (many clients have multiple diagnoses). These researchers also found that the physical demands of the work were actually less difficult and tiring than dealing with the emotional and technical demands of handling the huge amounts of information generated by the care given.

Sources: Bulechek GM, Butcher HK, Dochterman JM. *Nursing Interventions Classification (NIC)* (5th ed.). St. Louis, MO: Mosby Elsevier, 2008; Moorhead S, et al. *Nursing Outcomes Classification (NOC): Iowa Outcomes Project* (3rd ed.). St. Louis, MO: Mosby, 2004; Scherb CA, Weydt AP. Work complexity assessment, nursing interventions classification, and nursing outcomes classification: Making connections. *Creative Nursing*, 15(1):16–22, 2009.

foundation of new methods to define nursing practice and measure the outcomes of client care. The need to increase client satisfaction and achieve successful outcomes of nursing care is a key element in the Affordable Care Act (ACA), which was passed in 2010. Even more than in the past, these elements will be the basis of reimbursement for health-care providers.

Using the NIC as a starting point, the Work Complexity Assessment (WCA) was developed so that nurses could identify specific interventions they routinely perform for various client populations. Taking the process one step further, the Nursing Outcomes Classification system closes the loop by providing a means for nurses to evaluate whether the outcomes were achieved.[2]

Although initially used primarily to help nurses with the delegation of duties to unlicensed personnel by linking skills with performance requirements, WCA is now an important tool in the improvement of the quality of nursing care. When nurses analyze the care they provide and actually look at the various interventions they use, they increase their understanding of both the methods and rationales for care. WCA also fits nicely into the use of evidence-based practice when nurses share with other nurses what they have learned about improving care.

This type of research helps identify the important contributions made by nursing to the health and well-being of clients. It also demonstrates the complex and demanding nature of the nursing profession. Much of the public, and even many physicians and nurses, do not really understand what nurses do for clients on a daily basis. Using classification systems aids in clarifying what nurses bring to client care, makes what they do measurable, and validates the importance of the nursing profession.

Nursing Competencies

One way in which the nursing profession identifies what nurses do is by looking at **competencies**. In nursing, the word *competence* is often defined as the combination of skills, knowledge, attitudes, values, and abilities that support the safe and effective practice of the nurse. A nurse practices competently when he or she has mastered a range of skills and decision-making processes demonstrated in the care of clients. All the major nursing organizations have developed lists of competencies for nurses. These are usually general, broad statements rather than catalogues of specific skills. (See "Issues Now: The Pew Commission Final Report" in this chapter.)

Nursing competencies are currently under close scrutiny due to the large number of medication and other types of errors in the health-care setting that have led to numerous clients being injured or killed. The Institute of Medicine's (IOM) document on the future of nursing contains recommendations and lists of competencies for nursing school graduates to help improve the quality of care. The Quality and Safe Education for Nurses (QSEN) project, built upon the IOM recommendations, is in the process of developing a framework for nursing schools' curricula (see IOM and QSEN in Chapter 4).

Nursing researchers have attempted to develop specific lists of skills based on the general

> *" The need to increase client satisfaction and achieve successful outcomes of nursing care is a key element in the Health Care Reform Act, which was passed in 2010. Even more than in the past, these elements will be a basis of reimbursement for health-care providers. "*

competency statements from the various nursing organizations. These skills lists help differentiate the various levels of nursing practice. One such list of skills is presented in Table 3.1.

KEY CONCEPTS COMMON TO NURSING MODELS

Although nursing models vary in terminology and approach to health care, four concepts are common to almost all of them: Client or patient (individual or collective), health, environment, and nursing. Each nursing model has its own specific definition of these terms, but the underlying definitions of the concepts are similar.

Client

The concept of client (or patient) is central to all nursing models because it is the client who is the primary recipient of nursing care. Although the term *client* usually refers to a single individual, it can also refer to small groups or to a large collective of individuals (e.g., for community health nurses, the community is the client).

A Complex Relationship

The concept of client has changed over the years as knowledge and understanding of human nature have developed and increased. A client constitutes more than a person who simply needs **restorative care** and comes to a health-care facility with a **disease** to be cured. Clients are now seen as complex entities affected by various interrelating factors, such as the mind and body, the individual and the **environment,** and the person and the person's family. When nurses talk about clients, the term *biopsychosocial* is often used to express the complex relationship between the body, mind, and environment. These elements are at the heart of preventive care that has been an emphasis of professional nursing since the time of Florence Nightingale. The prevention of disease and promotion of health are key provisions in the health-care reform bill passed in 2010 and open the door for nurses to practice what has always been a part of their educational history.

(Text continued on page 51)

Table 3.1 **Competencies for Nursing Skills**

Associate Degree RN	Baccalaureate Degree RN
Administering Blood Products	
Obtain and document baseline vital signs according to agency policies and procedures.	Same
Obtain blood transfusion history. Initiate administration of blood products according to agency policies and procedures.	Same
Evaluate and document client response to administration of blood products.	Same
Admission, Transfer, Discharge	
Admit client to a health-care facility, following facility's policies and procedures.	Same
Transfer client within a health-care facility, following facility's policies and procedures.	Same
Assist client in exiting a health-care facility, following facility's policies and guidelines.	Manage the discharge planning process.
Assess client to determine readiness for discharge.	Same
Facilitate the continuity of care within and across health-care settings.	Same
Assessment of Vital Signs	
Monitor and assess oral, rectal, and axillary temperature.	Same
Measure and record temperature using an electronic or tympanic thermometer.	Same
Monitor and assess peripheral pulses.	Same
Monitor and assess apical pulse.	Same
Monitor and assess apical-radial pulse.	Same
Monitor and assess blood pressure.	Same
Monitor and assess respiratory rate and character.	Same
Bowel Elimination	
Document characteristics of feces.	Same
Perform test for occult blood.	Same
Administer enemas for cleansing or retention.	Same
Remove a fecal impaction.	Same
Provide and teach colostomy and ileostomy care.	Same
Administer a rectal suppository.	Same
Administer a rectal tube.	Same
Develop client's bowel retraining protocol.	Same
Care of the Dying Client	
During the dying process, provide measures to decrease client's physical and emotional discomfort.	Same
Evaluate final progress note on client's chart to determine completeness of information.	Same
Notify appropriate people and departments, according to agency's policies and procedures.	Same

Table 3.1 **Competencies for Nursing Skills—cont'd**

Associate Degree RN	Baccalaureate Degree RN
Evaluate family's response to client's death and make referrals as appropriate.	Develop services that support dying clients and their families.
Provide care for the body after client's death, according to agency's policies and procedures.	Same
Circulatory Maintenance	
Evaluate fetal heart rate pattern.	Same
Apply antiembolism stockings.	Same
Obtain cardiopulmonary resuscitation certification.	Same
Client Teaching	
Assess and document client's and/or family member's knowledge of specific procedure or health problem.	Assess client's readiness to learn.
Assess client and significant support person(s) for learning strengths, capabilities, barriers, and educational needs.	Develop materials to provide client and/or family member with information concerning procedure or health problem.
Develop an individualized teaching plan based on assessed needs.	Same
Modify teaching plan based on evaluation of progress toward meeting identified learning outcomes.	Same
Provide client and significant support person(s) with the information to make choices regarding health.	Same
Teach client and significant support person(s) the information and skills needed to achieve desired learning outcomes.	Same
Evaluate progress of client and significant support person(s) toward achievement of identified learning outcomes.	Using multiple teaching strategies, teach heterogeneous groups of clients, accounting for individual differences.
Implement teaching plan using individualized teaching and learning strategies with clients and/or groups in unstructured settings.	Implement teaching plan using individualized teaching and learning strategies with clients and/or groups in structured settings.
Communication	
Effectively use communication skills during assessment, intervention, evaluation, and teaching.	Same
Express oneself effectively using a variety of media in different contexts.	Same
Adapt communication methods to clients with special needs (e.g., sensory or psychological disabilities).	Same
Produce clear, accurate, and relevant writing.	Same
Use therapeutic communication within the nurse–client relationship.	Same
Maintain confidentiality of nurse–client interactions.	Same
Appropriately, accurately, and effectively communicate with diverse groups and disciplines using a variety of strategies.	Evaluate effectiveness of communication patterns.

(continued)

Table 3.1 **Competencies for Nursing Skills—cont'd**

Associate Degree RN	Baccalaureate Degree RN
Elicit and clarify client preferences and values.	Same
Evaluate dynamics of family interactions.	Same
Evaluate data concerning coping mechanisms of client/family/support system.	Same
Provide emotional support to client/family/support system.	Same
Evaluate strengths of client and family/significant other.	Same
Evaluate need for alternative methods of communicating with client.	Same
Use assertive communication skills in interactions with clients and other health-care providers.	Teach assertive communication skills to clients, unlicensed assistive nursing personnel, and other licensed nurses.
Communicate data concerning client to appropriate members of the health-care team.	Same
Communicate the need for consultation/referral to interdisciplinary care team.	Identify and plan for services to ensure continuity in meeting health-care needs during transition from one setting to another.
Collaborate with other health-care team members to provide nursing care.	Collaborate with community members in planning care for the community.
Critical Thinking	
Within acquired knowledge base, create alternative courses of action, develop reasonable hypotheses, and develop new solutions to problems.	Same
Develop an awareness of personal values and feelings and examine basis for them.	Same
Evaluate credibility of sources used to justify beliefs.	Same
Examine assumptions that underlie thoughts and behaviors.	Same
Seek out evidence and give rationale when questioned.	Use critical thinking to further develop working hypotheses, using patterns and inconsistencies in data.
Delegation and Supervision	
Provide assistive personnel with relevant instruction to support achievement of client outcomes.	Specify aspects of nursing care that can appropriately be delegated to unlicensed health-care providers and assistive personnel.
Coordinate the implementation of an individualized plan of care for clients and significant support person(s).	Coordinate and/or implement plan of care for clients with multiple nursing diagnoses, especially both physiological and psychosocial diagnoses.
Delegate aspects of client care to qualified assistive personnel.	Delegate performance of nursing interventions.
Supervise and evaluate activities of assistive personnel.	Delegate nursing care given by others while retaining accountability for the quality of care given to the client.
	Supervise performance of nursing interventions.

Table 3.1 **Competencies for Nursing Skills—cont'd**

Associate Degree RN	Baccalaureate Degree RN
	Supervise nursing care given by others while retaining accountability for the quality of care given to the client. Manage community-based care for a group of clients. Direct care for clients whose conditions are changing. Direct care for clients in situations with a potential for variation in client condition. Supervise implementation of a comprehensive client-teaching plan.
Documentation Maintain privacy of client's record.	Same
Accurately document data according to agency's policies and procedures.	Same
Use common abbreviations and nomenclature for recording information in the client's record.	Same
	Establish a reporting and recording system to provide for continuity and accountability of programs in designated structured and unstructured settings (e.g., school health, occupational health, community).
Health Assessment Using a systematic process, perform a head-to-toe assessment.	Perform a holistic assessment of the individual across the life span.
Assess physical, cognitive, and psychosocial abilities of individuals in all developmental stages.	
Assess family structure, roles of family members, and family's strengths and weaknesses.	Perform a risk assessment of the individual and family, including lifestyle, family and genetic history, and other risk factors.
Evaluate an individual's capacity to assume responsibilities for self-care.	Same
	Perform assessment of using a family genogram.
Assess community resources to determine possible referral sources.	Perform a community assessment for diverse populations. Perform an assessment of the environment in which health care is being provided. Establish processes to identify health risks in designated structured and unstructured settings (e.g., school health, occupational health, community). Integrate data from client, other health-care personnel, and other systems to which client is linked (e.g., work, church, neighborhood).

(continued)

Table 3.1 **Competencies for Nursing Skills—cont'd**

Associate Degree RN	Baccalaureate Degree RN
	Modify data collection tools to make them appropriate to client's situation (e.g., language and culture, literacy level, sensory deficit).
Use assessment findings to diagnose and evaluate quality of care and to deliver high-quality care.	Perform family assessment.
Evaluate family's emotional reaction to client's illness (e.g., chronic disorder, terminal illness).	Same
Evaluate client's emotional response to treatment.	Same
Evaluate adequacy of client's support systems.	Same
Assist in diagnostic procedures used to determine client's health status.	Same
Health Promotion	
Facilitate parental attachment with newborn.	Same
Determine the need for a health promotion program.	Develop and implement a health promotion program.
Evaluate risk factors related to client's potential for accident/injury/disease.	Same
Evaluate client's knowledge of disease prevention.	Same
Evaluate client's knowledge of lifestyle choices (e.g., smoking, diet, exercise).	Same
Heat and Cold Therapy	
Evaluate client's response to heat therapy.	Same
Evaluate client's response to cold therapy.	Same
Evaluate client's response to sitz bath.	Same
Monitor and evaluate client's response to hypothermia blanket.	Same
Monitor and evaluate infant's response to radiant warmer.	Same
Home Care Management	
Evaluate ability of family/support system to provide care for client.	Same
Evaluate client's home environment for self-care modifications (e.g., doorway width, accessibility for wheelchair, safety bars).	Develop criteria to evaluate client's home environment for self-care modifications (e.g., doorway width, accessibility for wheelchair, safety bars).
Infection Control	
Use aseptic practices: Hand washing, donning and removing a face mask, gowning, donning and removing disposable gloves, bagging articles, managing equipment use for isolation clients, assessing vital signs.	Same
Use universal precautions.	Same
Use body substances isolation procedures.	Same

Table 3.1 **Competencies for Nursing Skills—cont'd**

Associate Degree RN	Baccalaureate Degree RN
Evaluate client's immunization status.	Same
Use surgical aseptic practices: scrubbing hands, donning and removing a sterile gown, donning and removing sterile gloves, preparing and maintaining a sterile field.	Same
Assist with a sterile procedure.	Same
Information and Health Care Technology	
Use technology, synthesize information, and select resources effectively.	Use technology, analyze information, and select resources effectively.
Demonstrate competence with current technologies.	Same
Use computers for record-keeping and documentation in health-care facilities.	Same
	Use data-management system to evaluate a comprehensive program for monitoring health of populations in designated structured and unstructured settings (e.g., school health, occupational health, community).
IV Therapy	
Perform venipuncture to obtain blood specimens.	Same
Perform venipuncture with an over-the-needle device.	Same
Prime tubing and hang IV fluids.	Same
Load and discontinue a PCA pump.	Same
Administer and document IV piggyback medications.	Same
Administer and document IV push medications.	Same
Calculate IV flow rates.	Same
Document medications administered through IV.	Same
Discontinue an IV and document procedure.	Same
Monitor and maintain an IV site and infusion.	Same
Change IV tubing and container.	Same
Prime tubing and hang IV fluids.	Same
Determine amount of IV fluid infused and left-to-count each shift	Same
Assess implanted infusion devices.	Same
Maintain implanted infusion devices.	Same
Medication Administration	
Assess family members' knowledge of medication therapy: reasons for taking medication, daily dosages, side effects.	Same
Instruct clients and their families in the proper administration of medications.	Same
Accurately calculate medication dosages.	Same

(continued)

Table 3.1 Competencies for Nursing Skills—cont'd

Associate Degree RN	Baccalaureate Degree RN
Gather information pertinent to the medication(s) ordered: actions, purpose, normal dosage and route, common side effects, time of onset and peak action, nursing implications.	Same
Administer and document administration of enteral and parenteral medications per order.	Same
Administer and document administration of topical medications per order.	Same
Evaluate client's response to medication.	Same
Perform eye and/or ear irrigation according to agency guidelines.	Same
Meeting Mobility Needs	
Evaluate client's need for range-of-motion exercises.	Same
Evaluate client's level of mobility.	Same
Manage care of client who uses assistive devices.	Same
Provide client or family member with list of resources to contact when mobility or body alignment is impaired.	Evaluate client's need for range-of-motion exercises.
Evaluate client and/or family members' ability to perform range-of-motion exercises.	Evaluate client's level of mobility.
	Manage care of client who uses assistive devices.
	Provide client or family member with list of resources to contact when mobility or body alignment is impaired.
	Evaluate client and/or family members' ability to perform range-of-motion exercises.
Nursing Process	
Analyze collected data to establish a database for client.	Perform comprehensive assessment to determine client's ability to manage self-care, including physiological, psychosocial, developmental, and cognitive factors and their interaction with each other.
Identify client health-care needs to select nursing diagnostic statements.	Formulate individualized nursing diagnoses, based on a synthesis of knowledge from nursing, biological and behavioral sciences, and humanities, that reflect a health problem and its etiology.
	Consider complex interactions of actual and potential nursing diagnoses (e.g., two or more physiological and/or psychosocial nursing diagnoses).
Consider complex interactions of actual and potential nursing diagnoses.	Same
Identify client goals and appropriate nursing interventions.	Same
Develop and communicate nursing care plan.	Develop comprehensive plan of care in collaboration with client.

Table 3.1 **Competencies for Nursing Skills—cont'd**

Associate Degree RN	Baccalaureate Degree RN
Implement and document planned nursing interventions.	Same
	Implement a care plan for individuals, families, and communities with complex health problems that have unpredictable outcomes.
	Use preventive, supportive, and restorative measures to promote client comfort, optimum physiological functioning, and emotional well-being.
	Base care planning on knowledge of primary, secondary, and tertiary levels of prevention.
Establish priorities for nursing care needs of clients.	Same
Evaluate and document the extent to which goals of nursing care have been achieved.	Participate in obtaining collective data concerning client outcomes.
	Deliver care that reflects an understanding of interactions among potentially conflicting nursing interventions.
	Initiate a comprehensive plan for discharge of client at time of admission.
	Care for clients in an environment that may not have established protocols.
	Care for clients in situations requiring independent decision-making (e.g., community-based practice settings).
Pain Management	
Evaluate data from comprehensive pain history.	Same
Evaluate and document client's response to pharmacological and nonpharmacological interventions.	Same
Document client's response to interventions used to prevent or reduce pain.	Same
Assess client when pain is not relieved through ordered pharmacological and nonpharmacological methods.	Collaborate with other members of health-care team to identify alternative interventions.
Evaluate appropriateness of any pain medication taken by clients.	Same
Educate clients on correct use of medications.	Same
Manage and monitor client receiving epidural analgesia.	Same
Teach client to use a PCA device.	Same
Perioperative Care	
Preoperatively, assess client's risk for postoperative respiratory complications.	Same
Postoperatively, assess client's ability to perform respiratory exercises.	Same

(continued)

Table 3.1 **Competencies for Nursing Skills—cont'd**

Associate Degree RN	Baccalaureate Degree RN
Preoperatively, assess client's risk for postoperative thrombus formation.	Same
Postoperatively, assess client's ability to perform passive range-of-motion exercises.	Same
Preoperatively, assess client's willingness and capability to learn exercises.	Same
Preoperatively, assess family members' willingness to learn and to support client postoperatively.	Same
Postoperatively, assess client's condition during operative procedure, including range of vital signs, blood volume or fluid loss, fluid replacement, type of anesthesia, type of airway, and size and extent of surgical wound.	Same
Personal Hygiene of Clients	
Provide or assist with personal hygiene on developmental and/or chronological age basis.	Same
Provide or assist with personal hygiene needs as determined by physical limitations and/or diagnosis.	Same
Provide or assist with personal hygiene needs with respect to client's culture and/or religious values.	Same
Provide or assist with personal hygiene care in hospital, nursing home, or client's home.	Same
Assess and maintain chest tubes.	Same
Safety and Comfort	
Implement measures to protect the immunosuppressed client.	Same
Protect the client from injury.	Same
Verify identity of the client.	Same
Implement agency policies and procedures in the event of client injury.	Same
Follow policies and procedures for agency fires and safety measures.	Same
Follow procedures for handling biohazardous materials.	Same
Assess need for restraints or other safety devices.	Develop protocols for use of restraints or other safety devices.
Implement nursing measures to reduce the risk for falls, poisoning, and electrical hazards.	Same
Prepare for internal and external disasters.	Same
Develop a plan for reducing environmental stressors (e.g., noise, temperature, pollution).	Same
Evaluate client's orientation to reality.	Same
Evaluate need for measures to maintain client's skin integrity.	Same
Vascular Access Devices	
Assist with insertion of central venous catheters.	Same

Table 3.1 **Competencies for Nursing Skills—cont'd**

Associate Degree RN	Baccalaureate Degree RN
Change a central venous catheter dressing.	Same
Monitor administration of medications/nutrients via a vascular access device.	Same
Measure and monitor central venous pressure.	Same
Maintain central vein infusions in adults and children.	Same
Change parenteral hyperalimentation dressing and tubing.	Same
Wound Care and Dressings	
Assess and manage wounds, including irrigation, application of dressings, and suture/staple removal.	Same

PCA = patient-controlled analgesia.

Sources: Cowan DT. Competence in nursing practice: A controversial concept—a focused review of literature. *Accident & Emergency Nursing*, 151(1):20–26, 2007; Dickey C, et al. Nursing Skills Identified as Required Competencies. Helene Fuld Educational Mobility Grant. Oklahoma Nursing Articulation Consortium, Kramer School of Nursing, Oklahoma City University; Levett-Jones TL. Facilitating reflective practice and self-assessment of competence through the use of narratives. *Nurse Education in Practice*, 7(2):112–119, 2007.

Modeling a Healthy Client

A client, in many of the nursing models, does not have to have an illness to be the central element of the model (this explains the preference for using the term *client* over the term *patient*). This is also one of the clearest distinctions between medical models and nursing models. Medical models tend to be restrictive and reactive, focusing almost exclusively on curing diseases and restoring health after the client becomes ill. Nursing models tend to be proactive and **holistic.** Like medical models, they are certainly concerned with curing disease and restoring a client's health, but they also focus on preventing disease and maintaining health. A healthy person is just as important to many nursing models as the person with a disease.

> " *Although nursing models vary in terminology and approach to health care, there are four concepts that are common to almost all of them: Client or patient (individual or collective), health, environment, and nursing.* "

Health

Like the concept of client, the concept of health has undergone much development and change over the years as knowledge has increased. Traditionally, health was originally thought of as an absence of disease. A more current realistic view is that of health as a continuum, ranging from a completely healthy state in which there is no disease to a completely unhealthy state, which results in death. At any given time in our lives, we are located somewhere along the health continuum and may move closer to one side or the other, depending on circumstances and health status.[7]

Health is difficult to define because it varies so much from one individual to another. For example, a 22-year-old bodybuilder who has no chronic diseases perceives health differently than an 85-year-old who has diabetes, congestive heart failure, and vision problems. The perception of health also varies from one culture to another and at different historical periods within the same culture. In some past cultures, a sign of health was pure white skin, whereas in the modern American culture, a dark bronze tan has been more desirable as a sign of health—although research has shown how harmful ultraviolet light is to the skin.

Environment

The concept of environment is another element in most current nursing models. Nursing models often broaden the concept of environment from the simple physical environment to elements such as living conditions, public sanitation, and air and water quality. Factors such as interpersonal relationships and social interactions are also included.

Some internal environmental factors that affect health include personal psychological processes, religious beliefs, sexual orientation, personality, and emotional responses. It has long been known that individuals who are highly self-motivated and internally goal directed (i.e., type A personality) tend to develop ulcers and have myocardial infarctions at a higher rate than the general population. Medical models, which are primarily illness oriented, may not consider it to be treatable. Nursing models that consider personality as one of the environmental factors affecting health are more likely to attempt to modify the individual's behavior (internal environment) to decrease the risk for disease.

Like the other key concepts found in nursing models, the concept of environment is used so that it is consistent within a particular model's overall context. Nursing models try to show how various aspects of environment interrelate and how they affect the client's health status. In addition, nursing models treat environment as an active element in the overall health-care system and assert that positive alterations in the environment will improve the client's health status.

Nursing

The culminating concept in all the various nursing models is nursing itself. After consideration of what it means to be a client, what it means to be healthy, and how the environment influences the client's health status (either positively or negatively), the concept of nursing delineates the function and role of nurses in their relationships with clients that affect the client's health.

Historically, the profession of nursing has been interested in providing basic physical care (i.e., hygiene, activity, and nourishment), psychological support, and relief of discomfort. Modern nursing, although still including these basic elements of client care, has expanded into areas of health care that were only imagined a generation ago.

Client as Partner

In the modern nurse–client relationship, the client is no longer the passive recipient of nursing care. The relationship has been expanded to include clients as key partners in curing and in the health-maintenance process. In conjunction with the nurse, clients set goals for care and recovery, take an active part in achieving those goals, and help in evaluating whether those actions have achieved the goals.[8]

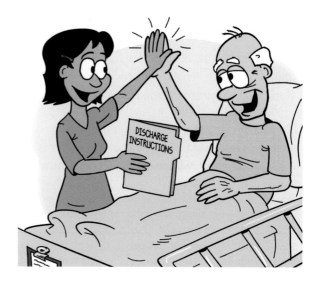

What Do You Think?

How do you define nursing? What competencies are important for you to practice safely when you graduate?

Because of the broadened understanding of environment, several nursing models include manipulation of environmental elements that affect health as an important part of the nurse's role. The environment may be directly altered by the nurse with little or no input from the client, or the client may be taught by the nurse to alter the environment in ways that will contribute to curing disease, increasing comfort, or improving the client's health status.[9]

Four Key Concepts

To analyze and understand any nursing model, it is important to look for these four key concepts: client, health, environment, and nursing. These concepts should be clearly defined, closely interrelated, and mutually supportive. Depending on the particular nursing model, one element may be emphasized more than another. The resultant role and function of the nurse depend on which element is given greater emphasis.

GENERAL SYSTEMS THEORY

A widely accepted method for conceptualizing and understanding the world and what is in it derives from a systems viewpoint. Generally understood as an organized unit with a set of components that interact and affect each other, a system acts as a whole because of the interdependence of its parts.[10] As a result, when part of the system malfunctions or fails, it interrupts the function of the whole system rather than affecting merely one part. The terminology and principles of systems theory pervade U.S. society. Humans, plants, cars, governments, the health-care system, the profession of nursing, and almost anything that exists can be viewed as a system.

A Basis in Thought

Although general systems theory in its pure form is rarely, if ever, used as a nursing model, its process and much of its terminology underlie many nursing models. Elements of general systems theory in one form or another have found their way into many textbooks and much of the professional literature. General systems theory often acts as the unacknowledged **conceptual framework** for many educational programs. An understanding of the mechanisms and terminology of general systems theory is helpful in providing an orientation to understanding nursing models.

> *The culminating concept in all the various nursing models is nursing itself. After consideration of what it means to be a client, what it means to be healthy, and how the environment influences the client's health status (either positively or negatively), the concept of nursing delineates the function and role of nurses in their relationships with clients that affects the client's health.*

Manageable Fragments

General systems theory, sometimes referred to simply as **systems theory,** is an outgrowth of an innate intellectual process. The human mind has difficulty comprehending a large, complex entity as a single unit, so it automatically divides that entity into smaller, more manageable fragments and then examines each fragment separately. This is similar to the process of deductive reasoning in which a single complex thought or theory is broken down into smaller, interrelated pieces. All scientific disciplines, from physics to biology and the social sciences (e.g., sociology and psychology), use this method of analysis.

Reassembling the Fragments

Systems theory takes the process a step further. After analyzing or breaking down the entity, systems theory attempts to put it back together by showing how the parts work individually and together within the system. This interrelationship of the parts makes the system function as a unit. Often, particularly when the system involves biological or sociological entities, the system that results is greater than the sum of its parts.

For example, a human can be considered to be a complex, biosocial system. Humans are made up of many smaller systems such as the endocrine system, neurological system, gastrointestinal system, urinary system, and so forth. Although each of these systems is important, in and of themselves they do not make a human. Many animals have the same systems, yet the human is more than the animal and more than the sum of the systems.

A Set of Interacting Parts

Although the early roots of general systems theory can be traced as far back as the 1930s, Ludwig von Bertalanffy is usually credited with the formal development and publication of general systems theory around 1950.[11] His major achievement was to standardize the definitions of the terms used in systems theory and make the concept useful to a wide range of disciplines. Systems theory is so widely applicable because it reflects the reality that underlies basic human thought processes.

Very simply, a system is defined as a set of interacting parts. The parts that compose a system may be similar or may vary a great deal from each other, but they all have the common function of making the system work well to achieve its overall purpose.

A school is a good example of how the dynamics and connections of a system work. A school as a system consists of several units, including buildings, administrators, teachers, students, and various other individuals (e.g., counselors, financial aid personnel, bookkeepers, and maintenance persons). Each of these individuals has a unique job but also contributes to the overall goal of the school, which is to provide an education for the students and to further the development of knowledge through research.

All systems consist of four key parts: the system itself (i.e., whether it is open or closed), input and output, throughput, and a feedback loop.

Open and Closed Systems

A system is categorized as being either open or closed. Very few systems are completely open or completely closed. Rather, they are usually a combination of both.

Open Systems

Open systems are those in which relatively free movement of information, matter, and **energy** into and out of the system exists. In a completely open system, there would be no restrictions on what moves in and out of the system, thus making its boundaries difficult to identify. Most systems have some control over the movement of information, energy, and matter around them. This control is maintained through the semipermeable nature of their boundaries, which allows some things in and keeps some things out, as well as allowing some out while keeping others in. This control of input and output leads to the dynamic equilibrium found in most well-functioning systems.

Closed Systems

Theoretically, a **closed system** prevents any movement into and out of the system. In this case, the system would be totally static and unchanging. Probably no absolutely closed systems exist in the real world, although some systems may tend to be closed to outside elements. A stone, for example, considered as a system, seems to be almost perfectly closed. It does not take anything in or put anything out. It does not change very much over long periods. In reality, though, it is affected by several elements in nature. It absorbs moisture when it is damp, freezes when cold, and becomes hot in the summer. Over long periods, these factors may cause the stone to crack, break down, and eventually become topsoil.

Systems with which nurses deal frequently are relatively open. Primarily, the client can be categorized as a highly open system that requires certain input elements and has output elements too. Other systems that nurses commonly work with (e.g., hospital administrators and physicians) are generally considered to be open, although their degree of openness may vary widely.

Input and Output

The processes by which a system interacts with elements in its environment are called **input and output.**

Input is defined as any type of information, energy, or material that enters the system from the environment through its boundaries. Conversely, *output* is defined as any information, energy, or material that leaves the system and enters the environment through the system's boundaries. The end product of a system is a type of output that is not reusable as input. Open systems require relatively large amounts of input and output.

Throughput

A third term sometimes used in relationship to the system's dynamic exchange with the environment is **throughput.** Throughput is a process that allows the input to be changed so that it is useful to the system.

For example, most automobiles operate on some form of liquid fossil fuel (input) such as gasoline or diesel fuel. However, going to the gas station and pouring liquid fuel on the roof of the car will not produce the desired effects. If the fuel is put into the gas tank, it can be transformed by the carburetor or fuel-injection system into a fine mist, which when mixed with air and ignited by a spark plug burns rapidly to produce the force necessary to propel the car. Without this internal process (throughput), liquid fuel is not a useful form of energy.

Feedback Loop

The fourth key element of a system is the **feedback loop.** The feedback loop allows the system to monitor its internal functioning so that it can either restrict or increase its input and its output and maintain the highest level of functioning.

Positive Feedback

Two basic types of feedback exist. Positive feedback leads to change within the system, with the goal of improving

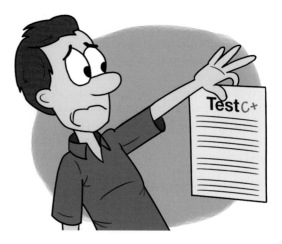

the system. For example, students in the classroom receive feedback from the teacher in several ways; it may be through direct verbal statements such as "Good work on this assignment" or through examination and homework grades. Feedback is considered positive if it produces a change in a student's behavior, such as motivating him or her to study more, spend more time on assignments, or prepare more thoroughly for class.

Negative Feedback

Negative feedback maintains stability—that is, it does not produce change. Negative feedback is not necessarily bad for a system. Rather, when a system has reached its peak level of functioning, negative feedback helps it maintain that level. For example, if a person on a weight-loss regimen has reached the target weight, he or she knows what type of diet and exercise is needed to stay at the ideal weight. Negative feedback—in the form of numbers on the bathroom scale—indicates that no changes in diet or exercise patterns are required.

The feedback loop is an important element in systems theory. It makes the process circular and links the various elements of the system together. Without a feedback loop, it is virtually impossible for the system to have any meaningful control over its input and output.

> *The feedback loop is an important element in systems theory. It makes the process circular and links the various elements of the system together.*

Feedback loops are used at all levels in a hospital. Nurses get feedback about the care they provide both from clients and their supervisors. The hospital administration gets feedback from clients and accrediting agencies. Physicians get feedback from clients, nurses, and the hospital administration. Since the passage of the ACA with its emphasis on quality of care, feedback from clients about the care they received while in health-care facilities is an important part of the facilities' economic survival. Systems theory is present, if sometimes unseen, in almost all health-care settings. Professional nurses need to be able to understand and identify the components of systems theory when they are encountered to improve their nursing practice and quality of care.

MAJOR NURSING THEORIES AND MODELS

At least 15 published nursing models (or theories) have been used to direct nursing education and nursing care.[12] The six nursing models discussed here (Table 3.2) have been selected because they are the most widely accepted and are good examples of how the concepts of client, health, environment, and nursing are used to explain and guide nursing actions. Discussion of these theories is not intended to be extensive but rather to provide an overview of the main concepts of the nurse theorist. It is important to understand the terms used in the theories as defined by their authors and to see the interrelationship between the elements in each theory as well as the similarities and differences among the various models.

The Roy Adaptation Model

As developed by Sister Callista Roy, the Roy Adaptation Model of nursing is very closely related to systems theory.[13] The main goal of this model is to allow the client to reach his or her highest level of functioning through adaptation.

Client

The central element in the Roy Adaptation Model is man (a generic term referring to humans in general, or the client in particular, collectively or individually). Man is viewed as a dynamic entity with both input and output. As derived from the context of the four modes in the Roy Adaptation Model, the client is defined as a biopsychosocial being who is affected by various stimuli and displays behaviors to help adapt to the stimuli. Because the client is constantly being affected by stimuli, adaptation is a continual process.[13]

Inputs are called *stimuli* and include internal stimuli that arise from within the client's environment and stimuli coming from external environmental factors such as physical surroundings, family, and society. The output in the Roy Adaptation Model is the behavior that the client demonstrates as a result of stimuli that are affecting him or her.

Output, or behavior, is a very important element in the Roy Adaptation Model because it provides the **baseline data** about the client that the nurse obtains through assessment techniques. In this model, the output (behavior) is always modified by the client's internal attempts to adapt to the input, or stimuli. Roy has identified four internal adaptational

Table 3.2 **Comparison of Selected Nursing Models**

Nursing Theory	Client	Health	Environment	Nursing
Roy Adaptation Model	Human being—a dynamic system with input and output	A continuum with the ability to adapt successfully to illness	Both internal and external stimuli that affect behaviors	Multistep process that helps the client adapt and reach the highest level of functioning
Orem Self-Care Model	Human being—biological, psychological, social being with the ability for self-care	Able to live life to the fullest through self-care	The medium through which the client moves	Assistance in self-care activities to help the client achieve health
King Model of Goal Attainment	Person—exchanges energy and information with the environment to meet needs	Dynamic process to achieve the highest level of functioning	Personal, interpersonal, and social systems and the external physical world	Dynamic process that identifies and meets the client's health-care needs
Watson Model of Human Caring	Individual—has needs, grows, and develops to reach a state of inner harmony	Dynamic state of growth and development leading to full potential as a human being	The client must overcome certain factors to achieve health	Science of caring that helps clients reach their greatest potential
Johnson Behavioral System Model	Person—a behavioral system; an organized, integrated whole composed of seven subsystems	A behavioral system able to achieve a balanced, steady state	All the internal and external elements that affect client behavior	Activities that manipulate the environment and help clients achieve the balanced state of health
Neuman Health-Care Systems Model	An open system that constantly interacts with internal and external environment	An individual with relatively stable internal functioning of a high state of wellness (stability)	Internal and external stressors that produce change in the client	Identifies boundary disruption and helps clients in activities to restore stability

activities that clients use and has called them the four adaptation modes:

1. The physiological mode (using internal physiological process)
2. The self-concept mode (developed throughout life by experience)
3. The role function mode (dependent on the client's relative place in society)
4. The interdependence mode (indicating how the client relates to others)

Health

In the Roy Adaptation Model, the concept of health is defined as the location of the client along a continuum between perfect health and complete illness. In this model, health is rarely an absolute. Rather, "a person's ability to adapt to stimuli, such as injury, disease, or even psychological stress, determines the level of that person's health status."[13] For example, a client who broke her neck in an automobile accident and was paralyzed but who eventually went back to college, obtained a law degree, and became a practicing lawyer would, in the Roy Adaptation Model, be considered to have a high degree of health because of the ability to adapt to the stimuli imposed.

Environment

The Roy Adaptation Model's definition of environment is synonymous with the concept of stimuli. The environment consists of all those factors that influence the client's behavior, either internally or externally. This model categorizes these environmental elements, or stimuli, into three groups: (1) focal, (2) contextual, and (3) residual.

Focal stimuli are environmental factors that most directly affect the client's behavior and require most of his or her attention. Contextual stimuli form the general physical, social, and psychological environment from which the client emerges. Residual stimuli are factors in the client's past, such as personality characteristics, past experiences, religious beliefs, and social norms, that have an indirect effect on the client's health status. Residual stimuli are often very difficult to identify because they may remain hidden in the person's memory or may be an integral part of the client's personality.

Nursing

In the Roy Adaptation Model, nursing becomes a multistep process, similar to the nursing process, to aid and support the client's attempt to adapt to stimuli in one or more of the four adaptive modes. To determine what type of help is required to promote adaptation, the nurse must first assess the client.

Assessment

The primary nursing assessments are of the client's behavior (output). Basically, the nurse should try to determine whether the client's behavior is adaptive or maladaptive in each of the four adaptational modes previously defined. Some first-level assessments of the client with pneumonia might include a temperature of 104°F, a cough productive of thick green sputum, chest pain on inspiration, and signs of weakness or physical debility, such as the inability to bring in wood for the fireplace or to visit friends.

A second-level assessment should also be made to determine what type of stimuli (input) is affecting the client's health-care status. In the case of the pneumonia client, this might include a culture and sensitivity test of the sputum to identify the invasive bacteria, assessment of the client's clothes to determine whether they were adequate for the weather outside, and an investigation to find out whether any neighbors could help the client upon discharge from the hospital.

Analysis

After performing the assessment, the nurse analyzes the data and arranges them in such a way as to be able to make a statement about the client's adaptive or maladaptive behaviors—that is, the nurse identifies the problem. In current terminology, this identification of the problem is called a **nursing diagnosis.** The problem statement is the first part of the three-part PES (problem–etiology–signs and symptoms) formulation that completes the nursing diagnosis (Fig. 3.1).

Setting Goals

After the problem has been identified, goals for optimal adaptation are established. Ideally, these goals should be a collaborative effort between the nurse and the client. A determination of the actions needed to achieve the goals is the next step in the process. The focus should be on manipulation of the stimuli to promote optimal adaptation. Finally, an evaluation is made of the whole process to determine whether the goals have been met. If the goals have not been met, the nurse must determine why, not how, the activities should be modified to achieve the goals.[11]

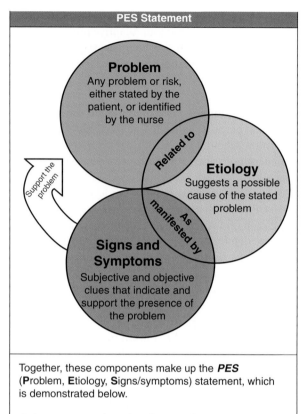

PES Statement

Problem
Any problem or risk, either stated by the patient, or identified by the nurse

Related to

Etiology
Suggests a possible cause of the stated problem

Support the problem

As manifested by

Signs and Symptoms
Subjective and objective clues that indicate and support the presence of the problem

Together, these components make up the **PES** (**P**roblem, **E**tiology, **S**igns/symptoms) statement, which is demonstrated below.

Pain, acute, may be **related to _surgical wound_, as manifested by _facial grimacing_, _increased heart rate_,** and **_verbal complaints_** of pain at the incision site.

Figure 3.1 Together, these components make up the **PES** (**p**roblem–**e**tiology–**s**igns and symptoms) statement: Pain, acute, may be related to _surgical wound_, as manifested by _facial grimacing, increased heart rate_, and _verbal complaints_ of pain at the incision site.

The Orem Self-Care Model

Dorothea E. Orem's model of nursing is based on the belief that health care is each individual's own responsibility. The aim of this model is to help clients direct and carry out activities that maintain or improve their health.[14]

Client

As with most other nursing models, the central element of the Orem model is the client, who is a biological, psychological, and social being with the capacity for self-care. _Self-care_ is defined as the practice of activities that individuals initiate and perform on their own behalf to maintain life, health, and well-being. Self-care is a requirement for maintenance of life and for optimal functioning.

Health

In the Orem Self-Care Model, health is defined as the person's ability to live fully within a particular physical, biological, and social environment, achieving a higher level of functioning that distinguishes the person from lower life-forms.

Quality of life is an extremely important element in this model of nursing. A person who is healthy is living life to the fullest and has the capacity to continue that life through self-care. An unhealthy person is an individual who has a self-care deficit. This group of unhealthy individuals also includes adults with diseases and injuries, young and dependent children, elderly people, and disabled people. This deficit is indicated by the inability to carry out one or more of the key health-care activities. These activities have been categorized into six groups:

- Air, water, and food
- Excretion of waste
- Activity and rest
- Solitude and social interactions
- Avoiding hazards to life and well-being
- Being normal mentally under universal self-care

Self-Care

In the Orem model, self-care is a two-part concept. The first type of self-care is called _universal self-care_ and includes those elements commonly found in everyday life that support and encourage normal human growth, development, and functioning. Individuals who are healthy, according to the Orem model, carry out the activities listed in order to maintain a state of health. To some degree, all of these elements are necessary activities in maintaining health through self-care.[15]

The second type of self-care comes into play when the individual is unable to conduct one or more of the six self-care activities. This second type of self-care is called _health deviation self-care_. Health deviation self-care includes those activities carried out by individuals who have diseases, injuries, physiological or psychological stress, or other health-care concerns. Activities such as seeking health care at an emergency department or clinic, entering a drug **rehabilitation** unit, joining a health club or weight-control program, or going to a physician's office fall into this category.

Environment

Environment, in the self-care model, is the medium through which clients move as they conduct their daily activities. Although less emphasized in this model, the environment is generally viewed as a negative factor in a person's health status because many environmental factors detract from the ability to provide self-care. Environment includes social interactions with others, situations that must be resolved, and physical elements that affect health.

Nursing

The primary goal of nursing in the Orem model is to help the client conduct self-care activities in such a way as to reach the highest level of human functioning. Because there is a range of levels of self-care ability, three distinct levels, or systems, of nursing care are delineated, based on the individual's ability to undertake self-care activities. As clients become less able to care for themselves, their nursing care needs increase.

Wholly Compensated Care

A person who is able to carry out few or no self-care activities falls into the wholly compensated nursing care category, in which the nurse must provide for most or all of the client's self-care needs. Examples of clients who require this level of care include comatose and ventilator-dependent clients in an intensive care unit, clients in surgery and the immediate recovery period, women in the labor and delivery phases of childbirth, and clients with emotional and psychological problems so severe as to render them unable to conduct normal activities of daily living (ADLs).

> *The primary goal of nursing in the Orem model is to help the client conduct self-care activities in such a way as to reach the highest level of human functioning.*

Partially Compensated Care

Clients in the partially compensated category of nursing care can meet some to most of their self-care needs but still have certain self-care deficits that require nursing intervention. The nurse's role becomes one of identifying these needs and carrying out activities to meet them until the client reaches a state of health and is able to meet the needs personally. Examples of this level of nursing care include postoperative clients who can feed themselves and do basic ADLs but are unable to care for a catheter and dressing, and clients with newly diagnosed diabetes who have not yet learned the technique of self-administered insulin injections.

Supportive Developmental Care

Clients who are able to meet all of their basic self-care needs require very few or no nursing interventions.

These clients fall in the supportive developmental category of nursing care, in which the nurse's main functions are to teach the client how to maintain or improve health and to offer guidance in self-care activities and provide emotional support and encouragement.

What Do You Think?

Based on your experiences with the health-care system, write your own definition of client (patient). What factors led you to this definition?

Also, the nurse may adjust the environment to support the client's growth and development toward self-care or may identify community resources to help in the self-care process.[15] Conducting prenatal classes, arranging for discharge planning, providing child screening programs through a community health agency, and organizing aerobic exercise classes for post-coronary clients all are nursing actions that belong in the supportive developmental category of care.

A Three-Step Process

In the Orem model, nursing care is carried out through a three-step process. Step 1 determines whether nursing care is necessary. This step includes a basic assessment of the client and identification of self-care problems and needs. Step 2 determines the appropriate nursing care system category and plans nursing care according to that category. Step 3 provides the indicated nursing care or actions to meet the client's self-care needs.

Step 3—the provision of nursing care (implementation phase)—is carried out by helping the client through one or a combination of five nursing methods:[12]

- Acting for or doing for another person
- Guiding another person
- Supporting another person (physically or psychologically)
- Providing an environment that promotes personal development
- Teaching another person

Orem, by focusing on the individual's ability to perform self-care, was many years ahead of her time. Current trends in health care reinforce her belief that individuals can take responsibility for care of themselves and others. The capacity for self-care is a key premise of the ACA and the more than 8000 apps that are available that deal with self-care. It might even be referred to as "Digital Orem."

The King Model of Goal Attainment

The current widely accepted practice of establishing health-care goals for clients, and directing client care to meet these goals, has its origins in the King Model of Goal Attainment developed by Imogene M. King. It is also called the King Intervention Model.[16]

The King model also notes that nursing must function in all three system levels found in the environment: Personal, interactional, and social. The primary function of nursing is at the personal systems level, where care of the individual is the main focus. However, nurses can effectively provide care at the interactional systems level, where they deal with small to moderate-sized groups in activities such as group therapy and health-promotion classes. Finally, nurses can provide care at the social systems level through such activities as community health programs. In addition, the role of nursing at the social systems level can be expanded to include involvement in policy decisions that have an effect on the health-care system as a whole.

Client

As in other nursing models, the focal point of care in the King model is the person or client. The client is viewed as an open system that exchanges energy and information with the environment—a personal system with physical, emotional, and intellectual needs that change and grow during the course of life. Because these needs cannot be met completely by the client alone, interpersonal systems are developed through interactions with others, depending on the client's perceptions of reality, communications with others, and transactions to reduce stress and tension in the environment.

Environment

Environment is an important concept in the King model and encompasses a number of interrelated elements. The personal and interpersonal systems or groups are central to King's conception of environment. They are formed at various levels according to internal goals established by the client.

Personal Systems

At the most basic level are the personal systems, where an interchange takes place between two individuals who share similar goals. An example of such a personal system is a client–nurse relationship.

Interpersonal Systems

At the intermediate level are the interpersonal systems that involve relatively small groups of individuals who share like goals, for example, a formal weight-loss program in which the members have the common goal of losing weight. Human interactions, communications, role delineation, and stress reduction are essential factors at this level.

Social Systems

At the highest level are social systems, which include the large, relatively homogeneous elements of society. The health-care system, government, and society in general are some important social systems. Common goals of these social systems are organization, authority, power, status, and decision. Although the client may not be in direct interaction with the social systems, these systems are important because the personal and interpersonal systems necessarily function within larger social systems.

Invoking the principle of nonsummativity,* whenever one part of an open system is changed, all the other parts of the system feel the effect. For example, a decision made at the governmental level to reduce Medicare or Medicaid payments may affect when and how often a client can use health-care services such as doctor's office visits, group therapy, or emergency department care. The King model also includes the external physical environment that affects a person's health and well-being. As the person moves through the world, the physical setting interacts with the personal system to either improve or degrade the client's health-care status.

Health

Viewed as a dynamic process that involves a range of human life experiences, health exists in people when they can achieve their highest level of functioning. Health is the primary goal of the client in the King model. It is achieved by continually adjusting to environmental stressors, maximizing the use of available resources, and setting and achieving goals for one's role in life. Anything that disrupts or interferes with people's ability to function normally in their chosen roles is considered to be a state of illness.

*Nonsummativity is the degree of connection among the systems parts. The higher the degree of nonsummativity, the greater the interdependence of parts.

Nursing

The King model considers nursing to be a dynamic process and a type of personal system based on interactions between the nurse and the client. During these interactions, the nurse and the client jointly evaluate and identify the health-care needs, set goals for fulfillment of the needs, and consider actions to take in achieving those goals. Nursing is a multifaceted process that includes a range of activities such as the promotion and maintenance of health through education, the restoration of health through care of the sick and injured, and preparation for death through care of the dying.[11]

The process of nursing in the King model includes five key elements considered central to all human interactions:

- Action: A sequence of behaviors involving mental and physical activities
- Reaction: The resulting behaviors produced by the process of action
- Interaction: The client and nurse communicating together to establish goals
- Transaction: A life situation in which perceivers and things perceived are encountered and entered into as active participants
- Feedback: Change that occurs as a result of the interaction and transaction process.

With some modifications, the King model has been successfully implemented in a variety of health-care settings ranging from rural clinics to acute urban care centers. Its focus on the one-on-one interaction between the nurse and the client is at the heart of all nursing practice. Establishing goals with the client rather than for the client raises the success level of the interventions and promotes better outcomes.

The Watson Model of Human Caring

Although the concept of caring has always been an important, if somewhat obscure, element in the practice of nursing, the Watson Model of Human Caring defines caring in a detailed and systematic manner. In the development of her model, Jean Watson used a philosophical approach rather than the systems theory approach seen in many other nursing models. Her main concern in the development of this model was to balance the impersonal aspects of nursing care that are found in the technological and scientific aspects of practice with the personal and interpersonal elements of care that grow from a humanistic belief

in life. Watson is also one of the very few theorists who openly recognizes the client's and family's spiritual beliefs as an essential element of health.[17]

Client

The concept of client or patient in the Watson model is developed closely with the concept of nursing. The individuality of the client is a key concern. The Watson model views the client as someone who has needs, who grows and develops throughout life, and who eventually reaches a state of internal harmony.

The client is also seen as a gestalt, or a whole entity, who has value because of inherent goodness and capacity to develop. This gestalt, or holistic, view of the human being is a recurring theme in the Watson model; it emphasizes that the total person is more important to nursing care than the individual injury or disease process that produced the need for care. "The Watson model views the client as someone who has needs, who grows and develops throughout life, and who eventually reaches a state of internal harmony."[17]

Environment

Environment in the Watson model is a concept that is also closely intertwined with the concept of nursing. Viewed primarily as a negative element in the health-care process, the environment consists of those factors that the client must overcome to achieve a state of health. The environment can be both external (physical and social elements) and internal (psychological reactions that affect health).

Health

To be healthy according to the Watson model, the individual must be in a dynamic state of growth and development that leads to reaching full potential as a human. As with other nursing models, health is viewed as a continuum along which a person at any point may tend more toward health or more toward illness.

Illness, in the Watson model, is the client's inability to integrate life experiences and the failure to achieve full potential or inner harmony. In this model, the state of illness is not necessarily synonymous with the disease process. If the person reacts to the disease process in such a way as to find meaning, that response is considered to be healthy. A failure to find meaning in the disease experience leads to a state of illness.

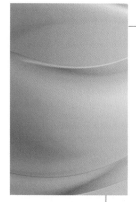

Issues Now

The Pew Commission Final Report

Projected estimates of the nursing shortage based on data collected by the U.S. Bureau of the Census Current Population Survey, Division of Nursing, the Pew Commission, and the Buerhaus and Staiger data collection agency in 1998 are now considered woefully inadequate. Current projections of the nursing shortage range from 400,000 to as many as 1,000,000 by the year 2015. The Pew Commission's final report addressed the competencies that nurses in the future will need.

Twenty-One Competencies for the 21st Century

1. Embrace a personal ethic of social responsibility and service.
2. Exhibit ethical behavior in all professional activities.
3. Provide evidence-based, clinically competent care.
4. Incorporate the multiple determinants of health in clinical care.
5. Apply knowledge of the new sciences.
6. Demonstrate critical thinking, reflection, and problem-solving skills.
7. Understand the role of primary care.
8. Rigorously practice preventive health care.
9. Integrate population-based care and services into practice.
10. Improve access to health care for those with unmet health needs.
11. Practice relationship-centered care with individuals and families.
12. Provide culturally sensitive care to a diverse society.
13. Partner with communities in health-care decisions.
14. Use communication and information technology effectively and appropriately.
15. Work in interdisciplinary teams.
16. Ensure care that balances individual, professional, system, and social needs.
17. Practice leadership.
18. Take responsibility for quality of care and health outcomes at all levels.
19. Contribute to continuous improvement of the health-care system.
20. Advocate for public policy that promotes and protects the health of the public.
21. Continue to learn and help others to learn.

The Pew Commission also went on to identify five key areas for professional education:

1. Change professional training to meet the demands of the new health-care system.
2. Ensure that the health profession workforce reflects the diversity of the nation's population.
3. Require interdisciplinary competence in all health professionals.

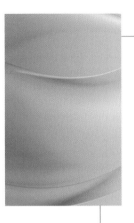

Issues Now _{continued}

4. Continue to move education into ambulatory practice.
5. Encourage public service of all health-professional students and graduates.

    The changes that will occur over the next decade may take some health-care professionals out of their comfort zone, but they will also open up a vista of opportunities for those willing to look creatively into the future. Nursing has to recognize that it will grow only to the extent that it is able to contribute to the needs of an evolving health-care system. These needs will change with time. The Pew Report, although broad in scope, provides the nursing profession with a blueprint for dealing with these changes as they occur. It is a call to action that nurses and the nursing profession need to hear.

Sources: Bellack JP, O'Neil EH. Recreating nursing practice for a new century: Recommendations of the Pew Health Professions Commission's Final Report. *Nursing and Health Care Perspectives*, 21(1):14–21, 2000; Brady M, et al. A proposed framework for differentiating the 21 Pew Competencies by level of nursing education. *Nursing and Health Care Perspectives*, 22(1):30–36, 2001; Pontious M. Where have all the nurses gone? *Oklahoma Nurse*, 47(1):1, 18, 2002; More than one million new nurses needed by 2010. *American Nurse*, 34(1):5, 2002; Critical Challenges: Revitalizing the health professions for the 21st century. Pew Health Professions Commission, San Francisco, 1995.

Nursing

Watson makes a clear distinction between the science of nursing and the practice of curing (medicine).[12] She defined nursing as the science of caring in which the primary goal is to assist the client to reach the greatest level of personal potential. The practice of curing involves the conduct of activities that have the goal of treatment and elimination of disease.

The process of nursing in the Watson model is based on the systematic use of the scientific problem-solving method for decision-making. To best understand nursing as a science of caring, the nurse should hold certain beliefs and be able to initiate certain caring activities.

Values

Basic to the beliefs necessary for the successful practice of nursing in the Watson model is the formation of a humanistic, altruistic system of values based on the tenet that all people are inherently valuable because they are human. In addition, the nurse should have a strong sense of faith and hope in people and their condition because of the human potential for development.

The Johnson model sees human behavior as being goal directed, which leads the person to constant growth and development beyond the maintenance of a mere steady state.

Caring

According to Watson's caring way, several activities are important in the practice of nursing. These include establishing a relationship of help and trust between the nurse and the client; encouraging the client to express both positive and negative feelings with acceptance; manipulating the environment to make it more supportive, protective, or corrective for the client with any type of disease process; and assisting in whatever way is deemed appropriate to meet the basic human needs of the client.

The Johnson Behavioral System Model

By integrating systems theory with behavioral theory, Dorothy E. Johnson developed a model of nursing that considers client behavior to be the key to preventing illness and to restoring health when illness occurs. Johnson holds that human behavior is really a type of system in itself that is influenced by input factors from the environment and has output that in turn affects the environment.[12]

Client

Drawing directly on the terminology of systems theory, the Johnson model describes the person, or client, as a behavioral system that is an organized and integrated whole. The whole is greater than the sum of its parts because of the integration and functioning of its subsystems. In the Johnson model, the client as a behavioral system is composed of seven distinct behavioral subsystems. In turn, each of these seven behavioral subsystems contains four structural elements that guide and shape the subsystem.

Security

The first behavioral subsystem is the attachment, or affiliate, subsystem. Its driving force is security. For the most part, the type of activity that this subsystem undertakes is inclusion in social functions, and the behavior that is observed from this subsystem is social interaction.

Dependency

The second behavioral subsystem is dependency; its main goal is to help others. The primary type of activity involved is nurturing and promoting self-image. The observable behaviors that are a result of this activity include approval, attention, and physical assistance of the person.

Taking In

The third behavioral subsystem is the ingestive subsystem. Its motive is to meet the body's basic physiological needs of food and nutrient intake. Correspondingly, its primary activity is seeking and eating food.

Eliminative Behavior

The fourth behavioral subsystem is the eliminative; its goal is removing waste products from the system. Its primary activity is means of elimination, which is observed as the behavior of expelling waste products.

Sexual Behavior

The fifth behavioral subsystem is sexual behavior, which is found in the Johnson model's description of the person. The sexual subsystem has gratification and procreation of the species as its goals. It involves the complex activities of identifying gender roles, undergoing sexual development, and participating in sexual activity. It manifests itself in courting and mating behaviors.

Self-Protection

The sixth behavioral subsystem is the aggressive subsystem; its main goal is self-preservation. All of the actions that individuals undertake to protect themselves from harm, either internal or external, derive from this subsystem and are shown in actions toward others and the environment in general.

Achievement

The seventh, and final, behavioral subsystem is achievement. Exploration and manipulation of the environment are the objectives of this subsystem. Gaining mastery and control over the environment is the primary activity; it can be demonstrated externally when the individual shows that learning has occurred and higher-level accomplishments are being produced.[18]

As with all open systems, the behavioral system that makes up the person seeks to maintain a dynamic balance by regulating input and output. This regulation process takes the form of adapting to the environment and responding to others. However, the Johnson model sees human behavior as being goal oriented, which leads the person to constant growth and development beyond the maintenance of a mere steady state.

Health

According to the Johnson model, a state of health is achieved when balance and a steady state exist within the behavioral systems of the client. Under normal circumstances, the human system has enough inherent flexibility to maintain this balance without external intervention. At times, however, the system's balance may be disturbed to such a degree by physical disease, injury, or emotional crisis as to require external assistance. This out-of-balance state is the state of illness.

Environment

In the Johnson model, the environment is defined as all those internal and external elements that have an effect on the behavioral system. These environmental elements include obvious external factors, such as air temperature and relative humidity;

sociological factors, such as family, neighborhood, and society in general; and the internal environment, such as bodily processes, psychological states, religious beliefs, and political orientation.

All seven behavioral subsystems are involved with the client's relationship to the environment through the regulation of input and output. The client is continually interacting with the environment in an attempt to remain healthy by maintaining an internal dynamic balance.

Nursing

In the Johnson model, nursing is an activity that helps the individual achieve and maintain an optimal level of behavior (state of health) through the manipulation and regulation of the environment.[11] Nursing has functions in both health and illness. Nursing interventions to either maintain or restore health involve four activities in the regulation of the environment:

- Restricting harmful environmental factors
- Defending the client from negative environmental influences
- Inhibiting adverse elements from occurring
- Facilitating positive internal environmental factors in the recovery process

As a professional, the nurse in the Johnson model provides direct services to the client. By interacting with, and sometimes intervening in, the multiple subsystems that are found in the client's environment, the nurse acts as an external regulatory force. The goal of nursing is to promote the highest level of functioning and development in the client at all times.

Nursing actions include helping the client act in a socially acceptable manner, monitoring and aiding with biological processes that are necessary for maintaining a dynamic balance, demonstrating support for medical care and treatment during illness, and taking actions to prevent illness from recurring. In this model, nursing makes its own unique contribution to the health and well-being of individuals and provides a service that is complementary to those provided by other health-care professionals.

The Neuman Health-Care Systems Model

As envisioned by Betty Neuman, the Health-Care Systems Model focuses on the individual and his or her environment and is applicable to a variety of health-care disciplines apart from nursing. Drawing from systems theory, the Neuman model also includes elements from stress theory with an overall holistic view of humanity and health care.[16]

Client

In this model, the client is viewed as an open system that interacts constantly with internal and external environments through the system's boundaries. The client-system's boundaries are called *lines of defense* and *resistance* in the Neuman model and may be represented graphically as a series of concentric circles that surround the basic core of the individual. The goal of these boundaries is to keep the basic core system stable by controlling system input and output.

Neuman classifies these defensive boundaries according to their various functions. The internal lines of resistance are the boundaries that are closest to the basic core and thus protect the basic internal structure of the system. The normal lines of defense are outside the internal lines of resistance; they protect the system from common, everyday environmental stressors. The flexible line of defense surrounds the normal line of defense and protects it from extreme environmental stressors. The general goal of all these protective boundaries is to maintain the internal stability of the individual.

Health

Health, then, in the Neuman model is defined as the relatively stable internal functioning of the client. Optimal health exists when the client is maintained in a high state of wellness or stability.

As in other nursing models, health is not considered an absolute state, but rather a continuum that reflects the client's internal stability while moving from wellness to illness and back. It takes a considerable amount of physical and psychological energy to maintain the stability of the person who is in good health.

The opposite of a healthy state, illness, exists when the client's core structure becomes unstable through the effects of environmental factors that overwhelm and defeat the lines of defense and resistance.

> *In the Johnson model, nursing is an activity that helps the individual achieve and maintain an optimal level of behavior (state of health) through the manipulation and regulation of the environment.*

These environmental factors, whether internal or external, are called **stressors** in this model.

Environment

The environment is composed of internal and external forces, or stressors, that produce change or response in the client. Stressors may be helpful or harmful, strong or weak.

Stressors are also classified according to their relationship to the basic core of the client-system. Stressors that are completely outside the basic core are termed *extrapersonal* and are either physical, such as atmospheric temperature, or sociological, such as living in either a rural or an urban setting. Interpersonal stressors arise from interactions with other human beings. Marital relationships, career expectations, and friendships are included in this group of interpersonal stressors. Those stressors that occur within the client are called *intrapersonal* and include involuntary physiological responses, psychological reactions, and internal thought processes.

Nursing

The nurse's role in the Neuman model is to identify at what level or in which boundary a disruption in the client's internal stability has taken place and then to aid the client in activities that strengthen or restore the integrity of that particular boundary. The Neuman model expands the concept of client from the individual to include families, small groups, the community, or even society in general.

Identifying Stressors

Nursing's main concern in this model is either to identify stressors that will disrupt a defensive boundary in the future (prevention) or to identify a stressor that has already disrupted a defensive boundary, thereby producing instability (illness).[16] The Neuman model is based on the nursing process and identifies three levels of intervention: primary, secondary, and tertiary.

Types of Intervention

The main goal of a **primary intervention** is to prevent possible symptoms that could be caused by environmental stressors. Teaching clients about stress management, giving immunizations, and encouraging aerobic exercise to prevent heart disease are examples of primary interventions.

A **secondary intervention** is aimed at treating symptoms that have already been produced by stressors. Many of the actions that nurses perform in the hospital or clinic (e.g., giving pain medications or teaching a client with cardiac disease about the benefits of a low-sodium diet) fall into this secondary intervention category.

A **tertiary intervention** seeks to restore the client's system to an optimal state of balance by adapting to negative environmental stressors. Teaching a client how to care for a colostomy bag at home after discharge from the hospital is an example of a nursing activity at the tertiary level. It occurs after the client has received a secondary intervention and offers support to the client so that he or she can continue to recover or prevent further deterioration in health.

What Do You Think?

Which of these major theories appeals to you most? Why? How would you apply it to an actual client you have seen in the clinical setting or to a sick family member?

TRENDS FOR THE FUTURE IN NURSING THEORY

Although the search for the perfect nursing model continues, the emphasis in recent years has shifted from developing new theories to applying existing theories to nursing practice. Also, the new theorists seem to be more interested in expanding existing nursing theories by including such concepts as cultural diversity, spirituality, family, and social change rather than starting all over again from the beginning. A good example of this trend is the cultural meaning–centered theory that was published by Mendyka and Bloom.[19] This theory expands the King model by adding a cultural perspective.

A More Recent Theory

One of the more recent of the established nursing theories is the Man-Living-Health Model proposed by Rosemary Rizzo Parse. Although her original work started in 1981, a more developed form of her theory was published in 1987.[20–22] Parse's theory stresses the elements of experience, personal **values**, and lifestyle choices in the maintenance of health.

A Matter of Choice

In this theory, the client can be any person or family who is concerned with the quality of their life situation. The client is viewed as an open, whole being who is influenced by past and present life experiences. The ability to make free choices is essential in this theory. The client, through choices he or she makes, interacts with the environment to influence health either positively or negatively.

For Parse, health is an ongoing process. Because clients make free choices, their health status is continually unfolding. In addition, health is determined by lived experiences, synthesis of values, and the way the client lives.[23]

Finding Meaning

The main role of nursing in the Parse model is to guide clients in finding and understanding the meaning of their lives. Once the client chooses a healthy life situation, the nurse can further increase the quality of the client's life and improve his or her health status. The ability to change the client's health-related values is an important skill for nurses to master in this model.

Parse never really defines the concept of environment in relationship to her theory. Specifically, it seems to be any health-related setting, but it can also be expanded to include past and present experiences.

MIDDLE-RANGE THEORIES AND MODELS

Middle-range theories and models have been present in nursing research for many years. Over 50 have identified themselves as middle range, although there are many more that fit into the category.[24] A **middle-range theory** is a set of relatively concrete concepts or propositions that lie between a minor working hypothesis found in everyday nursing research and a well-developed major nursing theory, like those previously discussed.[24,25] Middle-range theories are less comprehensive and more focused than the major nursing theories but are not as specific or concrete as situation-specific practice theories. Middle-range models develop from middle-range theories, although not all middle-range theories have a model.

Middle-range theories generally contain only a few basic ideas or concepts that researchers are attempting to prove or illustrate. They do not have a large number of variables and tend to focus on one or two problems that are linked, like the major theories, to human beings, environment, health care, or nursing. They are less abstract than the major theories and are much more easily applied to practice hypotheses. However, when several middle-range theories are used to investigate the same or similar concepts over a period of time, they can be woven together to reinforce or even form the fabric of a new major nursing theory.[24]

Middle-range theories should be socially significant, meaning that they deal with people or populations with health-care conditions. They should also have theoretical significance, meaning that they develop a new set of facts or data that adds to the theoretical knowledge base of nursing.[25] The whole movement toward evidence-based practice (EBP) depends on this type of research. Middle-range theories often form the theoretical framework for a research project.

Two Middle-Range Nursing Theories

Formulated in 1987, Dr. Nola Pender's Health Promotion Model is widely used as the theoretical framework for research on prenatal care and pregnancy. It was based on her conceptualizations on Orem's Self-Care model. Pender proposes that there are several key factors that provide the primary motivation for individuals to adopt behaviors that maintain and improve their health. These factors include the person's perception of:

• How important it is to be healthy
• How much control they have over their health
• How much control they have over the health-care system
• What it means to them to be healthy
• What their current health status is
• What the benefits and barriers are to health improvement

The goal of the individual is to move toward a balanced state of positive health and well-being.[26] Health is up to the individual, not the health-care system; although the health-care system can be an important part, it will always be secondary to the individual.

Swanson's Theory of Caring, first published in 1991, was inspired by the writings of Jean Watson and by Kristen M. Swanson's own experiences as a nurse providing care for clients and families. As she observed how clients used their internal strengths to overcome their illnesses and transition to a state of health, Swanson began to see a pattern of how clients who successfully made the transition to wellness related to other individuals and how those individuals affected the final health status of the client.[27]

As the elements of the theory became more defined, Swanson conducted three studies that reinforced the underlying assumptions of her theory. The data from these three studies were used to better clarify the key concepts of her theory: person, environment, health/well-being, and caring actions. Based on additional research, Swanson was able to develop instruments to measure key concepts and identify concrete interventions to use in implementing her theory of caring.[28] She identified five "caring processes" that were essential to the successful transition to health experienced by clients: knowing, being with, doing for, enabling, and maintaining belief.[29]

The role of the nurse in the Theory of Caring is to guide the client through discussions of their experiences so they believe that their problems are understood by the nurse. Additionally, they are being kept informed with key information, their needs are being met, their lives are being validated, and the nurse believes in the client's ability to move toward wellness. The anticipated outcome is that the clients are better able to integrate their sufferings and losses into their lives.[27] Although originally studied in the perinatal setting, the Theory of Caring has been adopted into many other health-care settings, including critical care, mental health, public health, hospice, gerontology, and oncology.

Some other middle-range theories that are commonly used in nursing research include Mishel's uncertainty in illness theory, Reed's self-transcendence theory, Thomas's women's anger theory, Jezewski's cultural brokering theory, Auvil-Novak's chemotherapeutic intervention for postsurgical pain theory, Good and Moore's balance between analgesia and side effects theory, and Huth and Moore's acute pain management theory.

New Challenges to Nursing Theory

As with any developing science, nursing will continue to change and respond to the dynamic trends of society. Older nursing models will be either replaced by new ones or modified to include developing concepts. Indeed, one of the hallmarks of a sound nursing theory or model is its flexibility and ability to adapt to new discoveries.

An increasing number of **independent nurse practitioners** and other advanced practice nurses are testing nursing theories as they have never been tested before. The theories that are flexible, realistic, and usable in practice will survive and remain as the pillars of professional nursing.[23] Those that are too theoretical or rigid will fall by the wayside and become mere footnotes in nursing texts.

Conclusion

As nursing takes its rightful place among the other helping professions, nursing theory will take on additional importance. Nursing theories and models are the systematic conceptualizations of nursing practice and how they fit into the health-care system. Nursing theories help describe, explain, predict, and control nursing activities to achieve the goals of client care. By understanding and using nursing theory, nurses will be better able to incorporate theoretical information into their practice to provide new ways of approaching nursing care and improving nursing practice.

The development of nursing theory and models indicates a maturing of the profession. As the knowledge associated with the profession increases and becomes unique, more complex, and better organized, the general body of nursing science knowledge also increases and EBP becomes a reality. When nursing becomes a well-developed body of specialized knowledge, it will be fully recognized as a separate scientific discipline and take its rightful place as a true profession.

Critical Thinking Exercises

Mrs. M is an 88-year-old woman who has been a resident of St. Martin's Village, a lifetime care community, since her husband died 8 years ago. Her health status is fair. She has adult-onset diabetes controlled by oral medication and a scar from a tumor behind her left ear that was removed surgically. The wound from this tumor removal has never healed completely, and it has continuously oozed a serous fluid, requiring a dressing.

At St. Martin's Village, Mrs. M has her own apartment, which she maintains with minimal assistance. She receives one hot meal each day in a common dining room and has access to a full range of services such as a beauty shop, recreational facilities, and a chapel. She is generally happy in this setting. She has no immediate family nearby, and the cost of the facility was covered by a large, one-time gift from her now-deceased husband. Recently, she has become much weaker and has had difficulty walking; attending activities, including meals; and changing the dressing on her ear. The nurse at St. Martin's Village is sent to evaluate this client.

• Select two nursing models and apply their principles to this case study. Make sure you include the concepts of client, health, environment, and nursing.

References

1. McCrae N. Whither Nursing Models? The value of nursing theory in the context of evidence-based practice and multidisciplinary health care. *Journal of Advanced Nursing*, 68(1): 222–229, 2012.

2. Brokel JM. Iowa e-health project: Planning for health information exchange with nursing standardized language with health information technology tools. *Iowa Nurse Reporter*, 22(3):1, 21–22, 2009.

3. Scherb CA, Weydt AP. Work complexity assessment, nursing interventions classification, and nursing outcomes classification: Making connections. *Creative Nursing*, 15(1):16–22, 2009.

4. Bulechek GM, Butcher HK, Dochterman JM. *Nursing Interventions Classification (NIC)* (5th ed.). St. Louis: Mosby Elsevier, 2008.

5. Moss J, Saba V. Costing nursing care: Using the clinical care classification system to value nursing intervention in an acute-care setting. *Computers, Informatics, Nursing*, 30: Topical Collection 3: TC149-54, 2012.

6. McCloskey JC, Bulecheck GM, Donohue W. Nursing interventions core to specialty practice. *Nursing Outlook*, 46(3):67–76, 1998.

7. Mitchell PR, Grippando GM. *Nursing Perspectives and Issues*. Albany, NY: Delmar, 1993.

8. McCann-Flynn JB, Heffron PB. Nursing. In: *Concept to Practice*. Bowie, MD: Robert J. Brady, 1984.

9. Miles KS, Vallish R. Creating a personalized professional practice framework for nursing. *Nursing Economic$*, 28(3):171–180, 189, 2010.

10. Putt A. *General Systems Theory Applied to Nursing*. Boston: Little, Brown and Company, 1978.

11. Stevens BJ. *Nursing Theory: Analysis, Application, Evaluation*. Boston: Little, Brown and Company, 1984.

12. Fawcett J. Conceptual models and nursing practice: The reciprocal relationship. *Journal of Advanced Nursing*, 17(2):224–228, 1992.

13. Clarke PN, Barone SH, Hanna D, Senesac PM. Roy's Adaptation Model. *Nursing Science Quarterly*, 24(4):337–344, 2011.

14. Allison SE. Self-care requirements for activity and rest: An Orem nursing focus. *Nursing Science Quarterly*, 20(1):68–76, 2007.

15. Leininger MM (ed). *Cultural Care Diversity and Universality: A Theory of Nursing*. New York: National League for Nursing, 1992.

16. Beryl Pilkington F. Envisioning nursing in 2050 through the eyes of nurse theorists: King, Neuman, and Roy. *Nursing Science Quarterly*, 20(2):108–128, 2007.

17. Watson J. *Nursing: Human Science and Human Care. A Theory of Nursing*. Norwalk, CT: Appleton-Century-Crofts, 1985.

18. Schaefer KM, Pond JB. *Levine's Conservation Model: A Framework for Nursing Practice*. Philadelphia: F. A. Davis, 1991.

19. Khowaja K. Utilization of King's interacting systems framework and theory of goal attainment with new multidisciplinary model: Clinical pathway. *Australian Journal of Advanced Nursing*, 24(2):44–50, 2007.

20. Aquino-Russell C. Living attentive presence and changing perspectives with a Web-based nursing theory course. *Nursing Science Quarterly*, 20(2):128–134, 2007.

21. Ursel KL, Aquino-Russell CE. Illuminating person-centered care with Parse's teaching-learning model. *Nursing Science Quarterly*, 23(2):118–223, 2010.

22. Chen H. The lived experience of moving forward for clients with spinal cord injury: A Parse research method study. *Journal of Advanced Nursing*, 66(5):1132–1141, 2010.

23. Manojlovich M. The Nursing Worklife Model: Extending and refining a new theory. *Journal of Nursing Management*, 15(3):256–263, 2007.

24. Fawcett J, Garity J. Chapter 6: Evaluation of middle-range theories. In: *Evaluating Research for Evidence-Based Nursing*. F. A. Davis, 2009.

25. Liehr P, Smith MJ. Middle range theory: Spinning research and practice to create knowledge for the new millennium. *Advances in Nursing Science*, 21(4):81–91, 1999.

26. Pender NJ. *Health Promotion Nursing Practice* (2nd ed.). Norwalk, CT: Appleton & Lange, 1987.

27. Andershed B, Olsson K. Review of research related to Kristen Swanson's middle-range theory of caring. *Scandinavian Journal of Caring Sciences*, 23(3):598–610, 2009.

28. Tesfamichael A. A pivotal caring experience for a nursing student. *International Journal for Human Caring*, 15(1):65–67, 2011.

29. Swanson KM. What is known about caring in nursing science. A literary meta-analysis. In Hinshaw AS, Shaver J, Feetham S (eds): *Handbook of Clinical Nursing Research*. Sage: Thousand Oaks, CA, 1999.

4

The Process of Educating Nurses

Joseph T. Catalano

EDUCATIONAL PATHWAYS

Unlike many other professions, nursing has several related, but unique, educational pathways that lead to licensure and professional status. Indeed, the current system of nursing education creates a great deal of confusion about nursing not only among the public but also among nurses. Perhaps the belief that "a nurse is a nurse is a nurse" developed because, even though registered nurses (RNs) may be trained in educational programs that vary in length, orientation, and content, the graduates all take the same licensing examination and, superficially, all seem able to provide the same level of care. The licensure examination measures knowledge at the minimal level of safe practice. The workplace, in general, has not provided pay differences to distinguish levels of education despite studies showing performance differences.

PARADIGM SHIFTING

As in times past, the current profession of nursing faces many difficult challenges and extraordinary opportunities. Future trends in health care are being driven by several powerful societal forces that are producing an inevitable reshaping of health-care delivery. Traditionally somewhat insulated from the forces of change, nursing educators have been made to recognize that graduates need to be prepared with knowledge and skills that are in tune with a rapidly evolving health-care system (Box 4.1). The most powerful of these forces of change are:

- Health-care reform that will increase the availability of health care to more clients and ethnic groups who previously were shut out of the health-care market.

Box 4.1

$$$$ for Nursing Students!

If you are a nursing student, you know firsthand how expensive nursing school can be. The good news is that there is now significantly more money available through federal grants and loans than there has been in the past 8 years. Barack Obama has been a champion for nurses since his time in the Illinois state senate, when he served on the Public Health Committee. As a U.S. Senator, he sponsored the Safe Nursing and Patient Care Act of 2007, which limits mandatory overtime for nurses except in major emergencies. He recognizes the value of nurses in the health-care system and the key role they will play in the recently passed Health Care Reform Act. He is also well aware of the nursing shortage and its effect on quality of care and the safety of clients.

In 2009, shortly after taking office, President Obama wrote an executive order that reversed the reduction in funds for nursing students implemented by the previous administration in a misguided attempt to cut spending. In 2009, he signed into law a $15 million increase for nursing grants and scholarships, bringing the total to $171 million, the highest amount since 2000.

Some grants and loans available through the Title VII Workforce Development Program include:

- *Workforce diversity grants.* These grants are aimed specifically at individuals who come from a disadvantaged background. They benefit students with very low incomes, ethnic and racial minorities, and groups that are under-represented in the nursing profession. These are outright grants directly to the student and do not need to be repaid.
- *Nurse education, practice, and retention grants.* These grants go to schools of nursing and other entities that educate nurses or work to improve the quality of health care. Students benefit from these grants indirectly with better facilities, additional faculty, and improved learning. For example, some schools have received money to purchase PDAs or iPads for all their students to enhance electronic learning.
- *Nurse student service corps.* These grants go directly to nursing students to repay loans after they graduate if they decide to work in a designated shortage area for 2 years after graduation. They generally will pay off 60 to 85 percent of any loans used during nursing school.
- *Comprehensive geriatric education grants.* These grants go directly to nursing students who make a commitment to care for elderly clients after graduation. The grants can also be obtained by faculty who wish to increase their knowledge of working with elderly clients and to schools of nursing that provided continuing education in elder care.

This is only a partial list of funds that have become available since 2009. As with all government-related funding, considerable forms and paperwork need to be completed. However, the effort of spending an hour or so filling out forms can reap great rewards.

Sources: Mali M. Obama signs $1.1 omnibus spending bill. Retrieved August 2014 from http://washingtonexaminer.com/obama-signs1-trillion-omnibus-spending-bill/article/2542403; Ebner AL. What nurses need to know about health care reform. Nursing Economic$, 28(3):191–194, 2010; Cardillo D. Three easy steps to finding a nursing scholarship . . . plus five great scholarships to get you started. *American Nurse Today,* 5(6), 2010.

- The wider use of capitated managed care for financing coverage and a market-driven system.
- The increasing age and diversity of the U.S. population.
- The shortage of RNs.
- The shortage of qualified nursing faculty.
- The rapid leaps forward in health care and information technology.
- The government's attempt to increase health-care coverage for large numbers of uninsured citizens.

Since the year 2000, about 60 percent of nurses have been employed in acute care hospitals.[1] Hospitals have attempted to slow the drain to other employment settings by seeking Magnet Status certification, which identifies the facility as being "nurse friendly" and a place where the nurse turnover rate is low.[2] The other 40 percent of nurses are employed in a wide variety of settings, including private practice, public health agencies, home health care, primary nursing school–operated nursing centers, **ambulatory care centers,** insurance and managed-care companies, education, and health-care research. There is also an ever-growing group of **emerging health occupations** that have not yet been officially recognized by professional organizations.

What Nursing School Graduates Must Know and Be Able to Do

It has always been a challenge for nursing educators to decide what nursing students need to learn before they graduate. Some of the curricular content is dictated by the licensure examination, but high-quality nursing programs recognize that this test knowledge is the minimum required for safe practice at an entry level. The health-care marketplace demands more than the minimum. In this regard, the consumers of the products of nursing education—that is, the health-care entities that hire nursing school graduates—have had an important if somewhat unstructured role in determining curricular content.

The Pew Report

The Pew Health Professions Commission Report, or Pew Report, was published in the late 1990s. It was the first comprehensive study to systematically address which competencies nursing students should possess upon graduation.[3] A few of the 21 recommendations for all schools preparing health-care professionals are:

- Expanding the scientific basis of the programs.
- Promoting interdisciplinary education.
- Developing cultural sensitivity.
- Establishing new alliances with managed-care companies and government.
- Increasing the use of computer technology and interactive software.

The Pew Report also recommends a differentiated practice structure to simplify and consolidate the titles that are used for the different practitioner levels so that there is just one title for each level.

Nursing educators are continually challenged to evaluate whether the graduates of their programs are adequately prepared to meet the demands of all areas of care. Nursing educators also need to evaluate whether their own educational and skill

> *Nursing educators are continually challenged to evaluate whether the graduates of their programs are adequately prepared to meet the demands of all areas of care.*

preparation is sufficient to meet the needs of diverse health-care settings.

Required Skills and Knowledge

In an attempt to structure the input from the facilities, a study was conducted to survey administrators who worked at hospitals, home health-care agencies, and nursing homes. They were asked to rank 45 skills or knowledge-based competencies they expected to see in the baccalaureate-level graduate nurses they hired. The results showed a mix of skills and knowledge competencies that were most sought after. Those that ranked the highest included:

- Teaching clients health promotion and prevention.
- Teaching clients about how lifestyle affects health.
- Effectively supervising fewer educated staff.
- Effectively delegating and monitoring staff.
- Efficiently organizing routine daily tasks.
- Safely administering medications.
- Having competency using computer databases and charting.
- Having the ability to organize nursing care for 6 to 10 clients at the same time.

Overall, the expectations for new graduates cluster around the ability to initiate and adapt to change, use critical thinking in problem-solving, attain a basic level of skills, and be able to communicate with clients and staff. It is interesting to note that the basic competencies have not changed much since Nightingale organized her first nursing school. Like her students, current students still need to master basic skills and learn to communicate effectively.

The IOM Competencies and the Future of Nursing

In 2010, a report by the American Nurses Association (ANA) and the Constituent Member Associations (CMA) moved the discussion to a new level by outlining the key messages from the IOM's (Institute of Medicine) report on the future of nursing. This report is part of an ongoing project aimed at using evidence-based practice to advance the nursing profession so that nursing can keep pace with health-care reform activities. Although not entirely new, the four key messages from the report are the following:

- *Nurses should practice to the full extent of their education and training.* A fundamental element of this goal is to revise states' nurse practice acts by removing unnecessary scope-of-practice restrictions. Work initiated in the 111th Congress is continuing and will promote this issue in various health-care settings.

- *Nurses should achieve higher levels of education and training through an improved education system that promotes seamless academic progression.* Fundamental to this message are the goals of increasing the number of RNs with baccalaureate degrees to at least 80 percent by 2020 (up from the current 50 percent), doubling the number of nurses with doctorates by 2020, and having nurses commit to lifelong learning. Another goal is to increase the diversity of nurses to better meet the needs of an increasingly diverse U.S. population. Expanded residency programs, focused on easing the transition into practice, are fundamental to the progression of newly licensed nurses into successful professionals.
- *Nurses should be full partners with physicians and other health professionals in redesigning health care in the United States.* For a long time, nurses have needed expanded opportunities to demonstrate their leadership and management skills as key members of the health-care team. In collaboration with physicians and other team members, nurses need to be involved in redesigning the health-care system through such activities as conducting research, improving practice environments, developing care systems, and improving quality of care.
- *Effective workforce planning and policy-making require better data collection and an improved information infrastructure.* Collaboration between national, state, and local initiatives in collecting and analyzing data can make the data more useful to all health-care providers.
- *Nursing education has long strived to be relevant and vibrant in a rapidly changing health-care system.* The shift in recent years to a consumer-driven health-care system is shaping what nurses need to be able to accomplish in their practice.

Out of these guiding principles, the IOM developed five key competencies that nursing students must be able to achieve upon graduation:

- Client-centered care
- Interdisciplinary teamwork

- Evidence-based practice
- Quality improvement
- Informatics

Although the IOM competencies can be used to form the curricular framework for a nursing program, the demands for an increased level of safety and high-quality nursing care at all times led to use of the IOM competencies in the development of the Quality and Safety Education for Nurses (QSEN) competency model for nursing curricula.[4,5]

QSEN Competencies Guide for Nursing Curriculum

Current leaders in nursing education have built on the Nightingale, Pew, and IOM principles and developed the QSEN competencies to help guide what is being taught in nursing programs. However, health-care technology has advanced so rapidly in recent years that it has put a strain on both the faculty teaching nursing students and the students attempting to master it.

The push for an improved nursing curriculum began with recognition of the large numbers of medication and medical errors that occur in today's health-care system. These errors lead to the injury and death of as many as 90,000 clients per year. Driven by community and professional concerns, the Robert Wood Johnson Foundation undertook a three-phase project to improve the quality and safety of client care by focusing nursing education on student competency. The project, QSEN, is built on the five competencies developed initially by the IOM.

Phase I began in 2005 with a $590,000 grant to the University of North Carolina at Chapel Hill School of Nursing. The goal of Phase I was to develop the theoretical foundations for QSEN, including student competencies; the knowledge, skills, and abilities (KSAs) necessary to maintain a safe health-care system; and measurable outcomes for graduates of nursing programs. During Phase I, an additional competency (safety) was added to the five IOM competencies, bringing the total to six. These competencies are:

- Client-centered care.
- Teamwork and collaboration.
- Evidence-based practice (EBP).
- Quality improvement (QI).

> *Health-care technology has advanced so rapidly in recent years that it has put a strain on both the faculty teaching nursing students and the students attempting to master it.*

- Safety.
- Informatics.

A thorough and extensive set of KSAs was developed for each competency for undergraduate students. In addition, Phase I established an electronic resources center, supported by the grant, which contains materials on client safety and quality initiatives.

Although Phase I was still ongoing, Phase II kicked off in 2007 with the goals of developing KSAs for graduate students and developing QSEN-based curricula in 15 selected schools. The 15 pilot schools are exploring the difficulties in implementing QSEN in their programs.

Phase III began in 2009 and is still ongoing. The goals of Phase III are:

- Developing nursing faculty knowledge and skills in teaching QSEN competencies.
- Writing textbooks that include the six competencies.
- Working with licensing, accreditation, and certification agencies to develop standards that reflect QSEN competencies.
- Developing ongoing innovative methods to implement QSEN.

Phase III will be in development for many years to come. Some of the pilot schools are beginning to publish information about their experiences implementing QSEN as their curricular model. Overall, the conversion seems to be going smoothly and successfully. However, nursing faculty resistance to change is an ever-present challenge.[6]

One issue troubling some nursing leaders is that the QSEN competencies are based on a model developed by the IOM (i.e., a medical model). All agree on the need for quality and safety measures to reduce harm to clients, and QSEN certainly meets that need. However, for many years, the AACN's *Essentials of Baccalaureate Education for Professional Nursing Practice* has been the gold standard for nursing program outcomes. Is there a clear-cut advantage in using the QSEN competencies over the *Essentials* as a curricular model?

Some nursing leaders believe that by conforming to QSEN-based curricula, they will transform the professional identity of nursing into something other than nursing. What about the competencies of caring, integrity, and client advocacy? What about research and scholarship? Where does prevention—a key nursing role since the time of Florence Nightingale—fit in? Those who support QSEN believe that if a nurse is providing safe, high-quality care, then caring and integrity are already included. Others believe that a seventh competency, "professional person," should be added to include those aspects of nursing that make it unique and separate from the medical profession[7] (see Box 4.2).

It has always been a challenge to measure competency in the health-care professions. The current interest in positive client outcomes as a measure of performance reinforces the need to better measure competency. It is by no means a new issue. The Competency Outcomes Performance Assessment (COPA) model, developed in the early 1990s, has been used by medical schools and some schools of nursing to validate the skills and knowledge of their graduates. It is designed to promote competency for clinical practice at all levels. With a few modifications, the COPA model fits well with QSEN and can be used as the evaluation tool for graduates of these schools. It can be used with both schools of nursing that have competency-based curricula and in schools that have more traditional curricula to enhance student learning and make curricular revisions appropriate for the demands of the health-care system of today and of the future.

> *Nurses of the future will need to practice with self-reliance, independence, and flexibility. They will be required to have well-developed decision-making skills on the basis of critical-thinking ability, a working knowledge of community resources, and computer and technical competencies.*

NURSES OF THE FUTURE

Nurses of the future will need to practice with self-reliance, independence, and flexibility. They will be required to have well-developed decision-making skills on the basis of critical-thinking ability, a working knowledge of community resources, and computer and technical competencies. Just as important, they will need to deliver high-quality care and client education while working within the constraints of a managed-care system with tight cost-control measures.

Will nursing education ever be able to prepare a graduate who fulfills all the qualities required

Box 4.2

Competency/Outcome Comparison: IOM, QSEN, AACN Essentials

IOM Competencies	QSEN Competencies	AACN Essentials
Client-centered care	Client-centered care	Liberal education for baccalaureate generalist nursing practice
Interdisciplinary teamwork	Teamwork and collaboration	Basic organizational and systems leadership for high-quality care and client safety
EBP	EBP	Scholarship for EBP
QI	QI	Information management and application of client-care technology
Informatics	Safety	Health-care policy, finance, and regulatory environments
	Informatics	Interprofessional communication and collaboration for improving health outcomes
		Clinical prevention and population health
		Professionalism and professional values
		Baccalaureate generalist nursing practice

AACN = American Association of Colleges of Nursing; EBP = evidence-based practice; IOM = Institute of Medicine; QI = quality improvement; QSEN = Quality and Safety Education for Nurses.

Sources: American Association of Colleges of Nursing. Essentials of baccalaureate education for professional nursing practice: Faculty tool kit, 2009. Retrieved August 2010 from http://www.AACN.nche.edu; Armstrong GE, Spencer TS, Lenburg CB. Using quality and safety education for nurses to enhance competency outcome performance assessment: A synergistic approach that promotes patient safety and quality outcomes. *Journal of Nursing Education,* 48(12):686–693, 2009; Nursing Workforce Centers: ANA and CMA activities reflected in the IOM recommendations. Retrieved October 2010 from http://www.nursingworkforcecenters.org

of nurses of the future? Nursing education responds with a yes, but only with curricular revisions that provide graduates with the tools to continue to learn as they advance in their careers.

Hospital Skills and More

Hospital-based acute care nursing practice will always have an important place in any health-care system. Highly skilled acute care nurses will always find a place to practice. It is generally accepted that the older population requires more health care of all types—acute, chronic, and community based. Although the current system experienced a decrease in the use of acute care beds, a gradual reverse in this trend is beginning as the baby boomers become the senior citizens who require more care for acute problems.

Paradigm shifting in nursing education does not need to be an either/or proposition. It is

sometimes felt that nursing education is either acute care focused or community focused. Nursing education needs to combine the two so that the graduate can practice with competence in either or both settings. The skills are similar, but the emphasis may be different. Although some hospital skills are being done by non-nurses at a cheaper cost, nursing education must still teach such important skills as critical thinking, therapeutic relationship, **primary care,** and **case management**, as well as how to be comfortable with a consumer-driven health-care system.

Critical Thinking

Critical thinking has been an important element in nursing practice for many years. It is generally recognized as the ability to use basic core knowledge and decision-making skills in resolving situations with a relatively small amount of data and a high degree of risk and ambiguity. Critical thinking is the basis for clinical judgment used by nurses in making decisions about client care and is a key part of the nursing licensure examination. Nursing has long been concerned with the ability to make good judgments and decisions about client care.

At a fundamental level, the nursing process is a type of critical thinking. Unfortunately, in the health-care system of the future, a nurse's critical-thinking skills will have to go far beyond those of the basic nursing process. Nursing education will need to prepare students for more advanced critical thinking by exposing them to real-life situations that require the use of creativity, intuition, analysis, and deductive and inductive reasoning. These situations are introduced in the classroom as case studies and are reinforced in the clinical setting through guided experiences and mentoring.

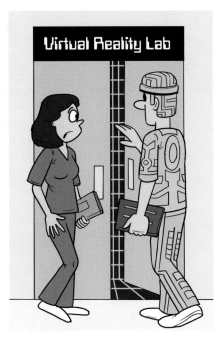

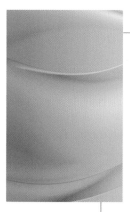

Issues Now

e-Nursing Education

The nursing shortage is expected to get worse. Projected shortages for RNs range from 200,000 to 800,000 over a 10-year period from 2012 to 2022. Compounding the nursing shortage is a deficiency of nursing staff qualified to educate new nurses. Many faculty are past retirement age and it is difficult to attract new staff due to the relative low wages in education as compared to hospitals and the private sector for nurses with similar degrees. However, a current trend viewed by some as a possible solution to the lack of nursing faculty is e-nursing education.

Almost all schools of nursing have incorporated more computer technology into their programs. However, full immersion into e-nursing education requires not only a total acceptance of technology but also a shift in fundamental thought processes and teaching techniques that go beyond what is currently accepted for the age of information. As a general rule, nurses find change difficult, and nursing faculty like change even less. Fortunately, the changes in technology have come in small doses, which are much more palatable than major upheavals in knowledge.

Both nursing students and nursing instructors can look forward to several key technologies in the not-too-distant future. "Intelligent" assistive health-care devices have spurred the growth of new industries that did not exist even 5 years ago. Artificial limbs that respond to computer-mediated signals from the brain are being used by those with amputations. Elderly people and those with mobility problems are being helped by intelligent walkers to ambulate and to change position from sitting to standing and vice versa. Nursing education will need to keep pace with these developments by teaching students how to use these devices and educate clients in their use.

All nursing faculty are aware that current nursing students are not like students of the past, even the recent past. Referred to as "Generation E" or "millennials" and raised with computers, cell phones, and a myriad of wireless devices, these students do not respond well to sitting in lecture classes. They like to be more interactive and adapt readily to new technologies. They are masters at electronic multitasking and are nonlinear in their thought processes. The challenge for nursing educators is to develop and use technologies that keep these students engaged while ensuring that they master the vast amount of material required to practice nursing safely in today's complex health-care environment. Several educational software companies are beginning to develop simulators and electronic learning games that address this need. One example is the Interactive Community Simulation Environment for Community Health Nursing, otherwise known as the Community Health Nursing Serious Game, which is based on the modular Synthetic Training Research Evaluation and Extrapolation Tool (mSTREET) platform to deliver computerized virtual training. In the game, students can investigate and respond to a variety of settings as they walk through the streets of a virtual city. The same mSTREET platform can be used for other health-care settings. Students will be able to walk into the room of an intensive care client and observe and manipulate the machines connected to the client, such as a ventilator, cardiac monitor, cooling blanket, and other commonly used devices.

(continued)

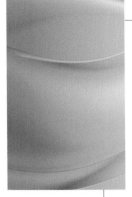

Issues Now continued

The Serious Games technology uses virtual reality to take learning one step beyond simulation. Although it is still developing as a learning methodology, it has great potential for education. It would allow students total participation in health-care scenarios, ranging from counseling sessions for clients with psychiatric disorders to advanced life support resuscitation of a client in cardiac arrest. Combined with simulation technology, virtual reality would allow students to use the equipment they will see in the work setting.

Wireless technology also has the potential to provide new learning opportunities and techniques. Access to the Internet is no longer tied to hard-wired devices. Through the cellular networks, anyone can access a whole world of information, from e-mail to video streaming. Students enrolled in online programs can now access them from almost any place where they can make a cell phone call. Some publishing companies have begun offering textbooks in electronic form (e-texts). Incorporated into these books are interactive exercises, videos, and simulation activities. Students can now read their textbooks on an iPad, a Kindle, or any one of the many tablets available on the market today.

What will the nursing classroom of the future look like? It is a sure bet that the whole experience will be different. In reality, there may be no centrally located classrooms at all. Classroom lectures and interactive discussions will be conducted electronically over wireless devices. The way students learn will not be as important as what they learn, and learning will be measured through outcome testing. Nursing education will be asynchronous and available to anyone anywhere. It has been proposed that sometime in the future there may be only one nursing program for the whole country that is located in the cloud and totally online. That possibility certainly requires major paradigm shifting!

Sources: Connors H. HIT plants SEEDS in healthcare education . . . Health Information Technology . . . Simulated E-Health Delivery System. Nursing Administration Quarterly, 31(2): 129–133, 2007; Newman L. Creating new futures in nursing education: Envisioning the evolution of e-nursing education. *Nursing Education Perspectives,* 27(1):12–15, 2006; Ornes LL: Computer competencies in a BSN program. *Journal of Nursing Education,* 46(2):75–78, 2007; Spalla TL. Technology. You've got mail: A new tool to help millennials prepare for the National Council Licensure Examination. *Nurse Educator,* 32(2):52–54, 2007.

The Therapeutic Relationship

Therapeutic relationship skills have long been stressed by mental health nursing faculty as a key element in the treatment of psychiatric problems. In reality, therapeutic relationship skills are essential for all nurses to fulfill their roles as health-care providers and healers. Although these skills are currently being taught in a limited and focused way in most nursing schools, they need to be expanded to involve directed services and relationship-centered nursing care.

Trust Is Essential

Relationship-centered nursing care is client focused and revolves around the client's trust in, value of, and understanding of the nurse's skills and role in the healing process. The client must be able to feel comfortable with the nurse and share his or her understanding of both illness and health.

Follow-up Care

Currently, in many licensed practical nurse and licensed vocational nurse (LPN/LVN) programs and schools offering the associate degree in nursing, clinical experiences consist of one-time, 8-hour provision of care for an acute or chronically ill client. Little time is spent in follow-up care. However, many bachelor of science in nursing (BSN) programs and some associate degree nursing (ADN) programs have expanded clinical experiences to include **discharge planning** and follow-up home health-care experiences.

> *Case management includes overseeing the clients' care while they are in the hospital and following clients through their rehabilitation at home, long-term follow-up, health-care practices, and developmental stages.*

To meet the demands of the future health-care system, all nursing education programs must be able to develop learning experiences for students that involve care for selected individuals or families over extended periods of time, perhaps ranging from several weeks to several semesters.

Case Management

Care management is a general term that refers to a method of coordinating care either with an individual client or on a system-wide basis. Case management, in a health-care system driven by the demand for better-quality and cost-effective care, usually is associated with coordinating care for individual clients as they move from one level to another through the health-care system. Case management is now a certified specialty; however, there is a lack of qualified nurses trained in case management. Almost all the proposals for revisions in the health-care system include the **case manager** as an important element in the overall management of care (see Chapter 27).

A Growing Need

With the changes introduced into the health-care system by the Affordable Care Act (ACA), the need for case managers will increase exponentially over the next decade. Currently, case managers do not have to be RNs; however, with the increased complexity of health-care technologies and demands for improved outcomes, RNs have the knowledge and skills to best fulfill the role. Perhaps the ideal situation would be to function as a **health-care team,** with both an RN and a social worker coordinating all aspects of the client's care.

A Wide Range of Skills

As case managers, nurses are responsible for developing clinical pathways and for directing and guiding the overall health care of a specific group of clients. Case management includes overseeing the clients' care while they are in the hospital and following them through their rehabilitation at home, long-term follow-up, health-care practices, and developmental stages.

The knowledge and thinking required by an effective case manager go far beyond what is currently required of new graduates. Nurses must be able to understand the immediate disease process and the long-term outcomes and factors that influence the disease. Case managers must also practice health-focused nursing and primary levels of intervention. Decisions will need to be made about care from a broad **database** as well as from an understanding of the client's abilities, knowledge level, and even financial status.

Nursing education will be severely challenged to provide experiences to prepare students for this role. Students must be allowed to experience the authority, accountability, and responsibility of guiding a client's health care over an extended period. It might be beneficial to combine the learning experiences mentioned earlier in establishing the therapeutic relationship with the managed-care experience.

The Consumer in Authority

A consumer-driven health-care system is the nurse's dream and nightmare. Many widely used nursing models or theories claim to be client centered, which translates into being consumer driven. Yet, when these models are put into practice, the care given is more provider driven than anything else.

Care as Requested

A client/consumer-driven health-care system means that the care given and the outcomes are both determined by the consumer. The nurse must be able to accept the authority of the group or community as a determinant of health care. The nurse's role becomes one of a partner in guiding, implementing, and overseeing ways to deliver requested health care for a given community.

Many nursing programs, particularly baccalaureate programs, include a course in community health and home health-care nursing. Often, a requirement of this course is to have the students perform a community survey in which they determine the needs of the community as they perceive them. Many of these courses have been modified so that the students learn the community members' perceptions of their own needs.

Paradigm shifting is never easy. Major paradigm shifts in thinking and acting are even more difficult. Nursing education is currently dealing with a huge paradigm shift. How educators are meeting these challenges will, to a large extent, shape the future of professional nursing.

> " *A consumer-driven health-care system is the nurse's dream and nightmare.* "

AMERICAN NURSES ASSOCIATION POSITION PAPER ON EDUCATION FOR NURSES

After evaluating the changes that occurred in the health-care system during the 1950s and studying the projected educational needs for nurses, the ANA published a paper in 1965 that took a stand on an issue that was, and still is, highly controversial. Although written some 50 years ago, this document is still relevant to many of the issues in nursing education today.

After World War II, there was an explosion of scientific and technological knowledge used in health care. The educational level of the population was also increasing, resulting in greater public demand for higher-quality health care. In reevaluating the nature and scope of nursing practice and the type and level of quality of education needed to meet these new demands, the ANA reached the conclusions that are presented in its position paper.

A Changing Role for Hospitals

Hospitals recognized that they would no longer retain their traditional role of preparing nurses for practice. Even though pressure to move nursing education from hospital-based diploma schools to institutions of higher education had been building for some time, in the mid-1960s, 75 percent of the graduating nurses were from hospital-based diploma programs.[8]

Colleges Under Pressure

Colleges and universities were pushed to quickly develop undergraduate and graduate curricula for increasing numbers of nursing majors. The relatively few baccalaureate programs in existence at the time were generally small and found it difficult to expand rapidly. It also became evident that a clear distinction between technical and professional programs needed to be made.

The Debate Continues

To this day, the ANA remains firmly committed to its stand that all nursing education should be housed in institutions of higher learning. More than 40 years have elapsed since this statement was made, and the profession of nursing is still trying to reach a consensus on the issue of basic educational preparation for entry into practice.

Over the past few years, several states have been looking at the "BSN in Ten" proposal, which would require graduates from ADN programs to obtain their BSN degrees within 10 years after graduating from the ADN program. Because of the strong lobbying efforts against this proposal on the part of the AD programs, there has been almost no movement on its implementation.[9]

Defining a Profession

A similar resolution defining entry into practice was proposed by the ANA in 1985, but it also met strong opposition and was never enacted. In 1996, the American Association of Colleges of Nursing

(AACN) presented its own position paper emphasizing the belief that the baccalaureate degree should be the minimal requirement for entry into the nursing profession. The discussion remains ongoing with seemingly little hope for resolution. The most influential reasons these proposals have not been adopted are economic, not conceptual. Although some experts believe it is time to leave the old debate behind and work toward developing a better-educated profession in general, many others see the issue as important to the definition of nursing as a profession.

DIPLOMA SCHOOLS

The Nightingale School of Nursing was a diploma school in the strict use of the term. When nurses graduated from this school, they were given a certificate or diploma noting their graduation, but no academic degree. The first graduates from the Nightingale School soon began to establish their own schools of nursing based on the Nightingale model and adhered to her philosophy of nursing education. These were also diploma schools.

An Improvement in Care

After an initial period of uncertainty and trepidation, both physicians and hospital administrators began to recognize that when the education of nurses improved, so, too, did the overall quality of the care provided by their hospitals. They also understood that these types of schools that were closely associated with hospitals could provide a source of free, or inexpensive, labor in the form of nursing students.

Diploma schools sprang up throughout Europe, and in time, each hospital had its own school of nursing. Many of Nightingale's principles and concerns about nursing education were abandoned during this period of growth.

Catching Up to Europe

In the United States, developments in nursing education, as with health care in general, lagged behind those in Europe. It was not until the mid-1870s that the first school of nursing was established in the United States. This was a diploma school attached to the New England Hospital for Women.[10]

As in Europe, the idea of diploma schools quickly caught on, and within 10 years almost every large hospital in the United States had its own diploma school of nursing. These schools had very little in common with the Nightingale School of Nursing. There was no uniformity in curriculum, length of program, or requirements. To guarantee adequate enrollment, candidates were again being recruited from the lowest levels of society.

A Source of Cheap Labor

In early hospital-based diploma schools of nursing, hospitals used the student nurses as a major source of free labor for their facilities. There was little or no classroom or theoretical study. The students learned exclusively by hands-on experience during their 12- to 14-hour, 7-day-a-week work shifts.

Most of the students were young, single women recruited just after they graduated from high school. They were confined to dormitories on the hospital property. The dormitories were monitored closely by a housemother who enforced the rigorous rules of behavior covering all aspects of the students' lives and dismissed students for even minor infractions of the rules. The early diploma schools of nursing were organized and administered on a model that was similar to the strictest of the religious orders.

> *The early diploma schools of nursing were organized and administered on a model that was similar to the strictest of the religious orders.*

Submission to Authority

The nurses who graduated from these schools were proficient in basic nursing skills and could assume positions in the hospital where they were trained or in home nursing, where they worked on a case-by-case basis without any additional orientation or education. Because of the 24-hour-a-day, 7-day-a-week socialization process administered by these schools, diploma graduate nurses tended to be very submissive to authority and willing to carry out any duty to please the physician, administrator, or head nurse. Before the advent of licensure examinations and standardization of practice, nurses from diploma schools were often limited to employment in their own training institutions or in home health-care settings.

A Move Toward Accreditation

Diploma schools of nursing remained relatively unchanged in the United States until 1949, when the

National Nursing Accrediting Service, working under the guidance of the National League for Nursing Education, became the licensing body for all schools of nursing that voluntarily sought accreditation. The first formal accreditation of nursing schools occurred in the early 1950s. In 1952, the National League for Nursing (NLN) assumed accrediting responsibilities for all schools of nursing.[11] Accreditation by the National League for Nursing Accrediting Commission (NLNAC) has always been and remains a voluntary undertaking.

Outcome Criteria

To be accredited by the NLN, schools of nursing had to meet specific **outcome criteria** and teach specific content in their curricula. Many of the diploma schools of nursing could not or would not submit to these criteria and eventually closed. Some of the requirements for the schools that did choose to comply with the NLN included:

- Implementing a 3-year course of study meeting the criteria established by the state board of nursing using only faculty with baccalaureate or higher degrees in nursing
- Developing a philosophy and demonstrating how that philosophy was implemented through learning objectives, course objectives, and outcome criteria
- Showing an adequate pass rate on the State Board or National Council Licensure Examination (NCLEX)

A Jump in Expense

One of the key factors that all state boards of nursing were concerned about was that the school should be able to demonstrate that the students were not being used as unpaid hospital personnel while they were in their education and training programs. When students could no longer be used as free labor, diploma nursing schools became very expensive to the hospitals, when previously they were virtually free.

Not only did the hospitals still have to pay for the room and board of the students, but they also now had to hire and pay additional staff because the students could no longer be included in the overall staff numbers. Due to the overwhelming financial burden to the hospitals, even more diploma schools closed. The schools that stayed open were forced to increase their tuition rates, which made nursing schools just as expensive as programs granting academic degrees.

CONVERTING THE CURRICULUM

During the 1960s and 1970s, many diploma schools became associated with universities and converted their curricula into degree-granting programs. According to recent data published by the NLN, approximately 100 accredited diploma programs remain open in the United States. They are of universally high quality and meet all the standards necessary for NLN accreditation. The main emphasis remains on preparing nurses who are highly competent in technical nursing skills through extensive hands-on practice in the clinical setting, but elements of leadership, humanities, and general sciences are also included in the classroom setting.[12]

ASSOCIATE DEGREE NURSING

> *Continuing the discussion and efforts to bring about collaborative agreement on nursing education is a goal that the profession must work toward.*

The **associate degree nursing (ADN) program** was developed by Mildred Montague as a short-term solution to the nursing shortage experienced after World War II.[13] Originally designed to prepare students for technical nursing practice, the 2-year ADN programs were offered through community colleges with an emphasis on developing the skills necessary to provide high-quality bedside care in less time than BSN programs.

Technical Orientation

A successful pilot program for ADNs was conducted by Montague at Teachers' College in Columbia University in New York City in 1952 to prepare technical nurses who could assist professional nurses. It demonstrated that community college–based programs could attract large numbers of students, prove cost-effective, and produce skillful technical nurses in half the time required for BSN programs.[14]

Which Exam to Take?

Early on, there was some heated debate concerning licensure and titling for this group of nurses. The technical orientation of the curriculum was very similar to that found in programs that prepare LPNs, but the location of the programs in the community college setting and the increased theoretical orientation seemed to elevate these programs to a higher educational plane. It was finally decided that the ADN graduates should take the RN licensure examination rather than the LPN/LVN examination.

A Proven Track Record

The emphasis on technical skills of the ADN programs met a need in the health-care system of the 1960s and 1970s. By the early 1980s, there were more than 800 ADN programs across the United States; as of 2012, the number was close to 1000, with more than 65,000 students attending; however, not all of the programs are accredited by a national agency.[15] Graduates from these programs exceeded the number of graduates from all the diploma, BSN, and LPN/LVN programs combined.

Although it is possible to complete the requirements for an ADN in 2 academic years, most programs take at least 3 years to complete for a new student who has no prior college credit.[16] ADN graduates have a proven track record for providing safe bedside care for clients from the first day they are hired. They function well as team members and, after a period of orientation, can assume responsibility for the care of clients who are more acutely ill.

> *ADN graduates have a proven track record for providing safe bedside care for clients from the first day they are hired.*

BACCALAUREATE EDUCATION

Early attempts at college-level nursing programs sometimes took the form of "prenursing" courses over a 1- or 2-year period that prepared students to enter upper-division schools of nursing. Generally acclaimed as the first university program to be completely conducted in the higher education setting, the University of Minnesota School of Nursing was opened in 1909. In 1923, the Yale School of Nursing began accepting students; it is considered the first autonomous college of nursing in the United States.

A Slow Increase

The development of schools of nursing in the university and college setting was a gradual process that extended over several decades. Only a few collegiate nursing programs were established during the years when the diploma programs were expanding. Some of these early collegiate programs were a hybrid of college-level classes and diploma school clinical experiences that still granted only a diploma rather than an academic degree.

The number of university-based nursing programs gradually increased over the years, and by the beginning of World War II, there were 76 programs granting baccalaureate degrees in nursing. These programs tended to specialize in preparing nurses for public health nursing, teaching, administration, and supervisory positions in hospitals. Although all of these programs included a clinical component, the emphasis was more on theoretical knowledge, development of critical thinking, decision-making skills, and leadership.

Universities in general enjoyed rapid growth immediately after World War II, and higher-education nursing programs expanded along with the universities. Many military nurses, prepared by the Cadet Nurse Corps during World War II, went back to school under the GI Bill to complete their baccalaureate degrees, thus providing the framework for current ADN to BSN programs.

Education for a Profession

During this rapid growth period, these **baccalaureate degree nursing programs** were plagued with problems similar to those found in the diploma programs during their own rapid expansion period. Primarily, the lack of uniformity in content, curriculum, and even length of programs was problematic. It was difficult to find qualified faculty because most of the nurses at this time had received their education in diploma programs. No doctorate degrees existed in nursing, few nurses had master's degrees, and only a smattering of nurses had baccalaureate degrees.

During the late 1940s and early 1950s, it was clearly necessary to start stratifying nursing education programs into technical levels and professional levels. It became apparent that all health-care professionals should have, at minimum, a baccalaureate degree.[17]

The NLN began to develop strict criteria for the accreditation of baccalaureate nursing programs. These criteria included courses in general education, general sciences, humanities, and language as well as specific nursing courses. They required a certain number of hours to be spent in the clinical setting practicing nursing skills, a faculty prepared at the master's degree level, and the availability of laboratory and library facilities for the students. Faculty-to-student ratios were limited, particularly in the clinical setting, and outcome criteria were required for the students.[18]

Different Approaches

Although all university-level baccalaureate degrees in nursing have the same number of required credit hours and educational requirements, there are three avenues for attaining this degree.

The Professional Degree

The BSN degree fulfills the criteria of a professional degree. It meets the overall requirements for a college baccalaureate degree (120 to 124 credit hours, 65 hours of nursing major, and most of the general education requirements) but does not meet all the general education requirements for an academic bachelor of science (BS) degree. Although a professional degree is usually obtained in a traditional college setting, it can also be obtained through an **external degree** program in which the student has to meet the criteria for the BSN.

The Full Academic Degree

The second approach is found in programs that offer a bachelor of science in nursing degree. This degree is a full academic college degree and guarantees that the person holding it has met all of the general education, science, and major subject requirements. According to statistics published by the NLN for the academic year 2012, there were more than 555 accredited programs offering baccalaureate degrees in nursing. A third avenue that may be pursued is sometimes called the career ladder program (see the "Ladder Programs" section later in this chapter).

PRACTICAL/VOCATIONAL NURSING

The practical/vocational nurse has been a part of the health-care system in the United States for well over 100 years. Although the earliest formal schools of practical/vocational nursing were started around 1890, informal training programs for this level of nursing probably existed well before that time—for example, in the Young Women's Christian Association (YWCA), particularly in New York City.

A Useful Trade

These programs took uneducated girls who had migrated from rural areas and farms to the cities in search of employment and taught them a useful trade with which they could support themselves. With no regulation or accreditation for the early practical/vocational nurse programs, there were wide variations in the quality, length, and focus of what was being taught. Generally, the students were taught to provide home care, similar to that given by private duty nurses, for clients ranging from newborns to elderly and invalid individuals.

The number of **practical nursing programs** gradually increased during the next 50 years. Graduates of these 3-month programs were beginning to find employment in hospitals and nursing homes as well as in areas of private duty. During the nurse shortage after World War I, many hospitals found that these relatively undereducated nurses, after receiving on-the-job training in the hospital, could function at a fairly high level of skill and at a much reduced cost. The word got around, and soon the number of these unlicensed nurses increased.

> *In early hospital-based diploma schools of nursing, hospitals used the student nurses as a major source of free labor for their facilities. There was little or no classroom or theoretical study.*

Compulsory Licensure

By the late 1930s, the ANA saw the need to regulate the quality of the practical/vocational nursing programs to protect public safety. It was not until 1938 that the state of New York took seriously the ANA's recommendation for compulsory licensure for practical/vocational nurses and enacted the first law requiring such licensure.

In 1960, all practical/vocational nurses were required to pass a licensure examination before they could practice. These nurses are now referred to as licensed practical nurses (LPNs). In Texas and California, these nurses are called licensed vocational nurses (LVNs).

The Importance of Technique

Although education for LPNs and LVNs varies slightly from one state to another, there are some common characteristics. Most of the programs are from 9 to 12 months and are measured in clock hours rather than academic hours. They are often offered in hospitals, high schools, vocational schools, or trade schools, although some programs are conducted in community colleges or even in universities.

Orientation of the curricula in these programs is highly technical and emphasizes the learning of skills in the hospital or nursing home setting, with less emphasis on theoretical knowledge. Because they are **technicians,** it is much more important for practical/vocational nurses to learn *how* to do something rather than *why* they are doing it.

Filling a Shortage

The stated scope of practice for the practical/vocational nurse involves providing care for clients in hospitals, nursing homes, or the home setting for those who have stable conditions. LPNs/LVNs are to be under the supervision of an RN or a licensed physician.

However, in the real world, LPNs/LVNs are often required to provide care well outside their scope of practice, leaving them vulnerable to lawsuits. They often function in leadership roles or provide care in acute settings with highly unstable clients. LPNs/LVNs are often hired when there are shortages of RNs to fill the gaps in client care.

Many associate degree RN programs have developed a ladder curriculum whereby an LPN/LVN can go back to school for a shorter period, often receiving credit for years of experience, complete the program in 1 year, and then take the RN licensure examination.

LADDER PROGRAMS

Career ladder, educational ladder, **articulation,** or educational mobility programs have become increasingly popular as a result of an interest in **upward mobility,** educational articulation, and **career mobility.**

Upward Mobility

A ladder program allows nurses to upgrade their education and move from one educational level to another with relative ease by granting credit for

previous course work and experience and without loss of credits from previous education.

Each ladder program is developed according to the philosophy of the particular nursing school, may use any one of a number of curricular patterns, uses one of several means of **advanced placement** or credit granted for previous education, and must meet NLNAC accreditation standards.

Ladder programs take several different forms. Some provide a **competency-based education** that allows the students to proceed at their own pace as long as they fulfill required educational outcomes. Ladder programs have become increasingly popular as colleges move toward Web-based courses and programs.

The Associate Ladder

The LPN/LVN-to-ADN ladder allows individuals who have been licensed as LPNs/LVNs to take a minimal number of courses in an associate degree program to obtain their ADN and then take the NCLEX-RN, CAT to become licensed as RNs. Programs vary widely as to how many credits they will accept from the LPN/LVN programs and how many courses the students take to complete the degree. Some of the requirements for number of hours are

> *"During the late 1940s and early 1950s, it was clearly necessary to start stratifying nursing education programs into technical levels and professional levels. It became apparent that all health-care professionals should have, at minimum, a baccalaureate degree."*

out of the control of the nursing programs because they have been established as general education requirements of the college or are state regent's requirements. These programs are highly compatible because of the similarity of curricula and the technical orientation of both types of programs.

The Baccalaureate Ladder

Some LPN/LVN-to-BSN ladder programs either allow licensed LPNs/LVNs to challenge a number of courses or grant them credit for nursing courses on the basis of previous experience and demonstrated competency. Students who enter these types of ladder programs usually spend more time in school than those in the LPN/LVN-to-ADN programs. In addition to meeting the requirements of the BSN, they also have to meet the general education requirements for a baccalaureate degree and complete 120 to 124 hours of college-level courses. One problem in developing these types of ladder programs is that many states' boards of regents do

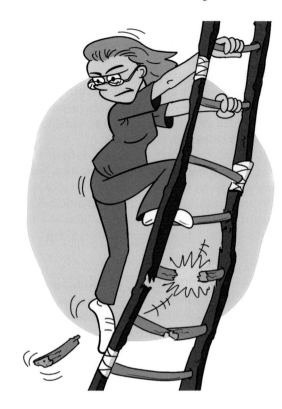

online format: Students take all of the classes on their home computers, with only minimal requirements for class attendance on campus. These types of classes work particularly well for students who work full-time and may have family responsibilities.

Other programs accept ADN or diploma graduates as students, in addition to generic students. These schools often have separate programs for ADNs or diploma RNs that allow them to take examinations to prove educational knowledge and nursing proficiency (**challenge examinations**) in specific classes, thus granting credit for their nursing experience. The RNs then take advanced-level nursing courses, such as Community Health/Home Health Care, Leadership, and Critical Care, which are not commonly found in diploma or ADN programs. Many of these programs are also online.

On completion of the degree requirements, these nurses are granted a baccalaureate degree. Some of these programs have an **open curriculum** that allows students to enter and leave the program freely. There are 418 such programs accredited by the NLNAC, and the number continues to grow.[19] The capacity to accept ADN graduates into these completion programs is almost unlimited. Should the "BSN in Ten" proposal ever gain a toehold, there will be more than enough spaces for students coming from ADN programs.

Fast-Track Options

Some nursing programs have gotten creative in their attempt to educate nurses at the baccalaureate level. One approach is to place students who have a BS or BA degree in another major, such as biology or English, in fast-track programs that allow them to obtain their nursing degree in 1 or 2 years. In many ways, these programs are similar to the RN-to-BSN programs, but they also teach the basic nursing skills that ADN graduates already have.

The Master's Ladder

A growing trend in educational ladder programs is the ADN-to-MSN programs. Schools that offer this type of ladder must have an MSN program in place. The ADN students who enter these programs are given credit for prior classes and work experience and take both undergraduate- and graduate-level courses, receiving a BSN along the way to obtaining the MSN.

For the ADN

These programs vary a great deal from school to school and may require from three to five semesters

not recognize courses taken at the vocational-technical level as higher education courses and therefore will not transfer them into the college setting. One way around this requirement is for students to take challenge examinations in both general education courses and nursing courses. Once the students pass the test, they are granted college-level credit for the course. These examinations tend to be difficult and are really a type of outcome-based learning. However, they do not require the student to attend classes and are much cheaper than a regular college course.

Two Plus Two

Nursing education has seen a marked increase in the number of ADN-to-BSN and diploma-to-BSN ladder programs, sometimes called **two plus two (2 + 2) programs.** These programs admit individuals who are already licensed as RNs but who have either a diploma or an associate degree.

These programs may take several different forms. Upper-division baccalaureate programs work exclusively with RNs, have no generic students, and are designed exclusively to meet the educational needs of students who are already RNs. Many of these programs have adopted or are moving toward a totally

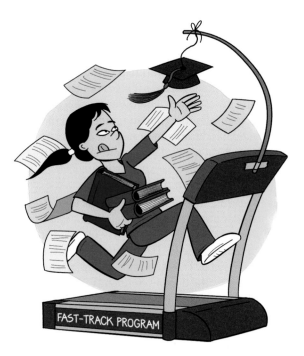

FAST-TRACK PROGRAM

of classes. Often they are offered on a part-time basis, with many evening and weekend classes or Web-based classes available to meet the needs of working students.

For the Nurse Practitioner

A less common type of educational ladder program is the nurse practitioner–to-MSN program. These programs admit nurse practitioners who graduated from programs that certified students but did not include enough credit hours for a master's degree. Again, the students are granted credit for past classes and work experience and often are allowed to challenge a certain number of core courses. Then they take the remaining required courses and are granted an MSN at graduation.

MASTER'S AND DOCTORAL-LEVEL EDUCATION

The baccalaureate degree is considered a generalist degree that exposes students to a wide range of subjects during the 4 years spent in college. The master's degree, on the other hand, is a specialist's degree.[20] Students who pursue a master's degree concentrate their study in one particular subject area and become expert in that given area.

Master's Degree Programs

Master's degree nursing programs have been in existence almost from the time baccalaureate-level nursing programs were started. Some early and current nurse leaders have stated that the master's degree in nursing should be the entry-level degree for the profession. The early master's degrees in nursing programs were designed for students who had baccalaureate degrees in other majors, such as biology, and wanted to become nurses. After completion of an additional 36 to 42 credit hours in nursing courses only, these students were awarded the MSN and could then take the licensure examination for RNs.

Experience Required

Today, most master's degrees in nursing programs are restricted to RNs who have a baccalaureate degree. Many of these programs require at least 1 year of clinical practice after the BSN and require an additional 36 to 46 college credit hours. Most students who enter master's degree programs attend classes on a part-time basis while they work and may take up to 5 years to complete the requirements. Many universities have recognized this trend and have tailored their programs to meet the needs of these part-time students. Universities now offer courses over the Internet, distance education in the evening and on weekends, or 1-day-a-week programs. There are 296 accredited master's degree programs in the United States.[21]

There are several available areas of study for those pursuing master's degrees in nursing. Some of the more popular areas include nursing administration; community health; psychiatric mental health; adult health; maternal–child health; gerontology; rehabilitation care; nursing education; and some more advanced areas of practice, such as anesthesiology, pediatric nurse practitioner (PNP), family nurse practitioner, geriatric nurse practitioner (GNP), and obstetric–gynecological nurse practitioner.[22]

Many of these programs require the student to pass a comprehensive written or oral examination. Some courses require the student to write an extensive research thesis before graduation, although some programs are now requiring a published journal manuscript in lieu of the thesis.

Professional and Academic Degrees

There are two basic types of the master's degree in nursing. The master's of science in nursing (MSN) is the professional degree, and the master's of science with a major in nursing degree (MS Nursing) is the formal academic degree.[23] In practice, however, little differentiation is made between the two. Almost all master's programs accredited by the NLNAC require the applicant to have at least a 3.0 grade point average and to demonstrate academic proficiency by achieving a satisfactory score on the Graduate Record Examination (GRE) or the Miller's Analogy Test before admission. The GRE is also used to recommend remedial coursework needed to correct deficiencies before the master's program is undertaken.

What Do You Think?

Have you ever been to an advanced practice nurse for care? How would you rate the quality of that care? If you have not been to an advanced practice nurse, would you consider going to one for care? Why or why not?

Doctoral Programs

In the evolution of the various levels of education, the baccalaureate degree is a generalist's degree, the master's degree is a specialist's degree, and the academic doctoral degree is a generalist's degree, although at a much higher academic level than the baccalaureate degree. The major purpose of early doctoral degrees was to prepare the individual to conduct advanced research in a particular area of interest. Nurses holding these degrees conduct much of the research used in evidence-based practice (EBP). Currently, doctoral degrees for nursing practice are becoming popular and are considered specialists' degrees.

Some early and current nurse leaders have stated that the master's degree in nursing should be the entry-level degree for the profession.

A Wide Range of Choices

Presently, there is a wide range of available doctoral degrees for nurses. The doctor of philosophy (PhD) degree is the most accepted academic degree and is designed to prepare individuals to conduct research. The doctor of education (EdD) degree is considered a professional degree, although in many programs there is little difference between the courses of study taken by the EdD and PhD candidates. In other programs, the PhD focuses primarily on research, whereas the EdD focuses more on administration in the educational setting. The classes and research credits differ somewhat between the two degrees.

Academic Doctorates

Almost all PhD in nursing programs have an additional focus on education because most PhD graduates will be teaching nursing in institutions of higher education. Nurses with PhDs learn about classroom teaching, curriculum development, and the evaluation process. Some programs require "nursing student teaching" for their candidates during their capstone courses to evaluate their teaching methodologies and techniques.

Professional Practice Doctorates

Since the 1970s, other doctoral programs for nurses have been developed to stress the clinical rather than the academic nature of nursing.[24] These include the doctor of nursing science (DNSc) and the doctor of science in nursing (DSN), which is a clinically oriented nursing degree. The doctor of nursing (DN or ND) degree is for the person with a BS or MS in a field other than nursing who wants to pursue nursing as a career. It is a generalist's degree at a basic level of education.

The doctor of nursing practice (DNP) degree was first granted almost 20 years ago at Case Western University. However, at that time very few schools of nursing granted it, and there was a great deal of confusion about what the degree was and what nurses holding it could do. A small number of nurses opted for the degree. The DNP is now being considered as the terminal degree for advanced practice nurses.

In recent years, there has been some discussion of making these degrees the basic entry-level degree into the profession of nursing. An additional degree for nurses who wish to pursue a career in higher education is the doctor of nursing education (DNEd) degree; however, it is considered a professional, not an academic, degree. Few nursing schools still offer this degree since the advent of the DNP. The corresponding academic degree is the EdD, which is available at many universities.

Few Programs, Tough Requirements

Despite the wide range of doctoral degrees in nursing, relatively few programs across the United States offer these degrees. Many nurses who seek them may obtain them in fields such as higher education, psychology, college teaching, and adult education. Fewer than 2 percent of nurses hold doctoral degrees.

The requirements for all doctoral education degrees are similar, even though the specific degrees being sought after may be different. The student must have attained a master's degree and must have achieved a satisfactory score on the GRE. Often candidates must go through an admission interview and preprogram examination before they can be formally admitted to the program. Doctoral programs are at least 60 college credit hours in length, require many statistics and research courses, and often have a residency requirement. Before the doctoral degree can be granted, the student must successfully complete both oral and written comprehensive examinations and must write a doctoral dissertation that explains how to conduct a major research project.

Many individuals now pursue doctoral degrees on a part-time basis while they are working full-time, whereas others attend classes full-time while working full-time, often completing the program in 3 to 4 years. Many programs have gone to a totally online format. Some programs require that the individual complete all the requirements within 10 years. Although this may seem like a long time, it is not unusual for the dissertation process itself to take 2 to 3 years.

> *In the evolution of the various levels of education, the baccalaureate degree is a generalist's degree, the master's degree is a specialist's degree, and the doctoral degree is a generalist's degree, although at a much higher academic level than the baccalaureate degree.*

Leaders in the Profession

Nurses with master's or doctoral degrees are regarded as leaders in the nursing profession. Many of the larger hospitals in the United States require their unit managers and supervisors to have master's degrees and their directors of nursing or vice presidents of nursing to have doctorates. Of course, in baccalaureate programs, the minimal requirement for teaching is the master's degree, and the doctorate is preferred. Nurses with these advanced degrees provide direction and leadership for the profession through their publications, research, and theory development. As health-care delivery becomes more complicated, facilities will require larger numbers of nurses with advanced degrees.

EDUCATION FOR ADVANCED PRACTICE

Advanced practice is one of those often misused terms in nursing that add to the public's confusion about educational levels of those in the profession. The advanced practice registered nurse (APRN) certification has become the recognized credential for nurses receiving a master's degree in a specialized expanded practice role. It is also sometimes referred to as expanded role or expanded practice. Nurses who obtain certification are allowed to practice at a higher and more independent level, depending on the nurse practice act of their individual state. Advanced practitioners diagnose illnesses, prescribe medications, conduct physical examinations, and refer clients to specialists for more intensive follow-up care. These nurses practice under their own licenses as independent practitioners but often work closely with a physician so that they can quickly refer clients who have medical problems that lie outside their scope of practice.

The Nurse Practitioner

The nurse practitioner levels of nursing are most widely accepted as advanced practice areas for nursing. These include the pediatric nurse practitioner (PNP), the neonatal nurse practitioner (NNP), the geriatric nurse practitioner (GNP), the obstetric–gynecological (OB-GYN) nurse practitioner, the family nurse practitioner (FNP), the rehabilitation nurse practitioner (RNP), the psychiatric nurse practitioner, and the nurse midwife.

The certified registered nurse anesthetist (CRNA) and nurse midwife are the oldest of the advanced practice specialties for nurses and are already well accepted in the medical community. Other advanced practice nurses experience varying levels of acceptance from physicians, although the public in general likes the care they receive from advanced practice nurses. All states now have granted some type of **prescriptive authority** to nurse practitioners.

In the past, nurses with baccalaureate degrees could attend highly concentrated courses of study for 1 to 2 years and increase their proficiency in a particular specialty area without obtaining an MSN. They could then take the certification examination and become certified as nurse practitioners. Currently, most nurse practitioner (NP) programs are offered in major universities, requiring students to complete the master's degree before allowing them to take the certification examination.[24]

The Clinical Nurse Specialist/Clinical Nurse Leader

Another level of nursing that falls under the umbrella of advanced practice is the **nurse specialist,** or **clinical nurse specialist** (CNS). Although relatively few schools offer specific CNS curricula, these nurses are self-classified as a CNS after completing a master's degree, or some additional education, in a particular clinical area. However, in a few states, such as Ohio, the CNS designation requires a master's degree and a special licensing examination. CNSs are usually hired by hospitals and often function as in-service educators for the hospital. The clinical nurse leader (CNL) is an emerging role that APRNs can assume. The CNL is a generalist with a master's degree who can coordinate care for clients, use EBP in care, focus on quality improvement, and oversee risk management and client safety.[25]

The Scope of Advanced Practice

In 1988, an amendment to the New York Nurse Practice Act established a separate scope of practice and title protection for NPs. Subsequent to the NP amendment, there has been some confusion regarding which of the advanced nursing practice categories are included within the scope of practice, particularly clinical nurse specialists, nurse midwives, and certified nurse anesthetists. This confusion, especially in psychiatric mental health nursing and nurse anesthesia, is related to the legal interpretations of the NP amendment. The resultant debate about this issue has led to a clearer definition and understanding of the term *advanced practice registered nurse* (APRN).

The career opportunities for advanced practice nurses are numerous.[26] Many nurse practitioners work for county health departments, for rural clinics, and on Native American reservations; others work in hospitals, with physicians in private practice, and in rehabilitation centers. Some have even established their own independent clinics. APRNs often provide primary health-care services in areas where there is a lack of primary care physicians. Although many of these areas are traditionally rural, today inner-city areas also often need this type of health care. With the passage of the Health Care Reform Act in 2010, the opportunity for APRNs will continue to grow. Health-care reform often requires that a client seeking entry into the health-care system be evaluated by a primary health-care practitioner before referral to a specialized practitioner.

Although the family practice physician, or general practitioner, is the most common primary health-care provider to evaluate the client, the nurse practitioner can also function in this role.

DNP for the APRN?

As the number of nursing schools granting the APRN increased and the number of APRNs grew, nursing leaders began to question whether all these NPs were prepared to meet the complexities of today's health-care system. Nursing leaders noticed that unlike dentists, physical therapists, or pharmacists, APRNs had no terminal degree. Because of the high level of skills and knowledge required for APRNs, many of whom can practice independently, they surmised that a clinical terminal degree focusing on practice expertise should be required for entry into the APRN level.[27]

Is the Master's Enough?

Out of the many practice-oriented doctoral degrees discussed previously, the DNP seems best suited to meet the requirements of a terminal advanced practice doctoral degree. As a result, the AACN decided in 2004 that all advanced practice nursing master's degrees should transition to the DNP by the year 2015.[26] Currently, practicing APRNs would not be affected, except to be exempted into the new status. More than 50 other nursing organizations and societies have endorsed the proposal. However, questions linger.

Does It Make Sense?

Those who favor the transition to the DNP point out that practitioners need the highest levels of education to care for clients in today's complex and demanding health-care system. Requiring the DNP is the only way to guarantee safe, high-quality care. Granting accreditation to all APRNs at the DNP level would provide better consistency in both the educational requirements and the titling of what is now a confusing array of programs and certifications. Those in favor also argue that current master's APRN programs have added so much practice and theoretical content in an attempt to keep current with the practice setting that they are almost at the doctoral level anyway.[22] Almost all professional practice specialty areas, except for nursing, now require a terminal degree. The DNP would seem the logical degree to demonstrate the high skill levels, knowledge, and expertise for nurses.

Those who do not support the DNP degree ask the questions: "How does the degree improve the practice of the APRN?" "Doesn't adding another degree only make it more confusing for the public?" Although no research has been conducted so far, it would be interesting to ask currently practicing APRNs if they believe they are practicing at the top levels of skills and knowledge and if an additional degree will make them "better." An additional degree does not necessarily make a higher-quality APRN.

Then there is the question of cost.[27] Again, no research has been conducted to date about how much more it will cost to obtain a DNP than a master's degree. If a program converts an MSN to a DNP and offers only the DNP, the additional cost may be onerous. However, this is not known at this time.

The Long-Term Effect

The bigger objection to the DNP degree is its long-term effect on nursing education. The PhD has been the gold standard for nursing education since the beginning of college-level nursing baccalaureate degrees. Deans and chairpersons of nursing programs had to hold a PhD to earn accreditation from a national organization. Currently, at some schools, nurses holding the DNP degree are being appointed to dean and chairperson positions. Also, nurses with the DNP are now being hired as faculty with a terminal degree.[27] The intent is not to imply that any particular individual is unqualified for his or her job. However, because the DNP is advertised as a "practice" degree and not an educational degree, the DNP programs are not providing the content required for teaching or administering nursing programs. Most college and university administrators do not understand the difference between a PhD and a DNP. To them, a doctoral degree is a doctoral degree is a doctoral degree. They do recognize how difficult it is to find nurses with any type of post-master's degree, so finding a nurse with any kind of doctorate is like finding hidden treasure.

The long-term impact on nursing education could be disastrous. In the short term, the negative effects are muted because all programs still have a mix of PhD and master's in nursing education faculty along with DNP faculty. However, as time goes on and the current aging PhD population is replaced by DNP deans and faculty, the expertise and knowledge in areas such as curriculum development, evaluation, and teaching methodologies will be lost. Also, because much of the research currently used as the basis for EBP is conducted by PhD-prepared nurses, over time the profession will lose the ability to maintain its body of knowledge at a rate that matches the growth in technology and in medical and nursing knowledge.

The debate will go on; however, the changeover to the DNP seems to be a certainty. It is extremely important for students who are thinking about obtaining advanced nursing degrees to consider the direction of their professional future. If they are truly interested in clinical practice as a lifelong career, the DNP is the degree to obtain. However, if they are even considering a career in education at some point in the future, the MSN in nursing education and the PhD are the way to go.[28]

INTERPROFESSIONAL EDUCATION

> " *Most college and university administrators do not understand the difference between a PhD and a DNP. To them, a doctoral degree is a doctoral degree is a doctoral degree.* "

Interprofessional education is defined as "two or more students from different professions learning about, from and with each other to enable effective collaboration and improve health outcomes."[29] It also goes by other names such as *transprofessional* and *interdisciplinary education*. Although interprofessional education has been an incidental part of nursing education for many years, it was first formally recognized as an element in health-care education in 1972 at the first IOM conference. There, over 120 leaders in many areas of health care—such as nursing, nutrition, physical therapy, pharmacy, dentistry, and medicine—recognized the necessity of learning centers to conduct interdisciplinary learning to improve the real-world outcomes for the well-being of clients.

More recently, along with the recognition that medication errors were a leading cause of injury and death for hospitalized clients, the Joint Commission (JC) also noted the poor communication and lack of teamwork among health-care professionals were major contributors to the increased number of medicine and other errors in the hospital setting. They surmised that increasing the communication skills between health-care professionals and promoting a spirit of teamwork would decrease errors and improve the quality of care.[30]

In 2011, in response to the JC findings, the AACN put together a blue ribbon panel (Interprofessional Education Collaborative Expert Panel [IECEP]) to study how nursing, in conjunction with other heath-care disciplines, could integrate teaching and learning to improve health-care outcomes. Their findings noted four key competencies related to interprofessional education efforts:

• Values and ethics for interprofessional practice
• Roles and responsibilities
• Interprofessional communication
• Teams and teamwork

They recommended that these competencies be emphasized throughout nursing and other professional health-care curriculums.[31]

The Medical Home

Passage of the ACA in 2010 further stimulated interest in interprofessional education. One of the new concepts to approach health care from this perspective is the medical home approach. The medical home focuses its interdisciplinary efforts on producing better outcomes for chronically ill and high-risk clients in the primary care arena. It takes the emphasis placed on primary care in the ACA and expands it to all areas of health care. The key components of the medical home model include:

• Expanded accountability for the management of chronic disease
• Joint efforts by acute and public health-care professionals to address prevention issues
• Making the maintenance of healthy environments the responsibility of health-care professionals in all settings

Although part of the emphasis in nursing care since the time of Nightingale, the medical home includes a community component along with the individual client. In the medical home, nurses coordinate care for clients and their families with cooperation from other health-care professionals in both urban and rural settings.[32]

New Models of Interprofessional Nursing Education

Over the past several years, several new models for nursing education have been developed that are built around interdisciplinary education. Three models in particular use a framework where interprofessional interaction is a key component.

The D'Amour and Oandasan model combines four key components: (1) health professional education, (2) interprofessional collaborative practice, (3) client needs, and (4) community-oriented care.[33] This model is linier in design and links the four concepts much in the same way as the systems model.

The World Health Organization (WHO) developed a "Framework for Action" that focuses on curriculum and the education process but also includes institutional support, the culture of the workplace, and the many environmental elements that affect collaborative practice. Some of the key factors included in this model that drive interprofessional practice include:

• Local health needs
• Fragmented health-care practices
• Present and future health-care needs
• Shortages in the health workforce
• Collaborative practice
• Improved health-care system

> *In response to the push from the ACA for a more comprehensive view of health care needs, the Commission on Education of Health Care Professionals in the 21st Century developed a model that focuses on social accountability and social equality.*

The model's goal is to produce a well-integrated health-care workforce that will improve the overall quality of health care.[34] The WHO model is not designed as a framework for a nursing curriculum but rather can be included as one element in a more detailed design.

Again, in response to the push from the ACA for a more comprehensive view of health-care needs, the Commission on Education of Health Care Professionals in the 21st Century developed a model that focuses on social accountability and social equality. They noted that current health-care education is fragmented and does not really respond to the needs of populations. Similar to the other two models, this model sees the need for integration of public health into the overall picture of health care. The model satisfies many needs in both the education and health-care systems. These include client and population needs, client and population demands, the actual provision of health care, labor market pressure for health-care workers, and the actual supply of health-care workers. They consider the current education system for health professionals a "silo," where the members interact only with themselves. Interprofessional or transprofessional education will force professionals to be collaborative and effective teams that are non-hierarchical, thus promoting better client care.[34]

Research Shortage

Only a few studies have been conducted that demonstrate the positive effects of interprofessional education for nurses and provide a limited EBP base. These studies are often hard to conduct, demonstrating the difficulty in implementing interprofessional education as a standard feature of health-care curricula.

Many of the studies focus on only one or two IECEP competencies. However, the results have been encouraging, particularly in the areas of teamwork and communication. Students involved in interprofessional research projects showed an increased awareness of client safety, particularly when they were caring for several clients with complex problems. In working with medical students, nursing students gained knowledge about when the physician should be notified, and conversely, medical students gained a clearer understanding of the need for more precise communication. Overall, communication became more effective with the members of the interdisciplinary team.[35]

More studies are needed to develop a solid foundation of real-world evidence-based knowledge that would support the extensive changes required to fully integrate interprofessional learning into the nursing curriculum. The benefits include decreasing errors in care, improving the quality of care, and increasing the satisfaction of health-care practitioners.

Conclusion

In today's rapidly changing health-care environment, there is an ever-increasing need for health-care professionals who are educated to practice at the highest levels.[1] It is imperative that the schools educating future nurses be responsive to the changes, challenges, and demands of an ever more sophisticated and technologically advanced health-care system. Nursing education is an important part of a much larger network of health-care systems, including the service and practice sector, government and regulatory agencies, and licensing and credentialing institutions. All of these interact with each other and together form the health-care system.

The nursing profession has, over the years, developed many different types of education programs in an attempt to meet the demands of a growing health-care system. Some of the programs developed for specific needs that no longer exist should be examined for their usefulness and viability in today's advanced health-care atmosphere. Perhaps their resources could be rechanneled to programs that are more in tune with current needs. Students

should carefully evaluate programs they might enter and decide which one best meets their career goals.

Meanwhile, nursing education continues to develop innovative approaches to help nurses meet the demands for more education, more technical skills, and more leadership ability. The ladder programs are a good example. By recognizing the dynamic state of nursing education and implementing changes that respond to or even anticipate changes in the health-care system, the nursing profession will continue as one of the pillars of the health-care system.

Educators in nursing have begun to recognize that it is impossible to teach nursing students everything they need to know in the short time allowed for formal education. The demands of the changing health-care system will make that goal even more difficult. However, it may not be necessary to teach nursing students everything. It is more important to teach these students the thinking, decision-making, and management skills that will allow them to adjust to an ever-changing and developing health-care system.

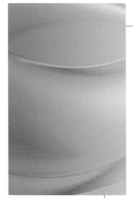

Issues Now

BS Degree = Lower Death Rates

Nurse educators have been insisting for many years that client outcomes will be better when more nurses have baccalaureate degrees. However, health-care policymakers and hospital administrators have not fully bought into the concept, as evidenced by their hiring practices. Part of the problem lies in the lack of empirical evidence that supports the supposition.

Over the past decade, only a few studies were conducted that demonstrated improved client outcomes when the nurses caring for them were educated at the baccalaureate level. Some studies even showed no significant improvements. However, a study conducted between 1999 and 2006 across Pennsylvania in 134 hospitals that examined discharge data from postoperative patients demonstrated that the BS degree does make a difference.

Conducted under the auspices of the Pennsylvania School of Nursing's Center for Health Outcomes and Policy Research, the researchers found that hospitals that increased the number of nurses with baccalaureate degrees by 10 or more percent had reductions in the death rates of postoperative clients by 2.12 for every 1000 undergoing surgery. Additionally, there was a reduction of 7.47 deaths for every 1000 clients who experienced either operative or postoperative complications. Although the study demonstrated a strong correlation between the increased number of baccalaureate RNs and the reduced death rates, it did not claim causality. A national study in 2010 reached the same conclusion that when more RNs were present to provide care, there were better outcomes and fewer medical errors.

The research design eliminated the effect of other variables such as staffing levels, nurses' years of experience, and variations in staff skill levels in affecting the outcome data. The research findings indicate that the reductions in death rates may be due to better assessment and monitoring of postoperative clients by baccalaureate prepared nurses. They were able to detect subtle changes in clients' conditions that were the first indicators of a deteriorating condition and then quickly initiate actions to reverse the decline.

This type of research is in line with the IOM's call for higher education levels for RNs. The research project was funded by grants from the Agency for Healthcare Research and Quality, the National Institutes of Health's National Institute of Nursing Research, and the Robert Wood Johnson Foundation.

Source: Kutney-Lee A, Sloane DM, Aiken LH. An increase in the number of nurses with baccalaureate degrees is linked to lower rates of post surgery mortality. *Health Affairs,* 32:3579–3586, 2013.

Critical-Thinking Exercises

- Discuss why the current educational system for nurses leads to confusion over the role and scope of practice for nurses.
- The literature reports that there will be a nursing shortage well into the 21st century. What aspects of health-care reform are likely to produce changes in nursing education? Identify possible changes that may occur in nursing education because of the projected nursing shortage. Will these changes be beneficial or harmful to the profession of nursing?
- Are nurses holding the DNP degree better practitioners than those with an MSN? Defend your position.

References

1. Kydd A. Counting nurses in a nursing shortage: What of the silent attrition? *Nursing Leadership,* 36(1):45–49, 2010.
2. Dumpel H. Hospital Magnet status: Impact on RN autonomy and patient advocacy. *National Nurse,* 106(3):22–27, 2010.
3. Greenwood B. Pew report highlights the impact of mobile technology. *Information Today,* 26(6):28, 2009.
4. Bleich MR. IOM report. The future of nursing: Leading change, advancing health: Milestones and challenges in expanding nursing science. *Research in Nursing and Health,* 34(3):169–170, 2011.
5. Jones D. Realizing the IOM future of nursing research within clinical practice. *Nursing Research,* 61(5):315, 2012.
6. Brown R, Feller L, Benedict L. Reframing nursing education: The Quality and Safety Education for Nurses Initiative. *Teaching and Learning in Nursing,* 5(3):115–118, 2010.
7. Cronenwett L, Sherwood G, Gelmon SB. Improving quality and safety education: The QSEN Learning Collaborative. *Nursing Outlook,* 57(6):304–312, 2009.
8. American Nurses Association. Position Paper on Education. Kansas City, MO, Author, 1965.
9. Fitzpatrick ML. *Prologue to Professionalism.* Bowie, MD: Robert J. Brady, 1983.
10. Jamieson EM, Sewell M. *Trends in Nursing History.* Philadelphia: WB Saunders, 1968.
11. Hegner BR, Caldwell E. *Nursing Assistant: A Nursing Process Approach* (6th ed.). Albany, NY: Delmar, 1995.
12. National League for Nursing: Trends in Education, 2010. Retrieved May 2014 from http://www.nln.org
13. Orsolini-Hain L, Waters V. Education evolution: A historical perspective of associate degree nursing. *Journal of Nursing Education,* 48(5):226–227, 2009.
14. Starr SS. Associate degree nursing: Entry into practice—link to the future. *Teaching & Learning in Nursing,* 5(3):129–134, 2010.
15. National League for Nursing: Statistics on Education, 2010. Retrieved April 2014 from http://www.nln.org
16. Matthias AD. The intersection of the history of associate degree nursing and "BSN in 10": Three visible paths. *Teaching & Learning in Nursing,* 5(1):39–43, 2010.
17. Forbes MO, Hickey MT. Curriculum reform in baccalaureate nursing education: Review of the literature. *International Journal of Nursing Education Scholarship,* 6(1):1–16, 2009.
18. Mills AC. Evaluation of online and on-site options for master's degree and post-master's certificate programs. *Nurse Educator,* 32(2):73–77, 2007.
19. Chornick N. Moving toward uniformity in APRN state laws. *Journal of Nursing Regulation,* 1(1):56–58, 2010.
20. Hathaway D. The practice doctorate: Perspectives of early adopters. *Journal of Nursing Education,* 45(12):487–496, 2006.
21. Hawkins R, Nezat G. Doctoral education: Which degree to pursue? *AANA Journal,* 77(2):92–96, 2009.
22. Brar K, Boschma G, McCuaig F. The development of nurse practitioner preparation beyond the master's level: What is the debate about? *International Journal of Nursing Education Scholarship,* 7(1):1–15, 2010.
23. Trossman S. Clarifying DNP versus CNL. *American Nurse,* 42(2):11, 2010.
24. Boland BA, Treston J, O'Sullivan AL. Climb to new educational heights. *Nurse Practitioner,* 35(4):34-–36, 2010.
25. Newland J. In defense of the DNP. *Nurse Practitioner,* 35(4):5, 2010.
26. Drinkert R. NP doesn't see need to pursue DNP. *Nurse Week,* 11(3):16, 2010.
27. Kutzin J. Other lessons learned completing a DNP program. *Journal of Nursing Education,* 49(4):181–182, 2010.
28. Sullivan L. Doctor of nursing practice degree: An era of change. *StuNurse,* 16:4–6, 2010.
29. World Health Organization (WHO). Framework for action on interprofessional education and collaborative practice. Geneva, WHO, Retrieved March 2013 from http://whqlibdoc.who.int/hq/2010/WHO_HRH_HPN_10.3_eng.pdf
30. Joint Commission. National patient safety goals. Retrieved March 2013 from http://www.jointcommission.org/standards_information/npsgs.aspx
31. Interprofessional Education Collaborative Expert Panel. (2011). Core competencies for interprofessional collaborative practice. Report of an expert panel. Retrieved March 2013 from http://www.aacn.nche.edu/education-resources/IPECReport.pdf
32. Henderson S, Princell CO, Martin SD. The patient-centered medical home. *American Journal of Nursing,* 112(12):54–59, 2012.
33. D'Amour, D, Oandasan I. Interprofessionality as the interprofessional practice and interprofessional education: An emerging concept. *Journal of Interprofessional Care,* 1(19):8–20, 2005.
34. Frenk J, Chen L, Bhutta ZA, Cohen J, Crisp N, Evans T. Health professionals for a new century: Transforming education to strengthen health systems in an interdependent world. *Lancet,* 376(9756):1923–1958, 2010.
35. Booth TL, McMullen-Fix K. Collaborative interprofessional simulation in a baccalaureate nursing education program. *Nursing Education Perspectives,* 2(33):127–129, 2012.

The Evolution of Licensure, Certification, and Nursing Organizations

5

Joseph T. Catalano

Learning Objectives

After completing this chapter, the reader will be able to:

- Identify the purposes and needs for nurse licensure
- Distinguish between permissive and mandatory licensure
- Explain why institutional licensure is unacceptable in today's health-care system
- Evaluate the importance of nurse practice acts
- Analyze the significance of professional certification
- Identify the key elements of the Licensure, Accreditation, Certification, and Education (LACE) model
- Discuss the long-term effects of the advanced practice registered nurse (APRN) Consensus Model on health care

MEETING EXPECTATIONS

Almost from the inception of nursing, societal needs and expectations have been the driving forces behind the establishment of the standards that guide the profession. In the early days of nursing, when health care was relatively primitive and society's expectations of nurses were low, there was little demand for regulations or controls over and within the profession. However, as technology and health care have advanced and become more complex, there has been a corresponding increase in societal expectations for nurses. All nurses now accept **licensure** and **certification** examinations as a given in today's health-care system. Where did these examinations come from, and what do they mean to the profession? This chapter explores the answers to these questions.

Rather than looking on the advent of the Affordable Care Act (ACA), growing information technologies, redesigned health-care organizations, and increasing **health-care consumer** demands with fear and trepidation, nurses should consider this an exciting time of growth and opportunity. In today's health-care system, nurses have an almost unlimited number of ways to provide new and creative nursing care for clients in all settings. As society's needs and expectations change, so will the regulations and standards that help define nursing practice. Through their professional nursing organizations, nurses can help shape health-care regulations that establish the most freedom to provide effective care while maintaining the goal of protecting the public. It is likely that in the future state boards of nursing will look very different, just as the profession of nursing will differ from that of its past.

THE DEVELOPMENT OF NURSE PRACTICE ACTS

A nurse practice act is state legislation regulating the practice of nurses that protects the public, defines the scope of practice, and makes nurses accountable for their actions. Nurse practice acts establish state boards of nursing (SBNs) and define specific SBN powers regarding the practice of nursing within the state. Rules and regulations written by the SBNs become **statutory laws** under the powers delegated by the state **legislature.**

Regulatory Powers

Although nurse practice acts differ from one state to another, the SBNs have many powers in common. These are considered regulatory powers because they provide the SBN with control over nurses according to rule, principle, or law. By legislative act, all SBNs have the power to grant licenses, approve nursing programs, establish standards for nursing schools, and write specific regulations for nurses and nursing practice in general in that state.

Of particular importance is the SBNs' power to deny or revoke nurse licenses (Box 5.1).[1] Additional functions of nurse practice acts include:

- Defining nursing and the scope of practice.
- Ruling on who can use the titles of registered nurse (RN) and licensed practical nurse/licensed vocational nurse (LPN/LVN).
- Setting up an application procedure for licensure in the state.
- Determining fees for licensure.
- Establishing requirements for renewal of licensure.

B o x 5 . 1

Reasons the State Boards of Nursing May Revoke a Nursing License

- Conviction for a serious crime
- Demonstration of gross negligence or unethical conduct in the practice of nursing
- Failure to renew a nursing license while still continuing to practice nursing
- Use of illegal drugs or alcohol during the provision of care for clients or use that carries over and affects clients' care
- Willful violation of the state's nurse practice act

- Determining responsibility for any regulations governing expanded practice for nurses in that particular state.

The Need for Licensure

Imagine what the quality of health care would be if anyone could walk into a hospital, claim to know how to care for clients, and be given a job as a nurse. This situation might sound impossible in today's health-care system, but in the past, it was the norm rather than the exception.

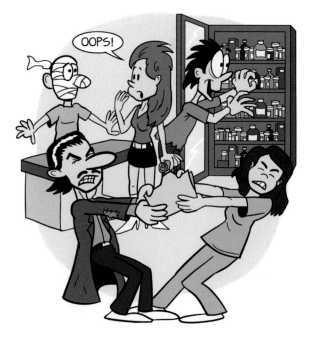

Throughout the last half of the 19th century and the first half of the 20th century, rapid growth in health-care technology led to the increasing use of hospitals as the primary source of health care. However, individuals who were qualified to provide this care were in short supply. There were wide variations both in the abilities of those who claimed to be nurses and in the quality of the care they provided. Paradoxically, nursing leaders who had always advocated some type of **credentialing** for nurses to ensure competency found that their attempts to initiate registration or licensure met with strong opposition from physician groups, hospital administrators, and practicing nurses themselves.

Early Attempts at Licensure

Although the idea of registering nurses had been in existence for some time, Florence Nightingale was the first to establish a formal list, or register, for graduates of her nursing school. In the United States and Canada, there was widespread recognition of the need for some type of credentialing of nurses as far back as the mid-1800s. The first organized attempt to establish a credentialing system was initiated in 1896 by the Nurses Associated Alumnae of the United States and Canada (later to become the American Nurses Association [ANA]). As with other early attempts at licensure, it was met with resistance and eventually failed.[2]

Several early American nursing leaders, including Lillian Wald and Annie Goodrich, recognized the inconsistent quality of nursing care and the need for licensure to protect the public. In 1901, after an extensive and lengthy campaign to educate the public, physicians, hospital administrators, and nurses themselves about the need for licensure, the International Council of Nurses passed a resolution that required each state to establish a licensure and examination procedure for nurses. It took 3 more years before the state of New York, through the New York Nurses Association, developed a licensure bill that passed the legislature (Box 5.2). Other states that followed New York's lead were North Carolina, New Jersey, and Virginia. Although these states had bills that were weaker than New York's nurse practice act, passage of such legislation was considered a major accomplishment for several reasons. Women did not even have the right to vote in general elections at the time these bills were passed. In addition, few licensure requirements and regulations of any type existed during this period in the United States, even for the medical profession.

The Importance of Licensure Examinations

The thought of having to take an examination that can determine whether or not one can practice nursing can make even the best student anxious. Adding to the tension is the fact that the examination is given outside of the academic setting, by computer, and is created by individuals other than the students' teachers. (See Chapter 9 for a detailed discussion of NCLEX-RN, CAT.)

A Measure of Competency

However, some type of objective method is necessary to prove that the individual is qualified to practice nursing safely; otherwise, the public is not protected from unqualified practitioners. Early attempts at creating licensure examinations for nurses were met with strong resistance. Although all states had some form of licensure examination by 1923, the format and length of the examinations varied widely. Some states required both written and practical examinations to demonstrate safety of practice; others added an oral examination.

Although licensure was and is a state-controlled activity, the major nursing organizations in the United States eventually realized that, to achieve consistency of quality across the country, all nurses needed to pass a uniform examination. The ANA Council of State Boards of Nursing was organized in 1945 to oversee development of a uniform examination for nurses that could be used by all state boards of nursing.

The NCLEX-RN, CAT

The National League for Nursing Testing Division developed a test that was implemented in 1950. Originally the test was simply called the State Board Examination, but it was renamed the National Council Licensure Examination (NCLEX) in 1987. In 1994, the computerized version of the examination was implemented—the National Council Licensure Examination Computerized Adaptive Testing for Registered Nurses (NCLEX-RN, CAT).

Licensure for nurses has undergone a major change. Some states implemented the Mutual Recognition Model for Nursing Licensure, which will allow nurses licensed in one state to practice nursing in other states that belong to their regional agreement. The eventual goal is to have a "universal" nursing

Box 5.2

Key Points in the New York State Licensure Bill (1904)

- Established minimum educational standards
- Established the minimum length of basic nursing programs at 2 years
- Required all nursing schools to be registered with the state board of regents (who oversee all higher education)
- Established a state board of nursing (SBN) with five nurses as members
- Formulated rules for the examination of nurses
- Formulated regulations for nurses that, if violated, could lead to the revocation of licensure

Source: Hirsh IL. Statement on nursing's scope describes how two levels of nurses practice. *American Nurse,* 20:13, 1988.

license that will allow nurses to practice in all states without having to become relicensed when they work in a different state.

REGISTRATION VERSUS LICENSURE

The terms *registration* and *licensure* are often used interchangeably, although they are not synonymous. They serve a similar purpose, but some technical differences exist.

Registration

Registration is the listing, or registering, of names on an official roster after certain preestablished criteria have been met. Before mandatory licensure by the states became the norm, the only way a health-care institution could find out whether an applicant had met the standards for the position was by calling the applicant's school to see if the person had graduated or passed an examination. The school would tell the institution whether the applicant's name appeared on the official roster or register—hence the origin of the term *registered nurse*. With the advent of state board examinations, an institution merely has to contact the SBN to find out whether the individual is registered or licensed.

> *Through their professional nursing organizations, nurses can help shape health-care regulations that establish the most freedom to provide effective care while maintaining the goal of protecting the public.*

Licensure

Licensure is conducted by the state through the enforcement powers of its regulatory boards to protect the public's health, safety, and welfare by establishing professional standards. Licensure for nurses, as for other professionals who deal with the public, is necessary to ensure that everyone who claims to be a nurse can function at a minimal level of competency and safety. There are several different types of licensure.

Permissive Licensure

Permissive licensure allows individuals to practice nursing as long as they do not use the letters *RN* after their names. Basically, permissive licensure only protects the "registered nurse" title but not the practice of nursing itself. Although most early licensure laws were permissive, all states now have mandatory

licensure. Under a permissive licensure law, anyone could carry out the functions of an RN, regardless of educational level, without having to pass an examination that indicates competency.

Health-care administrators seem to support the concept of permissive licensure because it allows them to employ less-educated and lower-paid employees rather than the more highly educated and better-paid RNs. However, they also recognize that the quality of care decreases when the education level of health-care providers is lower.

What Do You Think?

Should permissive licensure be reestablished because it will help reduce the cost of health care? Why? Why not?

Mandatory Licensure

Mandatory licensure requires anyone who wishes to practice nursing to pass a licensure examination and become registered by the SBN. Because different levels of nursing practice exist, different levels of licensure are necessary. At the technical level, the individual must take and pass the LPN/LVN examination; at the professional level, the individual must take and pass the RN examination.

Mandatory licensure forced SBNs to distinguish between the activities that nurses at different levels could legally perform. The scope of practice defines the boundaries for each of the levels: advanced practice registered nurse (APRN), RN, and LPN/LVN. As more levels of nursing education (e.g., the associate degree in nursing [ADN]) have been added, however, lines dividing the different scopes of practice have become blurred. In the current health-care system, it is not unusual to find LPNs/LVNs performing activities that are generally considered professional.

A particularly confusing element in today's health-care system is the use of unlicensed individuals to provide health care. The advent of certified nursing assistants (CNAs) and unlicensed assistive personnel (UAP) has led to widespread use of such individuals in all health-care settings. Although they must be supervised by an RN or LPN/LVN, these individuals are sometimes illegally assigned nursing tasks much more advanced than their levels of training. Even though permissive licensure is no longer legal, CNAs and UAP appear to fall under an unofficial type of permissive licensure.

Institutional Licensure

Although universally rejected by every major nursing organization, **institutional licensure** has become a reality for many other types of health-care workers, such as respiratory therapists and physical therapists.

Cut Corners, Cut Costs

Institutional licensure allows individual health-care institutions to determine which individuals are qualified to practice nursing within general guidelines established by an outside board. A back-door approach to allowing institutional licensure has been to allow **foreign graduate nurses** and nurses who are licensed in foreign countries to work in specific institutions without taking the U.S. licensure examination. Hospitals realize that the quality may not be the same as nurses licensed in the United States, but they believe the savings in lower wages to foreign nurses offset any decreases in quality care. Up to this point, bills that support this action have been stopped by the state nursing organizations before they could become law. Institutional licensure has been proposed periodically over the years as an alternative to governmental licensure.

A Lack of External Control

Probably the most critical problem is the lack of any external control to determine a minimal level of competency. The designations of RN and LPN/LVN would be virtually meaningless under institutional licensure. These nurses would not be under the control of a state licensing board and thus would not be held to the same standards of practice as nurses who were licensed by the states.

A second problem is that nurses who wished to move to a new place of employment would have to undergo whatever licensure procedure the new institution had established before being allowed to work there. Currently, nurses who move from one state to another can obtain licensure by endorsement by having the state recognize their nursing license from the original state of licensure. This process is generally referred to as **reciprocity.**

CERTIFICATION

At first glance, it may appear that there is not much difference between certification and licensure. Strictly defined, licensure can be considered a type of legal certification. However, in the more widely accepted use of the term, certification is a granting of credentials to indicate that an individual has achieved a level of ability higher than the minimal level of competency indicated by licensure.[3] As technology increases and the health-care environment becomes more complex and demanding, nurses are finding a need to increase their knowledge and skill levels beyond the essentials taught in their basic nursing courses.

Certification acknowledges the attainment of increased knowledge and skills and provides nurses with a means to validate their own self-worth and competence. Some certification also carries with it a legal status, similar to licensure, but in many cases, certification merely indicates a specific professional status. The public, employers, and even nurses have difficulty understanding what certification means.

Another element that adds confusion to the understanding of the process of certification is that a large number of groups can offer certification. These are usually professional specialty groups like the National Association of Pediatric Nurse Associates and Practitioners (NAPNAP) and the American Association of Critical-Care Nurses (AACN), but they can also be national organizations like the National League for Nursing (NLN) or the ANA.

Individual Certification

The most common type of certification is called *individual certification*. When a nurse has demonstrated that he or she has attained a certain level of ability above and beyond the basic level required for licensure in a defined area of practice, that nurse can become certified. Usually some type of written and practical examination is required to demonstrate this advanced level of skill.

The ANA has its own certifying organization, the American Nurses Credentialing Center (ANCC), that offers widely recognized certifications in more than 40 areas. Almost all nurses with individual certification are required to maintain their skills and competencies through continuing education and a specified number of continuing education units (CEUs). Recertification may be achieved by completing CEUs or retaking the certification examination.

Organizational Certification

Organizational certification is the certification of a group or health-care institution by some external agency. It is usually referred to as **accreditation** and indicates that the institution has met standards established either by the government or by a nongovernmental agency. Often the ability of the institution to collect money from insurance companies or the federal government depends on whether the institution is certified by a recognized agency. Most hospitals are accredited by the Joint Commission (formerly the Joint Commission on Accreditation of Healthcare Organizations, or JCAHO) as a minimum level of accreditation. Almost all baccalaureate and master degree programs are accredited by one of the two national nursing accrediting organizations, and many of the associate degree programs are also accredited. To work for any health-care facility run by the federal government (military, Indian health, Veterans Administration), nurses must be graduates of accredited programs.

Advanced Practice

Some state governments may either award or recognize certification granted to nurses in areas of advanced practice. In these cases, the certification becomes a legal requirement for practice at the APRN level. Depending on the individual state's nurse practice act, nurses thus certified fall under regulations in the state's practice act that control the type of activities nurses may legally carry out when they perform advanced roles.[4]

For example, many states recognize the position of nurse **midwife** as an advanced practice role for nurses. In these states, a nurse midwife may practice those skills allowed under the nurse practice act of that state after obtaining certification. Generally, nurse midwives are allowed to conduct prenatal examinations, do prenatal teaching, and deliver babies vaginally in uncomplicated pregnancies. They are not usually allowed to perform cesarean deliveries or other procedures that are surgical in nature.

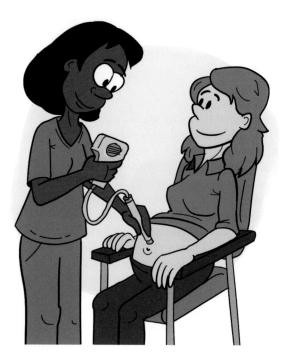

Varying Standards

In 1978, an independent certification center was proposed to establish uniform criteria and standards and to oversee all certification activities. This proposal received strong opposition from physicians and health-care administration groups for many years.

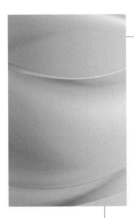

Issues Now

Health-Care Reform and Advanced Practice Nurses—Who's Driving the Bus?

Those who favor health-care reform see it as a giant step toward increasing health-care coverage for the some 56 million Americans who either don't have coverage or have only limited coverage. Those who oppose it see it as giant step toward socialization and an era of big government control. Either way, it is here, and one of the many issues that need to be worked out is the role of APRNs and how they will be regulated in the future.

Although nursing as a profession has consistently been ranked number one among the most trusted professions, the public still seems to have a very narrow view of what nurses can really do and the contributions they can make to health care. The role of APRN is even more obscure to the public, except for people who receive their care. For many years, APRNs have been quietly asserting their role as autonomous practitioners amid a swamp filled with confusing state regulations, multiple certifications, licensure issues, and political squabbling. Health-care reform will only fill the swamp with more alligators.

The American Medical Association (AMA) has always viewed APRNs as a threat to their scope of practice and even their livelihood, although study after study has shown this to be untrue. Their main concern on paper is the educational preparation of APRNs, and they have devoted significant research funds to comparing the education of APRNs to the education of MDs. Of course, it is the obligation of all professions to examine their preparation techniques and reflect on their growth and scope of practice. However, it seems strange that the medical profession is so concerned with how nursing educates its nurses. Nurses certainly do not expend the same amount of (if any) energy and resources to examining physician preparation.

Unfortunately, several major physician organizations see health-care reform as a back-door way to exert more influence over nursing practice, if not to control the regulation process of the nursing profession outright. The AMA has long held the belief that diagnosing, prescribing, and performing high-level clinical skills is the exclusive domain of physicians. APRNs, who graduate from accredited institutions of higher education and are certified by national organizations and licensed by their states, have shown that they, too, can successfully and safely carry out formerly exclusive physician practice areas, and usually more economically.

A more basic question is, who gave physicians the right to control the boundaries of the nursing profession? Professional groups such as nursing need to establish their own regulations to promote and achieve the outcomes of their profession. It is essential that all nurses, not just APRNs, control their own scope of practice and make their own decisions on how best to provide care for their clients. As health-care reform is fully implemented over the next several years, more and more clients will be seeing health-care providers for the first time. This situation is particularly suited for the skill set that APRNs bring to the table.

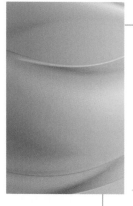

Issues Now continued

So, is there a rivalry between physicians and nurses? The answer is no. Both nurses and physicians will need the educational and skills preparation to work together to deal with the large influx of new clients in the near future. Will there be tensions between the two groups at the legislative and professional levels? As the situation exists today, it is hard to imagine there won't be. However, the nursing profession must stand its ground and vigorously guard against allowing other groups to regulate and define APRN practice. The ANA and most of the state organizations closely monitor legislation that deals with nursing practice. When a different health-care group is trying to change the scope of practice for nurses, they send out a warning. All nurses need to be politically tuned in to these attempts and quickly respond by contacting the appropriate legislators.

Sources: Rashid C. Benefits and limitations of nurses taking on aspects of the clinical role of doctors in primary care: Integrative literature review. *Journal of Advanced Nursing,* 66(8): 1658–1670, 2010; Traynor M, Boland M, Buus N. Autonomy, evidence and intuition: Nurses and decision-making. *Journal of Advanced Nursing,* 66(7):1584–1589, 2010; Ulrich CM. Who defines advanced nursing practice in an era of health care reform? *Clinical Scholars Review,* 3(1):5–7, 2010.

Some states recognized almost all certifications and had provisions in their nurse practice acts to help guide these practices. Other states had very little legal recognition of certification levels and thus few guidelines for practice. This confusion resulted from so many organizations offering certification in different areas. In some advanced practice specialties, such as nurse practitioner, two or more organizations may offer certification for the same title. The standards for qualifying for certification varied from organization to organization, and the method of determining certification may also be different.

A More Significant Role

The passage of the Affordable Care Act (ACA) of 2010 identified advance practice registered nurses (APRNs) as extremely valuable assets in the health-care system of the future. APRNs are in the perfect position to successfully move the country's health-care system into the 21st century. The ACA recognizes APRNs as equal partners in providing health care at multiple levels, but particularly in the area of primary care. In 2013, the ANA recommended that the Centers for Medicare and Medicaid Services (CMS), which is the organization that pays for health-care serves, must offer plans on state health insurance exchanges that include a minimum number of APRNs in each plan's network of health-care providers. That minimum number would be set in each state and should be equal to 10 percent of the number of APRNs recorded in the state as independently billing Medicare Part B. In 2011, there were 100,585 APRNs billing Medicare Part B independently.

APRNs will play an ever larger role in the rapidly evolving health-care system of the future. What that role will be depends on how well governmental organizations and the public understand the contributions of nurse practitioners and how hard APRNs work to meet the IOM's report recommendations that nurses must practice to the fullest extent of their education and at the top of their licenses.

APRN CONSENSUS MODEL (LACE)

As discussed above, the legal regulation and licensure of America's 267,000 APRNs is inconsistent and lacks steady definitions. Some states certify them as advanced practice nurses but do not have a separate license; other states recognize a licensing level for them but use different titles. If an APRN living in one state moved to another state, his or her scope of practice may be different and it is likely even the licensing process and title might also be different.

A Blueprint for the Future?

To address these and other related APRN issues, in 2008 the APRN Consensus Work Group and the National Council of State Boards of Nursing (NCSBN) APRN Advisory Committee issued a report on the Licensure, Accreditation, Certification, and Education (LACE) of APRNs. This statement addresses the lack of common definitions regarding APRN practice, the ever-increasing numbers of specializations, the inconsistency in credentials and scope of practice, and the wide variations in education for ARNPs.[5] The goal is to implement the APRN Model of Regulation in all states by 2015. As of early 2013, all national regulatory, educational, credentialing, and professional associations have agreed to promote the application of the model. In addition, 16 states are at or nearing completion of implementation of the model and several other states are in various stages of making the model part of their nurse practice act.

Definition and Roles

One of the first tasks accomplished by the NCSBN was to develop a uniform definition of the APRN role. According to the NCSN, the APRN is a nurse:

1. who has completed an accredited graduate-level education program preparing him/her for one of the four recognized APRN roles;
2. who has passed a national certification examination that measures APRN role and population-focused competencies and who maintains continued competence as evidenced by recertification in the role and population through the national certification program;
3. who has acquired advanced clinical knowledge and skills preparing him/her to provide direct care to patients, as well as a component of indirect care; however, the defining factor for **all** APRNs is that a significant component of the education and practice focuses on direct care of individuals;
4. whose practice builds on the competencies of registered nurses (RNs) by demonstrating a greater depth and breadth of knowledge, a greater synthesis of data, increased complexity of skills and interventions, and greater role autonomy;

5. who is educationally prepared to assume responsibility and accountability for health promotion and/or maintenance as well as the assessment, diagnosis, and management of patient problems, which includes the use and prescription of pharmacologic and nonpharmacologic interventions;
6. who has clinical experience of sufficient depth and breadth to reflect the intended license; **and**
7. who has obtained a license to practice as an APRN in one of the four APRN roles: certified registered nurse anesthetist (CRNA), certified nurse-midwife (CNM), clinical nurse specialist (CNS), or certified nurse practitioner (CNP).[5]

Some APRNs who have been in practice for many years are concerned that they will no longer be able to practice when the new requirements are implemented. The language of the consensus model includes a process called *grandfathering*, which allows the nurse to continue the same level of practice as long as he or she maintains an active license. The benefit of the model is that it would permit nurses to move to another state and still practice at the same level. However, it is up to each individual APRN to be knowledgeable about legislative issues that may affect their practice, monitor any additional requirements a state may add, and work to have the grandfathering language included in their state's practice act update.[6]

Titles for APRNs

The APRN Conesus Model requires that advanced practice nurses represent themselves with APRN and then specify a role. For example, an advanced practice nurse who is also a certified nurse practitioner would sign his or her name and then write *APRN, CNP* after it. The particular group of clients or specialty may also be included; for example, *APRN, CNP, pediatrics.* If the nurse was prepared and licensed in more than one role, he or she would include all the relevant roles. Employers of APRNs retain the responsibility for verifying the nurse's education and license.

Education for APRNs

Although there has been some movement by higher education for consistency in APRN programs, there remains a wide variation in length and requirements for the programs. The APRN Consensus Model expects that any educational program for advanced practice be preapproved by accrediting entities *before* the students enter the program. This will guarantee that the students will have met the prerequisites for licensure and certification upon graduation. The programs will have to meet established educational standards so that students can sit for national certification examinations when they graduate. Actually, these standards already exist, although not all programs currently meet them.[7]

Nurses currently in APRN educational programs need to keep up with proposed changes as they are applied to these programs. This begins with being aware of proposed legislation since the changes will first take place at the SBN and legislative levels. Generally, SBNs allow nursing programs 2 years to implement required changes after they become part of the practice act. It is imperative that students talk with the professors and the deans of their programs about how modifications will affect them. Again, the purpose of preapproval is to make sure the graduates meet the eligibility requirements for certification and licensure.

Even though specialization into areas such as oncology, nephrology, or palliative care do not fall into one of the four population focus areas of the APRN Consensus Model, nurses can still specialize in these areas. There are several ways to achieve this specialized education. The nurse can finish a preapproved APRN population-focused program, become certified and licensed, and then pursue additional education in the specialty of choice. Another option is to attend a program that will prepare the nurse for the population-focused APRN and the specialty he or she wishes to pursue at the same time. When the nurses graduate, they can take the certification/licensure exam for the APRN and then the certification exam for their specialty of choice. It is important to remember that specialty areas of practice are identified by professional organizations and are not specifically regulated by SBNs. The professional organizations establish the competencies for the specialization and usually have a separate certification examination and other requirements.[8]

The APRN Consensus Model does not require a program to offer a doctor of nursing practice (DNP) degree. A master's degree is the basic requirement. Programs do have the option to offer the DNP as long as it meets the requirements for the APRN as outlined in the model. With the current trend in nursing education being to promote the DNP as the terminal degree for advanced practice, it is likely that most programs will go this route.

LACE

LACE is not the same as the APRN Consensus Model, but rather an outgrowth of the process to put the model into practice. LACE serves as a means for those who are seeking to adopt the APRN Consensus Model to debate the concepts, requirements, and methods of execution. It is more inclusive and asks for input from parties who may be affected by changes in the legal status of APRNs or the scope of their practice, such as community groups, medical associations, and hospitals. The ultimate goal of LACE is to provide a general consensus for the implementation of the APRN Consensus Model.[9]

While states move forward on legislation to implement the APRN Consensus Model, it is important for nurses to watch for other proposed legislation and practices that politicians, medical associations, and health-care institutions are initiating. Many of these proposals and practices are covert ways of reintroducing permissive and institutional licensure, which reduces the control of nurses over their own practice and hinders attempts to provide higher quality health care to more of our citizens in the future.

NURSING ORGANIZATIONS AND THEIR IMPORTANCE

The establishment of a professional organization is one of the most important defining characteristics of a profession. An association is a group of people banding together to achieve a specific purpose. By working together for a specific purpose, an association or organization amplifies its impact, and by developing a strategic plan, it focuses that impact to achieve certain results. Many professions have a single major professional organization to which most of its members belong and several specialized suborganizations that members may also join. Professions with just one major organization generally have a great deal of political power.

Strength in Numbers

Nurses need and use power in every aspect of their professional lives, ranging from supervising unlicensed personnel to negotiating with the administration for increased independence of practice. Clearly, an individual nurse probably does not have much influence, but for nurses as a group, the potential is increased exponentially by the organization. The

dedication to high-quality nursing standards and improved methods of practice by the major nursing organizations has led to improved care and increased benefits to the public as a whole.[10]

Speaking With One Voice

National nursing organizations need the participation and membership of all nurses in order to claim that they are truly representative of the profession. A large membership allows the organization to speak with one voice when making its values about health-care issues known to politicians, physicians' groups, and the public in general.

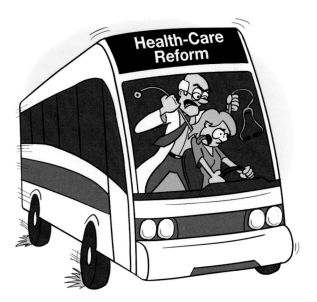

The National League for Nursing

The NLN is also a strong force in community health nursing, occupational health nursing, and nursing service activities. It was the first national nursing organization to provide accreditation for nursing programs at all levels.

Purposes

The primary purpose of the National League for Nursing (NLN) is to maintain and improve the standards of nursing education. Its bylaws state that its purpose is to foster the development and improvement of hospital, industrial, and public health; other organized nursing services; and nursing education through the coordinated action of nurses, allied professional groups, citizens, agencies, and schools so that the nursing needs of the people will be met.

Membership

Although membership is open to individual nurses, the primary membership of the NLN comes in the form of agency membership, usually through schools of nursing. One of the major functions of the NLN, through the organization formerly known as the National League for Nursing Accrediting Commission (NLNAC), but renamed the Accreditation Commission for Education in Nursing (ACEN), is to accredit schools of nursing through a self-study process. The schools are given a set of criteria, or **essentials for accreditation,** and are then required to evaluate their programs against these criteria. After the evaluation report is written and sent to the ACEN, site representatives visit the school to verify the information in the report and see whether the school has met the criteria. If the school meets the evaluation criteria, it is accredited for up to 8 years.

Accreditation of a nursing school by the ACEN indicates that the school meets national standards. In some work settings, a nurse must be a graduate of an ACEN-accredited school of nursing before he or she can be hired or accepted into many master's-level nursing programs.

Other services and activities that the NLN carries out include testing; evaluating new graduate nurses; supplying career information, continuing education workshops, and conferences for all levels of nursing; publishing a wide range of literature and DVDs covering current issues in health care; and compiling statistics about nursing, nurses, and nursing education.

The American Association of Colleges of Nursing

The American Association of Colleges of Nursing (AACN) was established to help colleges with schools of nursing work together to improve the standards for higher education for professional nursing. It serves the public interest by assessing and identifying nursing programs that engage in effective educational practices.

Purposes

The AACN, through the Commission on Collegiate Nursing Education (CCNE), has developed standards for the accreditation of baccalaureate schools of nursing and is poised to become a major accreditation agency, competing with the NLNAC. The AACN has developed and published a set of guidelines for the education of professional nursing students that is widely used as the theoretical basis for baccalaureate curricula.

Membership

Only deans and directors of programs that offer baccalaureate or higher degrees in nursing with an upper-division nursing major are permitted membership in the AACN.

The American Nurses Association

The American Nurses Association (ANA) grew out of a concern for the quality of nursing practice and the care that nurses were providing. In the early part of the 20th century, when the ANA was organized, there was little or no regulation for the requirements to practice as a nurse. ANA took some of the first steps in developing standards for the profession.

Purposes

The major purposes for the existence of the ANA, as stated in its bylaws, include improving the standards of health and access to health-care services for everyone; improving and maintaining high standards for nursing practice; and promoting the professional growth and development of all nurses, including economic issues, working conditions, and independence of practice.[6]

In 2012 and 2013, the ANA underwent a major structural reorganization. The ANA board of directors was reduced from 16 to 10, and all of the standing committees were disbanded. The traditional house of delegates that met every other year was restructured into a membership assembly model that reduced the representation at the convention to two elected members and one appointed member from each state with a weighted vote that now meets each year.[11] The goal of the restructuring is to streamline the organization and make it more responsive to a rapidly changing health-care system and society. Committees are now formed when needed to address a particular issue and then disbanded after the issue is resolved. For example, the Code of Ethics for Nurses was updated, so a committee was formed to deal with the changes that need to be made.

Membership

Membership in the ANA also changed with the restructuring. Currently, it is limited to 52 constituents: 50 state organizations; Washington, DC; and Puerto Rico. An individual joins a state organization and through the state organization indirectly is a member of the ANA. Certain discounts in membership are offered for new members and new graduate nurses. Various levels of membership are available for nurses who work part-time or those who are retired. The ANA makes every effort to encourage individual nurses to join the organization. The proposed changes to the governance and membership structure would not require nurses to join their states first. Rather, they would become direct members of the ANA. Unfortunately, most nurses do not belong to this potentially powerful, politically active, and very influential organization.

Each state has the opportunity to determine what is needed from each member to run the state association; the amount of the dues that is sent to ANA is predetermined. Although dues are not inexpensive (they change a little from year to year but are about $200 per year), the ANA offers various plans for payment, such as three equal payments over the course of a year or monthly payroll deductions. Because of the efforts of the ANA, nurses' salaries have risen to a point at which this sum is affordable.

Other Services

When nurses pursue advanced education and levels of practice, as many are doing today, the ANA ANCC is essential for testing and certification of many of these practice levels. Although other organizations offer advanced practice certification, without the ANCC, there would be even less standardization for and less recognition of these practitioners by the public, physicians, or lawmakers.

Entry Into Practice

Another important issue that the ANA has been involved in is the entry-level education requirement for professional nurses. The ANA has supported the baccalaureate degree as the minimum educational requirement for nurses since 1958. The ANA is always in the forefront of the debate over **entry into practice,** which has continued into the 21st century.

Standards of Practice

Additional functions carried out by the ANA include the establishment and continual updating of standards of nursing practice. These standards are the yardstick against which nurses are measured and held

> " *Clearly, an individual nurse probably does not have much power, but for nurses as a group, the potential is increased exponentially by the organization.* "

accountable by courts of law. The ANA also established the official code of ethics that guides professional practice.

Legislation

Many of the political and economic activities of the ANA are carried out in the halls of legislatures and offices of legislators. The ANA Political Action Committee (ANA-PAC) is one of the most powerful in Washington, DC. (See Chapter 20 for a more detailed discussion.) Such activities have a profound effect on the role that nurses play and will continue to play in health care well into the 21st century.

Successful PAC activities require money and the power of a large, unified membership. The ANA-PAC seeks to influence legislation about nurses, nursing, and health care in general. It has been and will be a strong voice in the formulation of current national health-care reform.

The National Student Nurses' Association

The National Student Nurses' Association (NSNA) is an independent legal corporation established in 1953 to represent the needs of nursing students. Working closely with the ANA, which offers services, an official publication, and close communication, the NSNA consists of state chapters that represent student nurses in those particular states.

Purposes

The main purpose of the NSNA is to help maintain high standards of education in schools of nursing, with the ultimate goal of educating high-quality nurses who will provide excellent health care.[12] The ideas, concerns, and needs of students are extremely important to nursing educators. Most nursing programs have committees in which students are asked to participate, including curriculum development and evaluation techniques. It is important that students belong to these committees and actively participate in the committees' activities.

Membership

Membership consists of all nursing students in registered nurse programs. Students can join at the local, state, or national level or at all levels if desired. Dues are low, with a discount for the first year's membership.

Other Services

Additionally, the NSNA is concerned with developing and providing workshops, seminars, and conferences that deal with current issues in nursing and health care, with a wide range of subjects, from ethical and legal concerns to recent developments in pharmacology, test-taking skills, and professional growth. Student nurses who belong to the NSNA and who take an active part in its functions are much more likely to join the ANA after they graduate. Professional identity and professional behavior are learned. By beginning the process during the formal school years, student nurses develop professional attitudes and behaviors that they will maintain for the rest of their careers.

Benefits for Students

Many benefits exist for student nurses who belong to the NSNA. Several scholarships are available through this organization to members of the NSNA. Members receive the official publication of the organization, *Imprint,* and the *NSNA News,* which keep the student nurse current on recent developments in health care and nursing.

Student members also have political representation on issues that may affect them now or in the future. Some of these issues include educational standards for practice, standards of professional practice, and health insurance. The NSNA is also concerned with the difficulty that many nursing students from minority groups experience in the educational process. The Breakthrough Project is an attempt by the NSNA to help such students enter the nursing profession.

Practicing Professionalism

Student nurses who join the NSNA experience first-hand the operation, activities, and benefits of a professional organization. In schools with active memberships, the NSNA can be a very exciting and useful organization for students.

Many NSNA chapters are involved in community activities that provide services at a local level and allow the student to practice "real" nursing. These services include providing community health screening programs for hypertension, lead poisoning, vision, hearing, and birth defects; setting up information and education programs; giving immunizations;

and working with groups concerned with drug abuse, child abuse, drunken driving, and teen pregnancy. All nursing students should be encouraged to belong to this organization.

The International Council of Nurses

Membership in the International Council of Nurses (ICN) consists of national nursing organizations, and the ICN serves as the international organization for professional nursing. The ANA is one member among 104 nursing associations around the world. Each member nation sends delegates and participates in the international convention held every 4 years. The quadrennial conventions, or congresses, are open to all nurses and delegates from all nations.

The goal of the ICN is to improve health and nursing care throughout the world. The ICN coordinates its efforts with the United Nations and other international organizations when appropriate in the pursuit of its goals.

Some issues that have been the focus of concern of the ICN are the social and economic welfare of nurses, the changing role of nurses in the present health-care environment, the challenges being faced by the various national nursing organizations, and how government and politics affect the nursing profession and health care. Overseeing the ICN is the Council of National Representatives. This body meets every 2 years and serves as the governing organization. ICN headquarters is located in Geneva, Switzerland.

Sigma Theta Tau

Sigma Theta Tau is an honors organization that was established in colleges and universities to recognize individuals who have demonstrated leadership or made important contributions to professional nursing. It is international, and candidates are selected from among senior nursing students or graduate or practicing nurses.

The organization has its headquarters in Indianapolis, where it has a large library open to members to use for scholarly activities and research. It also boasts the first online nursing journal, which can be accessed by any nurse with a computer anywhere in the world. Local chapters of Sigma Theta Tau collect and distribute funds to nurses who are conducting nursing research. The organization also holds educational conferences and recognizes those who have made contributions to nursing.

Grassroots Organizations

A growing trend in contemporary nursing has been the formation of grassroots nursing organizations. In reality, all nursing organizations start as the grassroots efforts of local nursing groups that are trying to solve a particular problem. Over time, these small grassroots organizations become more structured, larger, and eventually national or international when they spread to other areas across the country or around the world. Unfortunately, the large organizations tend to lose sight of the fundamental issues they were originally formed to solve, or they are unable to deal effectively with local problems.

Working to Bring About Change

Grassroots organizations usually have relatively small memberships; are localized to a town, city, or sometimes a state; and attempt to solve a problem or deal with an issue that the members feel is not being adequately handled by a large national organization. They may be created as a completely new and separate organization, or they may break away from a larger, established group. Because all the members of grassroots organizations are passionately concerned about only one or two issues at a time that affect them directly, they tend to work hard to effect change and can bring a great deal of concentrated power to bear on people, such as legislators, who make the decisions about the issues.

> *In reality, all nursing organizations start as the grassroots efforts of local nursing groups that are trying to solve a particular problem.*

Grassroots groups use a number of techniques that are often frowned upon by the more established organizations to attain their goals. In addition to the traditional techniques of writing letters, sending e-mails, and calling legislators, members of grassroots groups actively seek media attention, march on capitol buildings and state houses, introduce resolutions, and testify before committee hearings. Their success varies from issue to issue and location to location.

Successful Grassroots Efforts

Two examples of successful grassroots efforts are found in California and Pennsylvania. The California Nurses Association decided to break away from the ANA because it was not addressing some key state issues such as length of hospital stays, reduction in professional nursing staffs, and preoccupation with profit. The grassroots group in Pennsylvania formed a completely new organization, the Nurses of Pennsylvania (NPA), and focused their energies on the trend to replace licensed registered nurses with unlicensed technicians, sometimes called *downskilling*.

Special-Interest Organizations

The historical origins of special-interest organizations in nursing are even older than those of the main national organizations. For example, the Red Cross, established in 1864, is one of the oldest special-interest organizations that nurses have been involved with.

Why Do They Exist?

Most specialty organizations in nursing were founded when a group of nurses with similar concerns sought professional and individual support. These organizations usually start out small and informal, then increase in size, structure, and membership over several years. There were relatively few of these organizations until 1965, when an explosion in specialty organizations in nursing took place. During the next 20 years, almost 100 new organizations were formed, with the associated effect of diminishing membership levels in the ANA.

Clinical Practice

Specialty organizations are usually organized according to clinical practice area. Organizations exist for almost every clinical specialty and subspecialty known in nursing, such as obstetrics/gynecology, critical care, operating room, emergency department, and occupational health, as well as less known areas such as flight nursing, urology, and cosmetic surgery.

Education and Culture

Another focal area for these organizations is education and ethics. Organizations such as the AACN and the Western Interstate Commission for Higher Education fall into this category. Often organizations focus on the common **ethnic group** or cultural or religious backgrounds of nurses. The National Association of Hispanic Nurses and the National Black Nurses Association represent this type of specialty organization.

Education and Standards

Although many of these organizations promote the personal and professional growth of their membership, they also carry out many other activities. Particularly important among these activities is establishing the standards of practice for the particular specialty area. As much as the ANA establishes overall standards of practice for nursing in general, the specialty organizations establish standards for their particular clinical areas. Providing educational services for their members is another important activity of specialty organizations. Conferences, workshops, and seminars in the clinical area represented are important venues for nurses to keep current on new developments and to maintain high standards of practice.[7]

Should They Matter to You?

How many of these specialty nursing organizations are there? No one really knows. Many such organizations are informal and run by volunteers. Organizations are continually being formed, and others are being disbanded.

Should nurses belong to these organizations? The answer is yes, but only after they belong to the ANA. Many of the larger specialty organizations have recognized this fact and have established close ties with the ANA. The ANA is well aware of the membership bleed-off from the specialty organizations and has initiated efforts to become more involved in the specialty nursing areas.

Before nurses join a specialty organization, they should determine whether its purposes are at odds with those of the ANA. Many of the large specialty organizations have their own lobbyists in both state and national legislatures. Because the legislators really do not know the differences between the various nursing organizations, they can easily become confused over health-care issues if they are receiving pressure from two nursing groups representing opposing sides of the same issue. At this point, legislators may simply surmise that the professional opinions of those in the industry are too contradictory to consider and vote on an important issue without regard to nurses and nursing.

The tendency toward specialization has led to an ever-increasing number of nursing organizations, each focusing on a particular practice field within the profession. This trend has diluted the unity and ultimately lessened the power that nursing as a profession can exert in health-care issues. Although it is important to recognize the complexity of today's health-care system and the pluralism inherent in nursing, unity of opinion on major issues is essential if nursing is to have any influence on the future of the profession.

The challenge for nurses in the future is to use the diversity in the profession as a positive force and to unite as a group on important issues. Awareness of earlier development of nursing organizations provides a perspective for the current situation and can act as a framework for planning the future.

What Do You Think?

What type of power does the individual nurse have? Cite examples of individual nurses who have used their power to effect changes in health care and nursing.

Conclusion

Nursing, in its journey toward professionalism, has been propelled and shaped by its nursing organizations, which were the main vehicles for the development of educational and practice standards, initiation of licensure, promotion of advanced practice, and general improvement in the level of care nurses provided. From their beginnings, nursing organizations have served as channels of communication among nurses, consumers of health care, and other health-care professionals. In many cases, the nursing organizations have served as a focus of power for the profession to influence those important health policies that affect the whole nation. That continued unity is essential for the allegiance of nursing.

Licensure and certification are both methods of granting credentials to demonstrate that an individual is qualified to provide safe care to the public. Without proof of competency, the profession of nursing would become chaotic, disorganized, and even dangerous.

Issues in Practice

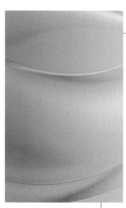

Juanita R, an RN at a large inner-city hospital, has been working on her off hours as a volunteer in a storefront clinic to treat the indigent and underserved population of that part of the city. The clinic clientele is primarily Mexican American, as are the majority of the 20 nurses working at the clinic. Because all the nurses, including a family nurse practitioner, volunteer their time and receive no pay, the small private grant that Juanita had managed to secure was adequate to cover the cost for rental of the building, basic supplies for the clinic, and a few medications. However, the grant is about to run out and is nonrenewable.

Juanita first tried to obtain money from the hospital to keep the clinic going, but she was told that the hospital was having its own financial problems because of managed care demands and could not spare any money. At a staff meeting of the nurses from the clinic, the nurses decided to band together and form a grassroots organization called the Storefront Clinic Nurses to focus their efforts on obtaining funds to keep the clinic open. They printed and passed out flyers, called local and city politicians, encouraged the patrons of the clinic to talk to people they knew, and even called the local television station for an interview about their plight.

Although most of the nurses' efforts went unrewarded, a large pharmaceutical company became aware of their plight and wanted to provide a sizable financial stipend to the clinic, in addition to supplying free medications, for a period of at least 5 years. In addition to their philanthropic interests, the pharmaceutical company also wanted to gather long-term data about a newly developed antihypertensive medication. The company would provide the medication free to the clients at the clinic, the majority of whom had some degree of hypertension, and all the nurses had to do was take and record the clients' blood pressure readings and complete "reported side effects" forms on each client. Client identifier codes, rather than names, would be used to maintain confidentiality. Juanita, as the group's coordinator, would be responsible for coordinating and preserving the data.

Although Juanita saw it as an answer to her prayers, she was concerned about the medication project. The pharmaceutical company said that no research consent forms were needed because the medication had already been through clinical trials and had received approval by the Food and Drug Administration. Juanita called another meeting of her nurses to discuss the issue. Without the grant, the clinic would close, but if they accepted the grant, they would have to participate in a medication research project that made Juanita feel uncomfortable.

Questions for Thought

1. What are the main issues in this case study?

2. What ethical principles are being violated? What is the ethical dilemma that Juanita is facing?

3. Are there any other solutions to this problem?

Critical-Thinking Exercises

- Develop a strategy for increasing the membership of the ANA.
- A labor union is attempting to organize the nurses at your hospital. Is it better for the professional nursing organization to represent the nurses? Why?
- A new graduate nurse is working in the intensive care unit (ICU) of a large hospital. She wants to join a nursing organization but has a limited amount of money to spend. Her coworkers in the ICU want her to join the AACN, but she would also like to join the ANA. Basing her decision on economic and professional issues, which organization should she join?
- Compare and contrast certification and licensure. Should certification be legally recognized? Justify your answer.

References

1. Romeo EM. Quantitative research on critical thinking and predicting nursing students' NCLEX-RN performance. *Journal of Nursing Education,* 49(7):378–386, 2010.

2. Smith CK. Professional perspective. Multistate licensure: Is your job putting you at risk? *Case in Point,* 7(2):24–25, 2009.

3. Eisemon N. Certification is an important part of nurse education, career growth. *American Nurse,* 42(2):6, 2010.

4. Snow T, Kendall-Raynor P. Why consensus proves elusive for advanced practitioner regulation. *Nursing Standard,* 24(36):12–13, 2010.

5. National Council of State Boards of Nursing. Consensus Model for APRN Regulation: Licensure, Accreditation, Certification and Education. Retrieved March 2013 from http://www.ncsbn .org/7_23_08_Consensue_APRN_Final.pdf

6. Madler B, Kalanek CB, Rising C. An incremental regulatory approach to implementing the APRN Consensus Model. *Journal of Nursing Regulation,* 3(2):11–15, 2012.

7. Stanley JM. Impact of new regulatory standards on advanced practice registered nursing: The APRN Consensus Model and LACE. Nursing Clinics of North America, 47(2):241–250, 2012.

8. Kleinpell RM, Hudspeth R, Scordo KA, Magdic K. Defining NP scope of practice and associated regulations: Focus on acute care. Journal of the American Academy of Nurse Practitioners, 24(1):11–18, 2012.

9. Goudreau, KA. LACE, APRN consensus . . . WIIFM (What's in it for me). Clinical Nurse Specialist. Retrieved March 2013 from http://www.cns-journal.com

10. Mata H, Latham TP, Ransome Y. Benefits of professional organization membership and participation in national conferences: Considerations for students and new professionals. Health Promotion Practice, 11(4):450–453, 2010.

11. American Nurses Association. Nursing's Social Policy Statement. Washington, DC: Author, 1995.

12. Smith TG. A policy perspective on the entry into practice issue. Online Journal of Issues in Nursing, 15(1):2, 2010.

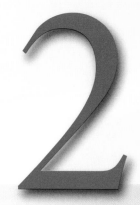

Making the Transition to Professional

Ethics in Nursing

6

Joseph T. Catalano

Learning Objectives

After completing this chapter, the reader will be able to:

- Discuss and analyze the difference between law and ethics
- Define the key terms used in ethics
- Discuss the important ethical concepts
- Distinguish between the two most commonly used systems of ethical decision-making
- Apply the steps in the ethical decision-making process

A LEARNED SKILL

Nurses who practice in today's health-care system soon realize that making ethical decisions is a common part of daily nursing care. However, experience shows that in the full curricula of many schools of nursing, the teaching of ethical principles and ethical decision-making gets less attention than the topics of nursing skills, core competencies, and electronic charting. As health-care technology continues to advance at a rapid pace, nurses will find it more and more difficult to make sound ethical decisions. Many nurses feel the need to be better prepared to understand and deal with the complex ethical problems that keep evolving as they attempt to provide care for their clients.[1]

There are many individuals who confuse ethics with social norms, religious beliefs, or the legal system. Some simply believe ethics are the same as morals. Although elements of ethics may be found in all these places, ethics itself is a stand-alone set of concepts and principles that guide humans in general, and professionals in particular, in making decisions about what types of behaviors will help or harm other members of society. Ethics generally presents broad concepts to guide decision-making and does not have specific rules such as are found in moral systems.

Ethical decision-making is a skill that can be learned. The ability to make sensible ethical decisions is based on an understanding of underlying ethical principles, ethical theories or systems, a decision-making model, and the profession's code of ethics. This skill, like others, involves mastery of the theoretical material and practice of the skill itself. This chapter presents the basic information required to understand ethics, the code of ethics, and ethical decision-making. It also highlights some of the important bioethical issues that challenge nurses in the current health-care system.

FOUR CATEGORIES

As a part of a philosophical system, ethics is generally divided into levels or categories:

Meta-Ethics: The abstract, overarching philosophical way of understanding ethics. One of the most important questions that philosophy in general addresses is the question of epistemology, or how we know that we know. In ethics, this question is refined to *how* do we know what is right and wrong. It also seeks to answer the question, "What is truth?" It is concerned with the meaning of ethical language and explaining the fundamental meaning of the words. The discussion below of the ethical terms is actually a meta-ethics approach to understanding ethics. Without meta-ethics, it is almost impossible to take the next step to normative ethics.

Normative Ethics: The use of the concepts and principles discovered by meta-ethics to guide decision-making about specific actions in determining what is right or wrong when interacting with other people. Normative ethics tends to be more prescriptive than meta-ethics and forms the basis for theories and systems of ethics (below). Both the codes of ethics and the deontological ethical system (below) find their underpinnings in meta-ethics and normative ethics

Applied Ethics: The application of the theories and systems of ethics developed by normative ethics to real-world situations. Applied ethics is broken into specialized fields such as health-care ethics, legal ethics, bioethics, or business ethics. This is the category of ethics that is used most by nurses and other health-care providers. It is used in resolving ethical dilemmas.

Descriptive Ethics: A bottom-up approach to ethics that starts with what society is already doing ethically and developing ethical principles based on the observed actions of people rather than starting with ethical principles and applying them to society such as normative ethics does. There are no preset values in descriptive ethics except for the consistent ethical decisions that are already being made by the majority of members of society. It is also sometimes called *comparative ethics* and forms the basis for situational ethics and the utilitarian system of ethics. Although widely used in politics, economics, and business, it creates additional issues for health-care providers when applied to difficult health-care decisions.

IMPORTANT DEFINITIONS

In Western cultures, the study of ethics is a specialized area of philosophy, the origins of which can be traced to ancient Greece. In fact, certain ethical principles articulated by Hippocrates still serve as the basis for many of the current debates. Like most specialized areas of study, ethics has its own language and uses terminology in precise ways. The following are some key terms that are encountered in studies of health-care ethics.

> " *Values are usually not written down; however, at some time in their professional careers, it may be important for nurses to make lists of their values.* "

Values

Values are ideals or concepts that give meaning to an individual's life. Values are derived most commonly from societal norms, religion, and family orientation and serve as the framework for making decisions and taking action in daily life. People's values tend to change as their life situations change, as they grow older, and as they encounter situations that cause value conflicts. For example, before the 1950s, pregnancy outside of marriage was unacceptable, and unmarried women who were pregnant were shunned and generally separated from society. Today this situation is more widely accepted, and it is not uncommon to see pregnant high school students attending classes.

Values are usually not written down; however, at some time in their professional careers, it may be important for nurses to make lists of their values. This value clarification process requires that nurses assess, evaluate, and then determine a set of personal values and prioritize them. This will help them make decisions when confronted with situations in which the client's values differ from the nurse's values.

Value conflicts that often occur in daily life can force an individual to select a higher-priority value over a lower-priority one. For example, a nurse who values both career and family may be forced to decide between going to work and staying home with a sick child.[2]

Morals

Morals are the fundamental standards of right and wrong that an individual learns and internalizes, usually in the early stages of childhood development. An individual's moral orientation is often based on religious beliefs, although societal influence plays an important part in this development. The word *moral* comes from the Latin word *mores*, which means "customs" or "values."

Moral behavior is often manifested as behavior in accordance with a group's norms, customs, or traditions. A moral person is generally someone who responds to another person in need by providing care and who maintains a level of responsibility in all relationships.[3] In many situations in which moral convictions differ, it is difficult to find a rational basis for proving one side right over the other. For example, animal rights activists believe that killing animals for sport, their fur, or even food is morally wrong. Most hunters do not even think of the killing of animals as a moral issue at all.

What Do You Think?

What type of value conflicts have you experienced in the past week? How did you resolve them? Were you satisfied with the resolution, or did it make you feel uncomfortable?

Laws

Laws can generally be defined as rules of social conduct made by humans to protect society, and these laws are based on concerns about fairness and justice. The goals of laws are to preserve the species and promote peaceful and productive interactions between individuals and groups of individuals by preventing the actions of one citizen from infringing on the rights of another. Two important aspects of laws are that they are enforceable through some type of police force and that they should be applied equally to all persons.

Ethics

The term *ethics* has its origins in the Greek word *ethos,* which is generally translated as "quality" or "character." It is a branch of traditional Western philosophy known as *moral philosophy* that studies moral behavior in humans and how humans should act toward each other individually and in groups. Ethics, as a system of beliefs and behaviors, goes beyond the law, which has as its primary underlying principle the preservation of society. Ethics is more focused on the quality of the society and its long-term survival. Similar to the legal system, ethical systems are only needed when there is a group of people living together. A hermit living in a cave on a mountain by himself does not need laws or ethical systems. Primitive societies that were composed of a small number of individuals had to have some basic laws for survival, such as not killing each other, and some basic ethical principles, such as distributive justice—for example, all members of the tribe get the same amount of food. As society increases in size and becomes more complex, there is a need for more laws and a stronger ethical system.

A System of Morals

Ethics are declarations of what is right or wrong and of what ought to be. Ethics are usually presented as systems of value behaviors and beliefs; they serve the purpose of governing conduct to ensure the protection of an individual's rights. Ethics exist on several levels, ranging from the individual or small group to the society as a whole. The concept of ethics is closely associated with the concept of morals in the development and purposes of both. In one sense, ethics can be considered a system of morals for a particular group. There are usually no systems of enforcement for those who violate ethical principles;[4] however, repeated and obvious violation of ethical precepts of a code of ethics by professionals can result in disciplinary action by the profession's licensing board.

A code of ethics is a written list of a profession's values and standards of conduct. The code of ethics provides a framework for decision-making for the profession and should be oriented toward the daily decisions made by members of the profession.

A Dilemma

An **ethical dilemma** is a situation that requires an individual to make a choice between two equally unfavorable alternatives. The basic, elemental aspects of an ethical dilemma usually involve conflict of one individual's rights with those of another, conflict of one individual's obligations with the rights of another, or combined conflict of one group's obligations and rights with those of another group.[5]

Principles in Conflict

By the very nature of an ethical dilemma, there can be no simple correct solution, and the final decision must often be defended against those who disagree with it. For example:

> A client went to surgery for a laparoscopic biopsy of an abdominal mass. After the laparoscope was inserted, the physician noted that the mass had metastasized to the liver, pancreas, and colon, and even before the results of the tissue biopsy returned from the laboratory, the physician diagnosed metastatic cancer with a poor prognosis. When the client was returned to his room, the physician told the nurses about the diagnosis but warned them that under no circumstances were they to tell the client about the cancer.
>
> When the client awoke, the first question he asked the nurses was, "Do I have cancer?" This posed an ethical dilemma for the nurses. If they were to tell the client the truth, they would violate the principle of fidelity to the physician. If they lie to the client, they would violate the principle of veracity.

KEY CONCEPTS IN ETHICS

In addition to the terminology used in the study and practice of ethics, several important principles often underlie ethical dilemmas. These principles include autonomy, justice, fidelity, beneficence, nonmaleficence, veracity, standard of best interest, and obligations.

Autonomy

Autonomy is the right of self-determination, independence, and freedom. It refers to the client's right to make health-care decisions for himself or herself, even if the health-care provider does not agree with those decisions.

As with most rights, autonomy is not absolute, and under certain conditions, limitations can be imposed on it. Generally these limitations occur when one individual's autonomy interferes with another individual's rights, health, or well-being. For example, a client generally can use his or her right to autonomy by refusing any or all treatments. However, in the case of contagious diseases (e.g., tuberculosis) that affect society, the individual can be forced by the health-care and legal systems to take medications to cure the disease. The individual can also be forced into isolation to prevent the disease from spreading. Consider the following situation:

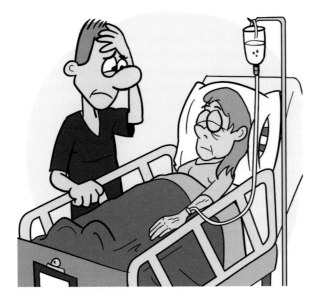

> June, who is the 28-year-old mother of two children, is brought into the emergency department (ED) after a tonic-clonic–type seizure at a shopping mall. June is known to the ED nurses because she has been treated several times for seizures after she did not take her antiseizure medications. She states that the medications make her feel "dopey" and tired all the time and that she hates the way they make her feel.
>
> Recently, June has started to drive one of her children and four other children to school in the neighborhood car pool 1 day a week. She also drives 62 miles one way on the interstate twice a week to visit her aging mother in a nursing home in a different city. The nurse who takes care of June this day in the ED knows that the state licensing laws require that an individual with uncontrolled seizures must report the fact to the Department of Motor Vehicles (DMV) and is usually ineligible for a driver's license. When the nurse mentions that she has to report the seizure, June begs her not to report it. She would have no means of taking her children to school or visiting her mother. She assures the nurse that she will take her medication no matter how it makes her feel.

The ethical issue in this case study is a conflict of rights and obligations. June has a right to autonomy to determine whether she will take her medication and whether she will self-report having seizures to the DMV. The nurse has an obligation to recognize and honor June's autonomy, but she also has an obligation to maintain public safety, including reporting June's seizures. This is a classical case of an ethical dilemma. Does June's right to autonomy supersede the nurse's obligation to public safety? Do the legal issues involved in the situation affect the ethical decision the nurse makes? How would you decide?

Justice

Justice is the obligation to be fair to all people. The concept is often expanded to what is called *distributive justice*, which states that individuals have the right to be treated equally regardless of race, gender, marital status, medical diagnosis, social standing, economic level, or religious belief. The principle of justice underlies the first statement in the American Nurses Association (ANA) Code of Ethics for Nurses (2014): "The nurse in all professional relationships practices with compassion and respect for the inherent dignity, worth, and uniqueness of each individual, unrestricted by considerations of social or economic status, personal attributes, or the nature of health problems."[4]

> " *By the very nature of an ethical dilemma, there can be no simple correct solution, and the final decision must often be defended against those who disagree with it.* "

What Do You Think?

Identify a situation in which a law is or may be unethical. Which system has higher authority? How do you resolve the conflict?

Distributive justice sometimes includes ideas such as equal access to health care for all. As with other rights, limits can be placed on justice when it interferes with the rights of others.[6] For example:

A middle-aged homeless man who was diagnosed with type 1, insulin-dependent diabetes mellitus demanded that Medicaid pay for a pancreas transplant. His health record showed that he refused to follow the prescribed diabetic regimen, drank large quantities of wine, and rarely took his insulin. The transplantation would cost $108,000, which is the total cost of immunizing all the children in a state for 1 year.

Fidelity

Fidelity is the obligation of an individual to be faithful to commitments made to himself or herself and to others. In health care, fidelity includes the professional's faithfulness or loyalty to agreements and responsibilities accepted as part of the practice of the profession. Fidelity is the main support for the concept of accountability, although conflicts in fidelity might arise from obligations owed to different individuals or groups. For example:

A nurse who is just finishing a very busy and tiring 12-hour shift may experience a conflict of fidelity when she is asked by a supervisor to work an additional shift because the hospital is short-staffed. The nurse has to weigh her fidelity to herself against fidelity to the employing institution and against fidelity to the profession and clients to do the best job possible, particularly if she feels that her fatigue would interfere with the performance of those obligations.

Beneficence

Beneficence, one of the oldest requirements for health-care providers, views the primary goal of health care as doing good for clients under their care. In general, the term *good* includes more than providing technically competent care for clients. Good care requires that the health-care provider take a holistic approach to the client, including the client's beliefs, feelings, and wishes, as well as those of the client's family and significant others. The difficulty in implementing the principle of beneficence is in determining what exactly is good for another and who can best make the decision about this good.[4]

Consider the case of the man involved in an automobile accident who ran into a metal fence pole. The pole passed through his abdomen. Even after 6 hours of surgery, the surgeon was unable to repair all the damage. The man was not expected to live for more than 12 hours. When the man came back from surgery, he had a nasogastric tube inserted, so the physician ordered that the client should have nothing by mouth (NPO) to prevent depletion of electrolytes.

Although the man was somewhat confused when he awoke postoperatively, he begged the nurse for a drink of water. He had a fever of 105.7°F. The nurse believed the physician's orders to be absolute; thus she repeatedly refused the client water. He began to yell loudly that he needed a drink of water, but the nurse still refused his requests. At one point, the nurse caught the man attempting to drink water from the ice packs that were being used to lower his fever. This continued for the full 8-hour shift until the man died. Should the nurse have given the dying man a drink of water? Why or why not? Or is it not that simple?

Again, the ethical dilemma in this situation is a conflict of rights and obligations. The client has a right to self-determination (autonomy) that would certainly include the right to have a drink of water. The nurse has an obligation of beneficence to do good for the client. She also has an obligation to carry out the physician's orders. However, is withholding water, which is an essential nutrient for life, really doing good for the client? On the other hand, she is fulfilling her obligation to follow the physician's order, which may be based on the physician's belief that withholding water is good for the client because giving it will harm him in some way or quicken his death. If the nurse believes that the physician is wrong, does her judgment supersede his?

What would you do? Is there something else the nurse could have done, such as calling the physician and asking him to change the order? Are physician's orders always absolute, even when they seem to be causing harm to the client?

Nonmaleficence

Nonmaleficence is the requirement that health-care providers do no harm to their clients, either intentionally or unintentionally. In a sense, it is the opposite side of the concept of beneficence, and it is difficult to speak of one term without referring to the other. In current health-care practice, the principle of nonmaleficence is often violated in the short term to produce a greater good in the long-term treatment of the client. For example, a client may undergo painful and debilitating surgery to remove a cancerous growth to prolong his life.[4]

By extension, the principle of nonmaleficence also requires that health-care providers protect from harm those who cannot protect themselves. This protection from harm is particularly evident in groups such as children, the mentally incompetent, the unconscious, and those who are too weak or debilitated to protect themselves. In fact, very strict regulations have developed around situations involving child abuse and the health-care provider's obligation to report suspected child abuse. (This issue is discussed in more detail in Chapter 7.)

> *Fidelity is the main support for the concept of accountability, although conflicts in fidelity might arise from obligations owed to different individuals or groups.*

Veracity

Veracity is the principle of truthfulness. It requires the health-care provider to tell the truth and not to intentionally deceive or mislead clients. As with other rights and obligations, limitations to this principle exist. The primary limitation occurs when telling the client the truth would seriously harm (principle of nonmaleficence) the client's ability to recover or would produce greater illness. Although the principle of veracity is not a law, it is one of the basic foundations for the trusting relationship between nurse and client that underlies any successful therapeutic relationship.

A Right to Know

Health-care providers often feel uncomfortable giving a client bad news, and they hesitate to give clients difficult information regarding their condition. But feeling uncomfortable is not a good enough reason to avoid telling clients the truth about their diagnosis, treatments, or prognosis. Although veracity is an obligation for nurses, it is a right of clients to know the information about their conditions.

One common situation in which veracity is violated is in the use of placebo medications. At some point during their careers, most health-care providers will observe the placebo effect among some clients. Sometimes, when a client is given a gel capsule filled with sugar powder and it seems to relieve the pain, the placebo has the same effect as a narcotic, but without the side effects or potential for addiction. Of course, if the client is told that it was just a sugar pill (veracity), it would not have the same effect. How should nurses feel about this practice?

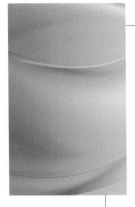

Issues in Practice

A Question of Distributive Justice

Jessica B was diagnosed with acute lymphocytic leukemia at age 4. She is now 7 years old and has been treated with chemotherapy for the past 3 years with varying degrees of success. She is currently in a state of relapse, and a bone marrow transplant seems to be the only treatment that might improve her condition and save her life. Her father is a day laborer who has no health insurance, so Jessica's health care is being paid for mainly by the Medicaid system of her small state in the Southwest.

The current cost of a bone marrow transplant at the state's central teaching hospital is $1.5 million, representing about half of the state's entire annual Medicaid budget. Although bone marrow transplants are an accepted treatment for leukemia, this therapy offers only a slim chance for a total cure of the disease. The procedure is risky, and there is a chance that it may cause death. The procedure will involve several months of post-transplant treatment and recovery in an intensive care unit far away from the family's home and will require the child to take costly antirejection medications for many years.

The family understands the risks and benefits. They ask the nurse caring for Jessica what they should do.

Questions for Thought

1. How should the nurse respond?

2. Does the nurse have any obligations toward the Medicaid system as a whole?

Costly Errors

Another issue that has come into the public eye recently is medical errors. According to an Institute of Medicine Report, the incidence of medical errors in the current health-care system is extremely high and accounts for as many as 98,000 deaths per year. Nurses are often involved in these incidents.[7] What is the nurse's ethical obligation to reveal this information? Some believe that if there is no injury to clients, the error need not be revealed; however, the reporting of errors or near errors has become a quality-control issue in the prevention of medical mistakes. (See Chapter 14 for more detail.)

Consider the following case study from the viewpoint of the principle of veracity:

Tisha S, a senior nursing student, was acting as the team leader during her final clinical experience. Jamie D, a close friend of Tisha's, was one of three junior nursing students on Tisha's team that day. Because of some personal problems, Jamie had been late and unprepared for several clinical experiences. She was informed by her instructor that she might fail unless she showed marked improvement during clinical training.

Claire B, a 64-year-old woman with diabetes and possible renal failure, was one of Jamie's clients. Mrs. B was having a 24-hour urine test to help determine her renal function. After the test was completed later that afternoon, she was to be discharged and treated through the renal clinic. Jamie understood the principles of the 24-hour urine test and realized that all the urine for the full 24 hours needed to be saved, but she became busy caring for another client and accidentally threw away the last specimen before the test ended. She took the specimen container to the laboratory anyway.

At the end of the shift, when Jamie was giving her report to Tisha, she confided that she had thrown away the last urine specimen but begged Tisha not to tell the instructor. This mistake meant that the test would have to be started over again, and Mrs. B would have to spend an extra day in the hospital. Out of friendship, Tisha agreed not to tell the instructor, rationalizing that they had collected almost all the urine and she was going to be treated for renal failure anyway. When the instructor asked Tisha for her final report for the day, she specifically asked if there had been any problems with the 24-hour urine test.

In this case, it is pretty clear that Jamie's and Tisha's obligation to veracity significantly outweighs Tisha's obligation of friendship to Jamie. The reporting of medical errors is important in identifying areas in the system that need to be corrected. In this case, the instructor should have supervised the student more closely.

> " *Using the standard of best interest requires that a good faith decision is made about what treatment(s) or actions would lead to the best results for the client after considering all the relevant information.* "

Standard of Best Interest

Originally designed as a standard of surrogate decision-making, the standard of best interest was first used by courts for making end-of-life decisions regarding incompetent clients. Using the standard of best interest requires that a good faith decision is made about what treatment(s) or actions would lead to the best results for the client after considering all the relevant information. The decision must be made in accordance with ethical and medical standards. This is generally considered a "quality of life" issue and is strongly opposed by groups who advocate for right to life at any cost.

The Client's Wishes

Standard of best interest describes a type of decision made about a client's health care when the client is unable to make the informed decision themselves. The standard of best interest is used on the basis of what health-care providers and the family decides is best for that individual. It is very important to consider the individual client's expressed wishes, either formally in a written declaration (e.g., a living will) or informally in conversation with family members.

A Designated Person

Individuals can also legally designate a specific person to make health-care decisions for them in case they become unable to make decisions for themselves. The designated person then has what is called durable power of attorney for health care (DPOAHC).[8] The Omnibus Budget Reconciliation Act (OBRA) of 1990 made it mandatory for all health-care facilities, such as hospitals, nursing homes, and home health-care agencies, to provide information to clients about the living will and DPOAHC.

In determining what is in the client's best interest, the DPOAHC, in consultation with medical professionals, should consider:

- the client's current level of physical, sensory, emotional, and cognitive abilities.
- the level of pain resulting from the client's disease process, treatments, or termination of the treatment.
- how much loss of dignity and humiliation the client will experience as a result of the illness and/or treatments.
- the client's life expectancy and chance for recovery both with and without the treatment.
- all the treatment options available to the client.
- the risks, side effects, and benefits of each of the treatment options.

The standard of best interest should be based on the principles of beneficence and non-maleficence. Unfortunately, when clients are unable to make decisions for themselves and no DPOAHC has been designated, the resolution of the dilemma can be a unilateral decision made by health-care providers. Health-care providers making a unilateral decision that disregards the client's wishes implies that the providers alone know what is best for the client; this is called *paternalism*.

Obligations

Obligations are demands made on an individual, a profession, a society, or a government to fulfill and honor the rights of others. Obligations are often divided into two categories: legal and moral.

Legal Obligations

Legal obligations are those that have become formal statements of law and are enforceable under the law. For instance, nurses have a legal obligation to provide safe and adequate care for clients assigned to them.

Issues in Practice

The nurse is caring for a critically ill client in the surgical intensive care unit (ICU) after radical neck surgery. The client is connected to a ventilator and is on a sedation protocol with continuous IV infusion of midazolam (Versed), a powerful sedative that requires constant monitoring and titration to maintain the required level of sedation. During the night shift, the nurse discovers that the medication bag is almost empty, and the pharmacy, which is closed, did not send up another bag. She looks the medication up in a drug guide and proceeds to mix the drip herself. The night charge nurse is busy supervising a cardiac arrest situation out of the ICU and is unavailable to double-check how the medication was mixed.

Inadvertently, the nurse mixes a double-strength dose of the medication. Thirty minutes after she hangs the new drip, the client's blood pressure is 44/20 mm Hg. The client requires a saline bolus and a dopamine drip to stabilize the blood pressure. The family is notified that the client has "taken a turn for the worse" and that they should come to the hospital immediately. In backtracking for the cause of the hypotension, the nurse realizes that she has mixed the sedative double strength and reduces the rate by half.

When the family arrives, the client's blood pressure has started to return to normal. They ask the nurse what happened and why their mother was on the new IV medication.

Questions for Thought

1. Should the family be told about the error?

2. Who should tell them? The nurse? The physician?

3. What approach should be used?

4. What ethical principles are involved in resolving this dilemma?

Source: Gallagher TH. Disclosing harmful medical errors to patients. *New England Journal of Medicine,* 356(26):2713–2719, 2007.

Moral Obligations

Moral obligations are those based on moral or ethical principles that are not enforceable under the law. In most states, for example, no legal obligation exists for a nurse on a vacation trip to stop and help an automobile accident victim.

Rights

Rights are generally defined as something owed to an individual according to just claims, legal guarantees, or moral and ethical principles. Although the term *right* is frequently used in both the legal and ethical systems, its meaning is often blurred in daily use. Individuals sometimes mistakenly claim things as rights that are really privileges, concessions, or freedoms. Several classification systems exist in which different types of rights are delineated. The following three types of rights include the range of definitions.

Welfare Rights

Welfare rights (also called **legal rights**) are based on a legal entitlement to some good or benefit. These rights are guaranteed by laws (e.g., the Bill of Rights of the U.S. Constitution), and violation of such rights can be punished under the legal system. For example, citizens of the United States have a right to equal access to housing regardless of race, sexual preference, or religion.

Ethical Rights

Ethical rights (also called **moral rights**) are based on a moral or ethical principle. Ethical rights usually do not need to have the power of law to be enforced. In reality, ethical rights are often privileges allotted to certain individuals or groups of individuals. Over time, popular acceptance of ethical rights can give them the force of a legal right.

An example of an ethical right in the United States is the belief in universal access to health care. In the United States, it has really been a long-standing privilege with many citizens left without health care, whereas in many other industrialized countries, such as Canada, Germany, Japan, and England, universal health care is a legal right.

Option Rights

Option rights are rights that are based on a fundamental belief in the dignity and freedom of humans. These are **basic human rights** that are particularly evident in free and democratic countries, such as the United States, and much less evident in totalitarian and restrictive societies, such as Iran. Option rights give individuals freedom of choice and the right to live their lives as they choose, but within a given set of prescribed boundaries. For example, people may wear whatever clothes they choose, as long as they wear some type of clothing in public.

ETHICS COMMITTEES

Physicians, nurses, and other staff members often encounter ethical conflicts they are unable to resolve on their own. In these cases, the interdisciplinary ethics committee can help the health-care provider resolve the dilemma. An increasing number of health-care facilities, particularly hospitals, have instituted ethics committees that make their consultation services available to health-care providers.

> *Health-care providers' making a unilateral decision that disregards the client's wishes implies that the providers alone know what is best for the client; this is called paternalism.*

The people who belong to the ethics committee vary somewhat from one institution to another, but almost all include a physician, a member of administration, a registered nurse (RN), a clergy person, a philosopher with a background in ethics, a lawyer, and a person from the community. Members of ethics committees should not have any personal agenda they are promoting and should be able to make decisions without prejudice on the basis of the situation and ethical principles.[4]

Depending on the institution, the scope of the ethics committee's duties can range widely, from very limited activity with infrequent meetings on an ad hoc basis to active promotion of ethical thinking and decision-making through educational programs. Other common functions of ethics committees include evaluating institutional policies in the light of ethical considerations, making recommendations about complex ethical issues, and providing education programs for medical and nursing schools as well as the community. It is extremely important that nurses participate in these committees and that the ethical concerns of the nurses are recognized and addressed.

Issues in Practice

When to Tell

A 48-year-old woman was scheduled for a below-the-knee amputation due to complications from diabetes. She was admitted to the preoperative area, signed a number of surgical permits, and was given her preoperative sedative medication. Because clients undergoing this type of surgery usually lose a significant amount of blood, several units of blood had been typed and cross-matched and placed on standby for her. After she was moved to the operating room and anesthetized, the nurse anesthetist rapidly administered the first unit of blood in preparation for the anticipated blood loss during surgery.

The circulating nurse was checking the paperwork before the beginning of the operation and noticed that there was no consent signed for the administration of blood products. In examining the chart further, she noted that "Jehovah's Witness" was written under the "Religion" section. The Jehovah's Witness religion does not allow blood transfusions or transplantation of any tissue or organs. The circulating nurse told the nurse anesthetist about the client's religion, and his response was, "Holy cow—I can't believe this is happening!"

The family did not know about the blood transfusion, and obviously the client, who was under anesthesia, did not know she had received a unit of blood. The nurse anesthetist announced that it was not his fault because he was never told about the client's religion and was not going to tell the family or client about the mistake. The circulating nurse felt that because she did not administer the blood, she should not be the one to inform the family. The unit manager was called in, and the consensus was that she should be the one to reveal the information because she was ultimately responsible for what occurred in the surgical unit. Her feeling was that because no physical harm was done to the client, the whole incident should just be kept quiet.

Questions for Thought

1. Using the ethical decision-making model listed, work through the decision-making process for this ethical dilemma.

2. What are the key ethical principles involved in this dilemma?

3. What are the possible solutions to the dilemma and their consequences?

4. How would you resolve the dilemma? How would you defend your decision?

ETHICAL SYSTEMS

An ethical situation exists every time a nurse interacts with a client in a health-care setting. Nurses continually make ethical decisions in their daily practice, whether or not they recognize it. These are called *normative decisions.*

Normative Ethics

Normative ethics deal with questions and dilemmas that require a choice of actions when there is a conflict of rights or obligations between the nurse and the client, the nurse and the client's family, or the nurse and the physician. In resolving these ethical questions, nurses often use just one ethical system, or they may use a combination of several ethical systems.[4]

The two systems that are most directly concerned with ethical decision-making in the health-care professions are utilitarianism and deontology. Both apply to bioethical issues: the ethics of life (or, in some cases, death).

Bioethics

Bioethics and **bioethical issues** are common terms that have become synonymous with health-care ethics and encompass not only questions concerning life and death but also questions of quality of life, life-sustaining and life-altering technologies, and biological science in general. It is in the context of bioethics that the following discussion of these two systems of ethics is undertaken.

Utilitarianism

Utilitarianism (also called **teleology,** *consequentialism,* or *situation ethics*) is referred to as the ethical system of utility. As a system of normative ethics, utilitarianism defines good as happiness or pleasure. It is associated with two underlying principles: "the greatest good for the greatest number" and "the end justifies the means." Because of these two principles, utilitarianism is sometimes subdivided into rule utilitarianism and act utilitarianism.

Rule Utilitarianism

According to rule utilitarianism, the individual draws on past experiences to formulate internal rules that are useful in determining the greatest good. With act utilitarianism, the particular situation in which a nurse finds himself or herself determines the rightness or wrongness of a particular act. In practice, the true follower of utilitarianism does not believe in the validity of any system of rules because the rules can change depending on the circumstances surrounding whatever decision needs to be made.

Act Utilitarianism

Situation ethics is probably the most publicized form of act utilitarianism. Joseph Fletcher, one of the best-known proponents of act utilitarianism, outlines a method of ethical thinking in which the situation itself determines whether the act is morally right or wrong. Fletcher views acts as good to the extent that they promote happiness and bad to the degree that they promote unhappiness. Happiness is defined as the happiness of the greatest number of people, yet the happiness of each person is to have equal weight.

Abortion, for example, is considered ethical in this system in a situation in which an unwed mother on welfare with four other children becomes pregnant with her fifth child. The greatest good and the greatest amount of happiness are produced by aborting this unwanted child.

> *Over time, popular acceptance of ethical rights can give them the force of a legal right. An example of an ethical right in the United States is the belief in universal access to health care. In the United States, it is really a long-standing privilege. . . .*

Because utilitarianism is based on the concept that moral rules should not be arbitrary but should rather serve a purpose, ethical decisions derived from a utilitarian framework weigh the effect of alternative actions that influence the overall welfare of present and future populations. As such, this system is oriented toward the good of the population in general and toward the individual in the sense that the individual participates in that population.

Advantages

The major advantage of the utilitarian system of ethical decision-making is that many individuals find it easy to use in most situations. Utilitarianism is built around an individual's need for happiness in which the individual has an immediate and vested interest. Another advantage is that utilitarianism fits well into a society that otherwise shuns rules and regulations.

A follower of utilitarianism can justify many decisions based on the happiness principle. Also, its utility orientation fits well into Western society's belief in the work ethic and a behavioristic approach to education, philosophy, and life.

Telling a Sad Truth?

The follower of utilitarianism will support a general prohibition against lying and deceiving because ultimately the results of telling the truth will lead to greater happiness than the results of lying. Yet truth telling is not an absolute requirement to the follower of utilitarianism. If telling the truth will produce widespread unhappiness for a great number of people and future generations, it would be ethically better to tell a lie that will yield more happiness than to tell a truth that will lead to greater unhappiness.

Although such behavior might appear to be unethical at first glance, the strict follower of act utilitarianism would have little difficulty in arriving at this decision as a logical conclusion of utilitarian ethical thinking.

> " *Another advantage is that utilitarianism fits well into a society that otherwise shuns rules and regulations. A follower of utilitarianism can justify many decisions based on the happiness principle.* "

Disadvantages
Who Decides?

Some serious limitations exist in using utilitarianism as a system of health-care ethics or bioethics. An immediate question is whether happiness refers to the average happiness of all or the total happiness of a few. Because individual happiness is also important, one must consider how to make decisions when the individual's happiness is in conflict with that of the larger group.

More fundamental is the question of what constitutes happiness. Similarly, what constitutes the greatest good for the greatest number? Who determines what is good in the first place? Is it society in general, the government, governmental policy, or the individual? In health-care delivery and the formulation of health-care policy, the general guiding principle often seems to be the greatest good for the greatest number. Yet where do minority groups fit into this system?

Also, the tenet that the ends justify the means has been consistently rejected as a rationale for justifying actions. It is generally unacceptable to allow any type of action as long as the final goal or purpose is good. The Nazis in the 1930s and 1940s used this aphorism to justify many actions that may be viewed by others to be considerably less than good.

What Is Good?

The other difficulty in determining what is good lies in the attempt to quantify such concepts as good, harm, benefits, and greatest. This problem becomes especially acute in regard to health-care issues that involve individuals' lives. For example, an elderly family member has been sick for a long time, and that course of illness has placed great financial hardship on the family. It would be ethical under utilitarianism to allow this client to die or even to euthanize her to relieve the financial stress created by her illness.

Utilitarianism as an ethical system in the health-care decision-making process requires use of an additional principle of distributive justice as an ultimate guiding point. Unfortunately, whenever an unchanging principle is combined with this system, it negates the basic concept of pure utilitarianism.

Pure utilitarianism, although easy to use as a decision-making system, does not work well as an ethical system for decision-making in health care because of its arbitrary, self-centered nature. In the everyday delivery of health care, utilitarianism is often combined with other types of ethical decision-making in the resolution of ethical dilemmas.[5]

Deontology

Deontology is a system of ethical decision-making based on moral rules and unchanging principles. This system is also termed the formalistic system, the principle system of ethics, or duty-based ethics. A follower of a pure form of the deontological system of ethical decision-making believes in the ethical absoluteness of principles regardless of the consequences of the decision.

The Categorical Imperative

Strict adherence to an ethical theory, in which the moral rightness or wrongness of human actions is considered separately from the consequences, is based on a fundamental principle called the *categorical imperative*. It is not the results of the act that make it right or wrong, but the principles by reason of which the act is carried out. These fundamental principles are ultimately unchanging and absolute and are derived from the universal values that underlie all major religions. Focusing on a concern for right and wrong in the moral sense is the basic premise of the system. Its goal is the survival of the species and social cooperation.

Unchanging Standards

Rule deontology is based on the belief that standards exist for the ethical choices and judgments made by individuals. These standards are fixed and do not change when the situation changes. Although the number of standards or rules is potentially unlimited, in reality—and particularly in dealing with bioethical issues—many of these principles can be grouped together into a few general principles.

> *Ethical theories do not provide recipes for resolution of ethical dilemmas. Instead, they provide a framework for decision-making that the nurse can apply to a particular ethical situation.*

These principles can also be arranged into a type of hierarchy of rules and include such maxims as the following: People should always be treated as ends and never as means; human life has value; one is always to tell the truth; above all in health care, do no harm; humans have a right to self-determination; and all people are of equal value. These principles echo such fundamental documents as the Bill of Rights and the American Hospital Association's Patient's Bill of Rights.

Advantages

The deontological system is useful in making ethical decisions in health care because it holds that an ethical judgment based on principles will be the same in a variety of given similar situations regardless of the time, location, or particular individuals involved. In addition, deontological terminology and concepts are similar to the terms and concepts used by the legal system.

The legal system emphasizes rights, duties, principles, and rules. Significant differences, however, exist between the two. Legal rights and duties are enforceable under the law, whereas ethical rights and duties are usually not. In general, ethical systems are much wider and more inclusive than the system of laws that they underlie. It is difficult to have an ethical perspective on law without having it lead to an interest in making laws that govern health care and nursing practice.

Disadvantages

The deontological system of ethical decision-making is not free from imperfection. Some of the more troubling questions include the following: What do you do when the basic guiding principles conflict with each other? What is the source of the principles? Is there ever a situation in which an exception to the rule will apply?

Although various approaches have been proposed to circumvent these limitations, it may be difficult for nurses to resolve situations in which duties and obligations conflict, particularly when the consequences of following a rule end in harm or hurt being done to a client. In reality, there are probably few pure followers of deontology, because most people will consider the consequences of their actions in the decision-making process.

APPLICATION OF ETHICAL THEORIES

Ethical theories do not provide recipes for resolution of ethical dilemmas. Instead, they provide a framework for decision-making that the nurse can apply to a particular ethical situation.

A Framework for Decisions

At times, ethical theories may seem too abstract or general to be of much use to specific ethical situations. Without them, however, ethical decisions may often be made without reasoning or forethought and may be based on emotions. Most nurses, in attempting to make ethical decisions, combine the two theories presented here.

Nursing Code of Ethics

A code of ethics is generally defined as a written statement or list of the ethical principles that govern a particular profession. Codes of ethics are presented as general statements and thus do not give specific answers to every possible ethical dilemma that might arise. However, these codes do offer guidance to the individual practitioner in making decisions.

A Lengthy Development Process

Although the term *code of ethics* is relatively new to health care, nurses have a long tradition of using ethical principles and basic values to guide the practice of the profession, starting with the writings of Florence Nightingale. Nightingale reflected the values of the society of her time and the place of women in that society. Her writings emphasize the need to follow the physician's orders and that nurses remain pure and inviolate as they carry out their duties in tending for the sick.

The history of the development of the current code of ethics is as follows:

- 1893—Nightingale Pledge: Although the Nightingale Pledge was written by Lystra E. Gretter and a committee at the Farrand Training School for Nurses in Detroit, Michigan, it was still called the *Nightingale Pledge* in recognition of the founder of modern nursing. The pledge is a statement of the ethics and principles that the nursing profession at that time held as important. It emphasizes keeping the nurse away from immoral and harmful situations and the need to seek out and treat the ill in any setting without regard for their social status (distributive justice). It also included the need to maintain confidentiality.
- 1926—The *American Journal of Nursing* (AJN), the official publication of the ANA, published a document that very much looked like a code of ethics but was not given that name. It was *not* accepted by the ANA as an official document or statement of ethics for nurses.
- 1935—The Nightingale Pledge was revised by adding a statement about nurses needing to help physicians and dedicating their lives "in service of human welfare."

- 1940—The *AJN* again published a list of statements that could be used to guide the ethical practice of nurses. Still not called a code of ethics, it was adopted by the NLN as a "statement of ethical principles."
- 1950—The ANA's statement of ethical principles began to look even more like a code of ethics, but it was still was not being called a code of ethics. Several revisions were made to include some of the rapid technological development of the postwar period.
- 1960—The statement of ethical principles was revised with an emphasis on the independence of practice for nurses. It still was not being called a code of ethics.
- 1968—The statement of ethical principles was again revised, making a distinction between public and private nursing. It still was not being called a code of ethics.
- 1985—A major revision of the statement of ethical principles was conducted to more accurately reflect the rapid growth in technology and society and to demonstrate that the profession of nursing was also growing to keep pace with the changes. It included statements about the need for all nurses to follow ethical principles, bioethical issues, and the social and international responsibilities of nurses. Although officially not called a code of ethics, many in the profession began referring to it as such and after a short time it was generally accepted as a code of ethics.
- 2001—The ANA Code of Ethics for Nurses was developed from the previous statements of ethical principles. The ANA identified it as a framework for ethical decision-making, and it included new statements on client's rights, focusing on the client's right to self-determination.
- 2011—The ANA approved the need for a new revision to be more reflective of society's changing values. A call was put out for a revision panel.
- 2014 - Revisions of the 2011 Code were accepted and it became the current code of ethics.

A Periodic Review

Ideally, codes of ethics should be reviewed periodically to reflect changes in values and technological advances in the profession and society as a whole. Although codes of ethics are not judicially enforceable as laws, consistent violations of the code of ethics by a professional in any field may indicate an unwillingness to act in a professional manner and will often result in disciplinary actions that range from reprimands and fines to suspension of licensure.

Although they are similar, there are several different codes of ethics that nurses may adopt. In the United States, the ANA Code of Ethics is the generally accepted code. After several years of work, the ANA revised the Code of Ethics in 2014 to be more reflective of the health-care challenges in the new century (Box 6.1). There is also a Canadian Nurses Association Code of Ethics.

Clearly Stated Principles

The ANA Code of Ethics has been acknowledged by other health-care professions as one of the most complete. It is sometimes used as the benchmark against which other codes of ethics are measured. Yet a careful reading of this code of ethics reveals only a set of clearly stated principles that the nurse must apply to actual clinical situations.

For example, the nurse involved in resuscitation will find no specific mention of **no-code orders** in the ANA Code of Ethics. Rather, the nurse must be able to apply general statements to the particular situation. For example:

> The nurse . . . practices with compassion and respect for the inherent dignity, worth, and uniqueness of every individual, unrestricted by considerations of social or economic status, personal attributes or the nature of health-care problems.

The nurse is responsible and accountable for individual nursing practice and determines the appropriate delegation of tasks consistent with the nurse's obligation to provide optimum patient care.

The ANA Code Revised, 2001

The 2001 Code of Ethics restates and reinforces the basic values and commitments that have been and remain essential to the profession of nursing (see Box 6.1). Traditional ethical principles such as confidentiality, veracity, justice, beneficence, and autonomy are reemphasized. The nurse is still expected to practice with cooperation, wisdom, compassion, honesty, courage, and respect for the client's privacy. However, the 2001 code, in response to changing health-care practices, defined the boundaries of duty and loyalty. Ethical challenges, such as cost containment, delegation, and information technology, require nurses to look at health care from new perspectives.

The 2001 code supported nurses in their attempts to upgrade their employment conditions and environment through measures such as collective bargaining. The 2001 code addressed and supported nurses who were involved in whistle-blowing when dealing with health-care team members who may be chemically impaired or otherwise incompetent in practice. It also supported nurses in their right to refuse to practice in treatments that violate their beliefs.[9]

The 2001 code also expanded nursing duties beyond individual nurse–client interactions. It recognized that professional nurses now work in multiple practice areas; therefore, they are responsible for developing and using their knowledge in these expanded areas through research and collaborative practice. The 2001 Code for Nurses is an important document that nurses need to be familiar with, both to help ensure ethical practice and to shape an improved future for the profession of nursing.

New Code of Ethics for Nurses

In 2011, the ANA began the process of reevaluating the 2001 Code of Ethics for Nurses. They sent an extensive survey to all ANA members to evaluate the 2001 code for relevancy and content. In 2013, they began the process of analyzing the survey information with an eye to updating the code in light of the recent sweeping changes in health care such as the Affordable Care Act and the APRN Consensus Model. Although this process took over a year, a revised ANA Code of Ethics was published in 2014. The revised code is a different type of code from those of the past. It is in electronic form and contains links embedded in the text to references, ethical situations, and other places where nurses can "click" and find additional information to help guide their ethical decision-making. Visit the ANA's website to see the revised code with interpretive statements at http://www.nursingworld.org/MainMenuCategories/EthicsStandards/CodeofEthicsforNurses/Code-of-Ethics.pdf.

THE DECISION-MAKING PROCESS

Nurses, by definition, are problem solvers, and one of the important tools that nurses use is the nursing process. The nursing process is a systematic step-by-step approach to resolving problems that deal with a client's health and well-being.

Although nurses deal with problems related to the physical or psychological needs of clients, many feel inadequate when dealing with ethical problems associated with client care. Nurses in any health-care setting can, however, develop the decision-making skills necessary to make sound

B o x   6 . 1

The American Nurses Association Code of Ethics (2001 and 2015 versions)

2001

1. The nurse in all professional relationships practices with compassion and respect for the inherent dignity, worth, and uniqueness of every individual, unrestricted by considerations of social or economic status, personal attributes, or the nature of health problems.
2. The nurse's primary commitment is to the patient, whether an individual, family, group, or community.
3. The nurse promotes, advocates for, and strives to protect the health, safety, and rights of the patient.
4. The nurse is responsible and accountable for individual nursing practice and determines the appropriate delegation of tasks consistent with the nurse's obligation to provide optimum patient care.
5. The nurse owes the same duties to self as to others, including the responsibility to preserve integrity and safety, to maintain competence, and to continue personal and professional growth.
6. The nurse participates in establishing, maintaining, and improving health-care environments and conditions of employment conducive to the provision of quality health care and consistent with the values of the profession through individual and collective action.
7. The nurse participates in the advancement of the profession through contributions to practice, education, administration, and knowledge development.
8. The nurse collaborates with other health professionals and the public in promoting community, national, and international efforts to meet health needs.
9. The profession of nursing, as represented by associations and their members, is responsible for articulating nursing values, for maintaining the integrity of the profession and its practice, and for shaping social policy.

2015

1. The nurse practices with compassion and respect for the inherent dignity, worth, and personal attributes of every person, without prejudice.
2. The nurse's primary commitment is to the patient, whether an individual, family, group, community, or population.
3. The nurse promotes, advocates for, and protects the rights, health and safety of the patient.
4. The nurse has authority, accountability, and responsibility for nursing practice, makes decisions, and takes action consistent with the obligation to provide optimal care.
5. The nurse owes the same duties to self as to others, including the responsibility to promote health and safety, preserve wholeness of character and integrity, maintain competence, and continue personal and professional growth.
6. The nurse, through individual and collective action, establishes, maintains, and improves the moral environment of the work setting and the conditions of employment, conducive to quality health care.
7. The nurse, whether in research, practice, education, or administration, contributes to the advancement of the profession through research and scholarly inquiry, professional standards development, and generation of nursing and health policies.
8. The nurse collaborates with other health professionals and the public to protect and promote human rights, health diplomacy, and health initiatives.
9. The profession of nursing, collectively through its professional organizations, must articulate nursing values, maintain the integrity of the profession, and integrate principles of social justice into nursing and health policy.

Source: Code for Nurses With Interpretive Statements. Washington, DC: American Nurses Publishing, American Nurses Foundation/American Nurses Association, 2001, p. 1, with permission.

ethical decisions if they learn and practice using an ethical decision-making process.

Modeling the Nursing Process

An ethical decision-making process provides a method for nurses to answer key questions about ethical dilemmas and to organize their thinking in a more logical and sequential manner. Although there are several ethical decision-making models, the problem-solving method presented here is based on the nursing process. It should be a relatively easy transition from the nursing process used in resolving a client's physical problems to the ethical decision-making process for the resolution of problems with ethical ramifications.

The chief goal of the ethical decision-making process is to determine right and wrong in situations in which clear demarcations are not readily apparent. This process presupposes that the nurse making the decision knows that a system of ethics exists, knows the content of that ethical system, and knows that the system applies to similar ethical decision-making problems despite multiple variables. In addition to identifying their own values, nurses need an understanding of the possible ethical systems that may be used in making decisions about ethical dilemmas.

The following ethical decision-making process is presented as a tool for resolving ethical dilemmas (Fig. 6.1).

Step 1: Collect, Analyze, and Interpret the Data

Obtain as much information as possible concerning the particular ethical dilemma. Unfortunately, such information is sometimes very limited. Among the important issues are the client's wishes, the client's family's wishes, the extent of the physical or emotional problems causing the dilemma, the physician's beliefs about health care, and the nurse's own orientation to issues concerning life and death.

What Do You Think?

Identify a health-care-related ethical situation that is currently in the news. What are the key elements of the dilemma? Discuss how to resolve it with your classmates.

Many nurses, for example, face the question of whether or not to initiate resuscitation efforts when a terminally ill client is admitted to the hospital. Physicians often leave instructions for the nursing staff indicating that the nurses should not resuscitate the client but should, instead, merely go through the motions to make the family feel better, which is sometimes referred to as a **slow-code order**.[10] The nurse's dilemma is whether to make a serious attempt to revive the client or to let the client die quietly. Important information that will help the nurse make the decision might include:

- The mental competency of the client to make a no-resuscitation decision.
- The client's desires.
- The family's feelings.
- Whether the physician previously sought input from the client and the family.
- Whether there is a living will or DPOAHC.

Many institutions have policies concerning no-resuscitation orders, and it is wise to consider these during data collection. After collecting information, the nurse needs to bring the pieces of information together in a manner that will give the clearest and sharpest focus to the dilemma.

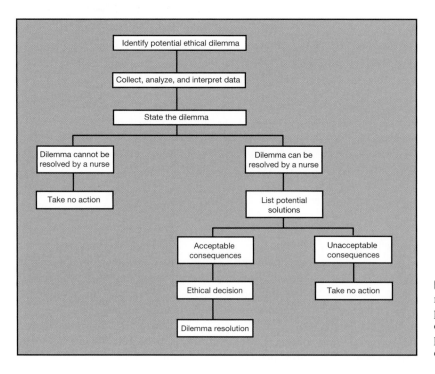

Figure 6.1 Ethical decision-making algorithm. (Adapted with permission from Catalano JT. Ethical decision making in the critical care patient. *Critical Care Nursing Clinics of North America*, 9(1):45–52, 1997.)

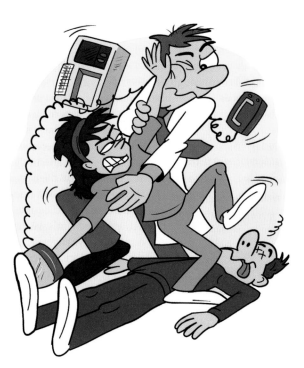

Step 2: State the Dilemma

After collecting and analyzing as much information as is available, the nurse needs to state the dilemma as clearly as possible. In this step, it is important to identify whether the problem is one that directly involves the nurse or is one that can be resolved only by the client, the client's family, the physician, or the DPOAHC.

Recognizing the key aspects of the dilemma helps focus attention on the important ethical principles. Most of the time, the dilemma can be reduced to a few statements that encompass the key ethical issues. Such ethical issues often involve a question of conflicting rights, obligations, or basic ethical principles.

In the case of a no-resuscitation order, the statement of the dilemma might be "the client's right to death with dignity versus the nurse's obligation to preserve life and do no harm." In general, the principle that the competent client's wishes must be followed is unequivocal. If the client has become unresponsive before expressing his or her wishes, the family members' input must be given serious consideration. Additional questions can arise if the family's wishes conflict with those of the client.

Step 3: Consider the Choices of Action

After stating the dilemma as clearly as possible, the next step is to attempt to list, without consideration of their consequences, all possible courses of action that can be taken to resolve the dilemma. This brainstorming activity may require input from outside sources such as colleagues, supervisors, or even experts in the ethical field. The consequences of the different actions are considered later in this chapter. Some possible courses of action for the nurse in the resuscitation scenario might include the following:

- Resuscitating the client to the nurse's fullest capabilities despite what the physician has requested
- Not resuscitating the client at all
- Only going through the motions without any real attempt to revive the client
- Seeking another assignment to avoid dealing with the situation
- Reporting the problem to a supervisor
- Attempting to clarify the question with the client
- Attempting to clarify the question with the family
- Confronting the physician about the question
- Consulting the institution's ethics committee

For nurses who are unsure about which issues can be referred to the ethics committee, the facility's policy and procedure manual can give direction.

Step 4: Analyze the Advantages and Disadvantages of Each Course of Action

Some of the courses of action developed during the previous step are more realistic than others. The identification of these actions becomes readily evident during this step in the decision-making process, when the advantages and the disadvantages of each action are considered in detail. Along with each option, the consequences of taking each course of action must be thoroughly evaluated.

Consider whether initiating a discussion might anger the physician or cause distrust of the nurse involved. Both these responses may reinforce the attitude of submission to the physician and could create difficulty in continuing to practice nursing at that institution. The same result may occur if the nurse successfully resuscitates a client despite orders to the contrary. Failure to resuscitate the client has the potential to produce a lawsuit unless a clear order for no resuscitation has been given. Presenting the situation to a supervisor may, if the supervisor supports the physician, cause the nurse to be considered a troublemaker and thus have a negative effect on future evaluations. The same process could be applied to the other courses of action.

When considering the advantages and disadvantages, the nurse should be able to narrow the realistic choices of action. Other relevant issues need to be examined when weighing the choices of action. A major factor would be choosing the appropriate code of ethics. The ANA Code of Ethics should be part of many client-care decisions affected by ethical dilemmas.

> *Recognizing the key aspects of the dilemma helps focus attention on the important ethical principles. Most of the time, the dilemma can be reduced to a few statements that encompass the key ethical issues.*

Step 5: Make the Decision and Act on It

The most difficult part of the process is actually making the decision, following through with action, and then living with the consequences. Decisions are often made with no follow-through because nurses are fearful of the consequences. By their nature, ethical dilemmas produce differences of opinion, and not everyone will be pleased with the decision.

In the attempt to solve any ethical dilemma, there will always be a question of the correct course of action. The client's wishes almost always supersede independent decisions on the part of health-care professionals. A collaborative decision made by the client, physician, nurses, and family about resuscitation is the ideal situation and tends to produce fewer complications in the long-term resolution of such questions.

Conclusion

The nursing profession has a long history of using ethical principles to guide its practice. Although society and society's values change and evolve over time, there are a number of unchanging ethical principles that nurses have been following since the development of modern nursing. These principles include maintaining confidentiality, treating the sick and injured regardless of their state in life, preventing injury, and doing good for clients. In the current era of concern for quality of care and economic responsibility in health care, nurses need to have a clear and comprehensive understanding of ethics and ethical principles. They must also know how to apply those principles to their daily professional setting so they can practice nursing ethically to the very best of their ability.

By definition, ethical dilemmas are difficult to resolve. Rarely will a nurse find ethical dilemmas covered in policy, procedure, and protocol manuals, but nurses can develop the skills necessary to make appropriate ethical decisions. The key to developing these skills is the recognition and frequent use of an ethical decision-making model and application of the appropriate ethical theories to the dilemma. As an orderly approach in solving the often disorderly aspects of ethical questions encountered in nursing practice, the decision-making model presented in this chapter can be applied to almost every type of ethical dilemma. Although each situation is different, ethical decision-making based on ethical theory can provide a potent tool for resolving dilemmas found in client-care situations.

Critical-Thinking Exercises

- Ask the facility where you work or have clinical rotations what code of ethics they use. How does that differ from the ANA Code?
- Ask your faculty what code of ethics is used for your evaluation.
- Compare and contrast ethics with laws by delineating the purposes, scopes, and methods of enforcement of each.
- Distinguish between the two types of obligations.
- Compare the three categories of rights.
- Analyze the following ethical dilemma case study using the ethical decision-making process:
    1. What are the important data in relation to this situation?
    2. State the ethical dilemma in a clear, simple statement.
    3. What are the choices of action, and how do they relate to specific ethical principles?
    4. What are the consequences of these actions?
    5. What decision can be made?

Bill L, a veteran ED nurse, called the resident physician about a client just admitted to the ED after a fall from a ladder. The client, a 52-year-old man, had been fixing his roof when the accident occurred. He had suffered a minor head injury, a twisted ankle, and a badly bruised arm. He also had a long history of asthma and heavy smoking. Not long after his admission to the ED, the client became cyanotic, dyspneic, and semiconscious. By the time the resident physician arrived, the nurse had prepared the client for endotracheal intubation and had already notified the personnel in the medical intensive care unit (MICU) that they would be receiving this client.

After a hasty evaluation of the client, the resident decided to perform an emergency tracheostomy before transporting the client to the MICU. While performing the tracheostomy, the physician severed a major blood vessel, and the client hemorrhaged profusely. After several tense minutes, the endotracheal tube was inserted, and the client was quickly transported to the MICU. The client remained cyanotic and had great difficulty breathing. Shortly after the client left the ED, the nurse realized that the oxygen tank connected to the client was empty. The client never regained consciousness and died 3 days after admission. His death was due to respiratory failure and not to the injuries sustained in the fall.

When the client's wife came to the unit to collect the deceased's belongings, the nurse was torn between telling her about the mistakes that were made in the treatment of her husband and remaining silent.

- What are the key ethical principles involved in this situation?
- Are there any statements in the ANA Code of Ethics that may help resolve this dilemma?
- What would be the consequences of informing the client's wife of the truth?
- What are the consequences of not informing her?

References

1. Park M, Kjervik D, Crandell J, Oermann MH. The relationship of ethics education to moral sensitivity and moral reasoning skills of nursing students. *Nursing Ethics,* 19(4):568–580, 2012.
2. Snellman I, Gedda KM. The value ground of nursing. *Nursing Ethics,* 19(6):714–726, 2012.
3. Park M, Kjervik D, Crandell J, Oermann MH. The relationship of ethics education to moral sensitivity and moral reasoning skills of nursing students. *Nursing Ethics,* 19(4):568–580, 2012.
4. What do I do now? Ethical dilemmas in nursing and health care. *Indiana State Nurses Association Bulletin,* 39(2):5–12, 2013.
5. Schneider DG, Ramos, FRS. Moral deliberation and nursing ethics cases: Elements of a methodological proposal. *Nursing Ethics,* 19(6):764–776, 2012.
6. Woods M. Exploring the relevance of social justice within a relational nursing ethic. *Nursing Philosophy,* 13(1):56–65, 2012.
7. Tzeng HM, Yin CY, Schneider TE. Medication error-related issues in nursing practice. *Medical-Surgical Nursing,* 22(1):13–50, 2013.
8. Nursing home admission: Daughter-in-law had no authority to sign, arbitration agreement void. *Legal Eagle Eye Newsletter for the Nursing Profession,* 21(1):3, 2013.
9. Thompson J. Getting the code of ethics off the shelf and into practice. *World Council of Enterostomal Therapists Journal,* 32(3):15–19, 2012.
10. Moulton B, King JS. Aligning ethics with medical decision-making: The quest for informed patient choice. *Journal of Law, Medicine & Ethics,* 38(1):85–97, 2010.

Bioethical Issues

7

Joseph T. Catalano

Sarah T. Catalano

Learning Objectives

After completing this chapter, the reader will be able to:

- Discuss the key ethical principles involved in:
  - Abortion
  - Genetic research
  - Fetal tissue research
  - Organ donation and transplantation
  - Use of scarce resources
  - Assisted suicide
  - AIDS
  - Children's issues
- Discuss the nurse's role in these ethical dilemmas
- Analyze and make a thoughtful ethical decision in a complex situation

THE CLIENT'S WELL-BEING

In the recent history of nursing, numerous biomedical and ethical dilemmas have arisen. Historically, nurses have been concerned with moral responsibility and ethical decision-making. The nursing code of ethics and its frequent revisions demonstrate the profession's concern with providing ethical health care.

The earliest codes of ethics made obedience to the physician the nurse's primary responsibility. Revisions of the code throughout the years have reflected changes in the values in society and the advancement of technology in health care. The 2001 Code of Ethics for nurses recognizes that the primary responsibility of the nurse is the client's well-being. This change in emphasis reflects the profession's increased self-awareness, independence, and growing accountability for its actions. Unfortunately, this new attitude has also heralded an era of increased tension, self-doubt, and ethical confusion for nurses. By examining the issues and identifying the key moral and ethical conflicts, nurses will be able to accept their moral responsibilities and make good ethical decisions.

In the course of their careers, nurses are likely to encounter any number of ethical dilemmas. Although a complete analysis of every issue is beyond the scope of this book, some of the more common situations and their important ethical features are presented as examples of ways to analyze such dilemmas and to make informed decisions. The resolution of ethical dilemmas is never an easy task, and it is likely that someone may disagree with the decision.

Abortion

Abortion is the termination of pregnancy before the fetus becomes viable. With the advances in neonatal care and technology, some babies born as early as 24 weeks can survive and eventually go home. Abortions that occur spontaneously—that is, without any outside intervention—are called *miscarriages*. When the termination of the pregnancy is intentionally caused by the mother or other persons, it is called an *induced abortion*. An elective abortion is an induced abortion that is performed when the mother, for a variety of reasons that change from case to case, no longer wishes to continue the pregnancy.

A Polarizing Issue

Few issues evoke as strong an emotional reaction as abortion. Because of its religious, ethical, social, and legal implications, the abortion issue touches everyone in one way or another. There seems to be very little middle ground. People are either strongly in favor of abortion or oppose it completely. Even in presidential elections, abortion has become a central issue, and the outcomes of some elections may very well be decided by the candidates' positions on the law that supports the practice.

What Do You Think?

Do you support or reject elective abortion? On what ethical principles do you base your belief? What advice would you give to a pregnant teenager who wanted to have an abortion?

A Matter of Convenience?

Elective abortion is the voluntary termination of a pregnancy before 24 weeks of gestation. An elective abortion may be either therapeutic or self-selected. Late-term abortion is the termination of a pregnancy after 24 weeks of gestation up to the day of delivery. A therapeutic abortion is one performed in consultation with and on the recommendation of a physician or psychiatrist, based on the conclusion that the mother's health or psychological state would be damaged otherwise.

Self-selected, or elective, abortions are those performed solely on the mother's own decision, without consultation with a physician or psychiatrist, often for economic or convenience reasons. In the case of *Roe v. Wade* in 1973, the Supreme Court changed the legal status of elective abortion in the United States, but the ethical basis and moral status of this decision remain controversial.

A careful reading of the court's decision in *Roe v. Wade* reveals that the justices made no decision about the ethics or morality of elective abortion. Rather, the court said that, according to the U.S. Constitution, all people have a right to determine what they can do with their bodies (i.e., the right to self-determination) and that such a right includes termination of a pregnancy.

> *In practice, ethical issues are always affected by the health-care provider's moral values. In the dilemma over abortion, nurses must analyze their own values and perceptions of their roles to make the best decisions.*

A Conflict of Rights?

The fundamental issues at the heart of the abortion debate center on the question of when life begins and the right of freedom of choice. Those who argue against abortion believe that life begins at the moment of conception and therefore hold that abortion is an act of killing. Proponents of abortion argue that the fetus is not really human until it reaches the point of development when it can live outside the mother's body (i.e., the age of viability, about 20 weeks). From a deontological standpoint, abortion represents a basic conflict of rights. On one hand, a woman's rights to privacy, self-determination, and freedom of choice are at issue. In the United States, these rights are fiercely held and are considered to be issues of public policy and **constitutional law.** Indeed, these rights form the basis of the *Roe v. Wade* decision.

The other side of the abortion dilemma is the fetus's right to life. In most Western civilizations, particularly those that are based on Judeo-Christian beliefs, the casual and intentional taking of a human life is strongly prohibited. Life is the most basic good because without it there can be no other rights. In general, the right to life is considered to be the most profound of the rights and is absolute in most situations.

When attempting to resolve the ethics and morality of abortion, these two conflicting rights need to be weighed against each other. Nurses are often placed in situations in which they must help clients make decisions about abortion. Just as frequently, they are asked to participate in the procedure itself.

Where Your Values Fit In

In practice, ethical issues are always affected by the health-care provider's moral values. In the dilemma over abortion, nurses must analyze their own values and perceptions of their roles to make the best decisions. As a client **advocate,** should a nurse be for or against abortion? How can a nurse avoid influencing the woman's decision about abortion? Can a nurse ethically and legally refuse to assist with abortions? Should the client's reason for wanting an abortion or her stage of pregnancy (i.e., first or second trimester, or later, requiring a partial-birth procedure) have any influence on the nurse's decision?

These questions are not easily answered, but understanding the underlying principles involved in the issue may help defuse some of the emotional impact that often surrounds this topic. As in all complicated ethical dilemmas, the nurse needs to remember that the client must receive competent, high-quality care regardless of the nurse's personal values or moral beliefs.

GENETICS AND GENETIC RESEARCH

The ability to alter genetic material to produce organisms that differ greatly from their original form has been a reality since the early 1900s. Scientific and popular literature is filled with reports of new ways to identify and change the genetic material of all types of living creatures.

The Future Is Now

Currently, genetically altered bacteria (e.g., *Escherichia coli*) are used to produce various medications, including a purer form of insulin. Genetically altered corn is now growing in very hot, dry places and is resistant to most insects. Abnormal genes that indicate individuals who are at risk for various types of cancer, Alzheimer's disease, Parkinson's disease, and Down syndrome have been identified. Recently, "artificial" bacteria have been produced in the laboratory by chemically generating DNA segments and then assembling them into larger structures. The process is called *homologous recombination* and has been used experimentally for several years to repair damaged chromosomes in yeast. Scientists view this process as the first step to understanding how life developed on earth and eventually as a way to create designer bacteria that can produce everything

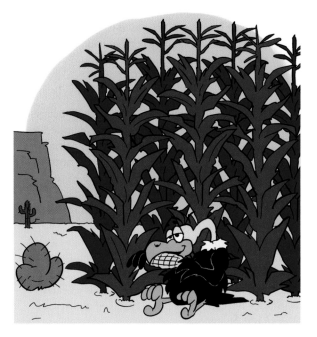

from medicines to biofuels. Detractors fear the development of bioweapons that will not have any antidotes and may spread worldwide, devastating the entire population of Earth.

In the 20th century, society became so accustomed to the idea that science should be allowed to do whatever it is capable of doing that very few questions were asked about the ethics of genetic engineering and research. As with most scientific research and techniques, the techniques of genetic engineering are ethically neutral. Procedures such as refining recombinant DNA, gene therapy, altering germ cells, and cloning other cells are neither good nor bad in themselves. However, the potential for misuse of these procedures is so great that it may permanently alter or even destroy the human species.

Ethics of Genetic Research

Several ethical issues need to be considered when genetic engineering and research are being conducted, including those involving the safety of genetic research, the legality and morality of genetic screening, and the proper use of genetic information. In 2008, the Genetic Information Nondiscrimination Act (GINA) was passed to help guide health-care workers in the use of genetic information and the protections for clients under the law. However, the law has several major limitations and does not protect all clients in all situations.[1] Other laws regulating genetic research have been proposed to prevent the production of a supervirus or superbacterium that could exterminate the entire human population.

Mandatory Screening

With current technology, it is possible to detect genetic patterns in newborn infants that are linked to breast and colon cancer, heart disease, Huntington's disease, and Parkinson's disease. Recently, home genetic testing kits that cost as little as $100 have become available. The person purchasing the kit swabs their mouth and sends in the sample. The results are returned in about 3 weeks, and all results are supposed to be confidential; however, in the age of electronic information, *confidentiality* is a nebulous term. The advantage to insurance companies, which may obtain these results or screen individuals as early as infancy for costly and potentially lethal diseases later in life, is obvious: these individuals could be excluded from health and life insurance coverage, thus saving the insurance companies a great deal of money.

What Do You Think?

Do you support genetic research? What restrictions, if any, would you place on this type of research? Are these restrictions plausible or enforceable?

Although this practice would most likely be unethical, the concept of mandatory genetic screening is not unrealistic. Because it requires just one blood sample from a person at some point during that person's life, it is possible that this type of screening could even be done without the individual's knowledge or consent.

Informed Consent

Informed consent is permission granted by a person with full knowledge of the risks and benefits of what is being done. The basic question is, Do parents violate the right of informed consent if they give permission to have gene testing performed on their newborn and have the results released to an insurance company? Do insurance companies violate informed consent if they somehow obtain the information without

the knowledge of the client? (Informed consent is discussed in detail in Chapter 8.)

Confidentiality

Similarly, confidentiality is at great risk for being violated by genetic screening. The confidentiality, trust, and fidelity that exist between the health-care provider and the client have been the basis of the therapeutic relationship since nursing began.

Sometimes individuals may be denied employment because of the results of genetic testing. In this time of the information superhighway and vast computerized databases, very little of a client's health history remains confidential.[2] Recently, various state and federal law enforcement agencies have compiled DNA databases for identifying criminals and are only a short step away from using genetic samples for disease screening and placing DNA samples in a national database.

> *The confidentiality, trust, and fidelity that exist between the health-care provider and the client have been the basis of the therapeutic relationship since nursing began.*

Emotional Impact

An important ethical implication for nurses is the emotional impact that genetic information may have on the client. Knowledge of the possible long-term outcome of one's health, particularly if that knowledge is negative, may cause a client **anxiety,** or the person may become depressed or suicidal. Nurses must further hone their teaching and counseling skills to assist clients in dealing with the implications of this type of information. Some women have opted for preventive mastectomies because genetic testing showed they had the gene for breast cancer.

Obstetric and pediatric nurses have been involved with genetic screening procedures for years. Some of the most important information obtained from amniocentesis deals with the genetic composition of the fetus. It is important that the mother understand the procedure and the type of information it may yield and that she give informed consent for this procedure. Pediatric nurse practitioners often observe abnormalities in the infant during follow-up well-child examinations that may indicate a genetic defect. These children are referred to a genetic clinic for testing.

Self-Determination

Nurses have a strict ethical obligation to refuse to participate in mandatory, involuntary screening programs and are strictly prohibited from revealing genetic test results to unauthorized individuals. Forcing testing on clients who are strongly opposed to finding out information about their genetic status is clearly a breach of those clients' right to self-determination.

However, as much as the current practice of routine screening for diseases such as tuberculosis, hepatitis, and blood lead levels promotes the general health of the population, so does the screening for genetic diseases. Clients who are strongly opposed to such genetic screening must be allowed the option to refuse it to maintain their right to self-determination.

Promise or Threat?

Now that the human genome has been decoded, a whole new world of possibilities—both positive and negative—has been opened for health-care providers. The impact of the Human Genome Project, cloning research, and other related genetic procedures is on par with the discovery of bacteria and antibiotics. The potential now exists for the cure of almost all known diseases, ranging from viral infections to cancer to the regeneration of spinal cord nerves.

On the other side of the issue, there is the potential for the development of superviruses that could wipe out our entire population. Nurses need to watch each development very closely and call their legal representatives when they believe science is moving into dangerous areas.[3]

The Genome Project was expanded in 2013 by decoding the entire genetic sequence of a great ape. The purpose is to examine the genetic structure of these animals, which is about 98 percent identical to humans, to see if there is a possibility of using animal DNA to repair or replace human DNA. Although this research is in its infancy, many believe it may hold the cure for cancer and many other diseases that currently stump scientists and health-care providers.

USE OF FETAL TISSUE

Fetal tissue research has been conducted since at least the early 1990s. Traditional fetal tissue research has been generally limited to taking living cells from an aborted fetus and transplanting them into people who have chronic or severe diseases. The procedure has been helpful to a limited extent in the treatment of Alzheimer's disease, Parkinson's disease, and spinal cord regeneration after traumatic injuries.

Growing Tissue on Demand

In the late 1990s, fetal tissue research was another hot-button issue with right-to-life proponents. Laws were passed restricting the research and then later were revised, removing most of the limitations. The fact is, fetal tissue research is a controversial initiative, which makes for passionate arguments both in favor and against.

Artificial Conception

From 1997 to 2000, the Human Genome Project added a new twist to this research. Rather than using tissue from aborted fetuses, scientists are now growing their own fetal tissue in the laboratory through **artificial insemination** and in vitro fertilization procedures. These test-tube fetuses are then dissected. Various fetal tissues are used for genetic and other types of research. The legal system became aware of the potential abuses of these procedures and has passed legislation to control their use, including limiting the age of in vitro fetuses to 6 weeks. After 6 weeks, such fetuses will have to be destroyed.

> *The potential now exists for the cure of almost all known diseases, ranging from viral infections to cancer to the regeneration of spinal cord nerves.*

Stem Cell Research

Stem cell research is a closely related issue. Stem cells are the very early cells present in the developing fetus that have not yet begun to differentiate—that is, all the cells are identical and contain all the genetic material needed to reproduce an identical individual. Stem cells can be separated and then placed in an environment where they will form more stem cells; the genetic material from the stem cell can be removed and replaced; or the genetic material can be removed, manipulated, and then replaced. Recent federal administrative acts have lifted many of the restrictions put in place by the Bush administration. However, the types of research that can be conducted are still tightly restricted. There are no restrictions on privately funded stem cell research.[4]

For a number of years, research in stem cell technology has demonstrated that umbilical cord blood contains significant levels of stem cells. Because the placenta and umbilical cord are discarded after a baby is born, this source of stem cells would seem to lack the ethical implications of in vitro fertilization and embryonic research, which require the destruction of embryos. However, several ethical questions to consider are, Who owns the placenta and umbilical cord after the baby is born? Does the mother own it? Should she receive payment for it? Is it the baby's? Or is it just considered medical waste, like a tumor that has been removed?

Like stem cells, fetal tissue is highly desirable for research and transplantation because it lacks some of the genetic material that makes more mature tissues and organs more likely to cause rejection in the host. These fetal tissues are also in a rapid growth mode and naturally develop more quickly than do tissues from other sources. Scientists involved in this research see fetal tissue as one of the most important means of curing diseases.

Adult stem cell research has yielded a new source of stem cells without the ethical issues that swirl around fetal stem cells. However, initial research results indicate that adult stem cells are useful in only a few disease processes.

The Source of the Material

Even a superficial consideration of these procedures necessarily raises many important ethical issues. The source of the research material is basic to the ethics of this type of research. In the past, much of the material came from elective abortions.

Potential for Abuse

Because of the immaturity and lack of differentiation of cells during the first trimester of pregnancy, the best fetal tissue comes from fetuses aborted during the second trimester. Most scientists agree that second-trimester fetuses have well-developed nervous, cardiovascular, gastrointestinal, and renal systems and are capable of feeling pain. Even though fetal tissue research has not led to an increase in abortions, the potential for abuse is tremendous.

Paying for Fetuses?

Another cause for concern is whether the fetal tissue research scientists are paying others for these aborted fetuses. If payment is being made for aborted fetuses, it would seem to violate both the laws that prevent payment for organs used in transplantation and the moral respect for humanity. Questions also arise concerning who is giving permission for the use of fetuses in transplantation procedures. Does anyone really own them?

In Vitro Fertilization

Another important ethical issue concerns the use of in vitro fertilization as a source for fetal tissue. Many religious groups question the morality of the procedure itself. Even if in vitro fertilization is considered ethical for procedures such as surrogate motherhood, is it ethical to create fetuses that are going to be used only for research and transplantation? From whom are the ova and sperm coming? Have these donors given permission for such use of their tissues? What about the rights of a fetus that was created in a test tube without ever having a hope of a normal life?

The Nurse's Role

The 1988 directive, which was extended indefinitely in 1990 to prevent the Department of Health and Human Services from using federal money for fetal tissue research, was amended in 2001 to allow this type of research on a very limited basis with federal funding. This regulation was reinforced by the Obama administration in 2009. Local biomedical ethical panels can make decisions about this type of research. Many of these panels, which consist mainly of research scientists, have ruled in favor of continuing research.

> *The American Academy of Pediatrics advises against private cord blood storage, unless there is a family history of specific genetic diseases.*

Nurses may have an important role to play in issues involving fetal tissue research. Although they will not likely be involved directly in research, nurses are often employed in facilities where elective abortions are performed. Nurses employed in such places must become aware of the issues involved in abortion. They also should know where the aborted fetuses are taken and how they are disposed of. Nurses should remain informed about developing procedures and techniques regarding fetal tissue research; they should support legal and ethical efforts to control its abuses.

CORD BLOOD BANKING

The potential use of the stem cells present in umbilical cord blood to treat disease has been steadily gaining public awareness and acceptance since the late 1990s.

It is worth noting that embryonic (pluripotent) stem cells come from fetal tissue, while cord blood supplies hematopoietic stem cells. These stem cells are responsible for the development of red blood cells, white blood cells, and platelets, thereby making cord blood a viable treatment option for blood and immune system diseases, cancers, and congenital defects.

Nurses caring for clients who are soon-to-be parents may encounter questions regarding cord blood banking, and it is important to remember there are two options to present to parents. Public cord blood banks will accept donations that can be used for anyone in need. For the most part, public cord blood banking is accepted by the general medical community, provided the entities involved in public cord blood banking follow the stringent guidelines set in place to allow the donated cord blood to be added to a public registry.[5–7] The National Marrow Donor Program has a list of public regional cord blood banks on their website.[8] It is important to note that most public banks do not charge processing or storage fees, and once cord blood is donated to a public bank, the family has no way to access the unit should it be needed again in the future.

Another option families have is a private cord blood bank, which can store the donated blood with a link to the donor so the unit can be accessed again if it is needed. Private banks charge processing and storage fees, as well as "biological insurance" premiums, so it is important to note that choosing to store cord blood in a private bank is a personal decision best made by both parents.[5] Additionally, many private cord blood banks use coercive marketing campaigns, designed to play on the fears of expectant parents.

Like transplantable human tissues, corneas, and bone, cord blood and cord blood banks are regulated by the Food and Drug Administration's Code of Federal Regulations under Title 21, Section 1271. All cord blood banks, both public and private, must comply with strict testing, storage, processing, and preservation guidelines.

Ethics in Cord Blood Banking

The medical community has varying opinions regarding cord blood banking; however, the general consensus is that public cord blood banking, because of its altruistic nature and low cost to the donors, is more widely accepted than private cord blood banking.[9] In fact, the American Academy of Pediatrics advises against private cord blood storage, unless there is a family history of specific genetic diseases.[6] Generally, autologous (self-to-self) transplants are discouraged because autologous cord blood samples may not be able to effectively treat some diseases. For example, if a child develops leukemia, it is possible cells containing the same defect also would be present in the autologous transplant.[10] In cases where a disease develops, the donated sample may not be enough to treat the disease. Private banks will store samples, but it is estimated that up to 75 percent of all cord blood samples do not contain enough stem cells to treat a small child.[11]

Nurses should encourage parents interested in cord blood banking to "read the fine print" before signing any contracts regarding processing and storage of their infant's cord blood. The contracts of many of the largest cord blood banks contain ambiguities that allow future uses of the cord blood that are not explicitly approved by the donor and the parents and do not provide the donors with reasonable ownership privileges.[12]

> *Transplantation centers and organizations involved in obtaining organs and tissues have developed complex procedures to cope with the ethical and legal issues involved in transplantation.*

ORGAN TRANSPLANTATION

Despite widespread public and medical acceptance of organ transplantation as a highly beneficial procedure, ethical questions still remain. Whenever a human organ is transplanted, many people are involved, including the donor, the donor's family, medical and nursing personnel, and the recipient and his or her family. Transplantation is the only health-care field in which actions taken by a group of medical professionals in one part of the country affect their counterparts in another part of the country.

Society as a whole is affected by organ transplantation, mainly because of the high cost of the procedures, which usually are covered by federal funding from taxes or reimbursement from private insurance, which in turn increases insurance premiums. Whether it occurs on a popular medically oriented television series or in a movie where organ donation is the primary focus, the general public is exposed to organ donation more frequently now than in decades past.[13] This popular exposure increases awareness of the need for organ donation and calls attention to people or groups of people who are affected by every aspect of donation and transplantation. Each one of these persons or groups has rights that may directly conflict with the rights of others.

The Good of the Donor

Currently, the three primary sources for organ and tissue donations are living related donors; living unrelated donors; and deceased donors, formerly called **cadaver donors.** Transplantation centers and organizations involved in obtaining organs and tissues have developed complex procedures to cope with the ethical and legal issues involved in transplantation. Despite these efforts, some ethical uncertainties still surround the issue of organ transplantation.

When the Donor Is a Child

Living pediatric organ donors exemplify a particularly sensitive issue. For example, when one sibling donates a kidney to another sibling, the procedure poses some serious risk for both donor and recipient. Parents are required to give consent for medical procedures for their children. By legal definition, a child younger than 18 years of age cannot give informed consent to such a procedure. However, it can be argued that ethically the donor child, as a participant, should have input in making such a decision. At what age should a child have a say in the decision? Can a child be forced, for example, to donate a kidney even if he or she refuses? (See the discussion of children's ethics later in this chapter.)

One situation that illustrates this dilemma is that of a teenage girl who developed leukemia. The only way to save her life was to find a bone marrow donor who matched her genetic type. When no donor could be found, the parents decided to have another baby in the hope that the bone marrow of the second child would match that of the first child. After the baby was born, it was found that the bone marrow did indeed match, and when the child was old enough to donate safely, the bone marrow was taken and transplanted into the older child.

Recently, a case in Pennsylvania of a 10-year-old girl with pulmonary hypertension who needed a bilateral lung transplant was being kept off the adult transplant list due to the "Under 12 Rule." This states that children under 12 years of age cannot be placed on the adult transplant list. The case was referred to a judge to decide whether the rule should be waived in this particular situation. The judge placed an injunction against the "Under 12 rule" and allowed the child to be placed on the adult transplant list. She is now on both the child and adult transplant lists. Soon after this decision, an 11-year-old child with cystic fibrosis also was allowed to waive the rule and is also on both lists.

What Do You Think?

How would you have decided this case if you were the judge? If you decided in favor of the children, where does distributive justice fit in? Should adults be allowed to be on the child lung transplant list also? Give a rationale for your decision.

> *Whenever a human organ is transplanted, many people are involved, including the donor, the donor's family, the medical and nursing personnel, and the recipient and his or her family.*

When Does Death Occur?

Despite the best efforts of the medical and legal community to establish criteria for death, some ethical questions still linger about what constitutes death. Because organs for transplantation such as the heart, lungs, and liver should ideally come from a donor whose heart is still beating, some clinicians fear that there will be a tendency for physicians to declare a person dead before death actually occurs. Many people also mistakenly believe that if they indicate they would like to be organ donors and become sick or injured and admitted to the hospital, physicians will not work as hard to "save their lives."

The most widely accepted criterion for determining death in deceased donors is death by neurological criteria, formerly called *brain death*. The definition of death by neurological criteria in conjunction with organ donation is very clear, and health-care professionals use proven procedures to test for and determine death by neurological criteria. Because death by neurological criteria is defined by the complete cessation of function of the brain stem, brain death can be declared even when an electroencephalogram (EEG) shows continued cortical brain activity. Some researchers and health-care professionals struggle with the perceived ramifications of this determination of death. Should some other criteria be examined in conjunction with the neurological criteria for death?

Since 2006, the use of organs from non-heart-beating donors, also known as donation after cardiac death (DCD), has become more readily accepted by the transplantation community as a viable alternative to narrowing the donation gap. DCD organ donation has its own set of ethical and legal considerations. Typically, only kidneys are recovered and transplanted from a DCD donor. However, progressive transplantation programs have been successfully transplanting DCD livers and lungs.

Selecting the Recipient

One of the most difficult ethical issues involved in organ transplantation is the selection of recipients. Because fewer organs are available than the numerous people who need them, the potential ethical dilemmas are great. To give some perspective of the disparity of need versus availability, as of December, 2014, 123,850 people were listed on the transplant waiting list, where as only 19,426 organ transplants were performed that same year.[14] (For more information, go to http://optn.transplant.hrsa.gov/.)

" Important criteria for ranking potential recipients include stage of disease process, length of time spent waiting, tissue and blood type compatibility, size matching, and geographic proximity to the donor. "

Legislating Donation

The Uniform Anatomical Gift Act, passed in 1968, made the donation of organs, eyes, and tissue for transplantation a legal transaction involving a prespecified recipient. Later legislation prohibited prespecification of recipients by creating a federal entity to regulate the transplantation industry and made the sale of human organs illegal. This legislation, the National Organ Transplant Act, created the United Network for Organ Sharing (UNOS) to regulate organ allocation and maintain the national organ transplant waiting list. UNOS created a database of all people wait-listed for an organ and listed potential recipients using a prioritized computerized algorithm designed to ensure each recipient will benefit the most from a transplant. Transplant professionals create match-run lists for

organ allocation based on the database and algorithm when a donor organ becomes available.

Additionally, each organ has its own requirements for allocation, and a match-run list for transplantation is generated according to the individual allocation policies for each organ. Important criteria for ranking potential recipients include stage of disease process, length of time spent waiting, tissue and blood type compatibility, size matching, and geographic proximity to the donor. The UNOS allocation policy is designed to provide organs for clients who have the greatest need as well as the best projected outcome for a successful transplantation. Despite widespread public beliefs, the amount of money a potential recipient has, or the amount of publicity generated by a recipient and his or her family, does not have any bearing on the way organs are allocated.

There are 46 states that have passed first-person consent (or donor designation) laws, which are strictly upheld by local organ recovery agencies.[15] Federal legislation known as the revised Uniform Anatomical Gift Act (UAGA) was designed to ensure the donor's wishes are honored at the time of death. This piece of legislation has created a myriad of ethical and legal issues, but all transplantation organizations agree that not accepting the donation from a medically suitable donor is a violation of this law. Additionally, failure to honor client wishes, in this case the donor's, may result in a risk management issue for the hospital in question. Recent revisions of the UAGA have strengthened the law to make the donor's wishes override all opposition and have given permission for organ procurement professionals to proceed with donation in the face of disapproving family members, many of whom threaten litigation (Box 7.1). A position paper from the National Organization for Transplant Professionals states, "From an ethical perspective, not accepting the donor's gift is a violation of their autonomy and a disregard for their wishes to help those in need."[16]

The Nurse's Responsibility

All states have passed laws requiring health-care workers to refer all potential organ donors to the local organization responsible for organ recovery. The most important function of nurses in the organ donation

B o x 7 . 1

Organ Donation

Have you ever called your hospital's attorney at 1 in the morning? I have. I also called my organization's lawyers, our medical director, and my executive director. The reason for all these early morning wake-up calls was that I had a brain-dead client on a ventilator who had declared her wish to be an organ donor on her driver's license and her heartbroken family was having none of it. They accepted her wish to be an organ donor, but they wanted the process to happen in 5 minutes. Despite what you see on television, that *never* happens in the world of organ donation. After learning that the donation would take time and that they could not override her wish, they became extremely upset and began yelling at me in the conference room of the unit. They were hostile to the hospital staff, and some family members were eventually escorted out by hospital security. Security also escorted me to my car when my shift ended at 8 a.m. because of threats made against me by the client's family.

I knew that I was doing the right thing by upholding the client's wish, but there were many times during the hours of confrontation with the family that I felt like backing down and "pulling the plug" on the whole situation. However, with every phone call I made, the answer was always the same: "Go ahead. Move forward. Proceed with the donation."

About 4 hours before taking the donor to the operating room, I called the client's family to see if they would like to return to the hospital to see her one last time before we took her away. Her husband, two sons, and one daughter returned to her bedside and said their tearful good-byes. After the surgical team took her to the operating room, I was able to have a sensible and more compassionate conversation with the family. Her husband dissolved into tears when I told him we were able to place her liver and both her kidneys. She saved three lives that day. Of course, they also had a lot of questions about her donor designation and why we had to do what we did.

This family was finally able to come to terms with the process of organ donation, and the fact that their loved one touched the lives of three others has been a great comfort to them in their grief. When I last spoke with them, they were working with an after-care specialist to facilitate a meeting with one of the kidney recipients. All because their wife and mother had a heart—on her driver's license.

Source: Sarah T. Catalano, University of New Mexico Hospital In-House Coordinator, New Mexico Donor Services.

process is to recognize and refer potential donors to the local organ procurement organization. Referral rates of potential organ donors within hospitals are tracked and reported to agencies such as the Joint Commission and the Centers for Medicare and Medicaid Services. Many nurses, particularly those who work in emergency departments and critical care units, care for clients who may potentially become organ donors. Such nurses should note that the referral of a client to the organ procurement organization for evaluation should not be viewed in any way as "giving up on the client" or "putting a nail in the coffin" for that client.

Organ donation professionals do not become involved in care of the client until after death has been declared by a physician or other designated health-care professional. Additionally, nurses should not hesitate to make a referral because of the physical or medical condition of the client. A referral is simply a notification of a client who meets or may meet

criteria for organ donation. It is up to organ recovery professionals to determine whether the client is medically suitable for donation and to facilitate the donation process.

When Should I Refer?

Although the exact requirements for referral vary by geographical service area, in general, clients meeting the following criteria should always be referred to the local organ procurement organization for evaluation for organ donation:

- Severe neurological insult or injury (i.e., hemorrhagic stroke, ruptured aneurism, head trauma such as gunshot wounds or motor vehicle accidents, and anoxic brain injury resulting from significant cardiac downtime)
- Glasgow Coma Scale score of 4 or less
- Intubated (on a ventilator) with a heartbeat
- When brain death evaluation is scheduled

• Before terminal extubation of a client meeting any of the above criteria[9]

Operating room nurses may help in surgical procedures to recover organs from a deceased donor and prepare them for transport and eventual transplantation into a recipient's body. Other nurses provide the postoperative care for clients who have received a transplant. Home health-care nurses give the follow-up care to such clients at home.

Many organ recovery agencies also train nurses to maintain the potential for organ donation in their clients and to deal with family members of potential donors in a compassionate, professional manner.

Nurses working with potential recipients should be sensitive to the potential for manipulation. Most people waiting for transplants are desperately ill or near death. They and their families can be easily manipulated or they themselves can become manipulative.

Obtain Permission Gently

On the other side, the families of potential organ donors are usually distraught about the sudden and traumatic loss of a loved one. They, too, are vulnerable to psychological manipulation. The emotionally fragile state of a trauma victim's family members predisposes them to feelings of guilt and grief. Health-care providers should avoid appealing to these emotions or becoming coercive when obtaining permission for organ donation. They are always welcome to participate in any discussion about donation with a potential donor's family. However, discussing organ, tissue, and eye donation and obtaining consent for these activities is generally best left to professionals who work exclusively for organ procurement organizations. They are specially trained, have time to spend with the families, and can make the organ donation process a positive experience for both the donor's family and the health-care professionals involved.

Nurses should avoid making statements or giving nonverbal indications of their approval or disapproval of potential recipients. Generally, neither the donor nor the family plays any part in selecting a recipient, and the identity of the recipient is carefully guarded by organ recovery professionals.

At times, organ recovery professionals can facilitate a process called *directed donation*, whereby a donor's family can indicate a particular recipient. Whether this process is successful depends on several factors, including geographical proximity, tissue and blood type compatibility, and whether the potential recipient is listed and has completed all the prerequisite tests to receive the organ. In cases in which directed donation is desired but not possible, the donated organs will be allocated according to UNOS policy.[17]

Tissue and Eye Donation

Although organ donation is done within a clinical setting, tissue and eye donation can take place in such venues as hospital morgues, funeral homes, and specialized recovery suites anywhere from 12 to 24 hours after cardiac death has occurred. Many families are approached regarding tissue and eye donation after they have left the hospital, if a death has occurred in a hospital, or on the arrival of the decedent's body at the funeral home. Recovery of donated tissue and corneas takes place in a sterile setting, and recovered tissues are often shipped to processors for storage and later dispersal.

> " *The most important function nurses perform in the organ donation process is the recognition and referral of a potential organ donor to the local organ procurement organization.* "

Tissue and eye donation differs from organ donation in several respects. First, donated human tissue is regulated by the FDA as a medical implant or device and is subject to stringent quality-control guidelines. Donated tissue undergoes rigorous testing before implantation to ensure the safety of the recipients. Tissue recovered from one cadaver can potentially be implanted in up to 2500 recipients, so testing for biohazards and infectious disease is of the utmost priority in tissue recovery and dispersal.

Second, recovered tissue typically does not have a predetermined recipient waiting on the other end for a transplant. Donated tissue, particularly bone, can be processed and stored for up to 10 years after recovery. Two exceptions to this rule are donated corneas, which can be transplanted up to 12 hours after recovery, and heart valves, particularly those recovered from children. Heart valves from pediatric donors go to pediatric recipients because heart valves must be implanted in a recipient heart of similar size.

Transplantation of Faces, Hands, and Other Body Parts

Bohdan Pomahac, MD, who has performed four face transplants at Boston's Brigham and Women's Hospital, has said, "There's [almost] nothing [about the human body] that could not be replaced by transplantation."[18] However, the question of how to maintain allocation procedures and waiting lists for less-commonly-transplanted body parts has quickly come to the forefront of national debate. Currently, waiting lists for faces, hands, feet, and possibly even a uterus or ovary are not regulated and tend to be localized. However, UNOS has agreed with federal agencies to look at new regulations for these transplantable tissues and hopes to eventually make these transplants part of the nationwide system currently in place to regulate organ and tissue transplantation. UNOS took public comment on the rules until February 14, 2013, and hopes to implement new rules later in the year.[18] At the time of publication, these rules were still in the development process.

The government regulates kidney, heart, and other organ transplants with waiting lists. What's next? Face and hand transplants. The nationwide system is intended to match and distribute body parts and donor testing to prevent deadly infections. It's a big step toward expanding access to these radical operations—especially for wounded troops returning home. More than 1,000 troops have lost an arm or leg in Afghanistan and are preparing to offer the operations.

> *Generally, neither the donor nor the family plays any part in selecting a recipient, and the identity of the recipient is carefully guarded by organ recovery professionals.*

"These body parts are starting to become more mainstream, if you will, than they were 5 or 10 years ago when they were first pioneered in this country," said Dr. James Bowman, medical director of the Health Resources and Services Administration, the government agency that regulates organ transplants.

Issues Now

Connie Culp, Recipient of First U.S. Face Transplant, Meets Donor Family

Since Connie Culp had her face torn off by a shotgun blast in 2004, she's measured her recovery with countless milestones. This weekend, Culp reached another, finally meeting the family of the donor who gave her a new face.

Culp, a 47-year-old mother and grandmother, underwent the first full face transplant surgery in the U.S. in December 2008 at the Cleveland Clinic. Before the surgery, Culp couldn't walk down the street without drawing stares, but the transplant has given her a new chance at life.

"I don't have little kids coming up saying, 'Eww, there's a monster,'" Culp said. "They think I'm amazing. I'm just normal, but we need more people like the donors to help people."

Until now, though, Culp knew little about the woman who provided her face. Doctors would tell her only the donor's age and nothing about the surviving family.

"They've never contacted me," Culp told ABC's Diane Sawyer this past August.

But two years after losing their beloved wife and mother, the family of donor Anna Kasper was finally ready to step forward. The Kasper family decided to break their silence and share their story, hoping to raise awareness for organ donation.

"My mom was my best friend," said 23-year-old daughter Becky Kasper. "You know, she did whatever she had to do to make sure we were always taken care of. . . . She taught me to be a very generous and forgiving person, just as she was."

"She was my wife. She was my friend," said Anna's husband, Ronald Kasper.

Two weeks before Christmas in 2008, Anna suffered a fatal heart attack.

"I got a call that she had fallen off the porch," said Ronald. "I thought maybe she had hurt her foot, but when I got to the hospital they explained to us that EMS was unable to resuscitate her."

"She had gone into cardiac arrest a couple of times while she was on life support," said Becky.

A day later, the family received devastating news. Though Anna's body was stable, she was brain dead. Following her wishes, Kasper's family agreed to donate her body, a decision which would help fifty strangers, including one with an unusual request: to transplant her face.

"I had never heard anything about a face transplant being done before," said Becky, "but her whole life, she always said, hell, if I can't use it and someone else can, you can take it!"

"It was the thing Anna would have wanted to do. She would've wanted to help Connie," said Ronald.

(continued)

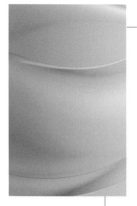

I s s u e s   N o w continued

Culp and Kasper Family Meet

Two years after the trauma of losing their loved one, the Kasper family decided that they wanted to meet Connie Culp, having seen her remarkable spirit in Culp's previous interviews.

"I just really want to hug her," said Becky, with tears in her eyes.

And though Culp felt some anxiety about finding words for a family that had given her a priceless gift, she was eager to meet the Kaspers in person.

"I don't know them, but I feel that I love them," said Culp. "To do something so wonderful for somebody. . . . What do you say? I mean, 'thank you' is not strong enough."

After waiting and wondering for so long, they finally met this weekend with tears and hugs.

"I'm so glad you did this for me," Culp told them with an emotional whisper.

And for the Kasper family comes the knowledge that despite their deep pain, there's comfort in helping someone else.

"This was the best day," said Becky. "I'm so happy I get to meet you."

At least 18 face transplants have been done around the world, starting in 2005 with a French woman mauled by her dog. The Cleveland Clinic did the first face transplant in the U.S. in 2008. The first successful hand transplant in the United States was performed in 1999, and more than three dozen have been performed worldwide.

The U.S. Department of Defense is providing money for more of these surgeries in Cleveland and Boston in hopes of helping soldiers disfigured in battle. The University of Pittsburgh, the University of California, Los Angeles, and other medical centers plan to offer face or hand transplants soon.

How do experts feel about the proposed expansion? "It's a huge step forward in the right direction. It will make it easier for programs to get started," Pomahac said.

The federal agency will accept public comments on the rules until Feb. 14 before making a final decision. The rules are expected to take effect later this year or early next year.

Sources: By Lana Zak (@LanaZak) and Bradley Blackburn. December 20, 2010. ABCNEWS.com.

Have a Heart

Since 2006, the world of organ donation has been quietly undergoing changes in functionality and technology. A movement solely focused on increasing the number of organ, tissue, and eye donors has gained significant momentum. As of 2011, 38 states, the District of Columbia, and Puerto Rico have donor registries that are classified as "effective" by UNOS. To be classified as "effective," the registries must be searchable by authorized recovery agency personnel and must ensure that donor designations are clearly documented and that the designations are legally binding.[8] In most cases, these databases are tied to the state's Department of Motor Vehicles (DMV), and the person's donor designation is indicated by a small red or pink heart or dot on the driver's license. In these states, donor designation is considered legally binding and includes consent for tissue and eye donation.

Nationally, almost 43 percent of people age 18 years and older have registered to be organ, tissue, and eye donors. These numbers vary from state to state, with Alaska and Montana topping the list at 79 percent of their populations registered as donors.[11] Although the creation of donor designation has succeeded in increasing the number of organ, tissue, and eye donors, legal and ethical considerations still arise—for example, what happens if a family objects strenuously to the donation?

The Maryland State Senate considered a law proposed in 2013 that would make presumed consent for organ donation legal with the issuance of a new driver's license. The bill, which bears the name of living kidney donor Pat Hanberry, would require those not wishing to be organ donors to "opt out" of the process, which is a reversal of the current process.[12] Maryland State Senator Ron Young has said he hopes this bill will increase the number of organ donors in the state, even though Maryland has one of the highest percentages of registered organ donors, at 46 percent.[13] Young also has garnered support for the bill in the Maryland House of Representatives. Pennsylvania passed a similar presumed consent law in 1994, and it increased the number of organs available for transplantation by 30 percent. However, several prominent religious groups are opposing this law on the grounds that it puts "man's will above God's will." This group managed to have a similar presumed consent law proposed in New York State defeated in 2010.

New experimental technologies are aimed at replacing humans as a source of organs for transplantation. In most cases, use of animal tissues and organs is not currently a viable option. The genetic protein structures of animal organs is so different from humans that the human immune system will identify them as a foreign substance and will try to destroy them (rejection) as it would a bacteria or virus. Advances in decoding and understanding the animal genome have the potential to alter animal DNA so it much more closely matches human DNA and therefore would not be rejected.

For a number of years, researchers have been "growing" human tissues and organs in the laboratory. Skin cells that are harvested from a person are placed in a special growth medium in a dish and will, within a few days or weeks, grow a new layer of skin. This process is currently being used for burn victims to grow new skin that is grafted onto third-degree burn areas of their bodies. Since the source of the skin is from the victims themselves, the DNA is a perfect match with no chance of rejection. Scientists have also been able to grow human ears on the backs of mice that were implanted with cells from a human donor ear.

The newest technology is from the world of electronics. Available on the market today, although very expensive, are 3-D printers. Also known as *additive manufacturing*, 3-D printing is a process of making a copy of a three-dimensional solid object in almost any shape or form from a digital model in a computer. In normal printing, there is just one layer of ink that is deposited on the paper. In the 3-D printing process, layers of material are laid on top of each other until a replica of the computerized shape is "printed." To print a shape, the 3-D printer reads the design from the computer and then lays down successive layers of liquid, powder, paper, or sheet material to build the form in series of cross-sectional layers. The process is being used in the architecture; construction; industrial design; and automotive, aerospace, military, and engineering industries. It has also been used to fashion jewelry, eyewear, educational material, and geographic information systems. The most common material used in the printing process is some form of plastic polymer, although other materials can be used if in the right form for the printer.

In the health-care industry, some items used in surgical procedures and dentistry are already being manufactured by the 3-D printing process. Someday soon, these 3-D printers might be able to "print" human organs that can be used in transplantation. It would require solving the problem of how to make human tissue cells acceptable to be used in the printer's layering process. One wonders if someday scientists will attempt to print an entire human being. However, once this problem is solved, there will be no more ethical or legal issue involved in obtaining organs for transplant. Or would there? (For more information on the printing of tissues and organs, go to http://www.cnn.com/2014/04/03/tech/innovation/3-d-printing-human-organs/; http://www.telegraph.co.uk/technology/news/10629531/The-next-step-3D-printing-the-human-body.html; or http://www.techtimes.com/articles/5236/20140405/3-d-3d-printed-human-organs-not-just-science-fiction.htm).

USE OF SCARCE RESOURCES IN PROLONGING LIFE

In these days of huge federal budget deficits and attempts to control them by shrinking the health-care budget, money for health care is becoming more difficult to obtain. It is recognized that most public money allocated for health care is spent during the last year of life for many elderly clients. Expensive procedures, therapies, technologies, and care are provided to terminally ill individuals to extend their lives by a few days or even a few hours. It is not unusual to spend as much as $5000 to $10,000 a day on a client receiving care in an intensive care unit.

Preserving Life at Any Cost

The traditional belief has been that life should be preserved at all costs and by any means available. Health-care providers feel uncomfortable when cost considerations are mentioned regarding treatments for terminally ill clients. Yet, in the context of current problems in society, such considerations are both economic and ethical realities. The necessity of conserving resources has forced society, through governmental action, to face this issue.

All proposed health-care plans, including the Patient Protection and Affordable Care Act and the Health Care and Education Reconciliation Act of 2010, take into consideration some type of cost-control measures related to restricting payment for client care. In addition, the **hospice care** movement and a growing number of physicians and other health-care professionals support **palliative** care for the terminally ill that provides pain relief and comfort measures but does not try to prolong the person's life.

In reality, the American health-care system has been rationing care to some degree for many years. People who are not covered by health insurance often do not seek health care. Groups such as the poor, who are covered by massive governmental programs, shy away from seeking health care because of the numerous restrictions placed on it. Individuals who are covered by insurance often have restrictions placed on them by the insurance companies.

> " *In reality, the American health-care system has been rationing care to some degree for many years.* "

The Ethics of Tube Feeding

The long-standing controversy over tube feedings periodically comes to public attention when the media become involved in cases such as those of Terri Schiavo, Karen Quinlan, and Nancy Cruzan. Tube feeding is a relatively simple procedure used in all areas of health care, from feeding premature infants in the neonatal intensive care unit to maintaining elderly postoperative clients under the supervision of home health-care staff. Additionally, it is a way of maintaining nutrition and hydration, two of the most basic needs of life. Nurses who work with terminally ill clients often believe that once a feeding tube has been inserted, it cannot be removed for any reason because that would constitute active euthanasia, or mercy killing.[19] But is that belief justified in all circumstances?

Issues in Practice

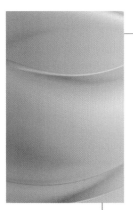

Mrs. Ada Floral, who is 82 years old, had just suffered a massive stroke that rendered her unresponsive. Her large family—consisting of her husband of many years, three sons, and two daughters—was very upset. Although she was breathing on her own, she had no voluntary movements and seemed to be completely paralyzed. Magnetic resonance imaging (MRI) showed a large area of bleeding around the midbrain and brain stem. Her pupils were constricted and unresponsive. The physician explained that the prognosis was extremely grave and that the likelihood of Mrs. Floral's survival was minimal.

However, the family members all agreed that "everything" should be done, so the physician reluctantly initiated aggressive medical therapy with intravenous (IV) glucocorticoids, osmotic diuretics, antihypertensives, and physical therapy. After a week, there was no change. The family wondered whether Mrs. Floral might be "starving to death" and asked the physician to have a feeding tube inserted and feedings started.

One month later, the still-unresponsive Mrs. Floral is being cared for at home by her family with the supervision of the local hospice and home health-care program. She is off all IV medications; however, she is receiving some medications, a commercially prepared feeding, and water through the feeding tube. Some of the family members are beginning to question whether they did the right thing by insisting that everything be done and wish to remove the feeding tube so that Mrs. Floral can die a peaceful and dignified death rather than just hanging on for months. Other family members feel that if they give permission for the tube's removal, they would be killing their mother and could not live with the guilt.

The hospice nurse in charge of the case has discussed the issue with the family. She, too, believes that once a feeding tube has been placed, it should not be removed, even if all the family agrees on its removal. She feels that it's not an issue a family can "just change their minds about." Although she is in frequent contact with Mrs. Floral's physician, she has not mentioned that the family is thinking about removing the feeding tube in fear that the physician might agree.

Questions for Thought

1. Is the hospice nurse correct in her belief about the removal of the feeding tube?

2. When do tube feedings stop being beneficial to clients?

3. What ethical rationales could be used for removing the feeding tube in this case?

4. Is there a right to death with dignity?

Should Care Be Restricted?

The use of public funds for health care is an ethical issue that revolves around the principle of distributive justice. In this context, distributive justice requires that all citizens have equal access to all types of health care, regardless of their income levels, race, gender, religious beliefs, or diagnosis. Many complex issues are involved in this dilemma.

These issues go far beyond the questions of who gets what type of care and where and how the care takes place. Although **universal health-care coverage** was not mandated for all Americans by the passage of the Health Care Reform Act, coverage has been expanded significantly. Is it fair that some individuals (taxpayers) pay for the health care of others? Should individuals who contribute to their own poor state of health by smoking, drinking, taking illicit drugs, or overeating be provided with the same type of care as those who do not put themselves at risk? Who is going to make the decisions about who gets expensive treatment such as organ transplantations, experimental medications, placement in intensive care units, or life-extending technologies?

The use of criteria such as age, potential for a high-quality life, and availability of resources for determining who receives life-extending technologies is gaining wider acceptance, but is this a valid ethical position? Nurses are often involved in situations in which terminally ill clients are brought to the hospital for end-of-life care. Nurses need to play an active role in helping formulate policies concerning the issues they face daily.

> " *The use of criteria such as age, potential for a high-quality life, and availability of resources for determining who receives life-extending technologies is gaining wider acceptance, but is this a valid ethical position?* "

What Do You Think?

Do all U.S. citizens have a right to health care? How can that be achieved? Discuss your rationale for your position.

THE RIGHT TO DIE

The right-to-die issue is an extension of the right to self-determination issue discussed in Chapter 8. It also overlaps with the dilemma of **euthanasia** and assisted suicide. Health-care providers often become involved in the decision-making process when clients are irreversibly comatose, vegetative, or suffering from a terminal disease. The choices that the families of such clients often face are either death or the extension of life using painful and expensive treatments.[20]

What Is Extraordinary?

One of the difficulties in resolving right-to-die issues is understanding the terminology used. Often clients who have living wills state that they want no extraordinary treatments if they should become comatose or unable to make decisions involving health care. But what constitutes extraordinary treatments? A general definition of ordinary treatments includes any medications, procedures, surgeries, or technologies that offer the client some hope of benefit without causing excessive pain or suffering.

By this definition, extraordinary treatments (sometimes called *heroic measures*) are those treatments, medications, surgeries, and technologies that offer little hope for curing or improving the client's condition. Although these general definitions provide some guidelines for making decisions about ordinary and extraordinary treatments, discerning the nature of the specific modalities remains difficult.

Ventilation

For example, a ventilator is a machine that assists a client's breathing. In intensive care units (ICUs), it is a common mode of treatment for many types of clients, including postoperative clients, clients with cardiac and respiratory diseases, and victims of trauma. Does its widespread and frequent use make the ventilator an ordinary mode of treatment? Many would say yes, whereas others would say it is still extraordinary because of its invasive nature and complicated technology.

Cardiopulmonary Resuscitation

Another issue often included in the right-to-die debate is that of codes and "do not resuscitate" (DNR) orders. Cardiopulmonary resuscitation (CPR) is widely taught to both health-care providers and the general public. It is often used to treat clients who have suffered heart attacks and gone into cardiac arrest, as well as clients suffering from electrical shock, drowning, and traumatic injuries.

In the hospital setting, the nursing staff is obligated to perform CPR on all clients who do not have a specific DNR order. This leads to situations in which terminally ill clients may be subjected to CPR efforts several times before it no longer is effective and they die.

Advance Directives

As an issue of self-determination, it is essential that the client's wishes about health care be followed. All client communication to the nurse about desires for future care should be documented. If at all possible, the client should be encouraged to designate an individual to act as a moral surrogate—a designated decision-maker—should the client become unable to make his or her own decisions. The expressed desires about future medical care are known as *advance directives*. They are the best means to guarantee that a client's wishes will be honored.

A Formal Document

Advance directives, in the form of a living will or durable power of attorney for health care, can and should specify which extraordinary procedures, surgeries, medications, or treatments can or cannot be used. These directives are often formal documents that need to be witnessed by two individuals who are not related to the client (Box 7.2). Living wills are also known as *personal directives* or *advance decisions*.

As useful as advance directives are in helping the client decide on future care, clients often are unable to anticipate all the possible types of treatments used. For example, an elderly client with a long history of cardiovascular disease specified in his living will that he did not want CPR performed and did not want a ventilator. When his heart developed a potentially lethal dysrhythmia that rendered him unresponsive, his physician decided to use electrical cardioversion because this mode of treatment was not specifically forbidden by the client's living will. Strictly speaking, the physician did not violate the letter of the living will, but did he violate its spirit? Similarly, would the administration of a potent and potentially dangerous IV antidysrhythmic medication be in violation of the client's living will?

Box 7.2

Checklist for Evaluating a Client's Living Will Document

1. Statement of intention: the document was written freely when the client was competent.
2. Statement of when the document goes into effect: usually when the client is no longer able to make decisions for himself or herself.
3. Section specifying general health-care measures to be excluded from care.
4. Open section for specific measures (e.g., ventilators, pacemakers, etc.) and any other specific instructions concerning care.
5. Proxy statement (sometimes called *durable power of attorney*): optional, but a strong addition. Allows another person to make decisions in situations not anticipated in the living will. (Check your state law concerning details of proxy selection.)
6. Substitute proxy: optional. Specifies who can make decisions if first-choice proxy is not available.
7. Legal statement that the proxy(s) may make decisions.
8. Witness selection statement. Many states require that witnesses not be related to or members of the health-care team.
9. Signature and date. Document must be signed and dated by the client. Some states have very specific regulations concerning how long the will is valid. It may range from a few months to 5 years.
10. Legal signatures of witnesses (required).
11. Notary seal, if required by state law. State laws differ on notary seal requirement. It is usually required if a proxy is selected.

A Legal Requirement

Advance directives, which include living wills, are now a required part of the health care of all clients. The Omnibus Budget Reconciliation Act of 1990 requires that all hospitals, nursing-care facilities, home health-care agencies, and caregivers ask clients about advance directives and provide information concerning living wills and durable power of attorney for health care (DPOAHC) to help clients make informed health-care decisions. However, the federal law mandates only the requirements and not the directives to implement the law. The actual implementation of the law is left to the individual states. Because of the law's vagueness, a great deal of confusion exists, particularly with regard to living wills.

Nurses play an important role in ensuring that clients understand the implications of their choices pertaining to decisions that may prolong their lives during medical emergencies. Because of their "frontline" position as caregivers within the health-care system, nurses must understand this role, specifically as it pertains to living wills.

Ethical Difficulties of Living Wills

In 2009, Barack Obama became the first U.S. president to announce publicly that he had a living will, and he encouraged others to obtain their own living wills. His announcement followed the misunderstood issue in the Affordable Care Act (ACA) that proposed reimbursement for physician time spent in talking to clients about advanced directives. (See Chapter 19 for more detail.)

What Did the Client Know?

Although a living will seems a simple solution to a complex care situation, there are some ethical difficulties inherent in its use about which nurses need to know. Primary among these ethical difficulties is the question of the person's level of knowledge of potential and future health-care problems at the time the will was formulated. Because living wills are often formulated long before they are to be used, there may later be serious questions about how informed the person was about the disease states and treatment modalities that might later affect care. If there is any indication that the person did not understand the full

implications of future therapies or potential medical problems, the validity of the living will is in question.

Additionally, living wills reflect a client's condition at a particular time during his or her life. Almost everyone knows or has heard about a person who was at "death's doorstep" and yet survived and later was living a normal life. As life situations change, living wills need to be updated to ensure that the actions taken by health-care providers are the actions the client really wishes.

A Moral Conflict

A second ethical difficulty for nurses encompasses the principles of beneficence and nonmaleficence. The principle of beneficence states that a health-care professional's primary duty is to benefit or do good for the client. The principle of nonmaleficence states that health-care providers should protect the client from harm. It is sometimes difficult to determine whether the primary duty is to produce benefit or prevent harm.

Generally, most health-care providers think that the duty to avoid harming the client outweighs the concerns for providing benefit. When evaluated from the beneficence and nonmaleficence viewpoints, living wills seem to violate the principle of providing benefit to the client. This perception makes many health-care providers ethically uncomfortable. In some situations, the implementation of a living will might actually involve the termination of some modes of treatments already in use. Termination of treatments would seem to constitute harm to the client.

In either case, respecting a living will might often appear to health-care providers to be a violation of their duty to help clients and preserve life. Nurses, as well as other health-care providers, often experience a sense of frustration when they are not allowed to use all the skills they have learned to preserve life.

Lack of Clarity

A third difficulty nurses and other health-care workers may have with living wills is their formulation and legal enforcement. In general, the language used in the standard living will document is broad and vague. Living wills are often not specific enough to include all the forms of treatments that are possible for the many types of illnesses that might render a person

> *The expressed desires about future medical care are known as advance directives. They are the best means to guarantee that a client's wishes will be honored.*

incompetent to make decisions. Health-care providers may have little direction as to the care they are to give if the circumstances at the time the living will was formulated are significantly different from the declared wishes of the client.

Furthermore, unless the particular state has enacted into law a special type of living will called a *natural death act*, the living will has no mechanism of legal enforcement. Also, when a client travels from one state to another, the legal effect of the living will may be in question. Does the nonresident state have an obligation to honor it?

In some states, a living will is considered only advisory, and the physician has the right to comply with the living will or treat the client as the physician deems most appropriate. There is no protection for nurses or other health-care practitioners against criminal or civil liability in the execution of living wills in states without a natural death act. Once a valid living will exists, it only becomes effective when the person who formulated it meets the qualifications for the natural death act. In most states, the individual must be diagnosed as having a terminal condition in which the continuation of treatment and life support would only prolong the client's dying process, but there is no clear consensus on the definition of *terminal condition*.

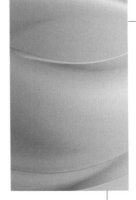

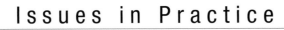

In the current health-care environment, nurses may encounter elderly clients who function independently at home and have not officially or legally been declared incompetent but whose behavior might indicate that they are unable to make rational decisions about their care. Consider the following situation:

A 74-year-old client, Buster Mack, had been a long-haul truck driver for most of his life and was still driving his big rig into his 60s. He had been in relatively good health until 5 years earlier, when he was diagnosed with lung cancer. A lobectomy was performed at that time, and he was treated with follow-up radiation and chemotherapy, but the cancer had slowly metastasized to the bone. His current hospitalization was because of a syncopal episode witnessed by a neighbor in the front yard of Mr. Mack's home, where he lives by himself.

During the admission assessment, the nurse observed that Mr. Mack had trouble focusing on the questions, and often the answer was unrelated to the question or in the form of a long rambling account of something that happened many years ago. Although he knew he was in a hospital (he could not remember the name), he had no idea where it was or what the date was. His demeanor was cooperative and pleasant, and he laughed easily when the nurse joked with him. He could not remember whether he had any family left living, although the name and address of a son in a distant city were listed on the old records.

Mr. Mack signed all the admission papers and consent forms placed in front of him for a number of neurological tests. His physician was fearful that the cancer might have spread to his brain and wanted to do an MRI, spinal tap, and brain scan. The MRI and brain scan showed a small tumor in an area of the brain where it could be removed rather easily. Mr. Mack's physician, in consultation with a neurosurgeon, felt that an immediate craniotomy with removal of the tumor was required. After explaining the procedure to Mr. Mack, the physicians placed the consent-to-operate form on his over-the-bed table and gave him a pen. He promptly signed and gave it back.

Later on that day during her shift assessment, the nurse checked on Mr. Mack. The neighbor who had found him unconscious was visiting at the time. When the nurse asked Mr. Mack whether he was ready for the surgery scheduled for the next morning, he had a blank look on his face. On further questioning, the nurse concluded that Mr. Mack had no idea what was going to happen to him the next day. The neighbor, who helped Mr. Mack with his bills and other paperwork at home, stated, "He'll pretty much sign anything that you put in front of him." At this point the nurse felt that Mr. Mack was incapable of making an informed decision about the craniotomy.

The nurse called both the primary physician and the neurosurgeon about her observations. She was told bluntly that the consent had been signed and that they were going to operate on Mr. Mack the next day for his own good. If she wanted what was best for the client, she would just drop the issue.

Questions for Thought

1. Should the nurse just drop the issue?

2. Is there anything she could do to resolve the problem?

3. What ethical principles are involved with this situation?

A Guide for the Care Provider

Despite all these difficulties, living wills are still a good way for a client to make health-care wishes known to providers. Documents that are specific about treatment modalities, that are written in a "legal" format, and that are signed by two or more witnesses tend to be treated with an increased level of respect by health-care providers. Because the laws on advance directives vary widely from state to state, there is no standard advance directive whose language conforms exactly with all states' laws. It is easy to download any particular state's form by going to the National Hospice and Palliative Care Organization's website at http://www.caringinfo.org/i4a/pages/index.cfm?pageid=3289 or the Partnership for Caring website at http://www.partnershipforcaring.org.

Nurses can help clients plan ahead for their care should they become unable to make decisions for themselves. Although the nurse should not make the decisions for the client, the nurse can provide important information about the various treatment modalities that the client is considering. The nurse also can help clients clarify their wishes and guide them through the process of formulating an advance directive (Fig. 7.1).

> " *Although the term euthanasia simply means a 'good' or peaceful death, it has taken on the connotation of some type of action that produces death.* "

EUTHANASIA AND ASSISTED SUICIDE

Although the term *euthanasia* simply means a "good" or peaceful death, it has taken on the connotation of some type of action that produces death. A distinction needs to be made between passive and active euthanasia. Passive euthanasia usually refers to the practice of allowing an individual to die without any extraordinary intervention. This umbrella definition includes practices such as DNR orders, living wills, and withdrawal of ventilators or other life support.

Active Euthanasia

Active euthanasia usually describes the practice of hastening an individual's death through some act or procedure. This practice is also sometimes referred to as *mercy killing* and takes many forms, ranging from use of large amounts of pain medication for terminal cancer clients to use of poison, a gun, or a knife to end a person's life.

The Case of Dr. Kevorkian

Assisted suicide—brought to public attention by Dr. Jack Kevorkian, a Michigan physician who publicly practiced it for many years—can be considered a type of active euthanasia or mercy killing. The central issue that Dr. Kevorkian demonstrated was whether it is ever ethically and legally permissible for health-care personnel to assist in taking a life. In most states, the practice is illegal. The legal definition of homicide—bringing about a person's death or assisting in doing so—seems to fit the act of assisted suicide. In the past, there has been a great deal of hesitation on the part of the legal system to prosecute persons who are involved in assisted suicide and on the part of juries to convict physicians who participate in the activity.

A Killing on TV

In the fall of 1998, Dr. Kevorkian raised the legal and ethical stakes. On a nationally broadcast network news show, *60 Minutes,* he not only admitted to administering a lethal medication to a client without the client's assistance, but he also played a videotape that showed the whole episode.

The client, who had Lou Gehrig's disease (amyotrophic lateral sclerosis), had requested that Dr. Kevorkian help him end his life. The client had signed a **consent** form and release and was even given an extra 2 weeks to "think about it." The client waited for only 3 days before making his final request for the lethal medication.

Under Michigan law, Dr. Kevorkian could have been charged with **manslaughter** or even first-degree murder. Dr. Kevorkian admitted that his **motivation** for the act was to be tried under these laws as a test case for active euthanasia. He was arrested 2 weeks after the tape was broadcast, on a charge of first-degree murder. However, he believed that a jury would never convict him. The jury found him guilty of second-degree murder, and he served 10 years of a 25-years-to-life prison term. He was released on probation in 2007 and died on June 3, 2011. This verdict reinforced the belief of most health-care professionals that mercy killing or assisted suicide is always ethically wrong.

The unfortunate fallout from Dr. Kevorkian's conviction is that many physicians have become even

INSTRUCTIONS	**PENNSYLVANIA DECLARATION**
PRINT YOUR NAME	I, _____, being of sound mind, willfully and voluntarily make this declaration to be followed if I become incompetent. This declaration reflects my firm and settled commitment to refuse life-sustaining treatment under the circumstances indicated below. I direct my attending physician to withhold or withdraw life-sustaining treatment that serves only to prolong the process of my dying, if I should be in a terminal condition or in a state of permanent unconsciousness. I direct that treatment be limited to measures to keep me comfortable and to relieve pain, including any pain that might occur by withholding or withdrawing life-sustaining treatment.

CHECK THE OPTIONS WHICH REFLECT YOUR WISHES	In addition, if I am in the condition described above, I feel especially strongly about the following forms of treatment:
	    I ( ) do ( ) do not want cardiac resuscitation.
	    I ( ) do ( ) do not want mechanical respiration.
	    I ( ) do ( ) do not want tube feeding or any other artificial or invasive form of nutrition (food) or hydration (water).
	    I ( ) do ( ) do not want blood or blood products.
	    I ( ) do ( ) do not want any form of surgery or invasive diagnostic tests.
	    I ( ) do ( ) do not want kidney dialysis.
	    I ( ) do ( ) do not want antibiotics.
	
	I realize that if I do not specifically indicate my preference regarding any of the forms of treatment listed above, I may receive that form of treatment.

ADD PERSONAL INSTRUCTIONS (IF ANY)	Other instructions:
© 2000 PARTNERSHIP FOR CARING, INC.	

Figure 4.1 Sample advance directive. Because the laws on advance directives vary widely from state to state, there is no standard advance directive whose language conforms exactly with all states' laws. (Reprinted with permission of Partnership for Caring, formerly Choice in Dying, 200 Varick Street, New York. For more information, visit http://www.partnershipforcaring.org.)

more reluctant to write DNR orders or comply with clients' or families' wishes to allow clients to be removed from life support. Clearly they do not understand the distinctions between active and passive euthanasia.

An Issue of Self-Determination

The fundamental ethical issue in these situations is the right to self-determination. In almost every other health-care situation, a client who is mentally competent can make decisions about what care to accept and what care to refuse. Yet, when it comes to the termination of life, this right becomes controversial.

A Last Act of Control?

Supporters of the practice of assisted suicide believe that the right to self-determination remains intact, even with regard to the decision to end one's life. It is the last act of a very sick individual to control his or her own fate. Many believe that medical personnel should be allowed to assist clients in this procedure, just as they are allowed to assist clients in other medical and nursing procedures.

An Unacceptable Practice?

Those who oppose assisted suicide find these arguments unconvincing. Legally, ethically, and morally, suicide in U.S. society has never been an accepted practice. Health-care staff goes to great lengths to prevent suicidal clients from injuring themselves. In addition, individuals in the terminal stages of a disease, who are overwhelmed by pain and depressed by the thought of prolonged suffering, might not be able to think clearly enough to give informed consent for assisted suicide. Also, because the termination of life is final, it does not allow for spontaneous cures or for the development of new treatments or medications.

Nonmaleficence is the term that describes the obligation to do no harm to clients. Whether assisting in or causing the death of a client violates this principle is most likely to be an issue that will continue to be debated for some time. Several states have passed laws permitting assisted suicide, but these states have very strict guidelines. The American Nurses Association (ANA) and other nurses' organizations oppose assisted suicide as a policy and believe that nurses who participate in it are violating the code of ethics. For similar reasons, the ANA opposes nurses participating in executions of convicted criminals.

> *The central issue that Dr. Kevorkian demonstrated was whether it is ever ethically permissible for health-care personnel to assist in taking a life.*

HIV AND AIDS

After several years of decrease, the number of HIV and AIDS cases has begun to rise again in the United States despite educational efforts on its prevention and spread. The Centers for Disease Control and Prevention (CDC) reports that the incidence of HIV infection rose from 56 percent in 2008 to 66 percent in 2011 in homosexual men. In the United States, more than 1.1 million people were HIV positive in 2010. The southern region of the United States has the highest incidence of HIV infection, with a rate of 20 percent per 100,000 people. The national average is 10.8 percent per 100,000 people. Several Asian

countries are also seeing a recent dramatic increase in cases of HIV/AIDS. In some parts of Africa, it is estimated that as much as 60 percent of the entire population is infected with the virus.

An Emotional Issue

HIV and AIDS have evoked strong emotions both in the public and in the medical community. Nurses, who for years held strongly to the ethical principle that all clients, regardless of race, gender, religion, age, or disease process, should be cared for equally, are questioning their obligation to take care of clients who have AIDS.

The Right to Privacy

Several ethical issues underlie the HIV/AIDS controversy. One of the most important is the right to privacy. Although there is a general requirement to report infection with HIV/AIDS to the CDC, many states have strict laws regarding the confidentiality of the diagnosis. Unauthorized revelation of the diagnosis of HIV/AIDS brings the possibility of a lawsuit against the health-care provider or institution. However, the right to privacy is not absolute. Diseases such as tuberculosis, gonorrhea, syphilis, and hepatitis, which are highly contagious and sometimes fatal, must be reported to public health officials.

If the right to privacy can be violated when the public welfare is at stake, does HIV/AIDS represent this type of threat? Is it unjust to ask health-care providers to care for clients with this disease without knowing that the client has it? Is it just to violate a client's privacy when the disease carries with it a potential for social stigma and isolation? Does the client have a right to know that a health-care provider is infected with HIV/AIDS?

The Right to Care

Another important ethical issue is the right to care. Can a nurse refuse to care for a client with HIV/AIDS? Obviously, a fundamental right of a client is to receive care, and a fundamental obligation of a nurse is to provide it.

The Nurse's Own Interest

The first statement of the 2014 ANA Code of Ethics for Nurses is that a nurse must provide care unrestricted by any considerations, including the "nature of the health problems." Most acute care facilities will make some exceptions for the treatment of clients with HIV/AIDS; for example, if the nurse is pregnant, is receiving chemotherapy, or has had other immunity problems. In most situations, however, the nurse is obligated to provide the best nursing care possible for all clients, including those with HIV/AIDS.

> *In most situations, however, the nurse is obligated to provide the best nursing care possible for all clients, including those with HIV/AIDS.*

What Cost to Society?

What about the tremendous cost involved in treating individuals who have HIV/AIDS? The medical cost of treating a client with HIV/AIDS from the time of diagnosis to the time of death can run into millions of dollars. In the face of this crisis, governmental agencies, which bear the brunt of paying for HIV/AIDS treatment, will have to make some difficult decisions concerning this issue. With more than 1 million U.S. citizens already infected with this disease, the cost to American society is becoming astronomical.

Nurses have the obligation to care for all clients, including those with HIV/AIDS, but should physicians, hospitals, or governmental agencies also be held to this same precept? Should our society regard health care as a right or a privilege?

Issues in Practice

Nurses Legally Protected for Reporting Child Abuse

A newborn was admitted to the nursery with signs of drug withdrawal and tested positive for cocaine, although the mother denied using the drug before delivery. Hospital personnel are required by law to report suspected child abuse, and illegal drugs in the circulatory system of a newborn are one of the indicators for mandatory reporting. On the basis of this finding, the nurses in the newborn nursery filed a report with the local Child Protective Services (CPS), which investigated the case.

CPS removed the child from the home shortly after discharge from the hospital. The mother went to court a few days after the child was removed to plead her case before a family court judge. The judge upheld the decision to remove the child. The mother then became even more irate, still insisting she had not used cocaine, and filed a lawsuit against the hospital, the physicians, the nurses, and CPS. She cited that these entities were conspiring to keep her from exercising her constitutional rights.

Over the past decade, courts have been recognizing the integrity of the family and are beginning to make rulings that support it as a constitutional right. Because of this trend, the mother's lawyer felt that the case had merit and might result in a ruling in her favor with a large punitive settlement.

Looking at all the evidence, the higher court decided that there had been no attempt on the part of the hospital and staff to deprive the mother of her constitutional rights—the mother had been given the opportunity to plead in a lower court shortly after the child's removal from the home. The court upheld the nurses' requirement to report suspected child abuse and their immunity from civil lawsuits for carrying out their obligations in good faith.

Questions for Thought

1. Did the court violate the mother's rights? If they did, why do you feel that way?

2. How do you feel about laws that require the mandatory removal of the infant from the mother when the infant tests positive for an illegal drug? Is there any alternative way to address this situation?

3. Common law seems to be moving in the direction of "giving the child back." Do you think this trend is moving in the right direction? Why?

Source: Stewart v. Jackson County, 2009 WL 2922940 S.D. Miss., September 8, 2009.

ETHICS INVOLVING CHILDREN

Although children are universally acknowledged as the hope of the future, many children remain poorly fed, inadequately clothed, in substandard housing, and educated below the minimal standard. They are in dire need of all types of health care, even in affluent countries such as the United States. In the past few years, there has been a marked increase in the reporting of incidents of child neglect and abuse by parents.

The Power of Parents

Our society generally acknowledges the tremendous decision-making power that parents have on behalf of their children; however, there are limits to how parents may decide to act. These limits are sometimes obvious, as in cases of physical abuse and cruelty to children; however, they may also be less conspicuous, such as in cases of neglect or decisions about withholding medical care for religious reasons. Health-care professionals often find themselves trying to make decisions about the appropriateness of a parent's actions toward a child.

The legal and ethical factors surrounding the decisions that health-care providers must make about child health issues are complicated and sometimes contradictory, ranging from laws about reporting suspected abuse to obtaining permission for treatment. This section focuses on child abuse and the ethical issues that it creates for nurses and on the issues of informed consent as it pertains to children.

Issues involving children have always been an important consideration in our society. Whereas the political attention seems to focus on education, drug and alcohol abuse, and child health-care issues, ethical concerns in **pediatrics** are never forgotten and often serve as the unspoken basis for the more visible issues.

Child health ethical issues are numerous and diverse, ranging from mass screening for diseases to withholding permission for treatment.

Child Abuse
Case Study

Emily, who is 8 months old, was brought to the hospital by her 17-year-old unemployed mother, who stated that the baby refused to eat at home and vomited a lot. Emily was very small for her age and was below the growth curve for weight. She was also neurologically introverted and showed little interest in her surroundings. She slept a great deal of the time. She was admitted to the hospital with a diagnosis of nonorganic failure to thrive.

During her stay in the hospital, Emily ate well and gained a significant amount of weight. Her neurological status also improved.

One nurse suspected that this was a case of neglect (a form of child abuse) and suggested to the physician that CPS be notified to evaluate the case. The physician resisted because there was not enough evidence to make a definitive case and thought that it was unfair to the parents to make such a claim. The other nurses felt that by reporting the case they would lose the trust of the mother and cause her to avoid health care for Emily in the future. They also cited a case in which nurses and the hospital were sued when they reported a teenage mother for neglect; the accusation later proved to be false.

Emily was sent home after 3 weeks but was readmitted 1 month later with the same complaints of poor feeding. She had lost weight since her discharge from the hospital, and she was again neurologically withdrawn. The physician still refused to notify CPS because of the lack of hard evidence. He thought that the available data did not warrant an investigation and possible removal of the child from the home. The nurse still believed that the mother should be reported on the basis of suspicions that could be substantiated legally.

Ethics Regarding Child Abuse

There is a general legal requirement in most states that suspected child abuse must be reported by health-care providers and by anyone who suspects that child abuse has occurred. Abuse is more obvious when the child has physical injuries that do not fit the medical history or are atypical for the age group. However, in cases of neglect, the evidence may be very minimal or even nonexistent. Often nurses and physicians who specialize in the care of children rely on their experience in making decisions to report or not report suspected abuse.

> "*Most acute care facilities will make some exceptions for the treatment of clients with AIDS; for example, if the nurse is pregnant, is receiving chemotherapy, or has had other immunity problems. In most situations, however, the nurse is obligated to provide the best nursing care possible for all clients, including those with AIDS.*"

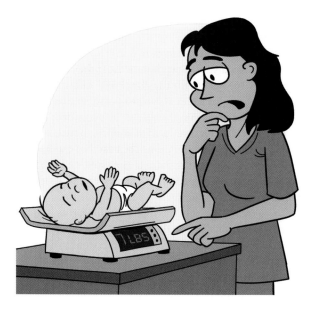

A conflicting ethical principle sometimes forgotten in the reporting of suspected child abuse is the family's right to privacy and self-determination. It is an equally fundamental right that Emily's parents be allowed to live their lives according to their own values, free from intrusions.

Decisions about reporting suspected child abuse or neglect rest on the underlying ethical principles of beneficence and protection of the best interests of the child. It is always difficult to decide how far ranging these concerns for "best interest" should be. However, when the child is a client in the hospital, beneficence usually outweighs fidelity and veracity.

Physicians tend to focus on solving the immediate problem. Nurses have a more holistic viewpoint and tend to see children in relationship to their environments and to the environments of the parents.

Resolving the Dilemma

How is the nurse going to resolve this dilemma? Should she report the case and go against the physician's decision? Should she just agree with the physician and defer to his greater experience? Should she submit the problem to the hospital ethics committee? Are there any other possible options for action in this case?

It is likely that the physician was correct in his decision about this case, although his ethical reasoning may leave something to be desired. Legally, it is unlikely that there would be sufficient proof to remove the infant from the mother because home monitoring could achieve the same results. Therefore, how can the ethical obligations for the best interest of the child be met?

One very plausible solution is to monitor the child closely through frequent follow-ups, either at the physician's office or at the local health department. In addition, a follow-up and home evaluation could be arranged through a home health-care agency, which could also make available other community resources to help in Emily's care. If the infant continued to fail to gain weight, or if it was later determined that Emily's mother was indeed unable to care adequately for her, the case could then be referred to CPS.

The role of the nurse who cares for the very young or abused child is one of client advocate. These children need help and protection, and at times, for their very survival, must be taken out of an abusive home setting. Nurses need to be aware of and use all the resources available in these situations, including the police, CPS, welfare, and home health-care agencies.

Informed Consent and Children

Case Study

Peter, one of a pair of 7-year-old identical twins, developed severe bilateral glomerulonephritis after a streptococcal (strep) throat infection. The renal involvement was so severe that it did not respond to any medical treatment, and both of his kidneys had to be removed. Paul, Peter's identical twin, was evaluated for kidney donation and, as expected, matched on all six antigens as well as blood type and size. Paul seemed to understand what had happened to his brother and agreed to donate one of his kidneys to keep his brother alive.

However, the children's parents were having some trouble agreeing on whether Paul should donate a kidney to Peter. The twins' mother felt that the donation and transplantation should be permitted because it would indeed help keep Peter alive and would also make Paul feel that he was an important part of the process. She argued that if Peter ever did die, Paul would be overcome with guilt knowing that he could have saved his brother but did not.

The twins' father was not as certain about the transplantation procedure. He thought that Paul was too young to make a truly free decision of that type and that he did not really understand the serious nature of a kidney removal operation. He thought that Paul, because he was so young, might have been unduly influenced by subtle yet powerful pressures from his family. No one had directly told Paul that he *must* donate one of his kidneys, yet the fact that his brother's survival might well depend on his decision could have had a major effect on his willingness to donate. Because Peter was being maintained on dialysis and seemed to be doing fairly well, the twins' father thought that he should be put on the transplant list to see whether a suitable nonrelated donor could be found.

The nurses on the unit where Peter was being cared for were equally divided about whether the transplantation should be performed. At various times during Peter's lengthy stay in the hospital, they had all been asked by the parents, usually one parent at a time, whether or not they should go ahead with the transplantation.

Case-Study Analysis

The question as related to the case study is, "Does a 7-year-old child have sufficient rational decision-making ability to decide to donate a kidney to his brother?" If, after careful assessment of the child, the answer is yes, then under the rights-in-trust doctrine, the right to self-determination can be turned over to the child, and he can make his own decision. If the answer is no, the child should not be permitted to donate the kidney.

Other ethical principles can be brought to bear on this decision. From a utilitarian viewpoint, the child should be allowed to donate the kidney because it would provide the greatest good or happiness for the greatest number of people. Similarly, love-based ethics, or the Golden Rule system of ethical decision-making, would also support the donation on the grounds that Paul identifies closely with his brother and appears to understand the issues involved in donation. However, from an egoistic or beneficent viewpoint, because the transplantation has little benefit for the donor and will surely cause pain and place him at risk for postoperative complications, the operation should not be permitted.

As with many ethical dilemmas, there is no perfect answer to this situation. The best that can be done is to ensure that the parents and children have as much necessary information as possible and to support their decisions (Box 7.3).

By recognizing the rights of children as individuals, we also recognize their importance to society. However, parents and health-care professionals also have the duty to nurture, support, and guide children as they grow into adolescence and adulthood. Nurses who work with children are challenged to support their independence by encouraging them to be responsible for and participate in their own health care.

Ethical Principles Regarding Child Health Care

One important difference between adults and children that always needs to be considered in ethical decisions about child health care is that children are dependents. As dependents, they generally are not attributed the right to self-determination that is fundamental to adult decision-making.

B o x 7 . 3
Determining the Greatest Good

Sherry is an RN who works for a rehabilitation center that deals mainly with developmentally delayed children. For several years, Sherry has been following the case of Margie N, who is now 8 years old and has Down syndrome and moderate retardation. Margie has made slow but steady progress in achieving basic motor and cognitive skills but still requires close supervision of all activities and care for all basic hygiene needs. Margie is still not advanced enough to participate in group activities at the center's day clinic.

Mrs. N, Margie's mother, a 42-year-old widow, has been providing a high level of care for Margie at home as well as meeting the child's demands for love and attention. Recently, Mrs. N has been diagnosed with systemic lupus erythematosus (SLE), which has displayed as its primary symptoms severe joint pain and stiffness. During the past several months, Mrs. N has been finding it increasingly difficult to care for Margie because of the progressive nature of the SLE.

Mrs. N is trying to make a decision about long-term care for Margie. She trusts Sherry's judgment completely and often relies on the information and teaching given by the nurse to make changes in Margie's care. Sherry is uncertain about what advice she should give. She recognizes that the high level of care and comfort provided by Mrs. N have been an essential part in the advances Margie has made up to this point, but she also recognizes that Mrs. N may soon reach a point where she can no longer provide care. It seems that to do what is good for Mrs. N (i.e., placing Margie in an institution) would be harmful to Margie, whereas doing what is good for Margie (i.e., leaving her at home) would be harmful to Mrs. N. What is the best course of action in this situation? Are there any alternative solutions to this dilemma?

A Three-Way Relationship

Whenever there is an ethical dilemma involving child health-care issues, a three-way relationship develops involving the child, the health-care professional, and the parents. Generally, the parents have the primary role in deciding health-care issues for their underage, dependent children on the basis of what they consider to be in the child's best interests.

Current routine child health practices reinforce this principle. Young children are given immunizations and medications, have blood drawn for tests, and even have operations such as tonsillectomies or myringotomies, all without anyone asking for their permission. This exemption to the principle of self-determination in children is based on the belief that young children do not yet have the capacity to make fully rational decisions. Yet the final expectation for children is that at some point in their lives they develop the capacity to make informed, correct decisions. The primary questions then become, "When do they develop this capacity for rational decision-making?" and "How should they be treated until they develop this capacity?"

Safeguarding the Child's Rights

The legal system has fixed the age for rational decision-making at age 18 years. Children who are younger than 18 years of age, with a few exceptions, require the permission of the parent for any and all medical procedures. Children older than 18 years of age can make their own decisions about health care.

The difficulty with fixing an age is that it is arbitrary and does not reflect the reality of the individual child's development. From experience, it can be observed that many children who are 9 or 10 years old exhibit rather advanced and adultlike decision-making skills, whereas other "children" who may be 18 or 19 years of age display a marked lack of this ability.

However, the more serious question is, "How should underage children be treated?" One solution is to deny, because of their age, that they have rights and then treat them as being incompetent by bringing to bear paternalistic, best-interest interventions. Another approach is to say that children do have the same rights as adults except that these rights are temporarily suspended until the child is sufficiently mature to exercise them. This is called *rights-in-trust*, and the rights are turned over to the child at the appropriate time. So, when is the appropriate time?

One way to proceed is to turn over all the rights to the child at the same time—for example, when he or she reaches 18 years of age. A more vigilant manner is to gradually release individual rights as the child grows older and is prepared to exercise them. In either case, appropriate adults, including nurses, have the role of safeguarding the child's rights and acting as guardians, protectors, and advocates of the children under their care.

> " *Whenever there is an ethical dilemma involving child health-care issues, a three-way relationship develops involving the child, the health-care professional, and the parents.* "

What Do You Think?

If you were the nurse, what would you suggest to the twins' parents? What ethical issues would be involved in your suggestions?

Conclusion

Ethical issues are a factor in the daily practice of all nurses. Any time a nurse comes in contact with a client, a potential ethical situation exists. In today's world, with rapidly advancing technology and unusual health-care situations, ethical dilemmas are proliferating. Nurses can be prepared to deal with most of these dilemmas if they keep current with the issues and are able to follow a systematic process for making ethical decisions. At some point, difficult decisions must be made, and we should not avoid making them. One of the worst elements of ethical decision-making is that it is very unlikely that everyone involved in the dilemma will be happy with the decision. However, if the decision is made after the situation has been analyzed and if it is made on the basis of sound ethical principles, it can usually be defended.

Critical-Thinking Exercises

CASE STUDY IN ETHICS

Analyze the following case study using the ethical decision-making process:

Sally Jones, registered nurse (RN), a public health nurse for a rural health department, was preparing to visit Mr. Weems, a 58-year-old client who was recently diagnosed with chronic bronchitis and emphysema. Mr. Weems was unemployed as a result of a farming accident and had been previously diagnosed with hypertension and extreme obesity. Ms. Jones was making this visit to see why Mr. Weems had missed his last appointment at the clinic and whether he was taking his prescribed antibiotics and antihypertensive medications.

As Ms. Jones pulled into the driveway of Mr. Weems's house, she noticed him sitting on the front porch smoking a cigarette. She felt a surge of anger, which she quickly suppressed, as she wondered why she spent so much of her limited time teaching him about the health consequences of smoking.

During the visit, Ms. Jones determined that Mr. Weems had stopped taking both his antihypertensive and antibiotic medications and rarely took his expectorants and bronchodilators. He coughed continuously, had a blood pressure of 196/122 mm Hg, and had severely congested lung sounds. Mr. Weems listened politely as Ms. Jones explained again about the need to stop smoking and the importance of taking his medications as prescribed. She also scheduled another appointment at the clinic in 1 week for a follow-up.

As she drove away to her next visit, Ms. Jones wondered about the ethical responsibilities of nurses who must provide care for clients who do not seem to care about their own health. Mr. Weems took little responsibility for his health, refused to even try to stop smoking or lose weight, and did not take his medications. She wondered whether there was a limit to the amount of nursing care a noncompliant client should expect from a community health agency. She reflected that the time spent with Mr. Weems would have been spent much more productively screening children at a local grade school or working with mothers of newborn infants.

- What data are important in relation to this situation?
- State the ethical dilemma in a clear, simple statement.
- What are the choices of action, and how do they relate to specific ethical principles?
- What are the consequences of these actions?
- What decisions can be made?

References

1. Clifton JM, VanBeuge SS, Mladenka C, Wosnik KK. The Genetic Information Nondiscrimination Act 2008: What clinicians should understand. *Journal of the American Academy of Nurse Practitioners,* 22(5):246–249, 2010.

2. Hodgkinson K, Pullman D. Duty to warn and genetic disease. *Canadian Journal of Cardiovascular Nursing,* 20(1):12–15, 2010.

3. Kaminskyy V, Zhivotovsky B. To kill or be killed: How viruses interact with the cell death machinery. *Journal of Internal Medicine,* 267(5):473–482, 2010.

4. Caulfield T. Stem cell research and economic promises. *Journal of Law, Medicine and Ethics,* 38(2):303–313, 2010.

5. Parents' guide to cord blood banking. Retrieved June 2013 from http://www.healthychildren.org/English/ages-stages/prenatal/decisions-to-make/Pages/Should-We-Store-Our-Newborns-Cord-Blood.aspx

6. Healthy children. American Academy of Pediatrics. Retrieved June 2013 from http://www.eurekalert.org/pub_releases/2005-02/plos-crc021605.php

7. Fisk R, Markwald M. Can routine commercial cord blood banking be scientifically and ethically justified? Retrieved June 2013 from http://bethematch.org/

8. National Marrow Donor Program website: Retrieved June 2013 from http://marrow.org/Get_Involved/Donate_Cord_Blood/How_to_Donate/Participating_Hospitals.aspx

9. Banking cord blood: More than a parent's responsibility? Retrieved June 2013 from http://bloodbanker.com/cord/banking-cord-blood-more-than-a-parent%E2%80%99s-responsibility

10. American Society for Blood and Marrow Transplantation (ASBMT). Retrieved June 2013 from http://www.asbmt.org

11. Blood pressures: The controversy over cord blood. Retrieved June 2013 from http://www.parents.com

12. Cord Blood Registry "Client Services Agreement." *Available prior to submitting payment information in account creation.* Retrieved June 2013 from http://www.cordblood.com

13. Quick B, Kim DK, Meyer K. A 15-year review of ABC, CBS, and NBC news coverage of organ donation: Implications for organ donation campaigns. *Health Communication,* 24(2):137–145, 2010.

14. U.S. Department of Health and Humans Services. Organ Procurement and Transplant Network, 2014 Retrieved December, 2014 from http://optn.transplant.hrsa.gov/

15. Bramstedt KA. Honoring first person consent. *Transplantation,* 86(11):163, 2008.

16. Organization for Transplant Professionals: Position statement: Adherence to first person consent. 2009, p 1. Retrieved May 2014 from http://www.natco1.org/public_policy/documents/FirstPersonConsent.pdf

17. National Council of Commissioners on United States Laws: The Uniform Anatomical Gift Act, Revised 2009.

18. Dr. Bohdan Pomahac changing lives with face transplants. Retrieved June 2013 from http://science.dodlive.mil/2014/01/09/changing-the-face-of-modern-medicine/

19. MacCormick IJ. Ruling on mercy killing: Suicide and euthanasia paradox. *British Medical Journal,* 14(341):318, 2010.

20. Mair J. Respect for autonomy; or the right to die? *Health Information Management Journal,* 39(1):46–50, 2010.

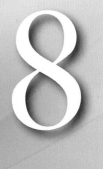

8

Nursing Law and Liability

Mary Evans

Tonia Aiken

Learning Objectives

After completing this chapter, the reader will be able to:

- Distinguish between statutory law and common law
- Differentiate civil law from criminal law
- Explain the legal principles involved in:
  - Unintentional torts
  - Intentional torts
  - Quasi-intentional torts
  - Informed consent
  - Do-not-resuscitate (DNR) orders
- Describe the trial process
- List methods to prevent litigation
- Identify the elements in delegation

THE LEGAL SYSTEM

For many nurses, the mere mention of the word *lawsuit* provokes a high level of anxiety. At first glance, the legal system often seems to be a large and confusing entity whose intricacies are designed to entrap the uninitiated. Many nurses feel that even a minor error in client care will lead to huge settlements against them and loss of their nursing license. In reality, even though the number of lawsuits against nurses has been increasing since the early 1990s, the number of nurses who are actually sued in court remains relatively small. However, many cases are settled out of court, often before any official legal action has been taken.

It is important to remember that the legal system is just one element of the health-care system. Laws are rules to help protect people and to keep society functioning. The ultimate goal of all laws is to promote peaceful and productive interactions among the people of that society.

An understanding of basic legal principles will augment the quality of care that the nurse delivers. In our litigious society, it is important to comprehend how the law affects the profession of nursing and the individual nurse's daily practice.

SOURCES OF LAW

There are two major sources of laws in the United States: statutory law and common law (Box 8.1). Most laws that govern nursing are state-level statutory laws because licensure is a function of the state's authority.

Box 8.1

Division and Types of Law

Statutory Law and Common Law
I. Criminal law
   A. Misdemeanor
   B. Felony
II. Civil Law
   A. Tort law
      1. Unintentional tort
      2. Intentional tort
      3. Quasi-intentional tort
   B. Contract law
   C. Treaty law
   D. Tax law
   E. Other

Statutory Law

Statutory law consists of laws written and enacted by the U.S. Congress; the state legislatures; and other governmental entities such as cities, counties, and townships. Legislated laws enacted by the U.S. Congress are called federal **statutes.** State-drafted laws are called *state statutes.* Individual cities and municipalities have legislative bodies that draft **ordinances,** codes, and regulations at their respective levels.

The laws that govern the profession of nursing are statutory laws. Most of these laws are written at the state level because licensure is a responsibility of the individual states. These laws include the nurse practice act, which establishes the state board of nursing, the scope of practice for nurses, individual licensure procedures, punitive actions for violation of the practice act, and the schedule of fees for nurse licensure in the state.

Common Law

Common law is different from statutory law in that it has evolved from the decisions of previous legal cases that form a **precedent.** These laws represent the accumulated results of the judgments and decrees that have been handed down by courts of the United States and Great Britain through the years.

Common law often extends beyond the scope of statutory law. For example, no statutes require a person who is negligent and causes injury to another to compensate that person for the injury. However, court decisions that have addressed the same legal issues, such as negligence, over and over have repeatedly ruled that the injured person should

receive compensation. The way in which each case is resolved creates a precedent, or pattern, for dealing with the same legal issue in the future. The common laws involving negligence or malpractice are the laws most frequently encountered by nurses.

Common law or case law is law that has developed over a long period. The principle of stare decisis requires a judge to make decisions similar to those that have been handed down in previous cases if the facts of the cases are identical. Common law decisions are published in bound legal reports. Generally speaking, common law deals with matters outside the scope of laws enacted by the legislature.

DIVISIONS OF LAW

In the U.S. legal system, there are many divisions in the law. A major example is the difference between criminal law and civil law, either of which may be statutory or common in origin.

Criminal Law

Criminal laws are concerned with providing protection for all members of society. When someone is accused of violating a criminal law, the government at the county, city, state, or federal level imposes a punishment that is appropriate to the type of **crime.** Criminal law involves a wide range of **malfeasance,** from minor traffic violations to murder.

Although most criminal law is created and regulated by the government through the enactment of statutes, a small portion falls under the common law. Statutes are developed and enacted by the legislature (state or federal) and approved by the executive branch, such as a governor or the president. Criminal law is further classified into two types of offenses: (1) **misdemeanors,** which are minor criminal offenses, and (2) **felonies,** which are major criminal offenses.

In the criminal law system, an individual accused of a crime is called the *defendant.* The prosecuting attorney represents the people of the city, county, state, or federal jurisdiction who are accusing the individual of a crime. A **criminal action** is rendered when the person charged with the crime is brought to trial and convicted. Penalties or sanctions are imposed on the violators of criminal law and are based on the scope of the crime. They can involve a range of punishments, from community service work and fines to imprisonment and death.

What Do You Think?

Do you know anyone who has filed a malpractice suit or a health-care provider who was the defendant in a malpractice suit? What was the situation that caused the case? How was it resolved? If you have never been involved with a malpractice suit or do not know anyone who has, how would you feel if a lawsuit were to be brought against you?

The Nurse's Involvement

Nurses can become involved with the criminal system in their nursing practice in several ways. The most common violation by nurses of the criminal law is through failure to renew nursing licenses. In this situation, the nurse is practicing without a license, which is a crime in all states.

Nurses also become involved with the illegal diversion of drugs, particularly narcotics, from the hospital. This is a more serious crime, which may lead to imprisonment. Recent cases involving intentional or unintentional deaths of clients and assisted suicide cases have also led to criminal action against nurses.[1]

Civil Law

Nurses are much more likely to become involved in civil lawsuits than in criminal violations. **Civil laws** generally deal with the violation of one individual's rights by another individual. The court provides the forum that enables these individuals to have their disputes resolved by an independent third party, such as a judge or a jury of the defendant's peers.

The individual who brings the dispute to the court is called the **plaintiff.** The formal written document that describes the dispute and the resolution sought is called the *complaint.* The individual against whom the complaint is filed is the defendant, who, in conjunction with his or her attorney, prepares the **answer** to the complaint. In civil cases, the **burden of proof** rests with the plaintiff.

Civil law has many branches, including contract law, treaty law, tax law, and tort law. It is under the tort law that most nurses become involved with the legal system.

> *The most common violation by nurses of the criminal law is through failure to renew nursing licenses. In this situation, the nurse is practicing nursing without a license, which is a crime in all states.*

Tort Law

A **tort** is generally defined as a wrongful act committed against a person or his or her property independently of a contract. A person who commits a tort is called the **tortfeasor** and is **liable** for **damages** to those who are affected by the person's actions. The word *tort*, derived from the Latin *tortus* (twisted), is a French word for "injury" or "wrong." Torts can involve several different types of actions, including a direct violation of a person's legal rights or a violation of a standard of care that causes injury to a person. Torts are classified as unintentional, intentional, or quasi-intentional.

Unintentional Torts

Negligence

Negligence is the primary form of **unintentional tort. Negligence** is generally defined as the **omission** of an act that a reasonable and prudent person would perform in a similar situation or the commission of something a reasonable person would not do in that situation. **Nonfeasance** is a type of negligence that occurs when a person fails to perform a legally required duty.[2]

Malpractice

Malpractice is a type of negligence for which professionals can be sued (professional negligence). Because of their professional status, nurses are held to a higher standard of conduct than the ordinary layperson. The standard for nurses is what a reasonable and prudent nurse would do in the same situation: Registered nurses must use the skill, knowledge, and judgment they have learned through their education and experience.[3]

For instance, it is reasonable and prudent that the nurse put the side rails up on the bed of a client who has just received an injection of a narcotic pain medication because the drug causes drowsiness and sometimes confusion. If the nurse gave an injection of a narcotic medication but forgot to put the side rails up and the client fell out of bed and fractured a hip, the nurse could be sued for the negligent act of forgetting to put the side rail up.

Four elements are required for a person to make a claim of negligence:

1. A duty was owed to the client (professional relationship).
2. The professional violated the **duty** and failed to conform to the standard of care (breach of duty).

3. The professional's failure to act was the **proximate cause** of the resulting injuries (causality).
4. Actual injuries resulted from the breach of duty (damages).

If any of these elements are missing from the case, the client will probably not be able to win the lawsuit (Box 8.2).

Box 8.2

Malpractice Considerations

Nursing malpractice is based on the legal premise that a nurse can be held legally responsible for the personal injury of another individual if it can be proved that the injury was the result of negligence.[2] Nursing malpractice is based on four elements: (1) duty, (2) breach of duty, (3) causation (the "but for" test), and (4) damage or injury.

Inappropriate work assignment and inadequate supervision are a breach of duty and could be the basis for finding a nurse's actions to be negligent. Failure or breach of duty to delegate is established by proving that a reasonably prudent nurse would not have made a particular assignment or delegated a certain responsibility or that supervision was inadequate under the circumstances.

The act of improper delegation of tasks or inadequate supervision must be evaluated in light of the "but for" test related to the injury. If the person who performed the injurious act had not been assigned or delegated to perform the task or had been adequately supervised, the injury could have been avoided. Consequently, the nurse is not being held liable for the negligent act of her subordinate, *but for the lack of competence in performing the independent duties of delegation and supervision.*

Off-Site Consideration

Registered nurses who practice in public health, community, or home-care settings must rely frequently on written or telephone communication when delegating patient care duties to assistive personnel. The nurse who must supervise from off-site has a particular duty to assess the knowledge, skills, and judgment of the assistive personnel before making assignments. Regular supervisory visits and impeccable documentation will help the registered nurse ensure that care provided by assistive personnel is adequate.

Source: Aiken TD. *Legal, Ethical, and Political Issues in Nursing*. Philadelphia: FA Davis, 1994, pp. 66–69.

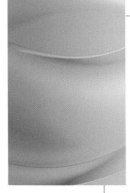

Issues in Practice

Case Study

Consider the following situation:

Mr. Fagin, a 78-year-old client, was admitted from a nursing home for the treatment of a fractured tibia after he fell out of bed. After the fracture was reduced, a fiberglass cast was applied, and Mr. Fagin was sent to the orthopedic unit for follow-up care. While making her 0400 rounds, the night charge nurse, a registered nurse (RN), discovered that Mr. Fagin's foot on the casted leg was cold to the touch, looked bluish purple, and was swollen approximately 1½ times its normal size. The nurse noted these findings in the client's chart and relayed the information to the day-shift nurses during the 0630 shift report.

The charge nurse on the day shift promptly called and relayed the findings to Mr. Fagin's physician. The physician, however, did not seem to be concerned and only told the nurse to "keep a close eye on him, and don't bother me again unless it is an absolute emergency." A short time later, Mr. Fagin became agitated, complained of severe pain in the affected foot, and eventually began yelling uncontrollably. The charge nurse called the emergency department (ED) physician to come check on the client. The ED physician immediately removed the cast and noted an extensive circulatory impairment that would not respond to treatment. A few days later, Mr. Fagin's leg was amputated. His family filed a malpractice lawsuit against the hospital, the physician, and both the night and day charge nurses.

Questions for Thought

- Are all the elements present in this case for a bona fide lawsuit?

- What could have been done to prevent this situation from happening?

- How should nurses deal with reluctant or hostile physicians?

Professional Misconduct

Malpractice is more serious than mere negligence because it indicates professional misconduct or unreasonable lack of skill in performing professional duties. Malpractice suggests the existence of a professional standard of care and a deviation from that standard of care. A professional **expert witness** is often asked to testify in a malpractice case to help establish the standard of care to which the professional should be held accountable.

A 1988 case in South Dakota presents an example of nursing malpractice. The nurse failed to question the physician's order to discharge a client when she discovered the client had a fever. In this case, a supervisory nurse provided expert testimony and reported to the judge that the general standard of care for nurses is to report a significant change in a client's condition, such as an elevated temperature. It is the nurse's responsibility to question the physician's order as to appropriateness of discharge.

The records on this case indicated that the client's elevated temperature was charted after the physician had completed his rounds. The nurse did not notify the physician of the client's fever, and the client was subsequently discharged. The client was readmitted a short time after discharge and died in the hospital. The nurse was found negligent. The court held that negligence can be determined by failure to act as well as by the commission of an act.

Many other types of actions by nurses can produce malpractice lawsuits. Some of the more common actions include:

- Leaving foreign objects inside a client during surgery.
- Failing to follow a hospital standard or protocol.
- Not using equipment in accordance with the manufacturer's recommendations.
- Failing to listen to and respond to a client's complaints.
- Not properly documenting phone conversations and orders from physicians.
- Failing to question physician orders when indicated (e.g., too large medication dosages, inappropriate diets).
- Failing to clarify poorly written or illegible physician orders.
- Failing to assess and observe a client as directed.
- Failing to obtain a proper informed consent.
- Failing to report a change in a client's condition, such as vital signs, circulatory status, and level of consciousness.
- Failing to report another health-care provider's **incompetency** or negligence.
- Failing to take actions to provide for a client's safety, such as not cleaning up a liquid spill on the floor that causes a client to fall.
- Failing to provide a client with sufficient and appropriate education before discharge.[3]

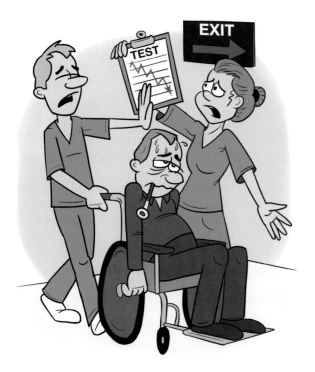

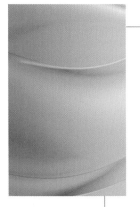

Issues in Practice

Nurse Malpractice in Client Fall

At a hospital in Washington State, a client with a recent leg amputation was still partially sedated after surgery. The nurse assigned to his care was called away from the room and failed to raise the bed rails. The client attempted to get out of bed, fell, and was injured.

The client sued the hospital for negligence. Using the hospital's own policies and procedures manual, the client's lawyer pointed out the requirement that satisfactory precautions be taken to restrain disabled or sedated clients.

The nurse's lawyer based the defense on the argument that the nurse was following the physician's standing orders to allow the client to ambulate postoperatively to hasten recovery and prevent complications.

The court agreed with the client and concluded that the nurse had an obligation, based on the hospital's policy and procedures, to assess the client's physical and mental condition. Nurses have an obligation not to leave clients unattended in an unsafe bed configuration.

All lawsuits alleging health-care provider negligence require expert witness testimony. Without this, courts will almost always dismiss a negligence case decided by a lay jury, even when it is as obvious as a fall from bed. In this case, the expert testimony not only supported the lawyer's contention that the hospital's policy and procedures upheld the suit but also emphasized the point that clients recently returned from surgery are disoriented from anesthesia and should never be left alone unless the bed rails are raised to their full upright position.

When the case was appealed, the court of appeals wrote the following ruling:

> *A lawsuit against a hospital for negligence does not necessarily have to involve medical malpractice committed by a physician. A hospital's nurses have their own independent legal duties in assessing and caring for their patients.*

A hospital is not relieved of its own legal liability for negligence just because the hospital's staff nurses followed the physician's orders. That is, a hospital's nursing staff cannot necessarily rely on a physician's standing orders for a patient to be up and out of bed and leave the bed rails down.

A patient freshly out of surgery who is taking pain and sedative medications must be evaluated continually by the staff. The patient's present physical and mental state is all that matters. The nurses may have to disregard the physician's standing orders and instead follow the hospital's policies and procedures for a restraint in the form of raised bed rails when necessary to insure the patient's safety.

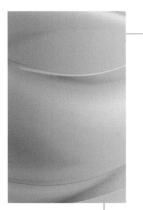

Issues in Practice continued

Questions for Thought

- Do you agree with the jury's decision against the nurse? Why?

- The nurse has a legal and ethical obligation (fidelity) to follow the physician's order. Is there ever a situation when the nurse can ignore a physician's order?

- Under what legal principle was the hospital held liable for the nurse's actions?

- What other actions might the nurse have taken, besides putting up the side rails, to prevent the patient from falling?

Source: Greenberg v. Empire Health Services Inc., 2006 WL 1075574 Wash. App., April 25, 2006. Court of Appeals of Washington, April 25, 2006.

If the Nurse Is Liable

If a nurse is found guilty of malpractice, several types of action may be taken. The nurse may be required to provide monetary compensation to the client for general damages that were a direct result of the injury, including pain, suffering, disability, and disfigurement. In addition, the nurse is often required to pay for special damages that resulted from the injury, such as all involved medical expenses, **out-of-pocket expenses,** and wages lost by the client while he or she was in the hospital.

Optional damages, including those for emotional distress, mental suffering, and counseling expenses that were an outgrowth of the initial injury, may be added to the total settlement. If the client is able to prove that the nurse acted with conscious disregard for the client's safety or acted in a malicious, willful, or wanton manner that produced injury, an additional assessment of punitive or exemplary damages may be added to the award.

Intentional Torts

An **intentional tort** is generally defined as a willful act that violates another person's rights or property. Intentional torts can be distinguished from malpractice and acts of negligence by the following three requirements: (1) the nurse must intend to bring about the consequences of the act, (2) the nurse's act must be intended to interfere with the client or the client's property, and (3) the act must be a substantial factor in bringing about the injury or consequences.

The most frequently encountered intentional torts are assault, battery, false imprisonment, abandonment, and intentional infliction of emotional distress. With intentional torts, the injured person does not have to prove that an injury has occurred, nor is the opinion of an expert witness required for adjudication. Punitive damages are more likely to be assessed against the nurse in intentional tort cases, and some intentional torts may fall under the criminal law if there is gross violation of the standards of care.

Assault and Battery

Assault is the unjustifiable attempt to touch another person or the threat of doing so. **Battery** is actual harmful or unwarranted contact with another person without his or her consent. Battery is the most common intentional tort seen in the practice of nursing.

For a nurse to commit assault and battery, there must be an absence of client consent. Before any procedure can be performed on a competent, alert, and normally oriented client, the client must agree or consent to the procedure being done. Negligence does not have to be proved for a person to be successful in a claim for assault and battery.

A common example of an assault and battery occurs when a nurse physically restrains a client against the client's will and administers an injection against the client's wishes.

False Imprisonment

False imprisonment occurs when a competent client is confined or restrained with intent to prevent him or her from leaving the hospital. The use of restraints alone does not constitute false imprisonment when they are used to maintain the safety of a confused, disoriented, or otherwise incompetent client. In general, mentally impaired clients can be detained against their will only if they are at risk for injuring themselves or others. The use of threats or medications that interfere with the client's ability to leave the facility can also be considered false imprisonment.

> *Because of their professional status, nurses are held to a higher standard of conduct than the ordinary layperson.*

Intentional Infliction of Emotional Distress

Intentional infliction of emotional distress is another common intentional tort encountered by the nurse. To prove this intentional tort, the following three elements are necessary: (1) the conduct exceeds what is usually accepted by society, (2) the health-care provider's conduct is intended to cause mental distress, and (3) the conduct actually does produce mental distress (causation). Any nurse who is charged with assault, battery, or false imprisonment is also at risk for being charged with infliction of emotional distress.

A 1975 case, *Johnson v. Women's Hospital,* is an example of infliction of emotional distress. A mother wished to view the body of her baby, who had died during birth. After she made the request, she was handed the baby's body, which was floating in a gallon jar of formaldehyde.[1] The *Johnson* case demonstrates a clear lack of respect shown to the mother. If the mother in this delicate situation had been treated with dignity and respect, the situation would have been avoided.

Client Abandonment

Because of the ongoing nursing shortage, **abandonment** of clients has become an important legal and ethical issue for health-care providers. Abandonment occurs when there is a unilateral severance of the professional relationship with the client without adequate notice and while the requirement for care still exists. The nurse–client relationship continues until it is terminated by mutual consent of both parties.

From an ethical standpoint, the issue of abandonment falls under the umbrella of beneficence. From the legal view, client abandonment can be considered an intentional tort, breach of contract, or in some cases in which injury occurs, malpractice. The key phrase to keep in mind when discussing client abandonment is *without adequate notice.* If the client knows that the nurse's shift is scheduled to end at 7 p.m., the client and the hospital both have adequate notice.

It is not uncommon for nurses in today's health-care system to be approached by nursing supervisors telling them, "Everyone else called in, so you will have to work a double shift or you could be charged with client abandonment." In this case, the abandonment becomes the hospital's responsibility, not the nurse's. Nurses sometimes feel uncomfortable about going on strike because it seems to imply client abandonment; however, if there is adequate notice about the strike and if the facility has had time to make arrangements for care or discharge of clients, there is no client abandonment. The growing practice of emergency client diversion, occurring when facilities can no longer safely care for emergency clients because of lack of space or staffing, can potentially fall under the legal definitions of abandonment.

Quasi-Intentional Torts

A **quasi-intentional tort** is a mixture of unintentional and intentional torts. It is defined as a voluntary act that directly causes injury or distress without intent to injure or to cause distress. A quasi-intentional tort does have the elements of volition and causation without the element of intent. Quasi-intentional torts usually involve situations of communication and often violate a person's reputation, personal privacy, or civil rights (Box 8.3).

Defamation of Character

Defamation of character, which is the most common of the quasi-intentional torts, is harmful to a person's reputation. Defamation injures a person's reputation

---

Box 8.3
Registered Nurse Licensure

The legislature of each state enacts laws that govern the practice of nursing. The purpose of licensing law is to ensure that the public is protected from unqualified practitioners by developing and enforcing regulations that define who may practice in the profession, the scope of that practice, and the level of education for the profession.

A fundamental premise of nursing practice is that a professional nurse is personally responsible for all acts or omissions undertaken within the scope of practice. The American Nurses Association defines delegation as "the transfer of responsibility for the performance of an activity from one person to another while retaining accountability for the outcome."[1] Additionally, the nurse is responsible for the adequate supervision of a task delegated to a subordinate. If the nurse fails to delegate appropriately or supervise adequately, any injuries resulting from the acts of the subordinate may result in licensure ramifications. The state licensing board may take disciplinary actions.

---

by diminishing the esteem, respect, good will, or confidence that others have for the person. It can be especially damaging when false statements are made about a criminal act or an immoral act or when there are false allegations about a client's having a contagious disease. In *Schessler v. Keck* (1954), a nurse was found liable for defamation of character when she told a friend that a client for whom she was caring was a caterer and was being treated for syphilis. Even though the statement was false, when the information became public, it destroyed his catering business.[2]

Defamation includes **slander,** which is spoken communication in which one person discusses another in terms that harm that person's reputation. **Libel** is a written communication in which a person makes statements or uses language that harms another person's reputation. To win a defamation lawsuit against the nurse, the client must prove that the nurse acted maliciously, abused the principle of **privileged communication,** and wrote or spoke a lie.[3]

Medical record documentation is a primary source of defamation of character. Through the years, the client's chart has been the basis of many defamation lawsuits. Discussion about a client in the elevators, cafeteria, and other public areas can also lead to lawsuits for defamation if negative comments are overheard.

Invasion of Privacy

Invasion of privacy is a violation of a person's right to protection against unreasonable and unwarranted interference with one's personal life. To prove that invasion of privacy has occurred, the client must show that (1) the nurse intruded on the client's seclusion and privacy, (2) the intrusion is objectionable to a reasonable and prudent person, (3) the act committed intrudes on private or published facts or pictures of a private nature, and (4) public disclosure of private information was made.[4] Examples of invasion of privacy include using the client's name or picture for the sole advantage of the health-care provider, intruding into the client's private affairs without permission, giving out private client information over the telephone, and publishing information that misrepresents the client's condition. Because of the Health Insurance Portability and Accountability Act (HIPAA) of 1996, health-care providers have become more aware than ever of the issue of confidentiality in the health-care setting.[5]

Breach of Confidentiality

Confidentiality of information concerning the client must be honored. A breach of confidentiality results when a client's trust and confidence are violated by public revelation of confidential or privileged communications without the client's consent.

Examples of invasion of privacy include using the client's name or picture for the sole advantage of the health-care provider, intruding into the client's private affairs without permission, giving out private client information over the telephone, and publishing information that misrepresents the client's condition.

Privileged Communication

Privileged communication is protected by law and exists in certain well-defined professional relationships—for example, physician–client, psychiatrist–client, priest–penitent, and lawyer–client. Privileged communication ensures that the professional who obtains any information from the client cannot be forced to reveal that information, even in a court of law under oath. Nurses do not have privileged communication with clients. However, they can be bound, by extension, under the seal of privileged communication if they are in a room with a physician when the client reveals personal information.

Most breach of confidentiality cases involve a physician's revelation of privileged communications shared by a client. Nurses who overhear privileged communication or information, however, are held to the same standards as a physician with regard to that information.

Privileged client information can only be disclosed if it is authorized by the client. In accord with the HIPAA regulations, all health-care facilities must have specific guidelines dealing with client information disclosure. Disclosure of information to family members violates HIPAA regulations unless the client is under 18 years of age or gives permission for the disclosure. For instance, a client may not wish to disclose to a family member a specific diagnosis, such as cancer. If this is the case, the nurse should honor this request; otherwise, it is considered a violation of HIPAA regulations.[5]

Electronic Pitfalls

Use of computerized documentation and telemedicine has led to several lawsuits based on breach of confidentiality and malpractice. (See Chapter 18 for examples.) The current widespread practice of texting on portable wireless electronic devices has also opened up a new world of possible confidentiality violations.[6] The HIPAA regulations on communication are the government's attempts to force the legal system to keep pace with the use of computers and electronic record-keeping. Cases exist in which medical records have been lost because of computer failure.

Other issues, such as correction of errors in **charting**, are complicated by use of computers. On paper charts, health-care providers had to draw a line through the erroneous entry, initial the entry, and date it. Many new computerized charting systems have attempted to address the "delete button" issue by including programs that track any changes made in the charting and indicate both the date and time of the change.[7]

FACING A LAWSUIT

Because of the rapid proliferation of lawsuits since the 1990s, there is now a higher probability that a nurse, at some time in her or his career, will be involved either as a witness or as a party to a nursing malpractice action. Knowledge of the litigation process increases nurses' understanding of the way in which their conduct is evaluated before the courts.

The Statute of Limitations

A malpractice suit against a nurse for negligence must be filed within a specified time. This period, called the **statute of limitations,** generally begins at the time of the injury or when the injury is discovered and lasts until some specified future time. In most states, the limitation period lasts from 1 to 6 years, with the most common duration being 2 years. However, in cases involving children, the statute of limitations extends until the person reaches 21 years of age. If the client fails to file the suit within the pre-scribed time, the lawsuit will be barred.

The Complaint

Filing the suit (also called the *complaint*) with the court begins the litigation process. The written complaint describes the incident that initiated the claim of negligence against the nurse. Specific allegations, including the amount of money sought for damages, are also stated in the **legal complaint.** The plaintiff, who is usually a client or a family member of a client, is the alleged injured party, and the defendant is the person or entity being sued (i.e., the nurse, physician, or hospital). The first notice of a lawsuit occurs when the defendant (nurse) is officially notified or served with the complaint. All defendants are accorded the right of **due process** under constitutional law.

The Answer

The defendant must respond to the allegations stated in the complaint within a specific time frame. This written response by the defendant is called the *answer.* If the nurse had liability insurance at the time of the negligent act, the insurer will assign a lawyer to represent the defendant nurse. In the answer, the nurse can outline specific defenses to the claims against him or her.

The Discovery

After the complaint and answer are filed with the court, the discovery phase of the litigation begins. The purpose of discovery is to uncover all information

relevant to the malpractice suit and the incident in question. The nurse may be required to answer a se-ries of questions that relate to the nurse's educational background and emotional state, the incident that led to the lawsuit, and any other pertinent information. These written questions are called **interrogatories.**

In addition, the plaintiff's lawyer may seek requests for production of documents. These are doc-uments related to the lawsuit, including the plaintiff's medical records, **incident reports,** card file, the insti-tution's policy and procedure manual concerning the specific situation, and the nurse's job description. The plaintiff is also required to disclose information as part of the discovery process, including the plaintiff's past medical history.

The Deposition

The next step in the process is the taking of a deposition from each party in the lawsuit, as well as any potential witnesses, to assist the lawyers in the trial preparation. A **depo-sition** is a formal legal process that involves the taking of testimony under oath and is recorded by a court reporter. These are usually wide ranging in scope and often include information not allowed in a trial, such as **hearsay** testimony. In some cases, videotaped depositions may be used. Nurses can prepare for a deposition by keeping some key points in mind (Box 8.4).

The deposition **testimony** is reduced to a written document called an **affidavit** for use at trial. If a witness during the trial changes testimony from that given at the deposition, the deposition can be used to contradict the testimony. This process is called *impeaching the witness.* Impeaching a witness on a specific issue can create doubt about that wit-ness's credibility and can thus weaken other areas in the witness's testimony. In some situations, witnesses can later be charged with **perjury** if it is proved that they gave false testimony under oath.

The Trial

The **trial** often takes place years after the complaint was filed. Once **jurisdiction** is determined, the voir dire process, more commonly called *jury selection,* begins. After jury selection, each attorney presents opening statements. The plaintiff's side is presented

> *Because of the rapid proliferation of lawsuits since the 1990s, there is now a higher probability that a nurse, at some time in his or her career, will be involved either as a witness or as a party to a nursing malpractice action.*

Box 8.4

Giving a Deposition

1. Do not volunteer information.
2. Be familiar with the client's medical record and nurse's notes.
3. Remain calm throughout the process and do not be intimidated by the lawyers.
4. Clarify all questions before answering; ask the lawyer to explain the questions if you do not understand.
5. Do not make assumptions about the questions.
6. Do not exaggerate answers.
7. Wait at least 5 seconds after a question is asked before answering it to allow objections from other lawyers.
8. Tell the truth.
9. Do not speculate about answers.
10. Speak slowly and clearly, using professional language as much as possible.
11. Look the questioning lawyer in the eye as much as possible.
12. If unable to remember an answer, simply state, "I don't remember" or "I don't know."
13. Think before answering any question.
14. Bring a résumé or curriculum vitae to the deposition in case it is requested.
15. Request a break if you are tired or confused.
16. Avoid becoming angry with the lawyers or using sarcastic language.
17. Avoid using absolutes in the answers.
18. If a question is asked more than once, ask the court recorder to read the answer given previously.
19. Be sure to read over the deposition just before the trial.

Source: Wagner KC, Hunter-Adkins D, Clifford R. Questions & answers. Effective preparation of the expert witness for deposition. *Journal of Legal Nurse Consulting,* 19(4):26–29, 34, 2009.

first. Witnesses may be served with **subpoenas** that require them to appear and provide testimony.

Each witness or party is subject to direct examination, cross-examination, and redirect examination. Direct examination involves open-ended questions by the attorney. Cross-examination is performed by the opposing lawyer, and questions are asked in such a way as to elicit short, specific responses. The redirect examination consists of follow-up questions to address issues that were raised during the cross-examination.

After both parties have presented their case, the lawyers deliver their closing arguments. The case then goes to a jury or a judge for deliberation. If the facts are not in dispute, the judge may render a **summary judgment.** If either party is not satisfied, the decision or ruling made about the case can be appealed. The party appealing the decision is called the **appellant.** There is almost always an appeal if a large sum of money is awarded to the plaintiff.

Monetary Awards

The primary reason clients sue physicians, nurses, and hospitals is to recover monetary compensation and other associated costs against the person or institution that harmed the client and secondarily to prevent additional malpractice by the defendant. Generally, when lawyers are evaluating a case as a potential malpractice suit, they look for the person or institution that has "deep pockets" (i.e., are backed by a large source of income or maintain a high payout insurance policy). Lawyers will generally refuse a case if there is not a good probability of substantial monetary rewards. There are several types of awards that a plaintiff may seek when a favorable decision is rendered by the jury:

Compensatory damages, also called *actual damages,* are awards that cover the actual cost of injuries and economic losses caused by the injury. These include all medical expenses related to the injury and any lost wages or income that resulted from extended hospitalization or recovery period.

General damages are monetary awards for injuries for which an exact dollar amount cannot be calculated. These awards include pain and suffering, loss of companionship, shortened life span, loss of reputation, and wrongful death. Some state legislatures have recently passed new tort reform laws that severely limit or completely eliminate general damage awards.

Punitive damages, also called *exemplary damages,* are awarded in addition to compensatory and general damages when the actions that caused the injury to the client were judged to be willful, malicious, or demonstrated an extreme measure of incompetence and gross negligence. The primary purpose of punitive damages is to "punish" the plaintiff and deter him or her from ever acting in the same way again. These awards are almost always extremely large, usually in the millions of dollars, and quickly gain the attention of other health-care providers to avoid the same types of actions. Some states have recently passed tort reform laws to limit punitive awards to much smaller amounts (less than 10 percent of a usual award) in belief that it will bring down the cost of malpractice insurance and, hopefully, the overall cost of health care.

Treble damages allow the judge, in certain instances, to triple the actual damage award amount as an additional form of punitive damages. Not all states allow judges this decision-making power and it, too, has been opposed by legislatures advocating tort reform.

Normal damages can be awarded when the law requires a judge and jury to find a defendant guilty but no real harm happened to the plaintiff. The award is usually very small, generally in the sum of $1000.

Special damages are awarded to the plaintiff for out-of-pocket expenses related to the trial. It would cover the expenses of taking a taxi back and forth to the courthouse, use of special assistive equipment, and special home health-care providers not covered under actual damages.

It is easy to understand why most malpractice suits are settled out of court by insurance companies. The expenses for lawyers and lengthy trials quickly become astronomical, and there is never any certainty about the way a jury will decide. On the plaintiff's side, although the money they receive from the insurance company may be significantly smaller than the award they might get from a jury, they get the money immediately rather than having to wait through a long appeals process that could take years. (For more information, go to http://www.lawfirms.com/resources/medical-malpractice/medical-negligence-lawsuits/why-sue-doctor-malpractice.htm or http://litigation.findlaw.com/filing-a-lawsuit/filing-a-lawsuit-should-you-sue.html or http://www.americannursetoday.com/article.aspx?id=8644.)

POSSIBLE DEFENSES TO A MALPRACTICE SUIT

Laws dealing with the awarding of damages vary from one state to another. The amount awarded also depends on the types of injuries sustained. Generally, the more severe the injuries, the greater the award due to the higher cost of treatment.

Contributory Negligence

In a state with contributory negligence laws, plaintiffs are not allowed to receive money for injuries if they contributed to those injuries in any manner. For example, a nurse forgot to raise the bed rail after administering an injection of a narcotic pain medication to a postoperative client but instructed the client to turn on the call light if he wanted to get out of bed. The client fell while attempting to go to the bathroom; because he did not use the call light, he contributed to his own injuries and thus could not receive compensation.

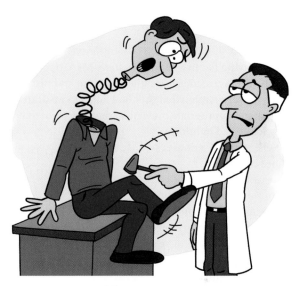

"I SUPPOSE THIS MEANS ANOTHER MALPRACTICE SUIT.

Comparative Negligence

In a state with comparative negligence laws, the awards are based on the determination of the percentage of fault by both parties. For example, in the aforementioned case, if $100,000 was awarded by the jury, it may be determined that the nurse was 75 percent at fault and the client was 25 percent at fault. In that case, the client would receive $75,000. In general, if the client is 50 percent or more at fault, no award will be made. Evidently, determination of these types of awards is highly subjective, and an **appeal** about the decision is almost always made to a higher court.

Case Study

Ms. Gouge, a 44-year-old client who weighed 307 pounds, was admitted to a large university medical center ED with complaints of chest pain and disorientation and a blood pressure of 208/154 mm Hg. She also displayed aphasia, hemiplegia, and loss of sensation and movement on her right side.

After an MRI scan of the head, it was discovered that she had an inoperable cerebral aneurysm. In addition to appropriate medical treatment for blood pressure and circulation, her family physician told her that she had to lose a significant amount of weight. The nurse in the physician's office instituted a weight loss teaching plan for Ms. Gouge, planned out a calorie-restricted low-fat diet, and gave her a large amount of information about a healthy diet and a DVD of low-impact aerobic exercises. At a follow-up visit 1 month later, Ms. Gouge weighed 315 pounds.

Six months later, Ms. Gouge's aneurysm ruptured, leaving her in a vegetative state. Ms. Gouge's family filed a lawsuit against the physician and his office nurse, claiming that they had failed to institute proper and appropriate preventive measures and that they had failed to inform the client of the seriousness of her condition.

Did the nurse's decisions or actions contribute to the filing of this suit? Is there any contributory negligence? What is the nurse's role in defending against this suit? What might the nurse have done to prevent the suit in the first place?

Assumption of Risk

When the client signs the informed consent form for a particular treatment, procedure, or surgery, it is implied that he or she is aware of the possible complications of that treatment, procedure, or surgery. Under the assumption-of-risk defense, if one of those listed or named complications occurs, the client has no grounds to sue the health-care provider. For example, a common complication from hip replacement surgery is some loss of mobility and range of motion of the affected leg. Even if a client, after having a hip replaced, is able to walk only using a walker, he or she still does not have any grounds for a lawsuit.

Good Samaritan Act

Health-care providers are sometimes hesitant to provide care at the scene of accidents, in emergency situations, or during disasters because they fear lawsuits. The **Good Samaritan Act** is designed specifically to

protect health-care providers in these situations. A health-care professional who provides care in an emergency situation cannot be sued for injuries that may be sustained by the client if that care was given according to established guidelines and was within the scope of the professional's education.

For example, a nurse who finds a person in cardiac arrest administers CPR to revive the person. In the process, she fractures several of the client's ribs. The client would not be able to sue the nurse for the fractured ribs if the CPR was administered according to established standards.

However, Good Samaritan laws do have some limitations. They do not cover nurses for grossly negligent acts in the provision of care or for acts outside the nurse's level of education. For example, in the case of a person choking on a piece of meat, the nurse initially attempts the Heimlich maneuver but without success. As the person loses consciousness, the nurse decides to perform a tracheostomy. The client survives but can sue the nurse for injuries from the tracheostomy because this is not a normal part of a nurse's education.

> *Health-care providers are sometimes hesitant to provide care at the scene of accidents, in emergency situations, or during disasters because they fear lawsuits. The Good Samaritan Act is designed specifically to protect health-care providers in these situations.*

Unavoidable Accident

Sometimes accidents happen without any contributing causes from the nurse, hospital, or physician. For example, a client is walking in the hall and trips over her own bathrobe. She breaks an ankle. There were no puddles on the floor or obstacles in the hall, and the client was alert and oriented. Because no one is at fault, there are no grounds for a lawsuit.

Defense of the Fact

Defense of the fact is based on the claim that the actions of the nurse followed the standards of care or that even if the actions were in violation of the standard of care, the actions themselves were not the direct cause of the injury.[4] For example, a nurse wraps a dressing too tightly on a client's foot after surgery. Later, the client loses his eyesight and blames the loss of vision on the nurse's improper dressing of his foot.

Going through the litigation process can produce high levels of anxiety. Placing every aspect of the nurse's conduct under scrutiny in a trial is very stressful. All aspects of the alleged negligent act will be examined and reexamined. Often events that happened years before can be brought in to establish a "pattern of behavior." Every word of the nurse's notes and the medical record will be closely analyzed and questioned. Nurses can survive the litigation process with the help of good attorneys and by being honest and demonstrating that they were acting in the best interests of the client. From this viewpoint, it is easy to see the importance of carrying nursing liability insurance.

ALTERNATIVE DISPUTE FORUMS

Although most lawsuits against nurses are settled through the court system, there are other methods of settling them. Because of the large number of cases and the resultant overload of the judicial system, different ways of resolving disputes have become increasingly more common. These alternative forums are being used for many types of conflict and are seen more frequently in the areas of torts, contracts, employment, and family law. Mediation and arbitration are the most commonly used alternatives to trial.

Mediation

Mediation is a process that allows each party to present his or her case before a mediator, who is an independent third party trained in dispute resolution. The mediator listens to each side individually. This one-sided session is called a *caucus*. The mediator's role is to find common ground between the parties and encourage resolution of the challenged matters by compromise and negotiation. The mediator aids the parties in arriving at a mutually acceptable outcome. The mediator does not act as a decision-maker but rather encourages the parties to come to a "meeting of the minds."

Arbitration

Arbitration, in contrast, allows a neutral third party to hear both parties' positions and then make a decision or ruling on the basis of the facts and evidence presented. Arbitration, by agreement or by statutory definition, can be binding or nonbinding. **Arbitrators**

> *Nurses can reinforce the physician teaching and even supplement the information but should not be the primary or only source of information for the informed consent. It is often difficult to draw a clear distinction between where the physician's responsibility ends and that of the nurse begins.*

or mediators are often retired judges who work on an hourly-fee basis or are practicing attorneys. In the family law area, they are frequently social workers or specially trained mediators. Negligence and malpractice issues are frequently resolved through arbitration and mediation.

COMMON ISSUES IN HEALTH-CARE LITIGATION

Nurses need to be aware of certain situations in the routine provision of care that constitute legal minefields. If the nurses are aware of these sensitive situations, they can exercise an extra degree of caution to make sure they are meeting standards of care and not violating a client's rights.

Informed Consent

Informed consent is both a legal and an ethical issue. Informed consent is the voluntary permission by a client or by the client's designated proxy to carry out a procedure on the client. Clients' claims that they did not grant informed consent before a surgery or invasive procedure can and do form the basis of a significant percentage of lawsuits.

Although these lawsuits are most often directed against physicians and hospitals, nurses can become involved when they provide the information but are not performing the procedure. The person who is performing the procedure has the responsibility to obtain the informed consent. However, some physicians habitually give the nurse the consent form and request him or her to "get the client to sign this." Informed consent can only be given by a client after the client receives sufficient information on:

- Treatment proposed.
- Material risk involved (potential complications).
- Acceptable alternative treatments.
- Outcome hoped for.
- Consequences of not having treatment.

The physician should provide most of this information. Nurses can reinforce the information given by the physician and even supplement the material but should not be the primary or only source of information for the informed consent.[8] It is often difficult to draw a clear distinction between where the physician's responsibility ends and that of the nurse begins.

What Do You Think?

Have you ever had a surgical procedure where you signed an informed consent form? Did it meet all five criteria listed? Which ones were missing?

Exceptions to Informed Consent

There are two exceptions to informed consent:

1. Emergency situations in which the client is unconscious, incompetent, or otherwise unable to give consent.
2. Situations in which the health-care provider feels that it may be medically contraindicated to disclose the risk and hazards because it may result in illness, severe emotional distress, serious psychological damage, or failure on the part of the client to receive lifesaving treatment.

Patient Self-Determination Act

The Patient Self-Determination Act of 1990, sponsored by Senator John Danforth, is a federal law that requires all federally funded institutions to inform clients of their right to prepare advance directives. The advance directives are meant to encourage people to discuss and document their wishes concerning the type of treatment and care that they want (i.e., life-sustaining treatment) in advance so that it will ease the burden on their families and providers when it comes time to make such a decision.

There are two types of advance directives: the living will and the medical durable power of attorney (Box 8.5). The **living will** is a document stating what health care a client will accept or refuse after the client is no longer competent or able to make that decision. The medical durable power of attorney, or health-care proxy, designates another person to make health-care decisions for a person if the client becomes incompetent or unable to make such decisions.

Each state outlines its own requirements for executing and revoking the medical durable power of attorney and living wills. These documents and rules can be accessed on the state's website, generally under the "Department of Health and Human Services" or a similar designation. Any particular state's living will

Box 8.5

Common Questions About Advance Directives

Q. Which is better—a living will or a medical durable power of attorney for health care or health-care proxy?

A. The documents are different and allow the nurse to do two different things. The living will states what health-care procedures a client will accept or refuse after the client is no longer competent or able to make that decision. The medical durable power of attorney or health-care proxy allows a client to designate another person to make health-care choices for him or her.

Q. If I change my mind and have a living will, can I cancel the living will or durable medical power of attorney?

A. Yes, each state has ways that your advance directives can be canceled or negated. Most states require an oral or written statement, destruction of the document, or notification to certain individuals, such as the physician. Again, each state's statute should be checked for the specific details required.

Q. If I have a living will in one state, is it good in all states?

A. It may or may not be, depending on that state's requirements for the living will. It is important that you have your living will checked by an attorney to determine whether or not it may be effective in the states in which you are traveling or working.

Q. If I have a living will and have a medical durable power of attorney, who should get copies?

A. Copies should be given to your next of kin, your physician, and your attorney so that more than one person has a copy and knows what your intentions are. Some states will allow you to register your living will with certain state agencies such as the Secretary of State. There are also national groups that will allow you to register your living will with them so that there is access to it.

form can be downloaded by going to the National Hospice and Palliative Care Organization's website at http://www.caringinfo.org/i4a/pages/index.cfm?pageid=3289 or the Partnership for Caring website at http://www.partnershipforcaring.org.

Incompetent Client's Right to Self-Determination

The courts are protective of incompetent clients and require high standards of proof before allowing a physician to terminate any life-sustaining treatment for that client. Consider the following example:

The issue before the U.S. Supreme Court was whether the state of Missouri could use its own standard of clear and convincing proof for removal of the tube or whether there was a 14th Amendment due process guarantee of a "right to die" that would override the state statute. It was decided that the constitutional right would not be extended and the state procedural requirement would be allowed, at which time the burden of proof was put on Cruzan's family to show that she would not have wanted to continue living in this manner.

Many aspects of the Terri Schiavo case in Florida parallel the Cruzan case. In the Schiavo case, after the feeding tube was removed by order of a Florida state judge, the U.S. Congress became involved and passed a bill, signed by President George W. Bush, that required the case be heard by the U.S. Supreme Court. The goal was to have the tube reinserted until the high court could rule on the case. It is interesting to note that not much progress has been made in developing legal solutions for this type of case during the 20-plus years since the Cruzan case.

> *Nancy Cruzan was 30 years old and in a persistent vegetative state. She had a gastrostomy feeding and hydration tube inserted to assist with feedings, which her husband consented to. Her parents, however, petitioned the court for removal of the tube. In the Cruzan case, the court held that the state had the right to err on the side of life. The U.S. Supreme Court recognized that a living will would have been sufficient evidence of Cruzan's wishes to sustain or to remove her feeding tube.*

The Nurse's Role in Advance Directives

Because laws vary from state to state, it is important that nurses know the laws of the state in which they practice that pertain to advance directives, clients' rights, and the policies and procedures of the institution in which they work. Nurses must inform clients of their right to formulate advance directives and must realize that not all clients can make such decisions.

It is important for the nurse to establish trust and rapport with a client and the client's family so that the nurse can assist them in making decisions that are in the client's best interests.[9] Nurses must also teach about advance directives and document all critical decisions, discussions with the client and client's family about such decisions, and the basis for the evaluation process. Also, it is essential to prevent discrimination against clients and their families based on their choices regarding their advance directives.

It is important that nurses determine whether clients have been coerced into making advance directive decisions against their will. Nurses need to become involved in ethics committees at hospitals or nursing specialty groups at local, state, or national levels to help clients come to a comfortable resolution about advance directives.

Do-Not-Resuscitate Orders

Although a DNR instruction may be included in an advance directive, DNR orders are legally separate from advance directives. For the health-care professional to be legally protected, there should be a written order for a "no code" or a DNR order in the client's chart.

Protection for the Nurse

Each hospital should have a policy and procedure that outlines what is required with regard to a client's condition for a DNR order. The DNR order should be reviewed, evaluated, and reordered. Different facilities have established different time periods for these reviews. Nurses must also know whether there is any law that regulates who should authorize a DNR order for an incompetent client who is no longer able to make this decision. Hospitals often have policies and procedures describing what must be done and which clients fit the requirements for a DNR order. The American Nurses Association (ANA) published a position statement on nursing care and DNR decisions.[10] The position statement stresses the need for nurses to talk with clients and their families about the DNR decision so that they are fully informed when they make the decision. It includes discussing the benefits and burdens of prolonged treatments, what comfort measures are possible, the effects of symptom palliation, and the understanding that aggressive life sustaining technology will be withdrawn if it does not meet the goals and wishes of the client and his or her family. Any decision about a DNR needs to be based on the client's right to self-determination in order to be ethical.

Nurses face many legal dilemmas when dealing with confusing or conflicting DNR orders. For example, it may be difficult to interpret a DNR order when it has been restricted—for instance, "do not resuscitate except for medications and defibrillation" or "no CPR or intubation." Often a lack of proper documentation in the medical records indicating how the DNR decision was reached can be a critical issue if a medical malpractice case is involved and it is disputed whether or not the client or family actually gave consent for the order.

Many facilities have developed DNR decision sheets. A DNR sheet may record information about DNR discussions or be dated and signed by the client and those family members who took part in the discussion. It then becomes a permanent part of the medical record.

Protection for the Client

It is very important that nurses not stigmatize clients by the use of indicators for DNR orders, such as dots on the wristband or over the bed. Health-care providers' attitudes often change because they feel that the client is "going to die anyway." This abandonment can jeopardize the care of a client designated with a DNR order. However, it is also important for the nurses and staff to know whether an order is to be honored and what the policies and procedures are with regard to transfer clients and DNR orders that accompany the incoming client.[10]

Information about the DNR status of a client should be obtained during shift reports. If there has not been a periodic review, is the order still in effect? If a client is transferred from one facility to another and has a DNR order that is time limited and has not been reordered, what should a nurse do?

Standards of Care

Standards of care are the yardsticks that the legal system use to measure the actions of a nurse involved in a malpractice suit. The underlying principle used to establish standards of care is based on the actions that would probably be taken by a reasonable person (nurse) in the same or similar circumstances.

> *Because laws vary from state to state, it is important that nurses know the laws of the state in which they practice that pertain to advance directives, clients' rights, and the policies and procedures of the institution in which they work.*

The standard usually includes both objective factors (e.g., the actions to be performed) and subjective factors (e.g., the nurse's emotional and mental state). Specifically, a nurse is judged against the standards that are established within the profession and specialty area of practice. The ANA and specialty groups within the nursing profession, such as the American Association of Critical-Care Nurses (AACN), publish standards of care that are updated continually as health-care technology and practices change. Recently, standards of care have become the concern of the U.S. government. The Affordable Care Act of 2010 addresses standards of care both directly and indirectly. Particular areas addressed are limiting readmissions, formation of Accountable Care Organizations (ACOs), and the review of the quality of care provided by physicians and hospitals.[11]

External Standards

Both external and internal standards govern the conduct of nurses. External standards include nursing standards developed by the ANA, the state nurse practice act of each jurisdiction, criteria from accrediting agencies such as the Joint Commission (JC), guidelines developed by various nursing specialty practice groups, and federal agency regulations. Nurses are encountering an increasing number of incidents in which conflicts occur between institutional and professional standards—for example, in staffing ratios. These disputes are difficult to resolve and may require deliberation and decisions from institutional committees. As a general rule, when a conflict exists, it is safer legally to follow professional standards.

Internal Standards

Internal standards include nursing standards defined in specific hospital policy and procedure manuals that relate to the nurse in the particular institution. The nurse's job description and employment contract are examples of internal nursing standards that define the duty of the nurse.

Criteria for Good Care

The rationale for advancing standards of care for the nurse is to ensure proper, consistent, and high-quality nursing care to all members of society. When nurses violate their duty of care to the client as established by the profession's standards of care, they leave themselves open to charges of negligence and malpractice. Until recently, nurses were held to the standards of the local community. National criteria have now replaced most **locality rule standards of care.** Individual nurses are held accountable not only to acceptable standards within the local community but also to national standards.

Although standards of care may seem to be specific, they are merely guidelines for nursing practice. Because every client's situation is different, the appropriate standard of care may be difficult to identify in a certain case. More than one course of nursing action may be considered appropriate under a proper standard of care. The final decision must be guided by the nurse's judgment and understanding of the client's needs.

The Nurse Practice Act

The nurse practice act defines nursing practice and establishes standards for nurses in each state. It is the most definitive legal statute or legislative act regulating nursing practice. Although nurse practice acts vary in scope from one state to another, they tend to have similar wording based loosely on the ANA model published in 1988. The nurse practice act provides a framework for the court on which to base decisions when determining whether a nurse has breached a standard of care.

> " *Nurses are encountering an increasing number of incidents in which conflicts occur between institutional and professional standards—for example, in staffing ratios.* "

Most state nurse practice acts define scope of practice, establish requirements for licensure and entry into practice, and create and empower a board of nursing to oversee the practice of nurses. In addition, nurse practice acts identify grounds for disciplinary actions such as suspension and revocation of a nursing license.[12]

The judicial interpretation of the nurse practice act and its relationship to a specific case provide guidance for decisions about future cases. Many state legislatures have responded to the expanded role of the nurse by broadening the scope of their nurse practice acts. For example, the addition of the term *nursing diagnosis* to many states' nurse practice acts reflects the legislature's recognition of the expansion of the nurse's role.

Although some states were beginning to include occupational roles such as nurse practitioner, **nurse clinician,** and clinical nurse specialist in their nurse practice acts, the process was inconsistent and confusing. To address this confusion, in 2008 the APRN Consensus Work Group and the National Council of State Boards of Nursing (NCSBN) APRN Advisory Committee issued a report on the Licensure, Accreditation, Certification, and Education (LACE) of APRNs. This statement addresses the lack of common definitions regarding APRN practice, the ever-increasing numbers of specializations, the inconsistency in credentials and scope of practice, and the wide variations in education for ARNPs. The goal is to implement the APRN Model of Regulation in all states by 2015 (for a more detailed discussion of the model, see Chapter 5). It is important to remember that as the nurse's role expands, so does the legal accountability of the role.[13]

PREVENTING LAWSUITS

What can the nurse do to avoid having to go through the stressful, sometimes financially and professionally devastating, process of litigation? The following guidelines provide some ways to avoid a lawsuit.

Effective Communication

After many years of collecting data and analyzing sentinel and critical events, the JC concluded that miscommunication among health-care workers is the leading cause of health-care-related errors leading to injury, death, and lawsuits. The Commission called for a communication strategy that would be concrete, would provide a framework for communication between caregivers, and would be easy for all health-care workers to remember. It would need to work in all situations, from end-of-shift reports to exchanges in high-pressure critical care areas, when a nurse's immediate responses and actions could make the difference between life and death. Care expectations could be communicated in a focused, simple way that allowed all team members to understand and respond quickly. The overall goal is to develop a "culture of client safety" that would permeate any organization.[14]

Situation, Background, Assessment, Recommendation (SBAR)

The SBAR system (pronounced "S-BAR") was initially developed by the U.S. Navy to improve communications on the nuclear submarine fleet. Refined and adopted by Kaiser Permanente of Colorado in the late 1990s, SBAR is being incorporated into health-care facilities and is working its way into the nursing education system. SBAR has proven useful when a client's status changes unexpectedly. A review of client charts in these emergency situations shows how confused the communication between the physician and the nurse can be. Fatigue, lack of experience, or reduced nursing education often leads to the omission of key information. In this type of situation, SBAR forms an outline for the communication of critical information.[15]

Each of the letters in SBAR stands for a step in the process:

Situation: Asks the question, "What is going on?" Information to provide or look for:
- Identify yourself, the hospital unit or health-care location, and the room number.
- Identify the client by name, age, gender, and date of birth.
- Describe the problem the client has that triggered the SBAR communication.

Background: Provides key information that will help determine what actions to take:
- Give a short summary of the client's relevant past medical history.
- Provide the client's diagnosis.
- Describe the client's current mental status, current vital signs, complaints, pain level, oxygen saturation, and physical assessment findings.

Assessment: Allows the nurse to analyze the situation and isolate the specific problem:
- Note what vital signs are outside of parameters.
- Give the nurse's clinical impressions of the client and additional concerns.
- Rank the severity of the client's condition.
- Identify specific client needs to resolve the situation.

Recommendation: Identifies what actions will resolve the situation:
- Identify what needs to be done to resolve the client's problem.

- Note how urgent the problem is and when action needs to be taken.
- Suggest what action should be taken.
- State the desired client response.[16]

Here is an example of how an SBAR communication could be used:

Situation: Hello, Dr. Nife, this is Alexis Zanetti, RN, in the step-down unit, calling about Mr. Jenkins. He is a 68-year-old male client born in October 1947. He had a femoral bypass graft done yesterday. He was undergoing cardiac monitoring according to protocol, and within the last 15 minutes went from a sinus rhythm to an atrial fibrillation of 165 beats per minute.

Background: As you know, Mr. Jenkins has a history of cardiac disease, including a myocardial infarction in 2005. He has type 1 diabetes and has had several deep vein thromboses over the past 3 years. He has an intravenous (IV) infusion of D5 half-normal saline running at 125 mL per hour. He is complaining of some slight chest pressure. His incision site is clean and dry, and he has +2 pedal pulses in both feet.

Assessment: His blood pressure normally runs 136/76, pulse 90, respiration 18, and O_2 saturation 96 percent. His current vital signs are: blood pressure, 98/54; pulse, 165; respirations, 26; O_2 saturation, 89 percent; and urine output, 82 mL per hour. This is the first time he has complained of chest pressure, but ranks it as only a 2 on a 1-to-10 scale. The vital sign changes all occurred shortly after the change in his cardiac rhythm. His neurological status is unchanged, and the femoral graft has not been affected by the cardiovascular changes. He has been taking sips by mouth and tolerating it well.

Recommendations: It appears that restoring Mr. Jenkins to normal sinus rhythm is the highest priority. What would you think about restarting him on Lanoxin, 0.25 mg, which was discontinued preoperatively? We could give it either by IV or by mouth because he is tolerating water.

In general, nurses feel uncomfortable making medical recommendations to physicians. Also, some physicians do not handle recommendations

> *The medical record is the single most frequently used piece of objective evidence in a malpractice suit. In preparation for the trial, the lawyers attempt to reconstruct the events surrounding the incident in a minute-by-minute time line.*

from nurses very well. However, recommendations are part of the SBAR process, and the physician can always just say no. Disguising the recommendations in the form of a question softens the impact and meets with more success.[17]

Medical Record

Charting in the medical record, whether it is still paper or, more likely, an electronic health record (EHR), is the best way to display the care provided and the communication between health-care workers. It is the single most frequently used piece of objective evidence in a malpractice suit. In preparation for the trial, the lawyers attempt to reconstruct the events surrounding the incident in a minute-by-minute time line. The client's **chart** is the most important source for this time line. Maintaining an accurate and complete medical record is an absolute requirement (Box 8.6).

In nursing and medical negligence claims, lawyers are beginning to ask whether the hospital has adopted the use of SBAR. They examine the materials used to educate the staff and any policies or procedures concerning the use of SBAR. They note any mention of SBAR communication in the medical record and see whether it is recorded properly.[17] Even if the facility has not adopted SBAR as a hospital-wide communication technique, nurses who know how can use it to help protect themselves in subsequent legal actions.

The old adage, "If it isn't written, it didn't happen" remains true in most situations; however, recent court trials have recognized some exceptions. Some judges and juries have begun to recognize that charting by exception is a valid form of health-care record-keeping. Charting by exception, very closely related to problem-oriented charting, was developed initially to save time for busy nurses and money for the facility by reducing the volume of documents created and stored. In institutions that use charting by exception, the nurse charts only those elements of client care that are abnormal or unusual or that constitute a health-care problem. If the client is stable and recovering as expected, there may be very little written in the chart about his or her physical or mental assessments.

Trying to recall specific events from 2 to 6 years ago without the benefit of written notes is almost impossible. In general, the client record should *not* contain personal opinion, should be legible, should be in chronological order, and should be written and signed by the nurse. Although opinions have a relatively low value in legal proceedings, the documentation should indicate the nursing judgments made. An entry should never be obliterated or destroyed. If a nurse questions a physician's order, a record must be made that the physician was contacted and the order clarified.

Rapport With Clients

Establishing a rapport with the client through honest, open communication goes a long way in avoiding lawsuits. Treating clients and their families with respect and letting them know that the nurse really cares about them may well prevent a lawsuit. Many people are willing to forgive a nurse's error if they have good rapport and a trusting relationship with a nurse who they believe is interested in their well-being.

> *Being direct, solving problems with the client, and helping the client become involved in his or her care are helpful in defusing this negative behavior.*

Current Nursing Skills

Keeping one's nursing knowledge and skills current is vital to preventing errors that may lead to lawsuits. It is better to refuse to perform an unfamiliar procedure than to attempt it without the necessary knowledge and skills. Taking advantage of in-service training, workshops, and continuing nursing education classes is an important part of maintaining the nurse's skill level.[18] Nurses must practice within their level of competence and scope of practice.

Knowledge of the Client

Recognizing the client who is lawsuit prone can help reduce the risk for litigation. Some common characteristics of this type of client include constant dissatisfaction with the care given, constant complaints about all aspects of care, and negative comments about other nurses. This client often complains about the poor care given by nurses on the previous shift and may also have a history of lawsuits against nurses.

Being direct, solving problems with the client, and helping the client become involved in his

B o x 8 . 6

Some Documentation Guidelines

Medications
- Always chart the time, route, dose, and response.
- Always chart prn medications and the client response.
- Always chart when a medication was not given, the reason (e.g., client in x-ray, physical therapy, etc.; do not chart that the medication was not on the floor), and the nursing intervention.
- Chart all medication refusals and report them to the appropriate source.

Physician Communication
- Document each time a call is made to a physician, even if he or she is not reached. Include the exact time of the call. If the physician is reached, document the details of the message and the physician response.
- Read verbal orders back to the physician and confirm the client's identity as written on the chart. Chart only verbal orders that you have heard from the source, not those told to you by another nurse or unit personnel.

Formal Issues in Charting
- Before writing on the chart, check to be sure you have the correct client record.
- Check to make sure each page has the client's name and the current date stamped in the appropriate area.
- If you forgot to make an entry, chart "late entry" and place the date and time at the entry.
- Correct all charting mistakes according to the policy and procedures of your institution.
- Chart in an organized fashion, following the nursing process.
- Write legibly and concisely and avoid subjective statements.
- Write specific and accurate descriptions.
- When charting a symptom or situation, chart the interventions taken and the client response.
- Document your own observations, not those that were told to you by another party.
- Chart frequently to demonstrate ongoing care and chart routine activities.
- Chart client and family teaching and the response.

Source: Tappen RM, et al. *Essentials of Nursing Leadership and Management* (2nd ed.). Philadelphia: FA Davis, 2001, p. 169, with permission.

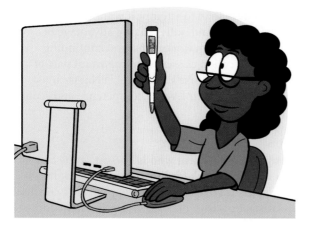

CHARTING VITAL SIGNS ASAP IS IMPORTANT.

or her care are helpful in defusing this negative behavior. Also, even more careful documentation of the care provided and the client's responses to the care can be helpful if a lawsuit is filed later.

Families can also be an important factor in lawsuits. Establishing a good relationship with family members when they are visiting, keeping them informed, recognizing that they are an important part of the recovery process, and providing them small comforts such as a cup of coffee or a soft drink while they are waiting goes a long way in softening the impact of bad news.

What Do You Think?

Think about being involved in a legal or courtroom activity as a defendant, complainant, witness, or juror. What would your role be in each situation?

LIABILITY INSURANCE

Maintaining proper liability insurance is a necessity. Nurses who do not carry liability insurance place themselves at high risk. The nurse's personal assets, as well as wages, may be subject to a judgment awarded in a malpractice action. Even if the client does not win at the trial, the litigation process, including hiring a lawyer and paying the costs of experts, can be financially devastating.

A professional liability insurance policy is a contract with an insurer who promises to assume the costs paid to the injured party in exchange for paying a premium (Box 8.7). There are two types of malpractice policies: claims made and occurrence. **Claims-made policies** protect only against claims made during the time the policy is in effect. **Occurrence policies** protect against all claims that occur during the policy period, regardless of when the claim is made. Generally, the occurrence type of liability insurance offers more protection. Claims-made policy coverage can be broadened by purchasing a tail—a separate policy that extends the time of coverage.

Some hospitals have liability insurance policies for the nurse as a part of the nurse's employment package with the institution. This hospital policy may be limited to claims arising from the nurse's employment and might not apply in a situation in which a nurse renders care outside the institution—for instance, at an automobile crash site.[19] It is preferable

---

Box 8.7

What to Look for in an Insurance Policy

The following factors should be reviewed to determine what is the best policy for your type of nursing practice:

1. Type of insurance policy (claims-made or occurrence basis)
2. Insuring agreement. The insurance company's promise to pay in exchange for premiums is called the *insuring agreement*. The insurance company agrees to pay a money award to a plaintiff who is injured by an act of omission or commission by a health-care provider who is insured by the company.
3. Types of injuries covered. The language must be scrutinized to determine whether it is broad or limiting. Some companies will agree to pay only if the insured nurse is sued for damages, which means the nurse must be sued for a money amount or award. If the nurse is sued for a specific performance lawsuit or an injunctive relief action, which means that the nurse will either have to perform something or discontinue doing something, that particular insurance policy may not be adequate. Also, most insurance policies do not cover the nurse for disciplinary actions.
4. Exclusions. Items that are not covered by a policy are called *exclusions*. It is important to review the exclusions. Some of the more common exclusions include sexual abuse of a client, injury caused while under the influence of drugs or alcohol, criminal activity, and punitive damages. Punitive damages are used to punish the defendant for egregious acts or omissions.

Who Is Covered Under the Policy
The purchaser is the named insured and can be an individual, institution, or group. Others who may be covered by the policy are nurses, employees, agents, and volunteers, among others.

Limitations and Deductions
In exchange for payment of the premium, the insurance company agrees to pay up to a certain amount on behalf of the insured. This amount is called the *limit of liability*. It is usually expressed in two ways: the amount that can be paid per incident (per occurrence) and the amount that will be paid for the entire policy year. For example, if you have a policy that states $1,000,000/$3,000,000, it means that the company will pay up to $1 million per incident and a total of $3 million per policy year. The insurance industry relies on the A. M. Best Company to evaluate both the financial size and relative strengths of insurance companies. An A. M. Best rating of A or better should be a prerequisite for purchase of any policy.

The Right to Select Counsel
Some insurance companies allow nurses to select their own attorneys to represent them in a medical negligence claim. Others retain attorneys or law firms, and the nurse does not have the opportunity to make that selection.

The Right to Consent to Settlement
Some policies allow the nurse to decide whether a case should be settled or go to trial, whereas others do not.

to have liability insurance coverage that includes all situations in which the nurse may be involved.

Individual indemnity insurance coverage independent of the facility's policy is recommended for all nurses. With passage of the **Federal Tort Claims Act** and similar state laws, nurses who were formerly protected from lawsuits by working at federal or state health-care facilities can now be sued for malpractice like nurses at any other facility.

REVOCATION OF LICENSE

One of the most severe punishments that a nurse can experience is revocation of the license to practice nursing. The nursing profession is responsible for monitoring and enforcing its own standards through the state licensing board. These actions may or may not be related to tort law, contract law, or criminal charges. Each state's licensing board is charged with the responsibility to oversee the professional nurse's competence.

The state's nursing board receives its authority to grant and revoke licenses from specific statutory laws. The underlying rationale for establishment of a licensing board is to protect the public from uneducated, unsafe, or unethical practitioners. If nurses fail to adhere to the standards of safe practice and exhibit unprofessional behavior, they can be disciplined by the state nursing licensing board.[20] One of the

remedies that these boards can use is suspension or revocation of a nurse's license.

The Disciplinary Hearing

A disciplinary hearing is held to review the charges of the nurse's unprofessional conduct. This hearing is less formal than the trial process, and the nurse is allowed to present evidence and be represented by legal counsel at the hearing. Due process requires that the nurse be notified in advance of the specific charges being made. The question of what constitutes unprofessional conduct is an issue frequently dealt with at the disciplinary hearing. Each respective state's nurse practice act provides guidance with regard to the specifics of unprofessional conduct.

Unprofessional conduct can be reported by a nursing peer, a supervisor, a client, or a client's family.[20] Many cases are dismissed before the hearing takes place if the board finds there is no support for the allegation being made against the nurse. If a hearing is necessary, it is in the best interest of the nurse to seek legal counsel because of the potential risk of license revocation.

License revocation is a serious consequence for the nurse because it removes the nurse's right to practice. Drug abuse, administering medication without a prescription, practicing without a valid license, and any singular act of unprofessional or unethical conduct can constitute grounds for losing a nursing license.

> " *The nursing profession is responsible for monitoring and enforcing its own standards through the state licensing board.* "

Conclusion

The legal system and its effects on the practice of nursing are ever-present realities in today's health-care system. Nurses need to be aware of the implications of their actions but should not be so overwhelmed by fear that it reduces their ability to care for the client. The more advanced and specialized the nurse's

practice becomes, the higher the standards to which the nurse is held. Nurses will be challenged throughout their careers to apply legal principles in the daily practice of nursing. An awareness of what constitutes malpractice and negligence will aid in the prevention of litigation.

Critical-Thinking Exercises

onsider the following case: *Thomas v. Corso* (MD 1982). The client was brought to the hospital emergency department (ED) after being involved in an automobile accident. The ED nurse assessed and recorded the client's vital signs and a complaint of numbness in his right anterior thigh. The client was able to move the right leg, and there was no discoloration or deformity. After he was given meperidine (Demerol) for his pain, his blood pressure (BP) dropped to 90/60 mm Hg, and the nurse notified the ED physician of the change. The physician ordered the nurse to arrange for admission to the hospital, which she did.

The client was transferred to a medical-surgical unit, but he could not be placed in a room because of an influenza epidemic. He was placed in the hall next to the nurses' station for close observation. A nurse checked the client's vital signs about 20 minutes after the transfer and noted that the BP was now 70/50, respiratory rate 40, and pulse 120. His skin was cool and diaphoretic, his breathing was deep and rapid, and he was asking for a drink of water. The client also complained of pain in his leg, but the nurse did not give him more pain medication because of his blood pressure.

The nurse assessed him about 30 minutes later and found his skin warmer, although he still complained of pain and thirst. The nurse also noted a strong odor of alcohol on the client's breath. An assistant supervisor also assessed the client's condition but refused to give him any water because he had obviously been drinking alcohol. She had been told about the low blood pressure by the client's nurse but attributed it to the alcohol and pain medication combination. The nurse checked his vital signs again and found a BP of 100/89. Thirty minutes later, it was 94/70, pulse 100, and respirations 28. When the nurse next assessed the client an hour later, he had a Cheyne-Stokes respiratory pattern, no pulse, and no blood pressure. She started CPR and called a "code blue," but after a lengthy attempt at resuscitation, the client died.

An autopsy was performed and showed that the client had a lacerated liver and a severe fracture of the femur with bleeding into the tissues. The coroner determined that traumatic shock, secondary to the fractured femur and lacerated liver, was the cause of death. His family sued the nurses for poor judgment and the hospital for malpractice and won.

- What mistakes were made by the nurses in this case?
- What legal liability did the nurses incur by their actions?
- How can the nurses best prepare for trial in this case?
- What actions could the nurses have taken with this client to prevent a lawsuit?
- What are your feelings toward inebriated clients? Did the nurses' attitudes about inebriation affect their judgment?
- Why are clients who are drunk at higher risk for injury and poor medical outcomes than other clients?

References

1. March AL, Ford CD, Adams MH, Cheshire M, Collins AS. The mock trial: A collaborative interdisciplinary approach to understanding legal and ethical issues. *Nurse Educator,* 36(2):66–69, 2011.

2. Guido G. *Legal and Ethical Issues in Nursing* (5th ed.). Upper Saddle River, NJ: Pearson Prentice Hall, 2009.

3. Aiken TD. *Legal and Ethical Issues in Health Occupations.* St. Louis, Saunders Elsevier: 2009.

4. Kopishke L, Peterson AM. *Legal Nurse Consulting: Principles and Practices* (3rd ed.). Medford, MA: Taylor & Francis, 2010.

5. McEwen DA, Dumpel H. HIPAA—the health insurance portability and accountability act: What RNs need to know about privacy rules and protected health information. *National Nurse,* 107(7):18–26, 2011.

6. Clinch T. Nursing practice question: Is texting/receiving patient information a HIPAA rules violation? *Nursing News,* 36(2):8, 2012.

7. Yee T, Needleman J, Pearson M, Parkerton P, Parkerton M, Wolstein J. The influence of integrated electronic medical records and computerized nursing notes on nurses' time spent in documentation. *Computers, Informatics, Nursing,* 30(6):287–292, 2012.

8. Mahjoub R, Rutledge DN. Perceptions of informed consent for care practices: Hospitalized patients and nurses. *Applied Nursing Research,* 24(4):276–280, 2011.

9. Watson E. Advance directives: Self-determination, legislation, and litigation issues. *Journal of Legal Nurse Consulting,* 21(1):9–14, 2010.

10. Abbo ED, Yuen TC, Buhrmester L, Geocadin R, Volandes AE, Siddique J, Edelson DP. Cardiopulmonary resuscitation outcomes in hospitalized community-dwelling individuals and nursing home residents based on activities of daily living. *Journal of the American Geriatrics Society,* 61(1):34–39, 2013.

11. Correia EW. Accountable care organizations: The proposed regulations and the prospects for success. *American Journal of Managed Care,* 17(8):560–568, 2011.

12. Russell KA. Nurse practice acts guide and govern nursing practice. *Journal of Nursing Regulation,* 3(3):36–42, 2012.

13. National Council of State Boards of Nursing. Consensus Model for APRN Regulation: Licensure, Accreditation, Certification and Education. Retrieved March 2013 from http://www.ncsbn.org/7_23_08_Consensue_APRN_Final.pdf, 2008.

14. Boaro N, Fancott C, Baker R, Velji K, Andreoli A. Using SBAR to improve communication in interprofessional rehabilitation teams . . . Situation-Background-Assessment-Recommendation. *Journal of Interprofessional Care,* 24(1):111–114, 2010.

15. Novak K, Fairchild R. Bedside reporting and SBAR: Improving patient communication and satisfaction. *Journal of Pediatric Nursing,* 27(6):760–762, 2012.

16. Beckett CD, Kipnis G. Collaborative communication: Integrating SBAR to improve quality/patient safety outcomes. *Journal for Healthcare Quality: Promoting Excellence in Healthcare,* 31(5):19–28, 2009.

17. Guhde J. Using high fidelity simulation to teach nurse-to-doctor-report: A study on SBAR in an undergraduate nursing curriculum. *Clinical Simulation in Nursing,* 6(3):115, 2010. Retrieved June 2013 from http://www.saferhealthcare.com/cat-shc/sbar-a-communication-technique

18. Brous E. Professional licensure protection strategies. *American Journal of Nursing,* 112(12):43–47, 2012.

19. Anselmi KK. Ethics, law, and policy. Nurses' personal liability vs. employer's vicarious liability. *Medical/Surgical Nursing,* 21(1):45–48, 2012.

20. Pugh D. A fine line: The role of personal and professional vulnerability in allegations of unprofessional conduct. *Journal of Nursing Law,* 14(1):21–31, 2012.

NCLEX: What You Need to Know

Joseph T. Catalano

Learning Objectives

After completing this chapter, the reader will be able to:

- Describe the NCLEX-RN, CAT test plan
- Discuss the NCLEX-RN, CAT test format
- Analyze and identify the different types of questions used on the NCLEX-RN, CAT
- Select the most appropriate means for preparing for the NCLEX-RN, CAT

I DON'T WANT TO TAKE THIS EXAM!

The primary purpose of licensure examinations is to protect the public from unsafe or uneducated practitioners of a profession. When you pass the National Council Licensure Examination (NCLEX), it indicates that you have the minimal level of knowledge or competency deemed necessary by the state to practice nursing without injury to clients. Licensure is a legal requirement for all professions that deal with public health, welfare, or safety.

Most people have varying levels of anxiety before taking an exam. The more important the examination, the higher the anxiety level. Anxiety is sometimes defined as fear of the unknown. This chapter presents key information about the NCLEX test plan to better help you understand and anticipate what you will encounter when you take the exam. It also includes some suggestions for study for the NCLEX and do's and don'ts for the exam. This information should help lower your anxiety about the NCLEX. Sample practice questions throughout the chapter give you an idea of how the NCLEX asks about different types of nursing information. This chapter should be used in conjunction with Bonus Chapter 1 on the Davis*Plus* site. Try to answer these questions as you read. The answers and rationales are found at the end of the chapter.

NCLEX TEST PLAN

The NCLEX is a computerized, **criterion-referenced examination** that you take after you graduate from nursing school. Unlike a **norm-referenced examination**, which bases a passing score on the scores of others who took the exam, criterion-referenced examinations compare your knowledge to a preestablished standard. If you meet or exceed the standard, you pass. The NCLEX measures nursing knowledge of a wide range of subject matter, but it mostly measures your ability to think critically and make sound judgments about nursing care. With computerized adaptive tests such as the NCLEX, the computer selects questions in accordance with the examination plan and how you answered the previous questions.

Changes in the Test Plan

Every 3 years, the National Council of State Boards of Nursing (NCSBN) undertakes an analysis of current nursing practice, with the most recent changes beginning April 1, 2013. An expert panel of nine nurses conducts a survey that asks approximately 12,000 newly licensed nurses about the frequency and importance of performing the 15 NCLEX-RN test plan nursing care activities. These activities are then analyzed in relation to the frequency of performance, impact on maintaining client safety, and client care settings where the activities are performed.

Because the findings of the NCSBN survey indicated an increase in the complexity of care, the difficulty level required to pass was increased by 0.05 logits (from minus 0.21 logits in 2009 to minus 0.16 logits in spring 2010). In the past, when the criterion difficulty level was increased, the national average pass rate decreased between 3 and 5 percent.

Questions Distributed by Category

In the past, the numbers of questions from each of the five categories were more or less equal. The percentages changed in 2010 and were again changed in 2013. Questions dealing with management and management issues have increased to 17 to 23 percent (increased by 1 percent) of the exam, the highest percentage of any single type of question. Pharmacology-related questions actually were decreased by 1 percent, to 12 to 18 percent of the exam. Both

of these increases reflect issues found in current nursing practice.

The NCLEX Computerized Adaptive Testing for Registered Nurses (NCLEX-RN, CAT) test plan is organized into three primary components: (1) client needs, (2) level of cognitive ability, and (3) integrated concepts and processes. The third component was expanded to include nursing process, caring, communication, cultural awareness, documentation, self-care, and teaching and learning. Alternative-format questions are now being used, and the length of time allowed to complete the exam is 6 hours.

Client Health Needs

The NCLEX asks questions about four general groups of material called *client health needs*:

- Safe and effective care environment
- Physiological integrity
- Psychosocial integrity
- Health promotion and maintenance needs

Safe and Effective Care Environment (21 to 33 percent)

a. Management of care: 17 to 23 percent of NCLEX questions
b. Safety and infection control: 9 to 15 percent of NCLEX questions

The questions in this category make up between 25 and 38 percent of the total questions on the NCLEX. These questions deal with overt safety issues in client care (e.g., use of restraints), medication administration, safety measures to prevent injuries (e.g., putting up side rails), prevention of infections, isolation precautions, safety measures with pediatric clients, and special safety needs of clients with psychiatric problems.

This needs category also includes questions about laboratory tests, their results, and any special nursing measures associated with them; legal and ethical issues in nursing; a small amount of nursing management; and quality assurance issues. Questions on these issues are interspersed with other questions throughout the examination.

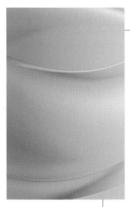

Issues Now

Handling Your Anxiety

It is perfectly reasonable to be slightly anxious about taking the NCLEX. You have expended plenty of blood, sweat, and tears to reach this point. As one diploma graduate told me, "I was in debt up to my ears and running out of money fast when I took the NCLEX. Passing was literally my meal ticket." Even if you're not in such dire financial straits, it's no small thing to be tested on years of accumulated knowledge. You would have to be comatose not to feel butterflies in your stomach at this point. Do not be anxious about being anxious.

Because you cannot go back and change answers, treat each question as an exam in itself; once you hit the "Next (N)" button, immediately turn your attention to the next question. Tell yourself not to be surprised by anything. You are at a psychological disadvantage if you expect the computer to turn off at a certain number and it doesn't. So if you can, avoid looking at the question number as you answer each question.

If you are distracted by the clicking of other people's computers or other such annoying sounds, you can ask for earplugs. The testing service provides them.

Finally, there are going to be other people close to you or next to you who may sit down at the computer at the same time as you do. They may get up before you, but ignore them. The testing centers administer many different tests, so you can realistically tell yourself that the person next to you who finished in 45 minutes was not even taking the NCLEX. Even if they were taking the NCLEX, you do not need to think about it.

Source: Dunham, KS. *How to Survive and Maybe Even Love Nursing School.* Philadelphia, FA Davis: 2008, pp. 101–115, with permission.

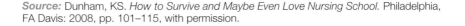

Physiological Integrity (38 to 62 percent)

a. Basic care and comfort: 6 to 12 percent of NCLEX questions
b. Pharmacological and parenteral therapies: 12 to 18 percent of NCLEX questions
c. Reduction of risk potential: 9 to 15 percent of NCLEX questions
d. Physiological adaptation: 11 to 17 percent of NCLEX questions

The physiological integrity needs are concerned with adult medical and surgical nursing care, pediatrics, and **gerontology**. This category comprises the largest groups of questions, with about 38 to 62 percent of the total number of questions on the NCLEX. The more common health-care problems, both acute and chronic conditions, that nurses deal with on a daily basis include:

- Diabetes.
- Cardiovascular disorders.
- Neurological disorders.
- Renal diseases.
- Respiratory diseases.
- Traumatic injuries.
- Immunological disorders.
- Skin and infective diseases.

There are also questions about nursing care of the pediatric client, including such topics as:

- Growth and development.
- Congenital abnormalities.
- Child abuse.
- Burn injury.
- Fractures and cast and traction care.
- Common infective diseases in children.
- Common childhood trauma such as eye injuries.

Psychosocial Integrity (6 to 12 percent)

a. Coping and adaptation: 6 to 12 percent of NCLEX questions
b. Psychosocial adaptation: 6 to 12 percent of NCLEX questions

Psychosocial integrity needs are health-care issues that revolve around the client with psychiatric problems. This material also deals with coping mechanisms for high-stress situations, such as acute illness and life-threatening diseases or trauma. These clients do not necessarily have any psychiatric disorders. This category constitutes at most 12 percent of the examination and includes questions about the care of clients with eating disorders, personality disorders, anxiety disorders, depression, schizophrenia, and organic mental disease. Also included in the psychosocial needs section are questions about therapeutic communication, crisis intervention, and substance abuse.

Health Promotion and Maintenance (6 to 12 percent)

a. Life span growth and development: 6 to 12 percent of NCLEX questions
b. Prevention and early detection of disease: 6 to 12 percent of NCLEX questions

Health promotion and maintenance needs deal with birth control measures, pregnancy, labor and delivery, the care of the newborn infant, growth and development, and contagious diseases, particularly sexually transmitted diseases. This section constitutes approximately 12 percent of the total examination. Teaching and counseling are important parts of the nurse's care during pregnancy, and knowledge of diet, signs and symptoms of complications, fetal development, and testing used during pregnancy is necessary.

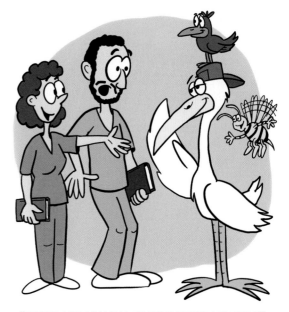

"THESE ARE MY HEALTH PROMOTION TUTORS."

Levels of Cognitive Ability

The level of cognitive ability is a component of the NCLEX that measures how information has been learned and how the nurse can use it. For the NCLEX, knowledge is tested at three different levels.

Level 1: Knowledge and Comprehension

Level 1 consists of knowledge and comprehension questions. Fewer than 10 percent of the questions are at this level, and there is a good chance that you may not even see a Level 1 question. These questions involve recalling specific facts and the ability to understand those facts in relation to a pathophysiological condition. They cover knowledge of specific anatomy and physiology, medication dosage and side effects, signs and symptoms of diseases, laboratory test results, and the elements of certain treatments and interventions.

Being able to remember and understand information is the most basic way of learning. Although this type of knowledge is important and underlies the other levels of knowledge, it is not sufficient to ensure safe nursing care. The following is an example of a Level 1 question:

1. A client is admitted to the medical unit with respiratory failure. Identify the normal range for the P_{O_2}.
   a. 10–30 mm Hg
   b. 35–55 mm Hg
   c. 10–20 cm H_2O
   d. 70–100 mm Hg

Level 2: Analyze, Interpret, and Apply

Level 2 questions add an additional step to the answering process. These questions presume that you have the basic information memorized and then ask you to analyze, interpret, and apply this information to specific situations. Analysis and application questions are more difficult to answer because they require you to do more than simply repeat the information you have read or heard in class. Analysis requires the ability to separate information into its basic parts, decide which of those parts are important, and then determine what the information is telling you. Application requires that you be able to use that information in making client-care decisions.

Some examples of this type of question involve interpreting electrocardiographic (ECG) strips, interpreting blood gas values, making a nursing diagnosis based on a set of symptoms, or deciding on a treatment plan. These questions provide a better indication of your ability to safely care for clients. An example of a Level 2 question is:

> *Being able to remember and understand information is the most basic way of learning. Although this type of knowledge is important and underlies the other levels of knowledge, it is not sufficient to ensure safe nursing care.*

2. A client is becoming progressively short of breath. The results of his arterial blood gas (ABG) tests are pH, 7.13; P_{O_2}, 48; P_{CO_2}, 53; and H_{CO_3}, 26. What do these values indicate?
   a. Metabolic acidosis
   b. Respiratory alkalosis
   c. Respiratory acidosis
   d. Metabolic alkalosis

Level 3: Synthesis, Judgment, and Evaluation

Level 3—synthesis, judgment, and evaluation—takes the process a step further. More than 95 percent of the questions on the NCLEX are at either Level 2 or 3. Questions at the synthesis and judgment level ask you to process information on more than one fact; apply rules, methods, principles, or theories to a situation; *and* make judgments and decisions about client care. You can identify these higher-level questions by recognizing that they require you to *process two or more* facts, concepts, theories, rules, or principles of care before you can answer the question.

One factor that adds to the difficulty of answering Level 3 questions is that there is often more than one correct answer. You may be asked to choose the best, or highest-priority, answer from among several correct answers. Questions at this level often ask about the priority of care to be given, the priority of nursing diagnosis formulated, how to best evaluate the effectiveness of care you are giving, and the most appropriate nursing action to be taken. Your ability to make decisions about nursing care at these higher levels is the best indication of your critical thinking ability and best demonstrates the ability to provide safe nursing care. Three examples of Level 3 questions are:

3. A client is becoming progressively short of breath. The results of his arterial blood gas (ABG) tests are pH, 7.13; P_{O_2}, 48; P_{CO_2}, 53; and H_{CO_3}, 26. What action should the nurse take first?
   a. Call a code blue and begin cardiopulmonary resuscitation.
   b. Call the physician and report the condition.
   c. Make sure the client's airway is open and begin supplemental oxygen.
   d. Give the ordered dose of 200 mg aminophylline intravenous piggyback (IVPB) now.

4. After receiving shift report at 0645, identify the client the nurse should assess first.
   a. 65-year-old man with stable angina
   b. 37-year-old woman with possible GI bleeding; vital signs stable
   c. 56-year-old woman with COPD and an oxygen saturation of 89%
   d. 19-year-old man with type 1 diabetes and a fasting blood sugar of 55 mg/dL

5. The nurse assesses a 7-month-old hospitalized girl and finds that the infant has a positive tonic neck reflex. What intervention would be most important for the nurse to include in the child's nursing care plan?
   a. Daily head circumference measurements
   b. Measure intake and weigh all diapers
   c. Position the infant on her back for naps
   d. Assess neuro/developmental levels each shift

Integrated Concepts and Processes

The integrated concepts and processes component includes the following:

- Nursing process
- Concepts of caring
- Therapeutic communication
- Cultural awareness
- Documentation
- Self-care
- Teaching and learning

These concepts are integrated throughout the examination and are included as elements in the four needs categories.

Nursing Process

The nursing process has traditionally been a very important part of the NCLEX. The NCLEX-RN, CAT uses the five-step nursing process: assessment, analysis, planning, intervention and implementation, and evaluation. Each of the questions you will be asked on the NCLEX falls into one of these five categories.

It is important that you keep in mind the steps of the nursing process when answering questions. Often questions that ask, "What should the nurse do first?" are looking for an assessment-type answer because that is the first step in the nursing process. Questions on the nursing process are no longer equally divided on the examination. Recent analysis has shown a higher percentage of questions in the implementation phase of the nursing process.

Assessment

The assessment phase primarily establishes the database on which the rest of the nursing process is built. Some components of the assessment phase include both subjective and objective data about the client, significant history, history of the present illness, signs and symptoms, environmental elements, laboratory values, and vital signs. Often the examination will ask you to distinguish between appropriate and inappropriate assessment factors. An example of an assessment phase question is:

6. What would be the most important information for the nurse to obtain when a client is admitted for evaluation of recurrent episodes of Stokes-Adams syndrome?
   a. Ability to perform aerobic exercises for 15 minutes
   b. Bradycardia and increases in blood pressure
   c. Changes in level of consciousness
   d. Ability to discuss fat and sodium diet restrictions

Analysis

The analysis phase of the nursing process involves developing and using a nursing diagnosis for the care of the client. The NCLEX uses the North American Nursing Diagnosis Association (NANDA) nursing diagnosis system. Questions concerning nursing diagnosis will often ask you to prioritize the diagnoses. (See Bonus Chapter 1 for detailed information about prioritization.) The basic rules for prioritization are to use Maslow's hierarchy of needs and the ABCs you learned in CPR (airway, breathing, and circulation). An example of an analysis phase question is:

7. A client is admitted to the unit with a diagnosis of bronchitis, congestive heart failure, and a fever. The nurse assesses him as having a temperature of 101.8°F, peripheral edema, dyspnea, and rhonchi. The following nursing diagnoses are all appropriate, but which one has the highest priority?
   a. Anxiety related to fear of hospitalization
   b. Ineffective airway clearance related to retained secretions
   c. Fluid volume excess related to third spacing of fluid (edema)
   d. Ineffective thermoregulation related to fever

Planning

The planning phase of the nursing process primarily involves setting goals for the client. Included in the planning phase are such factors as determining expected outcomes, setting priorities for goals, and anticipating client needs based on the assessment. These questions may ask you to identify the most appropriate goal or may ask you to identify the highest-priority goal from several appropriate goals. You can prioritize goals the same way you did the nursing diagnosis. Remember that a good goal is measurable, client centered, time limited, and realistic. An example of a planning phase question is:

8. A client is found to be in respiratory failure and is placed on oxygen. Which goal has the highest priority for this client?
   a. Walk the length of the hall twice during a nurse's shift.
   b. Complete his bath and morning care before breakfast.
   c. Maintain an oxygen saturation of 90 percent throughout the shift.
   d. Keep the head of the bed elevated to promote proper ventilation.

Intervention and Implementation

The intervention and implementation phase of the nursing process involves identifying nursing actions that are required to meet the goals stated in the planning phase. Some of the material in the intervention and implementation phase includes:

- Providing nursing care based on the client's goals.
- Preventing injury or spread of disease.
- Providing therapy with medications and their administration.
- Giving treatments.
- Carrying out procedures.
- Charting and record-keeping.
- Teaching about health care.
- Monitoring changes in condition.

An example of an intervention and implementation phase question is:

9. When the nurse ambulates a client who has been on bed rest for 3 days, he suddenly becomes very restless, displays extreme dyspnea, and complains of chest pain. Select the most appropriate nursing action.
   a. Call a code blue.
   b. Continue to help the client walk, but at a slower pace.
   c. Give the client an injection of his ordered pain medication.
   d. Return the client to bed and evaluate his vital signs and lung sounds.

Evaluation

The **evaluation** phase of the nursing process determines whether the goals stated in the planning phase have been met through the interventions. The evaluation phase also ties the nursing process together and makes it cyclic. If the goals have been achieved, it is an indication that the plan and implementation were effective, and new goals need to be established. If the goals were not met, then you have to go back and find the difficulty. Were the assessment data inadequate? Were the goals defective? Was there a deficiency in the implementation?

Evaluation is a continuous process. Material in the evaluation phase includes comparison of actual outcomes with expected outcomes, verification of assessment data, evaluation of nursing actions and client responses, and evaluation of the client's level of knowledge and understanding. Evaluation questions are often worded very similarly and are relatively easy to identify after you have experienced a few of them. An example of an evaluation question is:

10. A client is being prepared for discharge. He is to take theophylline by mouth at home for his lung disease. Which statement by the client indicates to the nurse that her teaching concerning theophylline medications has been effective?
    a. "I can stop taking this medication when I feel better."
    b. "If I have difficulty swallowing the time-released capsules, I can crush them or chew them."
    c. "If I have a lot of nausea and vomiting or become restless and can't sleep, I need to call my physician."
    d. "I need to drink more coffee and cola while I am on these medications."

> " *Contrary to rumor, no graduates are randomly selected to take all 265 questions.* "

NCLEX FORMAT

You will take the NCLEX examination on a personal computer at a Pearson Professional Center (Fig. 9.1). The majority of the questions are in a multiple-choice format and are constructed similarly. They include a client situation, a question stem, and four answers, or distracters, like the sample questions you have seen so far in this chapter.

All the multiple-choice questions on the NCLEX stand alone, although a similar situation may be repeated. Occasionally a single question may be included without a case situation.

Choosing the Right Answer

For the multiple-choice questions, you are asked to select the best answer from among the four possible choices. No partial credit is given for a "close" answer; there is only one correct answer for any particular question. The questions are totally integrated from the content areas that were previously discussed along with the approximate percentages that were identified. Each question carries an equal weight or value toward the final score.

When the question appears on the screen, read the question and answers using the process described in Bonus Chapter 1. When you decide what the correct answer is, place the cursor in the circle in front of the answer and click to select the answer (see Fig. 9.1). If you decide to change the answer (never a good idea), place the cursor on the answer you selected and click again. It will remove the indicator and you can move the cursor to another answer. When you are sure you have selected the correct answer, click the "Next (N)" button at the bottom of the screen. That question will disappear and a new one will appear. You cannot go back and change an answer after you click the "Next (N)" button.

Alternative Format Questions

In 2004, alternative format questions were first added to the exam; in 2010, three new types of alternative format questions were added. No new types were added with the 2013 revisions. The NCSBN states that there is no preset number of alternative format questions for each exam and that they are included as part of the overall test plan. In practice, there seems to be between 2 and 10 percent of the total number of questions that will be alternative format, and each graduate has at least two of them on the exam. There are several types of these questions. They are scored like the multiple-choice questions in that they are either correct or incorrect (no partial credit). They are also given a difficulty rating based on the same criteria as the multiple-choice questions. If you want more information on these types of questions, go to http://www.mightynurse.com/lp-practice-test-register-mightiest/?gclid=CIPXhsCXjsACFSMLMgodpEUAtw for an extensive question-and-answer presentation on alternative format questions. There are a number of books now in print that deal exclusively with alternative format questions. All of the general NCLEX review books now have samples of these questions for students to practice.

Fill in the Blank

These alternative format questions may ask for a range of information. They may be calculation

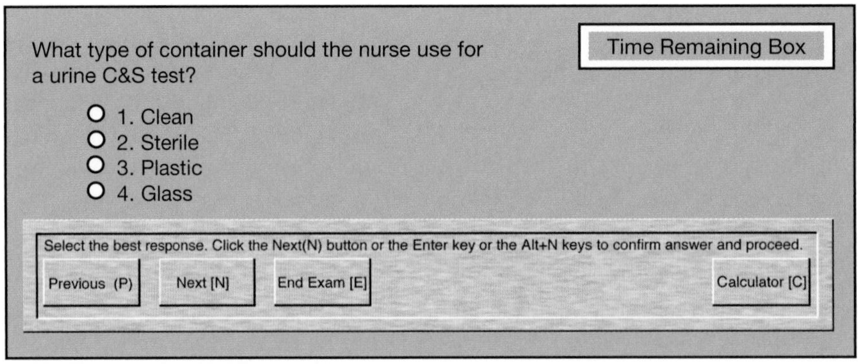

Figure 9.1 Sample multiple-choice question. Select the answer by placing the cursor in the circle and click or type in the answer. Change the answer by placing the cursor in a new circle and clicking. Move to the next question by clicking on the "Next (N)" button at the bottom of the screen.

An adult client with Hodgkin's disease who weighs 143 lb
is to receive vincristine (Oncovin) 25 mcg/kg IV.
Calculate the correct medication dosage.

Time Remaining Box

Type your answer in the box below.

Select the best response. Click the Next(N) button or the Enter key or the Alt+N keys to confirm answer and proceed.

Previous (P)   Next [N]   End Exam [E]   Calculator [C]

F i g u r e   9 . 2   Alternative format question. Fill in the blank by clicking on the
"Calculator (C)" button at the lower right corner of the bar.

questions or may ask for knowledge. After you read
the questions, you need to type the answer in the box
provided (Fig. 9.2). If it is a calculation question, you
may use the pop-up calculator, accessible by clicking
the cursor on the "Calculator (C)" button (Fig. 9.3).
After you have typed in your answer, you can go back
and change it. Once you have decided that it is
correct, click on the "Next (N)" button and a new
question will appear.

Multiple Answers

With the multiple-answer questions, you are given a
list of options or answers and must select all that are
correct. You must get them all correct in order to get
credit for the question. To select the options you
think are correct, place the cursor in the circle or box
before the option and click (Fig. 9.4). If you decide
that one of the options is not really the one you want,
you can click on the circle again and it will be removed. When you decide you have the options you
want, click on the "Next (N)" button and the next
question will appear on the screen.

Sequencing Items

Sequencing questions provide you with a question
and then four or more options (items) that are related
to the question. Your task with this type of question is
to place them in the proper sequence (Fig. 9.5). You
do this by selecting the circle or box in front of the
option you think is number one and typing in "1."
Then move to the option you believe is number two
and type that number in, and so forth. You can

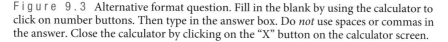

An adult client with Hodgkin's disease who weighs 143 lb
is to receive vincristine (Oncovin) 25 mcg/kg IV. Calculate
the correct medication dosage.

Time Remaining Box

VUE Calculator
File View Memory
1625

Backspace   CE   C

MC   7   8   9   /   sqrt
MR   4   5   6   X   %
MS   1   2   3   -   1/X
M+   0   +/-   .   +   =

Type your answer in the box below.

1625

Select the best response. Click the Next(N) button or the Enter key or the Alt+N keys to confirm answer and proceed.

Previous (P)   Next [N]   End Exam [E]   Calculator [C]

F i g u r e   9 . 3   Alternative format question. Fill in the blank by using the calculator to
click on number buttons. Then type in the answer box. Do *not* use spaces or commas in
the answer. Close the calculator by clicking on the "X" button on the calculator screen.

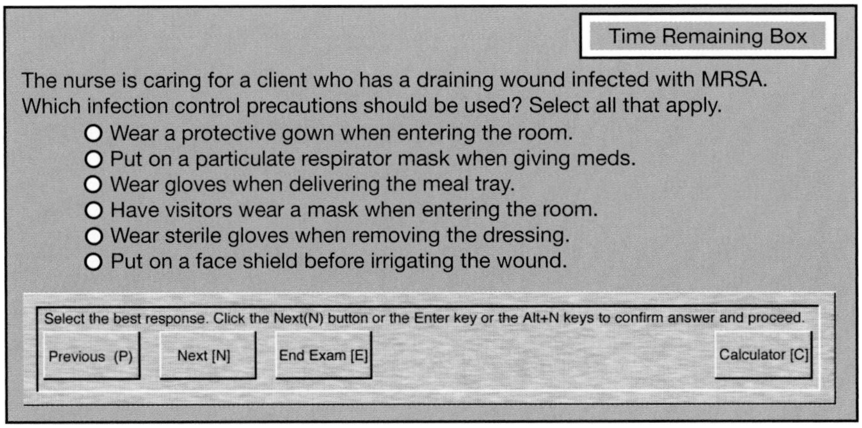

Figure 9.4 Alternative format question—multiple answer.

change the numbering by clicking on the boxes to re-move the numbers.

Some of the newer sequencing questions use a drag-and-drop answer system where you can click and hold on the answer you think is number 1, then drag it and drop in the number 1 box. There is a series of items in a box on the left side of the screen and a set of boxes on the right. The same method works for the rest of the answers. If you want to change an answer, click and hold and then drag it to another slot. When you have the options sequenced the way you think they should be, click on the "Next (N)" button and a new question will appear on the screen.

Identify the Area (or Hot Spot)

These types of questions provide you with a picture or diagram and then ask you to identify an area or a spe-cific element on the picture (Fig. 9.6). You place the cursor on the area that you think is correct and click.

An "X" will appear. If you decide that is not where you really want the "X," you can click on the "X" again to remove it and then place the cursor in a new spot and click again. Once you have it where you want it, click on the "Next (N)" button, and the next question will appear on the screen.

Chart/Exhibit Items (Type 1)

A chart or exhibit item will present you with a chart, graph, or some other picture or graphic item, or with a series of charts, graphs, or other pictures. You will need to be able to read the chart, graph, or picture to obtain the information to answer the question. Then you will be asked to select the correct answer from four or more options by using the information you gleaned from the chart, graph, or picture.

Exhibit Items (Type 2)

With this type of question, you are presented with either a question or a problem. To answer

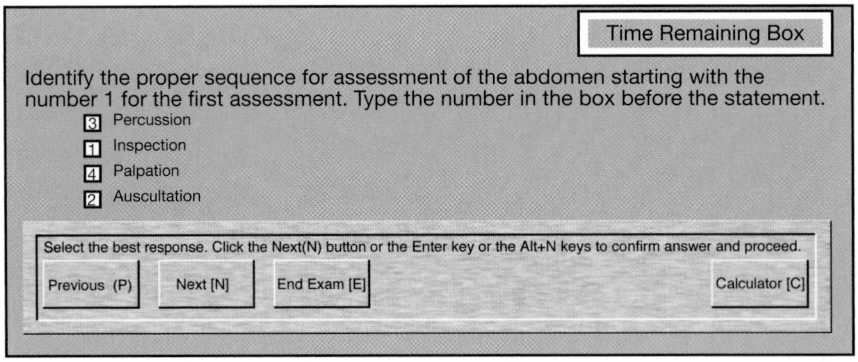

Figure 9.5 Alternative format question—sequencing items.

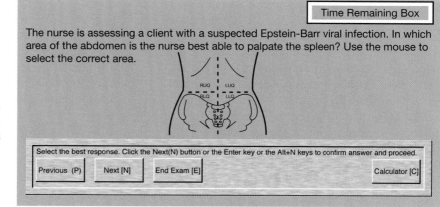

The nurse is assessing a client with a suspected Epstein-Barr viral infection. In which area of the abdomen is the nurse best able to palpate the spleen? Use the mouse to select the correct area.

Time Remaining Box

RUQ   LUQ
RLQ   LLQ

Select the best response. Click the Next(N) button or the Enter key or the Alt+N keys to confirm answer and proceed.

Previous (P)   Next [N]   End Exam [E]   Calculator [C]

Figure 9.6 Alternative format question—identify area. With this type of question, you are given a diagram or picture and asked to locate a structure or area. Place the cursor on the area you think is correct and click. An "X" will appear in that area. To deselect the answer, click on the "X" and move the cursor to the new area. When finished, click on "Next (N)."

the question or solve the problem, you must click on an "Exhibit Button." Each exhibit contains three tabs with drop-downs; you must click on each tab and read the information. The question will ask you to find some data provided by one of the tabs. Once you determine which tab has the correct information, you must select the one corresponding correct item from the four options provided. Then you click on the "Next (N)" button and move on to the next question.

Exhibit item questions test your ability to use information correctly. This type of question responds to the increase in the use of evidence-based practice in the health-care setting. If a nurse cannot understand and interpret research findings correctly, the safety of clients becomes an issue.

Audio Items

This type of question requires the use of a headset. When the question comes up, you will initially see what looks like the audio bar from a DVD with the usual symbols for play, pause, forward, stop, and reverse.

There will be four options (answer choices) underneath the bar. You must put on the headset and click on the arrow-shaped play button to listen to the audio clip. The volume can be adjusted using the volume slide bar. After listening to the clip, you must select the one correct option related to it. You can repeat the clip as often as you want, stop it, or pause it by clicking on the appropriate audio bar symbols. After selecting your answer, click the "Next (N)" button to move on to the next question.

The NCSBN has not indicated what you might find on these audio clips. Logically, it would

seem that anything a nurse usually "hears" in the course of a day's work could be included: heart sounds, breath sounds, bruits, and even client statements (is this client depressed, angry, anxious, or expressing echolalia?). These might be difficult.

Graphic Items

These questions are similar to the traditional multiple-choice questions in that there is a written question. However, the question presents four pictures or graphics, not written options, as answer selections. As with the audio items, the NCSBN has not provided any indication of the types of graphics you might encounter. They could be charts of disease frequencies, pictures of rashes or wounds, ECG strips, types of syringes, medication labels on bottles, or just about anything a nurse might see during a work shift.

How Many Questions?

You may take between 75 and 265 questions, depending on how you answer. Of the first 75 questions, only 60 count. The other 15 are "trial" questions that will be used on future examinations; however, they are completely integrated with the other questions, and there is no way to know which ones do not count, so do your best on all of them. The NCSBN is attempting to establish reliability and validity data on the new trial questions.

If you get a lot of questions in a particular category—for example, pediatrics—it may mean one of two things. The NCSBN may be testing pediatric questions on your exam, so you are receiving a lot of them, or you may be having some problems answering pediatric questions correctly. The computer will continue to give you questions in a particular content area until you meet the requirements of the test plan. The computer randomly draws the questions you are seeing from a pool of more than 4000 questions.

The NCSBN, which is responsible for designing the test, publicly states that no graduates are randomly selected by the computer to take all 265 questions. You can pass or fail the test with either 75 or 265 questions or any number in between. The average number of questions taken over the past 5 years is 119, and the average time is just over 2 hours.

How Long Does It Take?

There is a maximum time limit of 6 hours for the entire examination, although there is no minimum time limit. There is a mandatory break when the computer "locks up" about 2½ hours into the test. For 10 minutes, you will not be able to answer any questions. There is another optional break at about 4 hours into the test, although the computer will not lock up at this time. You can take breaks at any time during the exam if you need to use the restroom, but remember that you will lose this time off your total time for the exam.

The exam is not really timed except for the overall time limit. Theoretically you could sit at the computer for the full 6 hours with question number 1 on the screen. The computer does not make you take questions at any particular rate. Most people can answer a multiple-choice question in about 45 seconds. As a rule of thumb, if you are spending more than 2 minutes on any single question, put an answer down and move on to the next question.

If you calculate that you are going to take 265 questions in 6 hours, it comes out to about 80 seconds per question. Some of the alternative-format questions may take a little longer to answer, although some may take less time than the multiple-choice questions. Take a watch along and keep an eye on the "Time Remaining" box at the top of the screen.

How It's Graded

The NCLEX is graded on a statistical model that compares your responses with a preestablished standard. If you can demonstrate a knowledge level consistently above the standard, you will pass the examination.

Because the NCLEX-RN examination is given by computerized adaptive testing (CAT),

increases in the passing standard do not necessarily require you to answer a greater number of items correctly. However, the new passing standard does require that you answer questions correctly at a slightly higher difficulty level than the previous year's graduates (i.e., the examination is going to be a little more difficult to pass). Questions are assigned a difficulty value on a seven-logit (unit) scale called the NCLEX-RN logistic scale, ranging from the easiest (minus 3), which all graduates should answer correctly, to the most difficult (plus 3), which almost all graduates would be expected to miss (Box 9.1). It is important to keep in mind that a "logit" is *not* a percentage point, nor does it have anything to do with percentages. You might hear someone say you need a 50 percent or 60 percent or 70 percent on the NCLEX to pass it. Those numbers are meaningless to the NCLEX exam. The NCSBN reevaluates the difficulty level every 3 years. On April 1, 2013, the pass level was raised from minus 0.16 logits to 0.000 logits. The current pass criterion is exactly in the middle of the seven-point logit scale. In the past, whenever the pass standard was raised on the NCLEX, the national pass rate dropped by an average of 5 percentage points.

So What Is a Logit?

The term *logit* is an abbreviation for "log odds units." It was originally developed for use in mathematical probability calculations in which different-sized units of data are analyzed as if they were all the same size. On the NCLEX, ranking the questions to logit levels compares the difficulty of items (criterion referencing) rather than the answers different

Box 9.1

NCLEX-RN Logistic Scale

Logits	
3	Most difficult
2	
1	
0	Approximate pass level
−1	
−2	
−3	Least difficult

graduates might give (norm referencing). This establishes a more objective standard for passing the exam. So what percentage must you answer correctly to pass? It doesn't really matter. You must answer enough questions ranked above the pass criteria to demonstrate that you can practice nursing safely. If you do that, you pass the NCLEX. If you answer a lot of questions correctly below the passing standard, they do not help with the final calculation of your pass/fail status.

Level of Difficulty

The difficulty level of the questions is determined by the writers and question reviewers. It is based on such factors as when the material is usually presented in nursing programs (material presented earlier is considered less difficult) and the complexity of the material. To you, the test taker, difficulty level is somewhat relative. If you know the answer to a question, then it will seem relatively easy to you even if it is classified by the test writers as being of a higher difficulty level. Similarly, if you do not know the answer, that question will be difficult for you even if it is determined to be at a relatively low difficulty level.

> *Keep in mind that the NCLEX is designed so that no one can answer all the questions correctly. Even your most knowledgeable nursing instructor would not be able to answer some of the questions on the exam.*

No Happy Questions

Keep in mind also that there are no "happy" questions on the NCLEX. There is always something wrong, and if there is a problem in the question, you need to worry about it. Also, as a general guiding principle, anything you know really well from your classes will *not* be on the NCLEX, so anticipate difficult questions.

After you finish the mandatory tutorial on the use of the computer, the first real question you get will be at a medium difficulty level, probably a little above or a little below the pass criteria. If you answer it correctly, the next question will be a little more difficult. If you answer that one correctly, the next question will also increase in difficulty, and so forth, until you start missing questions. Then the computer will give you slightly less difficult questions until you start answering them correctly. The computer is trying to establish your "zone of knowledge." If that zone is above the pass standard, then you will pass the exam.

Your Zone of Knowledge

The first question you see will be at or slightly above the pass level. If you miss the first question, and many graduates do because of anxiety, the computer will give you a slightly easier question for number 2. If you answer that one correctly, the next one will increase in difficulty level, and so forth, until you start missing questions. If the computer can determine with a 95 percent accuracy that your zone of knowledge is above the pass criteria within the first 75 questions, it will stop the test and ask you to complete a short survey. The reason many graduates take more than 75 questions is because the computer is having difficulty establishing a clear zone of knowledge above or below the pass standard. It will keep giving questions until a 95 percent accurate determination of your knowledge level is made.

Graduates who take all 265 questions have answered questions above and below the pass standard throughout the whole exam. If you do have to take all 265 questions, it does not necessarily mean you failed.

Example: Low Difficulty Level

11. What blood test does the nurse evaluate as the best measure of a client's long-term control of diabetes mellitus?
    a. Fasting blood sugar
    b. Arterial blood gases
    c. Glucose tolerance test (GTT)
    b. Glycosylated hemoglobin (Hgb A_1C)

Example: Mid Difficulty Level (Pass Criteria)

12. While evaluating the results of a pulmonary function test, the nurse notes that an adult man who is short of breath has a vital capacity of 2800 mL, a tidal volume of 375 mL, and a residual volume of 2200 mL. Select the action the nurse should avoid implementing for this client.
    a. Position the client with the head of the bed elevated 45 degrees.
    b. Encourage fluid intake of 2 to 3 liters per 24 hours.

    c. Begin oxygen by non-rebreather mask.
    d. Encourage the client to cough and to breathe deeply every hour during the shift.

Example: High Difficulty Level

13. While monitoring a client with a pulmonary artery catheter, the nurse notes catheter fling artifact on the pressure tracing. Identify the nursing measure that best compensates for this problem.
    a. Record only mean pressures.
    b. Ask the physician to reposition the catheter.
    c. Irrigate the catheter forcefully with heparinized saline solution.
    d. Level and zero the transducer before taking readings.

Remember that it is probably a good sign that you are getting difficult questions. It means that you are answering questions above the pass standard. You do not want a lot of easy questions on the NCLEX. Also keep in mind that the NCLEX is designed so that no one can answer all the questions correctly. Even your most knowledgeable nursing instructor would not be able to answer some of the questions on the exam.

However, the NCLEX asks entry-level questions that tend to be very "textbookish." When you are answering NCLEX questions, look for the expected textbook-type knowledge. Don't look for exceptions. Each examination is different and unique to the person taking it because future questions depend on how you answered previous questions.

NCLEX BACKGROUND INFORMATION

After you graduate from your nursing program, you must apply to the state board of nursing for permission to take the NCLEX. Once you have been approved by the state board, that information is sent on to the NCSBN, which sends you an "authorization to test" card or document. You will receive your authorization document more quickly if you select the "e-mail" option on the application form for the examination.

You then call for an appointment at the center wherever is most convenient for you to take the test. Appointments are made on a first-come, first-served basis. The centers are required to schedule the examination within 30 days from the time you apply. Each state establishes its own maximum time interval for the graduate to take the exam after graduation, usually 1 year.

There are both morning and afternoon sessions of 6 hours' duration. Depending on the size of the center, between 8 and 15 graduates may be taking the test at the same time. Additionally, there may be other people at the center taking examinations in other disciplines at the same time as the nursing graduates.

Test Vendor and Logistics

The test vendor for the NCLEX is Virtual University Enterprises (VUE), a subsidiary of National Communication Systems (NCS) Pearson Professional Centers. The tests are given at Pearson Professional Centers. The test items and the format of the examination always stay the same, even if vendors change, because the exam is owned by the NCSBN, which contracts with vendors to administer the examination.

Testing by Computer

The computer skills required are minimal. The mouse is used for most of the examination, with minimal typing required. A digital picture is taken at the time you enter the exam room, and that picture, along with your information, appears on one of the computer screens in the room. A digital thumbprint and signature are also obtained when you enter the exam center.

You sit at the computer with your picture on it and complete a tutorial with the use of the mouse and computer. You have two attempts at completing the tutorial successfully. If you are unable to do so after the second try, a person who is working at the testing center will come and help you. After the examination is completed, you will be asked to complete a short computerized personal data questionnaire and an evaluation of the examination site.

Questions appear one at a time on the computer screen, with a button bar on the bottom of the screen and a "time remaining" box in the upper corner. After you select an answer, the question is replaced with another question and answer options. No question is ever repeated, nor are you able to change the answer once you have clicked on the "Next (N)" button.

An on-screen pop-up calculator is available for answering dosage and other questions that require calculations. Because of the increased emphasis on pharmacology and the concern about medication errors, it is probably safe to assume that the difficulty level of future calculation questions will increase markedly.

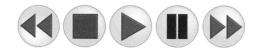

Security

Security is very tight at the examination sites. Lockers are provided and you must leave all your personal belongings at the door, so do not bring a lot of things with you. As of 2013, you can no longer take in cell phones or any type of electronic devices into the exam room. You will be required to place the device into a plastic bag and it will be secured until you finish the exam. If you refuse to secure your phone, you will not be allowed to take the exam and will forfeit your $200 examination fee.

All exam sessions are videotaped, and there is a proctor in the room monitoring all the test takers. Although cheating on the NCLEX is virtually impossible—every examination is different—it is important to not even look as if you are attempting to cheat. Do not talk to the person next to you. Keep your eyes on your own computer. Do not take out any papers or electronic devices during the exam. Magic slates are generally provided for use as "scrap paper," so you will not need any paper or pens during the exam.

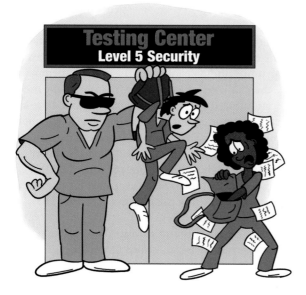

How the Test Is Graded

The NCLEX is graded on a pass/fail basis. The results are checked twice for accuracy. If the graduate fails, he or she must take the entire exam again. The

NCSBN requires a 45-day waiting period before repeating the test, and first-time takers are given preference over those who are repeating the examination. Several states have restricted the number of times the graduate can retake the test (usually up to three) or have placed a time limit on the retake of 1 or 2 years. Check with your state board of nursing for the particular regulations.

When the computer shuts off, it knows if you passed or failed, but it will not give you that information at that time. At the end of the day, after the last testing session, results are downloaded electronically to NCSBN in Chicago. The next business day, NCSBN notifies the state board of nursing electronically and sends a hard copy; then it is up to the state board of nursing to notify you.

The official exam results may be sent to you by mail, usually within 7 to 10 days after the exam has been completed, although this time frame varies from state to state. Most states now offer official online results within 72 hours after the exam. Check with your state board of nursing to make sure they offer this service and to find out how to access the site. The NCSBN offers a "quick results" service that allows you to obtain unofficial results 2 business days after you take the examination. Just go to the Pearson View website at http://www.pearsonvue.com/nclex and sign in with your user name and password. The cost is about $10. Not all states participate in the service, and your employment agency may or may not accept the results since they are unofficial.

Some graduates have found a very quick way to get unofficial results in as little as 2 or 3 hours, but more commonly by the next day. After you take the NCLEX and return home, log on to the Pearson VUE site. Attempt to register for the NCLEX again under your original login. Register for the exact same test just like you did when you originally registered. Continue through the registration process until you find the message where you are asked to pay for the exam. If the site allows you to put in your credit card information, it is an indication that you might have failed the exam. It is best not to do anything else until you get the official results from your SBN. If you get a message saying that you are unable to schedule the NCLEX because one is already on record, you most likely passed the exam. To double check, try this again later to see if you get the same message.

NCLEX STUDY STRATEGIES

There are several ways to prepare for examinations, including the NCLEX. To attempt to take the examination with an attitude of "If I don't know it by now, I never will" is to court failure. Carefully directed study and preparation will considerably increase the chances of passing the test. Review Bonus Chapter 1 for general tips on how to study for and take exams. Below is some specific information on preparing for the NCLEX.

The NCSBN and Pearson VUE Websites

You can access the NCBSN website at http://www.ncsbn.org. This website can provide significant help as you prepare to take the NCLEX. It offers the most recent information on any changes in the test and simply lays out the steps to register for the examination. The Pearson VUE site also has a wealth of information, including free sample examination questions (http://www.vue.com/nclex). The more you learn about the exam before you have to take it, the lower your anxiety will be and the better you will do.

Review Books

The material covered by review books is the key material found on the NCLEX. These books usually follow the NCLEX Test Plan very closely. However, a review book is just that; it reviews the material that you should already know. Reviewing is important to reinforce learning and recall of information you may not have used in a year or more.

What Do You Think?

When was the last time you sat in on a group study session? List three of the problems you encountered at the session. How could they be solved?

Review books are not really designed to present any new information about key material. If you are totally unfamiliar with the material in a particular section of the review book, reading a more comprehensive textbook on that particular subject area will be necessary.

Another important function of a review book is to point out areas of weakness. If you find a section that seems to contain "new" material, it is important to investigate that section in more detail. If you find most of the material familiar and easy to grasp, you are probably well on your way to passing the NCLEX.

Group Study

Group study can be an effective method of preparation for an examination such as the NCLEX. To optimize the results of group study sessions, several rules should be followed:

Rule 1: *Be very selective when choosing the members of the study group.* They should have a similar frame of mind and orientation toward studying. They should be graduates who are also going to be taking the NCLEX. The ideal size for a study group is between four and six people. Groups larger than six become difficult to organize and handle. After the group has been formed and has begun its study sessions, it may be necessary to ask an individual to leave the group for not participating or for being disruptive to the study process or displaying negative attitudes about the examination.

Rule 2: *Have each individual prepare a particular section for each group study session.* Study groups generally meet once or twice a week. For example, if next week the group is going to study the endocrine system, assign group member 1 the anatomy and physiology of the system, member 2 the pathological conditions, member 3 the medications used for treatment, and member 4 the key elements of nursing care. When the group comes together, have each individual present his or her prepared section. This type of preparation prevents the "What are we going to study tonight?" syndrome that often plagues group study sessions.

Following this process organizes the study group and allows for more in-depth coverage of the topic. It also permits the members of the group to ask questions of the other members, thereby reinforcing the information being discussed.

Rule 3: *Limit the length of the study session.* No single study session should be longer than 60 to 90 minutes. Sessions that go longer tend to get off the topic and foster a negative attitude about the examination. Try to avoid making group

> *" No matter what other study and preparation methods are used, individual preparation for the NCLEX is a necessity. "*

study sessions into party time. A few snacks and refreshments may be helpful to maintain the group's energy level, but a real party atmosphere will detract significantly from the effectiveness of the study session.

Rule 4: *Use role-playing to reinforce information.* The more senses you can involve in the learning process, the better the learning.

Rule 5: *Remain positive.* Although group study times should not be party times, relax and have some fun with the study.

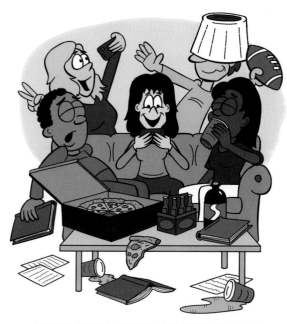

GROUP STUDY TIME IS NOT PARTY TIME!

Individual Study Tips

No matter what other study and preparation methods are used, individual preparation for the NCLEX is a necessity. This preparation can take several forms:

Tip 1: Use a review book. As previously discussed, use of a review book is valuable to indicate areas of deficient knowledge. Reading and studying the appropriate textbooks and study guides can be helpful if it is approached correctly. It is important that the graduate mentally organize the information being read into a format similar to that found in the NCLEX. After reading each page of a textbook or study guide, the graduate should be able to ask three or four multiple-choice questions about that information. These questions can be asked silently or written out and should answer the question, "How might the NCLEX test my knowledge of this material?"

Tip 2: Take practice exams on the computer and learn the format. Practice answering questions similar to those found on the exam you are going to take. Most of the review books come with a CD or a link to a website that has practice questions on it. It will help alleviate some of the unknowns, particularly if you have not had a lot of experience with computer-based exams. Experts recommend that you take between 3000 and 5000 practice questions before you take the NCLEX. Try to take at least 1000 questions using a computerized format and alternative format questions. Obviously, starting early in this process (6 months) is important, along with some planning and time management. Don't try to take 1000 questions at a time! For maximum learning, take 50 to 100 at a sitting and review the answers to understand why you missed the ones you missed.

When practice questions are answered, the following important mental processes occur:

Getting comfortable. First, you are becoming more familiar with and therefore more comfortable with the format of the examination. In research, this process is termed the *practice effect;* it must be accounted for when analyzing the results from pretest/post-test types of research projects. Individuals will have better results after a test, even without any type of intervention, because of having practiced answering questions on the pretest. Similarly, your score on the NCLEX may increase by as much as 10 percent through answering practice questions.

Reinforcing information. A second result of answering practice questions is that it reinforces the information already studied. Although it is unlikely that a question on the NCLEX examination will be identical to a practice question, there are many similarities. Realistically, only a limited number of questions can be asked about any given subject. After a while, the questions will begin to sound very similar.

Identifying weak spots. A third advantage of answering practice questions is that it quickly reveals subject areas that you will need to study. It is relatively easy to say, "I understand the renal system pretty well." It is quite another to answer correctly 10 or

15 questions about that system. If you answer the questions correctly, you can move on to the next topic. If you miss the majority of the questions, however, further review is required.

After you have answered the questions, you need to review them and compare your answers with the answers provided in the study book. You should also look at the rationales and the categories into which the questions fall. Try to understand why you missed the questions you did. Was it lack of knowledge? Didn't read the question carefully? Didn't use critical thinking?

Tip 3: Complete a 265-item test in one sitting in 6 hours. Many websites provide testing materials and sample examinations, such as http://www.4tests.com/nclex.

Tip 4: Take the NCLEX as soon as possible. The NCSBN has done some studies that show the following:

- The NCLEX taken less than 26 days after graduation has an 89 percent average pass rate.
- The NCLEX taken between 27 and 39 days after graduation has an 80 percent average pass rate.
- The NCLEX taken between 40 and 62 days after graduation has a 72 percent average pass rate.
- The NCLEX taken more than 62 days after graduation has a 45 percent average pass rate.

Formal NCLEX Reviews

The NCSBN does not endorse or sponsor any review courses for the NCLEX directly, but many companies offer reviews shortly after graduation. An online comprehensive review course for the NCLEX-RN examination on the NCSBN website is offered by an independent company (http://www.learningext.com). These review courses range from 2 to 5 days and basically cover the information found in review books. They are rather expensive, and the quality of NCLEX reviews varies. In general, they are only as good as the people who are presenting the material. Also, look at the reported pass rate of the graduates after they take the review. Courses with higher pass rates are probably better.

> *Experts recommend that you take between 3000 and 5000 practice questions before you take the NCLEX. Obviously, starting early in this process is important, along with some planning and time management.*

PREPARING FOR THE BIG DAY

Several Months to One Week Before the Exam

1. Get mentally and physically prepared. Eat a good healthy diet; emphasize foods with protein, vitamin K, and calcium. These foods have been shown to help control long-term stress. Exercise regularly. Drink lots of water (64 ounces per day) to rid your body of accumulated toxins. Avoid alcohol, street drugs, and even over-the-counter medications like antihistamines that can affect your ability to concentrate and think. Ease off on the caffeine and stop smoking.
2. Practice doing NCLEX-type questions—lots of them!
3. Avoid major life-altering activities, such as buying a car or planning a wedding, major vacation, or baby shower!

The Day Before the Exam

1. Don't work. Most employers understand that the NCLEX produces anxiety and are willing to let you have the day off. If your stress levels are high, it may be difficult for you to concentrate on your work, possibly compromising the health and well-being of your clients.
2. Do something fun and relaxing, but don't overdo it. Activities that involve some moderate exercise will help with anxiety levels.
3. Eat citrus fruits or drink liquids with vitamin C. Vitamin C has been shown to decrease short-term stress.
4. If you are unfamiliar with the area where the test center is located, drive to the test site. Note parking facilities and places where you can get a meal. This preparation will save you from getting lost the next day and help you be on time.

The Night Before the Exam

1. Make sure you have all the materials you will need for the exam, including two forms of picture ID, authorization to test card, and Social Security card.
2. Review formulas, common medications, and information that can be summarized in tables or on cards and lists. It is probably not a good time to pull out all your old textbooks and notes and try to

read them. Concentrate on things that are visual and may have caused you some problems in the past, like the list of cranial nerves or the glands and hormones in the endocrine system. Don't try to study everything. The "If I don't know it now, I never will" attitude is a negative thought process. You can always learn something.

3. Avoid strange or exotic foods that you have never eaten before. This can be a real temptation if you have to travel away from home and stay in a hotel the night before the exam. Stick to your usual diet. New or unusual foods may cause some gastrointestinal consequences that can be very distracting during the exam.

4. Go to bed at a reasonable hour. It is probably best to stick to your normal schedule. Staying up all night trying to study is counterproductive. You will be nervous and may have some problems sleeping, but stay away from sleep aids. They will interfere with your decision-making ability on the exam. Even if you are not sound asleep, the fact that you are resting will be helpful.

The Day of the Exam

1. Stick to your regular schedule and routine as much as possible. Avoid drinking excessive amounts of caffeine or sugary beverages to try to stay awake. They will only make you nervous and may increase the amount of time you need to spend on breaks in the restroom.

2. Eat breakfast, especially if you are scheduled for the morning session. Eat something with some glucose for a quick start (bread with jelly) and something with protein to get you through the morning (cereal and milk; egg and bacon). Drink some cinnamon tea, eat some lemon drop candies, or chew some peppermint gum. These flavors have been reported to enhance learning and sharpen thought processes! If you are taking the exam in the afternoon, eat lunch, but avoid a large meal with a lot of greasy food. It will make you sleepy and sit in your stomach like a lump.

3. Don't let the security at the site fluster you. They will take a digital picture, thumbprint, and signature. They will make you leave all your belongings in lockers at the door. Someone will be walking around the room during the exam. Just concentrate on your computer and answer the questions and you will do fine (see "Issues Now" box).

4. Wear comfortable clothes. You don't get extra points on the NCLEX for looking like a fashion model. Dress appropriately for the season, but keep in mind that some buildings are cool in the summer because of air conditioning and hot in the winter because of heating. Wear something you have worn before. Gym clothes are a good choice, particularly because you can dress in layers.

5. Think positively! If you truly believe you will do well, you will do well. If you go into the exam with an "I'm never going to pass this—I'm too dumb" attitude, you probably are not going to do as well.

Conclusion

Taking and passing the NCLEX-RN, CAT is a necessary step in the process of becoming a professional registered nurse. Like all licensure examinations, its purpose is to protect the public from undereducated or unsafe practitioners. The examination is comprehensive and includes material from all areas of the graduate's nursing education. Although most graduates have some anxiety about taking this test, knowledge about its format and content and strategies for taking it can lower anxiety.

Critical-Thinking Exercises

- Obtain an NCLEX-RN, CAT review book. Analyze the questions in the practice examination for type, cognitive level, and level of difficulty.
- Identify three to five other students in your class with whom you would feel comfortable working in a study group. Organize a study group session before the next major course examination.
- When you get the results of your next course examination, identify why you missed the questions you missed and what strategies might have been used to answer those questions correctly.

Answers to Questions in Chapter 9

1. **Correct answer: d.** You either have or do not have the knowledge for this particular laboratory test.

2. **Correct answer: c.** Not only do you need to know the normal values for each of the blood gas components given, but you must also be able to use that information in determining the underlying condition.

3. **Best answer: c.** Choices *b* and *d* are also actions that should be carried out, but at this time, opening the airway and oxygenating the client must receive highest priority. This question requires that you know the normal values and be able to interpret them, and it requires that a decision be made about the seriousness of the condition (analysis) and a selection of the type of care to be given from several correct options (judgment).

4. **Correct answer: d.** This question measures critical thinking and decision-making ability by asking you which of these clients is the sickest or least stable. Type 1 diabetic patients may have symptoms of hypoglycemia even when their blood glucoses are normal. This one is below normal, and all the other clients are stable.

5. **Correct answer: d.** This question requires you to know what a tonic neck reflex is and its significance. It is present in the newborn because of immaturity of the central nervous system and usually is gone by 1 month. If a child at 7 months still has it, it indicates a delay in neurological development.

6. **Correct answer: c.** Stokes-Adams syndrome is a suddenly occurring episode of asystole. The client becomes unconscious quickly.

7. **Correct answer: b.** Nursing diagnoses that deal with the airway always have highest priority.

8. **Correct answer: c.** Choice *a* is unrealistic for this client; choice *b* is not client-centered; choice *d* is a nursing intervention, not a goal. Maintaining an oxygen saturation of 90 percent is realistic, measurable, and within normal limits.

9. **Correct answer: d.** These are symptoms of a pulmonary embolism, which is a common complication of prolonged bed rest.

10. **Correct answer: c.** Answer *c* lists some side effects of theophylline medications that may indicate the onset of toxicity. The physician needs to know about these toxic side effects so that the medication can be stopped and the dosage of the medication reduced when it is restarted.

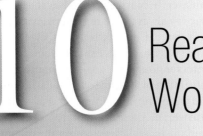

10 Reality Shock in the Workplace

Joseph T. Catalano

Leah Cullins

Learning Objectives

After completing this chapter, the reader will be able to:

- Describe the concept of reality shock
- Describe appropriate documents and procedures for job interviews
- List evidential artifacts used to develop professional nursing portfolios
- Define burnout and list its major symptoms
- Discuss the key factors that produce burnout
- List the important elements in personal time management
- Analyze how the nurse's humanity affects nursing practice
- List at least four health-care practices nurses can use to prevent burnout and to improve their professional performance

WHAT IS REALITY SHOCK?

"That is not how we do it in the real world." How many times do students and new graduate nurses hear that sentence? In many ways, that sentence is correct: In nursing school, students are instructed in the ideal theoretical, research-based, and instructor-supervised practice. Although demanding physically, mentally, and emotionally, nursing school shelters students from the realities of the real world, where nursing practice consists of not only theory and research but also heuristic practice, human emotion and response, policies, regulations, and the push and pull of life responsibilities. Things are different in the real world. The transition from nursing student to registered nurse is often referred to as **reality shock (transition shock)**.[1]

MAKING THE TRANSITION FROM STUDENT TO NURSE

At any point in their lives, most people fulfill several different roles simultaneously. Sometimes, role conflict occurs.[2] Role conflict exists when a person is unable to integrate the three distinct aspects of a given role: ***ideal, perceived,*** and ***performed role images.*** For nursing students, a significant role conflict may occur when they transition from the role of student to that of registered nurse.[3]

Ideal Role
In the academic setting, the student is generally presented with the ideal of what a nurse should be. The ideal role projects society's expectations of a nurse. It clearly delineates obligations and responsibilities as well as the rights and privileges that those in the role can claim. Although the

ideal role presents a clear image of what is expected, it is often somewhat unrealistic to believe that everyone in this role will follow this pattern of behaviors.

An Angel of Mercy

The ideal role of the nurse might require someone with superhuman physical strength and ability and unlimited stamina who possesses superior intelligence and decision-making ability, yet remains kind, gentle, caring, and altruistic and not concerned about money. This perfect nurse can communicate with any client at any time and can function independently and know more than even the physician. This angel of mercy is able to prevent grievous errors in client care while continuing to always be responsive to clients' needs and requests and carry out the physician's orders with accuracy and absolute obedience. Perceptive students soon begin to suspect that this ideal role of nurse does not exist anywhere in the real world.

Perceived Role

The perceived role is an individual's own definition of the role, often more realistic than the ideal role. When individuals define their own roles, they may reject or modify some of the norms and expectations of society that were used to establish the ideal role. Intentionally or unintentionally, though, the ideal role is often used as the intellectual yardstick against which the perceived role is measured.

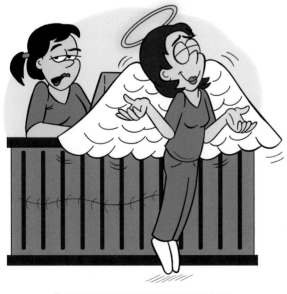

"THE NEW GIRL CERTAINLY HAS TAKEN ON AN IDEAL ROLE."

After a minimal amount of clinical experience, nursing students may realize that nurses do not possess extraordinary physical strength or intellectual ability but may continue to accept unconditionally, as part of their perceived role, that nurses must be kind, gentle, and understanding at all times with all clients and other health-care staff. The perceived role is the role with which the nursing student often graduates.

Performed Role

The performed role is defined as what the practitioner of the role actually does. Reality shock occurs when the ideal or perceived role comes into conflict with the performed role. Many new graduate nurses soon realize that the accomplishment of role expectations depends on many factors other than their perception and beliefs about how nursing should be performed. The environment has a great deal to do with how the obligations of the role are met.

In nursing school, where students are assigned to care for one or two clients at a time, there is plenty of time to practice therapeutic communication techniques; to provide completely for the physical, mental, educational, emotional, and spiritual needs of the client; and to develop an insightful care plan. However, the realities of the workplace may dictate that a nurse be assigned to care for six to eight clients at a time. In this situation, the perceived role of the nurse may have to be set aside for the more realistic performed role, from communicator to task organizer. Meeting all of the client's physical, psychological, social, and spiritual needs becomes less possible, and the care plan becomes more brief and to the point.

Heart, Hands, and Ears
I lost a baby I wanted more than anything
    He was stillborn at 35 weeks
        You sat on the edge of my bed and listened
        to me sob when no one else would

I am only 8 and have leukemia
    The chemo shots hurt really really bad
        You sang a silly song with me while you gave
        the shot and made me laugh

I crashed my motorcycle and ripped open my leg
    It got a raging infection that required constant
    treatment
        You changed the dressing with skill and
        compassion

I had a stroke long before I should have
   My hands no longer work the way they used to
      You taught me how to use the fork
      with the big handle and now I can feed
      myself

I stood by my father's bedside while the machines
he was connected to went straight line
   He was sick for a long time but I loved him
   with every fiber of my being
      You stood quietly beside me and
      your strength gave me the courage to
      go on

I asked you one day, "What does a nurse do?"
   I was wondering if it was something I could
   do too
      You answered:
      Nurses use their ears and compassion to
      listen
      Nurses use their hands and skills to
      heal
      Nurses use their hearts and
      souls to care
      Nurses take those who are
      at the crossroads of their
      lives,
      Who are battered and scarred
      with disease, and
      change their souls forever more with their
      hearts and their hands and their ears.

Joseph T. Catalano

Cognitive Dissonance

Such situations can produce what is called *cognitive dissonance* in many new graduate nurses. They know what they should do and how they should do it, yet the circumstances do not allow them to carry it out. The end result is increased apprehension. High levels of anxiety, left unrecognized or unresolved, can lead to various physical and emotional symptoms. When these symptoms become severe enough, a condition called **burnout syndrome** may result. In today's health-care climate and with the current nursing shortage, it is important that health-care agencies retain high-quality nurses and that nursing schools prepare graduates for their transition from student to nurse.

NURSING SHORTAGE CONTRIBUTES TO STRESS

A lack of qualified nurses has been present in the health-care system for so long that the term *nursing shortage* has become a truism. However, as recent history has demonstrated, the demand for nurses is cyclical and increases or decreases with changes in the health-care system. In addition, the demand for nurses is to some extent regional. Some areas of the country have a higher demand for registered nurses, and others may have fewer available jobs. However, studies about employment opportunities project that there will continue to be a shortage of nurses well into to the middle of this century.[4]

What Do You Think?

Is there a nursing shortage in your region? Does it affect the health care that you can obtain at your local hospital? How can the nursing shortage be "fixed"?

> *The Department of Health and Human Services currently projects a shortfall of up to 267,000 registered nurses by the year 2025.*

Nurses in Demand

The demand for nurses is finally being recognized by high school counselors and employment agencies. They are now encouraging young people to enter nursing schools, and enrollments in nursing schools are up after several years of decline in the mid-2000s that reduced the number of graduates by almost 30 percent nationally. Since 2009, nursing schools have experienced a steady increase in enrollment so that nationwide in 2013 there were 46,000 more applicants for registered nurse (RN) programs than there were places for them in the programs.

Drops in nursing program enrollments tend to occur when the economy is strong; however, this does not seem to be the case with the current economic recovery. Enrollment in higher education in general tends to decrease during periods of strong economic growth and increase when the economy takes a downturn. In short, when the economy is strong, there are more employment opportunities, which gives graduating high school students a broader spectrum of both professional and nonprofessional fields to choose from.

There are several reasons for the increased demand for registered nurses. One of the primary reasons is the ever-increasing demand for health care. As the population of the United States continues to age, and there is a recognition that an older population has increased health-care needs, the demand for well-educated, highly skilled nurses will continue to increase (Chapter 23). It is also important to note that a high percentage of the currently working registered nurses will retire within the next 10 years and therefore will not be an active part of the workforce. In addition, it is projected that some nurses will leave the profession after the economy recovers to seek more lucrative jobs.

A few consistent factors have contributed to the ongoing nursing shortage, including the unprofessional image of nurses portrayed in the media and believed by the public, the lack of equitable pay for equitable work, substandard working conditions such as short staffing and long hours and multiple shifts, and the inability of nursing programs to accept all the qualified applicants due to an extreme shortage of qualified nursing faculties.[5] Although the numbers vary, the Department of Health and Human Services currently projects a shortfall of up to 260,000 registered nurses by the year 2025.[6] Other research and health-care groups project a nursing shortage ranging from 800,000 to 1 million.

Preceptorships allow students to experience a more realistic employment situation before they graduate.

Periodically, some facilities try to cut costs by reducing the number of their most expensive personnel, the registered nurses. Most of these facilities eventually recognize that, although a reduction in RN positions may reduce the costs in the short-term, the long-term effects on the quality of health care are devastating. It is obvious that exchanging qualified nurses for lower-paid unlicensed technicians will eventually affect the quality of client care. With the current emphasis being placed on the delivery of quality client care from the Joint Commission (JC), the Institute of Medicine (IOM), the American Nurses Association (ANA), and the Affordable Care Act of 2010 (ACA), hospitals and other health-care facilities are recognizing that increasing the number of RNs they employ is the only way to increase the quality of care they provide. Unfortunately, in many areas of the country, facilities have been unable to fill their vacant RN positions.

Decentralized Care

Certain groups of nurses are in higher demand than ever; these include nurses who can practice independently in several different settings, multiskilled practitioners, home-care nurses, community nurses, and hospice nurses.[7] A major trend in health care today is to move the care out of the hospital and into the community and home settings. Provision of nursing services in these settings often requires that a nurse have at least a bachelor's degree or an even higher education. Fewer than 50 percent of all new graduate nurses today are graduating from bachelor's degree programs. The IOM report, "The Future of Nursing," established a goal of 80 percent baccalaureate-prepared nurses by 2020 to meet the needs of a health-care system that is constantly increasing in complexity.[8]

Although most nurse practitioners are currently based in community clinics, the ACA of 2010 is providing them with an ever-expanding opportunity to become involved in primary care and even the care of hospitalized clients. A key element in the ACA is that clients must be evaluated by a primary health-care provider before they can be referred to secondary health-care providers or specialists. The advanced-practice education of nurse practitioners would make them eminently qualified to fill this role of primary health-care provider.

Certain specialty areas with a high burnout rate such as transplant, intensive care, neonatal, oncology, and burn units are always seeking nurses. The nursing shortage has added to lower levels of satisfaction, increased stress levels, and high turnover rates of these nurses with highly specialized skills. Research has shown that as the perception of staffing shortages increases, so, too, does the number of nurses leaving these types of specialty units.[9] As with community nurses, nurses who provide care in specialty units must be able to work independently and use evidence-based practice by drawing from the large base of theoretical knowledge now available on the Internet.

The nursing profession and nursing educators need to increase their vigilance during nursing shortages to maintain the high standards of the profession and not fall into the "any warm body will do" trap. They must continue to recruit high-quality students and improve working conditions and salaries to keep the high-quality professional nurses they already have.

A POSITIVE TRANSITION TO PROFESSIONAL NURSING

The reality shock that new graduates often experience can be reduced to some extent. Some schools of nursing have instituted preceptor clinical experiences and other types of experiences during the last semester of the senior year. The main goal of preceptor clinical experience is to help the student feel more comfortable in the role of registered nurse.

Nurse Residency Programs

The IOM has recommended that nurse residency (NR) programs be established to help new nurses make the transition from the sheltered environment of nursing school to the practice setting. NR programs help develop new nurses' skills, increase their knowledge, and aid them in providing safer client care.[10] Researchers have calculated that it takes 1 or more years for a new graduate to master the skills necessary to be successful in their position. Specialty units generally take longer. In the past, many hospitals used a sink-or-swim approach, where the new graduate was placed on a unit soon after graduation and expected to perform at the same level as a skilled nurse. This is no longer acceptable. New graduate nurses often do not possess the knowledge or skills to make a quick transition to providing competent and safe bedside care.

Without residency programs, some hospitals experience a resignation rate of new nurses at or above 75 percent during their first year. A high turnover rate of nurses is equated with a high financial cost in recruiting and training more new nurses. A new graduate nurse who leaves his or her job within the first year will cost the institution between $22,420 and $77,200. That cost is then added to the expense of recruiting and orienting a new nurse, which has been estimated to range from a low of $8,000 to as much as $50,000 for nurses in specialty units.[11]

> *In the past, many hospitals used a sink-or-swim approach, where the new graduate was placed on a unit soon after graduation and expected to perform at the same level as a skilled nurse. This is no longer acceptable.*

The IOM has established some guidelines for NR programs. They believe it is important for state boards of nursing and state nurses associations to actively support and encourage facilities to develop programs that will ease the transition to safe clinical practice. The IOM encourages external funding for NR programs, which can be very expensive. This funding should be sought from major health-care organizations or groups that have a vested interest in improving health-care quality. Once the programs are established, they must be overseen and evaluated for effectiveness. Three key evaluation criteria include increased nurse retention, increased knowledge and competency of the nurses in the program, and an overall improvement in client satisfaction and outcomes.[10] Although the number of NR programs in the United States is relatively small at this time, the results have been extremely positive. The retention rate for new nurses completing 1-year NR programs was 95.6 percent in 2013. Evaluation data also showed that nurses felt a marked increase in their ability to provide safe, high-quality nursing care.[12]

Preceptorships

A student who works with a preceptor is assigned to one RN for supervision for most of the semester. The student experiences the role of the RN by working the same hours and on the same unit as the nurse to whom he or she is assigned. As the student absorbs the role expectations of the workplace during the preceptor experience, the student's perceived role expectations also change, allowing movement from the student role to that of practicing professional with less anxiety and stress.[13]

Another experience that lessens role transition shock may be an internship (sometimes called an *externship,* depending on the name used by the hospital). Internships or externships are available to students between the junior and senior years at some hospitals. These experiences allow students to work in a hospital setting as nurses' aides while permitting them to practice, with a few restrictions, at their level of nursing education. These experiences are invaluable for gaining practice in skills and for becoming socialized into the professional role.

Employment in Today's Job Market

Although the health-care industry is in dire need of registered nurses, employers are still looking for the best of the best for the positions they have available.

What Do You Think?

Have you ever been on a job interview? What were some of the mistakes you made? How can you correct those mistakes in the future?

Initial Strategies

Employers are looking for graduates who can function independently, require little retraining or orientation, and can supervise a variety of less-educated and unlicensed employees. The ability to use critical-thinking skills in making sound clinical judgments is a necessity in today's fast-paced, complicated, and highly technical health-care systems.

Although these requirements may seem daunting, some strategies can be used to increase the chance of being hired. Students should take advantage of preceptor and intern or extern experiences in their junior and senior years and should attempt to meet their clinical obligations in the institution where they want to be employed. In this way, the student can evaluate the hospital closely and observe its working conditions and the type of care provided to clients.

For its part, the hospital has the opportunity to examine closely the student's knowledge, skills, personality, and ability to relate to clients and staff. The hospital benefits by getting employees who are familiar with the hospital before employment starts, thus decreasing the overall time of paid adjustment (referred to as *orientation*).

The Résumé

In today's job market, the **résumé** is often the institution's first contact with the nurse seeking employment, and it has a substantial effect on the whole hiring process (Box 10.1). First impressions are important. Preparing a neat, thorough, and professional-looking résumé is worth the time and effort. If you have access to a computer, a good-looking résumé can be prepared at almost no cost. If a computer is not available, it is a good idea to spend a few dollars to have the résumé professionally prepared and reproduced.

Box 10.1

Sample Résumé

Mary P. Oak
100 Wood Lane, Nicetown, PA 22222 Telephone (333) 555-1234 (H) e-mail: moak@aol.com

Objectives
Obtain an entry-level position as a registered nurse; deliver high-quality nursing care; continue my professional development.

Skills
- Good organizational and time-management skills
- Communication and supervisory ability
- Sensitivity to cultural diversity

Education
Mountain University, Nicetown, PA
Bachelor of Science in Nursing, May 2013

Experience
Supercare Hospital, Hilltown, PA
Nursing Assistant, 2011 to present
    Responsibilities: Direct client care, including bathing, ambulation, daily activities, feeding paralyzed clients, assisting nurses with procedures, charting vital signs, and entering orders on the computer.
Big Bob's Burgers, Hilltown, PA
Assistant Manager, 2009–2011
    Responsibilities: Supervised work of six employees; counted cash-register receipts at end of shift; inventoried and ordered supplies.

Awards
Nursing Student of the Year, 2013
Mountain University, Nicetown, PA
Pine Tree Festival Queen, 2009
Hilltown High School, Hilltown, PA

Professional Membership
National Student Nurses Association, 2010 to present
Mountain University, Nicetown, PA

A Complete Picture

The goal of a résumé is to provide the hospital with a complete picture of the prospective employee in as little space as possible. It should be easy to read and visually appealing and have flawless grammar and spelling.[14] Although various formats may be used, all résumés should contain the same information. Each area of information should have a separate heading (see Box 10.1).

Many books available in local bookstores can serve as a guide in organizing the information in a résumé. Many new computers now come from the factory loaded with software that can prepare résumés in different formats. Keep an electronic copy of the résumé for future use or reference. The required information includes the following:

- Full name, current address (or address where the person can always be reached), telephone number (including area code), and e-mail address.
- Educational background (all degrees), starting with the most recent, naming the institution, location, dates of attendance, and degrees awarded. Usually high school graduation information is not necessary.
- Former employers, again starting with the most recent. Give dates of employment, title of position, name of immediate supervisor, supervisor's telephone number, and a short description of the job responsibilities. Should non-health-care-related work be included? Very basic jobs—for example, cooking hamburgers at Big Bob's Burgers—could probably be omitted unless it fills in a large gap in your employment history. However, if the job required supervision of other employees or demonstrated some higher degree of responsibility such as developing budgets,

> *First impressions are important. Preparing a neat, thorough, and professional-looking résumé is worth the time and effort.*

handling money, or preparing work schedules, it should be included and described.

- Describe any scholarships, achievements, awards, or honors that have been received, along with any professional development activities in which you participated, starting with the most recent.
- List professional memberships, offices held, and date of memberships.
- List any publications. If both books and journal articles were published, list the books separately, starting with the most recent.
- Include an "Other" category to describe any unpublished materials produced (e.g., an internal hospital booklet for use by clients), research projects, **fellowships**, grants, and so forth.
- Provide professional license number and annual number for all states where licensed, along with the date of license and expiration date.

References

References should be included on a separate sheet of paper. Most institutions require three references. After obtaining permission from the individuals listed as references, the nurse preparing the résumé should make sure to have current and accurate titles, addresses, e-mail addresses, and telephone numbers. Many facilities are now using e-mail or phone references in place of letters as a time-saving method.

Issues in Practice

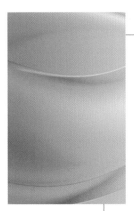

Compassion Fatigue Among Nurses

If you no longer really care about the clients to whom you are assigned, you may be suffering from compassion fatigue. Much like burnout, compassion fatigue results from long-term stress that generally revolves around the never-ending demands of caring for those with chronic diseases or those with terminal illness. Nurses with compassion fatigue also experience chronic physical fatigue, emotional distress, and feelings of apathy. Nurses can recognize the condition when they become calloused and withdraw from the delivery of health by merely going through the motions. Unfortunately, compassion fatigue can spread to other staff and ultimately produces negative client outcomes.

The first step in preventing compassion fatigue is taking care of yourself. You need to eat right, exercise, and get plenty of rest. There is no shame in reaching out to a professional counselor for advice and help. Staying in close contact with family and friends, looking after spiritual needs, developing fulfilling and fun hobbies, and participating in activities that are fun and renew the spirit are all important in dissipating the stress that leads to compassion fatigue. Also, rely on your coworkers. Working with a team you enjoy will help you stay connected with the reasons you entered the profession in the first place.

There are also courses and seminars available that can teach you ways to lower stress and deal with difficult situations. They will help you build up positive emotions to improve your attitude and enthusiasm levels.

Sources: Babbel C. Compassion fatigue. *Psychology Today*, 2012. Retrieved June 2013 from http://www.psychologytoday.com/blog/somatic-psychology/201207/compassion-fatigue; Krischke MM. Suffering from compassion fatigue, burnout or both? What a nurse can do. *Nursing News,* 2013. Retrieved June 2013 from http://www.nursezone.com/Nursing-News-Events/more-news/ Suffering-from-Compassion-Fatigue-Burnout-or-Both-What-a-Nurse-Can-Do_41375.aspx

An individual selected for a reference must know the applicant well in either a professional or a personal capacity, have something positive to say about the applicant, and be in some position of authority. The director of the nursing program, esteemed nursing faculty, supervisory-level personnel at a health-care facility, and even a physician make good references. It is best not to list relatives, unless the hospital is asking specifically for a personal reference.

Do not obtain letters of reference until the facility asks for them. Many facilities are now using e-mail or phone references in place of letters as a time-saving method.

Résumés via Institutional Website

Many health-care facilities want prospective employees to apply for positions and submit their résumés by the institution's website rather than in person or on paper. The first step is to find the link on the institution's website that will bring you to the employment application; the link will read something similar to "Prospective Employees" or "Job Opportunities." Under that heading there should be a subheading: "Apply for a Job." It is important that the job seeker read the instructions carefully and follow them to the letter. Comparable with the paper résumé, first impressions are important. If the person applying for a job cannot even follow the directions for applying, what kind of impression is that going to make on the human resources director? Each institution has its own format for applying. Some have boxes where a résumé can be pasted, some have a place to attach a résumé electronically, and some have a combination of the two. Others merely want the résumé attached to an e-mail and sent to a specific e-mail address.

A well-written paper résumé is a suitable place to start in creating an electronic résumé. However, the transition from a paper résumé created on a common word-processing program like Microsoft Word is anything but smooth and seamless. Many e-mail systems, scanners, or Web browsers will change how a document looks when it is opened in another system. These systems will change fonts for headings, delete punctuation, and even move text around. To have the best-looking electronic résumé, it is important to use the least amount of formatting possible and a letter font that is nonproportional. Generally, such features as tables, page borders, and multiple fonts should not be used. Keeping two versions of a résumé is a good idea—a "fancier" one for submitting by mail or taking to an interview and a second simpler electronic version that can be e-mailed or attached to an institutional website with minimal alterations.

The following steps for formatting an electronic résumé will work with most word-processing programs:

1. Open the résumé in the word-processing program normally used.
2. Click on FILE, then click on SAVE AS and select TEXT ONLY. (This will eliminate all nontext formatting.)
3. Close and then reopen the résumé using the new text-only version in Notepad or a similar plain-text editor.
4. Format the text-only résumé by:
   - Changing to a nonproportional font (i.e., a font where all the letters are the same size, such as Courier Brougham, Letter Gothic, Orator, Lucida Sans Typewriter, MonoTxt, Isocteur, Lucida Console, Courier, and Monospace 821). These fonts prevent the lines of text from varying in width across the page.
   - Do not indent by using tabs. Some Web browsers don't recognize them and might move the text around on the page.
   - Keep all lines justified to the left side of the page, and use line breaks (Enter key) to separate headings and sections. Using the spacebar to indent or center text has unpredictable results when read by another browser.
   - Use ALL CAPS rather than **bolding** or *italicizing* to emphasize a word or words or when starting a new section of the résumé.
   - Never use accent marks such as quotations (""), asterisks (***), or other characters ($#). These almost never come out like they were in the original document.
5. Save the edited résumé as a separate document from the original.
6. Send the electronic résumé by attaching it to an e-mail, posting it on the Internet, or copying and pasting it into an institution's Web page.[15]
7. These steps should also be followed when creating a personal website or electronic portfolio.

As with the paper résumé, there should be a separate cover document specifying what job the applicant is applying for and why they feel qualified for the position (see "cover letter" below). Some sites have a "Check which job you want" box that may eliminate the need for a cover letter; however, format the letter using the guidelines above and make it the first page of the résumé. This action will cover all possibilities.

Creating a Personal Website Summary

By the time students have completed their nursing education, they have looked at enough websites to know which ones grab their attention and which ones they quickly skip over. There are some general principles that all personal websites should follow, although creativity has a place as long as it is not too far out there! Then when the job applicant e-mails a prospective employer, a link can be attached to the site. Remember that first impressions count. What to include in a Web page:

1. A professional photo of the applicant on the first page. Grainy cell-phone shots with red eyes do not make a good initial impression. Each page should have a different, related photo. A résumé page should have a candid photo of you in a work setting. A personal page should have a tasteful photo of you at play.

> " *Harassing the personnel director or director of nursing about a job is not usually an effective employment strategy.* "

2. On the first page, use creative graphics or background photos that say something positive about you. A picture of a field of wildflowers behind the individual indicates a calm, attractive personality. A picture of a waterfall projects an image of power and direction. Be careful that the background is not so dark as to make the text hard to read.

3. Give a short summary of your personality and strengths on the home page. Use third-person descriptions. For example: "Julie's passion is to provide high-quality care to the most vulnerable of the population––premature infants and abused children." This page should also summarize your background. How did you become interested in nursing—through a specific event (e.g., a parent having cancer) or a person who inspired you? Did you have to overcome any difficult circumstances in nursing school? This page can also demonstrate your writing skills. Make sure an experienced writer or editor reviews it before you post it.

4. Write a career objective page. This page is like a résumé, but it can be longer and is in paragraph form. You can include portfolio images of your work to demonstrate your accomplishments visually—show pictures from that in-service presentation you gave as part of the leadership class assignment. Make sure you include information about your education, employment history, and a description of what you would consider the "perfect career." Describe in a few sentences what your dream job would be like and why. Describe your professional objectives and why they are important to you. Do you want to go back to school to become a nurse practitioner at some point in the future? Why?

5. Include a résumé page. This page should use the standard résumé format for professional résumés. It should be no longer than one page. Make sure you update the information on this page as it changes. You will be sending an electronic copy to the employer's Web page and using the hard copy when going for an interview.

6. Include a contact page with all your contact information: address, phone numbers, and e-mail addresses. Make sure these are kept current. Include a link on the contact page to the site you created, just in case the prospective employer is not adept at previewing job candidates electronically. Also include a link to the personal website.[16]

Where to Post It?

Several websites are generally recognized as locations for professional résumés. Web-savvy employers will often search these first. They include:

1. http://www.linkedin.com. This site contains more than 5 million professional résumés and is often used by professionals to track each other. Employers can use it for finding potential employees in specific fields of expertise.

2. http://www.blogger.com. Probably the easiest of the sites to use. It takes the user through the step-by-step process of setting up a blog in less than 30 minutes.

3. http://post.resumedirector.com/rd/default.asp. Posts your resume on up to 90 top resume sites with just one click—gets your resume in front of a large number of recruiters and employers all at one time. Also offers live help by phone or chat, resume building and job searching tips.

4. http://www.wordpress.com. This site is generally used by top-level professionals, although anyone can post on it. It has some advanced features in design and content generation.[5]

The Cover Letter

A cover letter should be sent with every mailed résumé (Box 10.2). Like the résumé, it should be neatly typed without errors and should be short and to the point. Although a friendly, rambling letter might provide insight into a prospective employee's underlying personality, most personnel directors or directors of nursing are too busy to read through the whole document. The letter should be written in a business letter format, be centered on the page, and include the name and title of the person who will receive the letter. Letters beginning with "To Whom It May Concern" do not make as favorable an impression.

Organizing the Letter

The statement of interest and name of the position should constitute the opening paragraph of the letter. The prospective employee should mention where he or she heard about the position. This information should be included in the first paragraph as well as a date when the applicant would be able to begin working.

The second paragraph should give a brief summary of any work experience or education that qualifies the applicant for this position. Newly graduated nurses will have some difficulty with this part, but they should include their graduation date, the name of the school they graduated from, the prospective date for taking the NCLEX, and the name of the director of the program. This paragraph should also state which shifts the applicant is willing to work.

The third paragraph should be very short. It should express thanks for consideration of the nurse's résumé, a telephone number, and an e-mail address. Both the letter and résumé should be sent by first-class mail in a 9 x 12 envelope so that the résumé will remain unfolded, thus making it easier to handle and read.

Box 10.2

Sample Cover Letter

Mary P. Oak
100 Wood Lane
Nicetown, PA 22222

May 25, 2015

Mr. Robert L. Pine
Director of Personnel
Doctors Hospital
Gully City, PA 44444

Dear Mr. Pine:

I am interested in applying for the registered nurse position in the General Medical-Surgical Unit. I have 5 years of experience in providing care for a variety of clients with medical-surgical health-care problems as a nursing assistant. I completed my baccalaureate degree in nursing on May 9 and am scheduled to take the NCLEX examination on June 3. Enclosed find my résumé.

I believe that my organizational and time-management skills will be a great asset to your fine health-care facility. I work well with all types of staff personnel, and having been a nursing assistant for the past 5 years, I can appreciate the problems involved in their supervision.

Thank you very much for consideration of my résumé and application. I will call you within the next few days to arrange a date and time for an interview. Feel free to call me at home anytime (333) 555-1234 or contact me by e-mail: moak@ol.com.

Sincerely,

Mary P. Oak

Will They Ever Answer?

Waiting for a reply can be the most difficult part of the process. Resist the urge to call the hospital too soon. Because most health-care institutions recognize the high anxiety levels of new graduates, they attempt to return calls within 1 to 2 weeks after receipt of the application. If no response is given after 3 weeks, the nurse should call the hospital to see whether the application was received. Mail does get lost. If the application has been received, the applicant should make no further telephone calls. Harassing the personnel director or director of nursing about a job is not usually an effective employment strategy.

The Portfolio

Today's current work climate requires recruiters to interview, screen, and hire the most qualified person for the job in a short amount of time. The nursing shortage and a workforce that embraces career portability have created the need to often recruit and hire nurses on a moment's notice.

Evidence of Positive Outcomes

Professional portfolios are being looked at closely by many nonartist professions to document skill qualifications, continued competency, accountability for professional development, and credible evidence to support employment claims during an interview. Nursing is one of the professions embracing this concept, and if the trend continues, student nurses of today will become the next generation of the 2.6 million registered nurses in the United States who use portfolios instead of résumés to interview for jobs, become certified, maintain certifications, and demonstrate competency.

Health-care employers today are looking for nurses who believe that high-quality performance on the job is more important than just having a job. Professional nurses can apply the nursing process to their own personal development, and evidence of positive outcomes is placed in the portfolio.

Constructing a portfolio requires looking at a career as a collection of experiences, which can be grouped and reordered to match the changing direction of one's career journey. A portfolio also offers an opportunity for nurses to evaluate their experiences, create new goals, create and implement a plan, and then evaluate it. The portfolio supports the lifelong process of self and career development.[16]

Assembling a Portfolio

Once a student has decided to initiate a portfolio as a professional vehicle for showcasing his or her experiences, education, skill sets, accomplishments, and potential for achievement, it will require time and effort to create it. However, the effort is well worth it in the long run.

The initial development of a portfolio may be somewhat time-consuming, but once it is developed, keeping it current should become part of a professional's routine activities. Converting it to an electronic format is a must in today's high-tech health-care system.[16] Whether the portfolio is paper or electronic, the content and purpose are the same. Many books and online resources are available that describe the format and organization of a portfolio; an example is also discussed here.

Portfolios are an excellent way to impress potential employers, reach a larger employment pool, and put the Internet to work for a prospective employee.

Use a Binder. One format that many experts agree on is a three-ring binder. This should include a table of contents, and the various sections should be separated by dividers.

Ask Yourself Questions. Questions to ask while you prepare to gather materials for your portfolio include: What do I want to do next in my career? Why do I think I am qualified for this job? What do I want to tell the employer about myself? Why should my employer promote me?

Interview a Professional. Once a decision has been made on an employment area of interest, it is helpful to discuss the needed skills and education with someone who is currently employed in that work setting. Personal interviews can provide information about what skills or education is required. It is a good idea to show a draft of the portfolio to the nurse being interviewed to see if it reflects the required knowledge or if there is a need to pursue further education or skill development.

Showcase Your Education. Box 10.3 lists work samples that can be included in the portfolio. Box 10.4 lists basic categories for organizing the portfolio. Remember, these are just examples, and each

B o x   1 0 . 3

Examples to Collect for a Professional Portfolio

1. Education and training examples
2. General work performance examples
3. Examples regarding using data or nursing informatics
4. Examples pertaining to people skills
5. Examples demonstrating skills with equipment

Items that may be collected to support these areas include, but are not limited to, the following:

Articles	Awards
Brochures	College transcripts and degrees
Drawings and designs	Forms
Flyers	Grants
Letters of commendation	Letters of reference
Manuals and handbooks	Merit reviews
Photographs	Military service and awards
Presentations	PowerPoint presentations
Proposals	Professional memberships
Résumés	Research
Technical bulletins	Scholarships
Videos	Training certificates

B o x   1 0 . 4

Categories to Organize Your Professional Portfolio

1. **Career Goals:** Where do you see yourself in 2 to 5 years?
2. **Professional Philosophy/Mission Statement:** What are your guiding principles?
3. **Traditional Résumé:** Concise summary of education, work experience, achievements.
4. **Skills, Abilities, and Marketable Qualities:** Examples that support skill area, performance, knowledge, or personal traits that contribute to your success and ability to apply that skill.
5. **List of Accomplishments:** Examples that highlight the major accomplishments in your career to date.
6. **Samples of Your Work:** See Box 10.3; you can also include CD-ROMs.
7. **Research, Publications, Reports:** Include examples of your written communication abilities.
8. **Letters of Recommendation:** A collection of any kudos you have received, including from clients, past employers, professors, and so on.
9. **Awards and Honors:** Certificates of award, honor, or scholarship.
10. **Continuing Education:** Certificates from conferences, seminars, workshops, and so on.
11. **Formal Education:** Transcripts, degrees, licenses, and certifications.
12. **Professional Development Activities:** Professional associations, professional conferences, offices held.
13. **Military Records, Awards, and Badges:** Evidence of military service, if applicable.
14. **Community/Volunteer Service:** Examples of volunteer work, especially as it may relate to your career.
15. **References:** A list of three to five people who are willing to speak about your strengths, abilities, and experience; prepared letters from same.

nurse needs to use a format that will best showcase his or her education, work experience, skill sets, and accomplishments.

Use the Internet. Creating a Web version of the portfolio can enhance the application process (see earlier). Links can be created to digitize versions of portfolio information, examples of presentations, or photos of accomplishments or events. Portfolios are only limited by the nurse's imagination and access to space on the Web. Portfolios are an excellent way to impress potential employers, reach a larger employment pool, and put the Internet to work for a prospective employee.[16] Even if the nurse has a Web version, it is a good idea to bring the paper portfolio and a copy to an interview.

As discussed in the previous section, a résumé is an excellent tool for allowing the prospective health-care recruiter or employer to receive a concise overview of a potential employee in as little space as possible, and it will serve as a frame of reference once the interview process is complete. A nurse who offers to share a portfolio during the interview process provides tangible evidence of skills, accomplishments, and future potential. Showing a well-prepared portfolio leaves a positive lasting impression with the interviewer and provides a foundation to build on as the nurse's career develops.

Interviews

The next important step in the process is the interview. The interview allows the institution to obtain a firsthand look at the applicant and provides an opportunity for the applicant to obtain important information about the institution and position requirements. The interview often produces high levels of anxiety in new graduates who are interviewing for what might be their first real job.

Make a Good Impression

Again, first impressions are important (Box 10.5). The interview starts the moment the applicant enters the office. Conservative business clothes that are clean, neat, and well pressed are an absolute necessity.

B o x 1 0 . 5

Fashion Do's and Don'ts of Interviews

The Do List
Men
1. Do shave or trim facial hair closely.
2. Do use aftershave and/or cologne sparingly (a little goes a long way).
3. Do carry a money clip or leather wallet and a small, plain functional briefcase.
4. Do wear leather shoes that are polished and in good repair. Lace-up or slip-on shoes are best.
5. Do wear calf-length dark socks.
6. Do wear a tailored suit (blue, gray, beige are best) with a dress shirt (lighter in color than the suit). Do wear a conservative tie.
7. Do shut off your cell phone or beeper.

Women
1. Do apply perfume or cologne sparingly (a little goes a long way).
2. Do invest in a good haircut. Clean, neat, and conservative is best.
3. Do wear shoes that are polished and in good repair. Plain pumps with medium heels are best.
4. Do carry a briefcase or simple (small) handbag that matches your shoes.
5. Do wear hose that coordinate in color, style, and texture with your shoes and outfit. Do take an extra pair for emergencies.
6. Do apply makeup lightly and carefully.
7. Do apply conservatively colored nail polish carefully.
8. Do dress conservatively.
9. Do wear colors that make a strong statement, such as shades of gray in medium to charcoal, or blue in a medium to navy.
10. Do wear small, conservative earrings.
11. Do shut off your cell phone and beeper.

Continued

B o x   1 0 . 5

Fashion Do's and Don'ts of Interviews—cont'd

The Don't List
Men
1. Don't overstuff wallet, money clip, or briefcase.
2. Don't carry a can of smokeless tobacco in your back pocket or pack of cigarettes in a shirt pocket.
3. Don't wear sandals, running shoes, or cowboy boots.
4. Don't wear socks that are a lighter color than your trousers.
5. Don't wear green or flashy colors.

Women
1. Don't wear sneakers, sandals, cowboy boots, or heels more than 1½ inches high.
2. Don't overstuff your handbag or briefcase.
3. Don't apply makeup so that it looks artificial and heavy.
4. Don't use black or bright or dramatically colored nail polish.
5. Don't wear skimpy or low-cut outfits, leather, or fringed apparel.
6. Don't wear large, dangling earrings or display other body piercings, such as nose rings, lip rings, tongue rings, or multiple earrings.

Sources: Doyle A. How to interview. Job Searching. Retrieved June 2013 from http://jobsearch.about.com/cs/interviews/a/aceinterview.htm; Interview Tips. Capella University. Retrieved June 2013 from http://msn.careerbuilder.com/msn/category.aspx?categoryid=iv

Similarly, a conservative hairstyle and a limited amount of accessories, jewelry, and makeup produce the best impression. Smoking, chewing gum, biting fingernails, or pacing nervously does not make a good first impression. The interviewer recognizes that interviews are stressful and will make allowances for certain stress-related behaviors, but do try to avoid the mistakes listed in Box 10.6.

Arriving a few minutes early allows time for last-minute touch-ups of hair and clothes and gives the applicant a chance to calm down. Carrying a small briefcase with a copy of the résumé, cover letter, references, and information about the hospital also makes a favorable impression.[17]

Come Prepared
Mental preparation is as important to a successful interview as physical preparation. Most interviewers will start with some "small talk" to try putting the interviewee at ease. Resist the temptation to launch into a long and rambling account of personal experiences. Next, the interviewer will usually ask about the résumé or portfolio, if one is used. A quick review just before the interview is helpful so that the interviewee is familiar with the information contained in the résumé or portfolio.

Expect questions about positions held for only a short time (less than 1 year), gaps in the employment record (longer than 6 months), employment outside the field of nursing (e.g., waitress, clerk), educational experiences outside the nursing program, or unusual activities outside the employment setting. Answer the questions honestly but briefly. Most personnel directors or directors of nursing are busy and do not appreciate long, detailed, chatty answers. Applicants can anticipate being asked:

- Why do you want this position?
- Why have you selected this particular facility?
- Why do you think you are qualified for the position?
- What unique qualifications do you bring to the job to make you more desirable than other applicants?
- Where do you see yourself 5 years from now? Ten years from now?[10]

Using the portfolio will help answer some of these questions. By showing tangible examples of qualifications and accomplishments, the interviewee can help the busy interviewer discern between actual performance and mere rehearsed answers.

Forbidden Topics
Because of the emphasis placed on political correctness and discrimination issues in recent years, there are a number of areas that prospective employers are not supposed to discuss but sometimes do anyway.

Box 10.6

Twenty Worst Job Interview Mistakes

1. Arriving late
2. Arriving too early (10–15 minutes is okay)
3. Dressing wrong (see Box 10.5)
4. Having your cell phone or beeper go off during the interview (and answering it)
5. Drinking alcohol or smoking before the interview
6. Chewing gum and/or blowing bubbles
7. Bringing along a friend, relative, or children
8. Not being prepared—not having an interview "dress rehearsal"
9. Calling the interviewer by his or her first name
10. Not knowing your strengths and weaknesses
11. Asking too many questions of the interviewer (a few are okay)
12. Not asking any questions at all
13. Asking about pay and vacation as the first questions
14. Accusing the interviewer of discrimination
15. Bad-mouthing your present or former boss or employer
16. Name-dropping to impress the interviewer
17. Appearing lethargic and unenthusiastic
18. Weak, "dead fish," or bone-crusher handshake
19. Looking at your watch during the interview
20. Losing your cool or arguing with the interviewer

Sources: Chun J. Questions to ask during a job interview. *Nursing Review,* 13(26):472, 2010; Clear J. 99 Interview tips that will actually help you get a job. Passive Panda, 2013. Retrieved June 2013 from http://passivepanda.com/interview-tips;

Marriott P. Quality in practice . . . get the best out of job hunting: Polish your CV and shine at interview. *Community Care,* 4(1808):34, 2010.

Smith LS. Are you ready for your job interview? *Nursing,* 40(4):52–54, 2010.

These include questions about sexual preferences or habits, age, race, plans for a family, personal living arrangements, **significant others**, and religious or political beliefs.

If these questions are asked, the applicant needs to consider the implications of not answering them. Although there is no legal obligation for the applicant to answer, refusal to do so or pointing out that the question should not have been asked in the first place may be unwise. If the graduate answers these personal questions, which violate an individual's right to privacy or seem discriminatory, and then is not hired for the position, there may be grounds for some type of legal action based on discrimination.

Ask Your Own Questions

At some point in the interview, usually toward the end, applicants are asked whether they have any questions. Although most do have questions, many applicants are afraid to ask. In fact, asking questions can be seen as a demonstration of independence,

initiative, and intellectual curiosity—all traits that are highly valued by health-care providers. It is important that the first questions are not about salary, vacations, and other benefits. Questions that indicate interest in the institution are included in Box 10.7.

Box 10.7

Questions Interviewees Should Ask

- What are the responsibilities involved in the position?
- Who are the other staff or personnel working on this unit?
- What is the typical client-to-staff ratio for the unit?
- Are there any mandatory rotating shifts, weekend obligations, overtime, or floating?
- Does the hospital offer opportunities for continuing education, clinical ladder, advancement, or movement to other departments?
- Please describe the facility's policies for employee health and safety.

After these questions have been answered, the applicant may want to ask about salary, raises, vacations, and other benefits. Some questions that the applicant should never ask include: "When will I get a promotion?" "When do I get my first raise?" "What sort of flex-time options do you have?" or any question that indicates they were not paying attention during the interview. It would also be wise to inform the interviewer of the dates scheduled for the NCLEX so that arrangements can be made for time off. The applicant should also ask for written material on the nurse's contract with the institution, including benefits and job descriptions. Often the interviewer will provide this information without being asked in the course of answering some of the other questions.

Take this scenario as an example: The job applicant had successfully fielded all the usual interview questions: "Why do you want this job?" "What are your qualifications?" "Why should I select you over other candidates?" Then the interviewer asked the question that all job applicants hate: "What do you consider to be your major weakness?" A good way to answer that question is to find a weakness that can be turned into a strength. The applicant might answer, "I tend to be a perfectionist and spend too much time trying to get things just right."

It is appropriate to close the interview by asking for a tour of the facility. A tour allows first-hand evaluation of the workplace and a chance to observe the staff and clients in a real work setting. The interviewer may not be able to provide a tour at that time and may ask another individual (e.g., a secretary) to take the applicant on the tour.

Beware of the Internet

Nothing Is Private

Savvy employers almost always Google the name of a prospective employee before an interview. Research has shown that 75 percent of employers look up candidates before the interview and up to 70 percent have rejected potential employees because of information online. Some employers go even further to find out about the candidate; often they can electronically locate unflattering pictures or video sequences, ill-advised comments or tirades, and even financial information.[17] Although somewhat slow to catch on in the health-care arena, this trend is taking hold.

It Never Goes Away

As a candidate for a job, especially as a new graduate, you need to be aware that the person sitting across

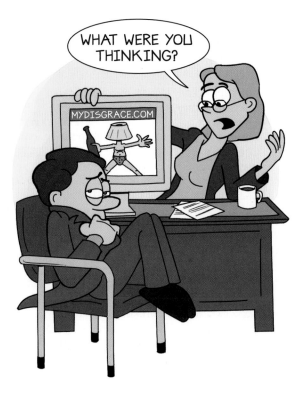

from you at the interview desk may well have run your name through an electronic search engine and found you on some social media format. The following situation is an example of what happened during one candidate's interview for a job. During an interview, after the candidate answered all the questions, the interviewer remarked, "I found a video segment of you on MySpace.com that was shot about 2 years ago showing you at a party appearing inebriated with very few clothes on. Would you mind commenting on that?"

Personal blogs can be deleted and after a time will become harder to access. However, the truth is that once something goes electronic, it never completely goes away. Search engines have improved to such a point that they can find information that is 5 or more years old.

Although you can use the Internet to your advantage, it can also be a tool of your own demise in the job market. You may feel secure and private in a chat room with your "friends," but in reality, anything you post on the Internet can end up on Facebook, YouTube, Xanga, Twitter, Instagram, Vine, or one of the other blog websites. You may feel safe using a pseudonym or password protection, but these are only as trustworthy as the people who have access to your information. A jilted boyfriend or girlfriend, a friend who thinks what you said was funny, someone with a large circle of electronic friends all have the power to reveal your most private information.[17]

You can offset negative information about yourself by generating as much positive information as possible. Eventually, the positive information will get more hits, and the negative information will be pushed to the end of the site, where people are less likely to see it. However, sites like wayback-machine.com can dig up information that has been sanitized and removed from a website even years before. Remember, nobody is perfect, and all people have information they would prefer to keep secret. If negative information about you does exist online, you can try to control it by spinning it in the best way possible. If there is a large amount of negative information and pictures, you might want to spend some money and have it professionally removed by sites like IronReputation.com, Reputation.com, or elixirinteractive.com, which can scrub and wipe clean even the most incriminating and damaging materials. These sites guarantee removal of ALL unwanted content and will also monitor your website for new postings of untoward pictures or information and automatically remove it.

Business Cards—Old School?

In some circles, business cards are considered old school. Electronic business cards are now taking the place of piles of paper business cards. One of the most commonly used electronic business cards on social media is BizEcards (https://www.facebook.com/bizEcards). It is an interactive business card that you can text. The site will help you develop the card and show you how to use it. Another format that is commonly used is vCard (http://vcardmaker.com/). It is an electronic business card that can be read by many formats including iPhone and e-mail. The site helps you develop the card and to make the most of the vCard. Another site that provides paperless business cards is http://mashable.com/2009/06/11/virtual-business-card/. This site can create as many nonpaper business cards as you want, and the cards will never run out. They can also be sent to anyone who has a computer or a mobile phone.

Follow-Up

As with the résumé, making frequent calls about the results of the interview is unwise. However, it is appropriate for the applicant to send a letter within 1 week after the interview to thank the interviewer for his or her time and express appreciation for being considered for the position (Box 10.8). The applicant should also

---

B o x   1 0 . 8
Sample Follow-up Letter

Mary P. Oak
100 Wood Lane
Nicetown, PA 22222

June 20, 2015

Mr. Robert L. Pine
Director of Personnel
Doctors Hospital
Gully City, PA 44444

Dear Mr. Pine:

Thank you very much for considering my résumé and for the interview on June 3, 2015. I learned a great deal from the interview and from my tour of the hospital after the interview.

   I am writing to let you know that I am still interested in the position and was wondering about the status of my application. If at all possible, I would appreciate it if you could either call me or write a note relating to my potential employment at your facility.

   Feel free to call me at home any time (333) 555-1234 or contact me by e-mail: moak@aol.com

Sincerely,

Mary P. Oak

acknowledge how much it would mean to him or her to become a member of the staff at such a high-quality agency or hospital, but avoid overdoing the compliments.

If the position is offered, a formal letter of acceptance or refusal should be sent to the institution. Health-care facilities will not hold positions indefinitely, and failure to accept the position formally in a timely manner may result in their offering the position to someone else.

WHEN NURSES BURN OUT

The burnout syndrome has existed for many years and has been recognized as a problem that can be reduced or even prevented. A widely accepted definition of burnout is a state of emotional exhaustion that results from the accumulative **stress** of an individual's life, including work, personal, and family responsibilities. The term *burnout* is used to describe a slow, continuous depletion of energy and strength combined with a loss of motivation and commitment after prolonged exposure to high occupational stress. Examples of occupational stress include heavy workload, lack of participation or social support, injustice, uncertainty, lack of incentive, wearing out role conflicts, job insecurity, job complexity, and structural constraints.

Although the term is not often applied to students, many of the symptoms of burnout can be observed in these aspiring nurses.[8]

Who Burns Out?

The people who are most likely to experience burnout tend to be more intelligent than average, hard-working, idealistic, and a perfectionistic. There are certain categories of jobs and careers that tend to produce a higher incidence of burnout: situations and positions in which there is a demand for consistent high-quality performance, unclear or unrealistic expectations, little control over the work situation, and inadequate financial rewards. These jobs or careers tend to be very demanding and stressful, with little recognition or appreciation of what is being done. Also, jobs in which there is constant contact with people (i.e., customers, clients, students, or criminals) rank high on the burnout list.

Even with the most superficial knowledge of nursing, it is easy to see that many of these elements are present in the nurse's work situation. It is possible to recognize nurses who are in the early stages of burnout by identifying some classic behaviors (Box 10.9).

How It Starts

One of the earliest indications of burnout is the attitude that work is something to be tolerated rather than eagerly anticipated. Nurses in the early stages of burnout often are irritable, impatient, cynical, pessimistic, whiny, or callous toward coworkers and clients. These nurses take frequent sick days, are chronically late for their shifts, drink too much, eat too much, and often are not able to sleep.

Eventually, as their idealism erodes, their work suffers. They become careless in the performance of their duties, uncooperative with their colleagues, and unable to concentrate on what they are doing, and they display a general attitude of boredom and **apathy**. If allowed to continue, burnout may lead to feelings of helplessness, powerlessness, purposelessness, and guilt.[9]

Complications of Burnout

A new study published by the *American Journal of Infection Control* has found that nurses experiencing burnout may be contributors to the spread of infection, especially when working long hours and caring for too many clients at a time. When client-to-nurse ratios are increased, there is a corresponding increase

B o x   1 0 . 9
Symptoms of Burnout

- Extreme fatigue
- Exhaustion
- Frequent illness
- Overeating
- Headaches
- Sleeping problems
- Physical complaints
- Alcohol abuse
- Mood swings
- Emotional displays
- Anxiety
- Poor-quality work
- Anger
- Guilt
- Depression

in rates of infection in hospitals. Increased client loads lead to external mental demands, such as interruptions, divided attention, and feeling rushed. Just the addition of one extra client per shift per nurse was related to a 10 percent increase in rates of urinary catheter and postoperative infections. The study showed that the extra time out of the nurse's day to monitor, administer medication, and provide care for an additional client is sufficient to reduce infection control measures such as hand washing. The study noted that reducing burnout by 10 percent could prevent thousands of hospital-acquired infections per year and save $41 million per hospital. By decreasing nurses' workloads, there is an increased likelihood of following through on infection control procedures. It would also create a better atmosphere for nurse and client safety.[10,11]

Nurses suffering from burnout have also been linked to increases in client clinical errors, such as medication mistakes, missing treatments, and missing signs and symptoms of serious changes in condition. Burnout has also been linked to failure to complete documentation and errors in documentation.[11]

Recognizing Burnout

The first step in dealing with burnout is recognizing its signs. Here are some of the key signs that a nurse may be experiencing burnout:

- Continuous physical exhaustion and excessive illnesses
- Strong feelings of being taken advantage of and unappreciated
- A feeling of impending doom when preparing to go to work
- Pulling back at work—spending as little time as possible doing tasks and communicating
- Lack of empathy for clients[12]

Despite this bleak picture, nurses do not have to fall victim to the burnout syndrome. Many nurses practice their profession for many years, manage to deal with the stress, and find great personal satisfaction in what they do. These satisfied and motivated nurses have developed ways to deal with the stress of their careers while maintaining their goals and purpose as nurses.

Nurses experiencing burnout usually go through four progressive stages with some overlap between them. These include physical and mental exhaustion; self-shame and doubt; cynicism about work and lack of empathy for clients; and a sense of personal failure, feelings of helplessness, and an overwhelming sense of crisis.[12] Many nurses who are burning out use denial and rationalization to block recognition of burnout because it is just too painful for them to think they put so much time, money, and effort into preparing for a career they no longer want or enjoy.

It is important to realize that burnout can be halted in any one of the four phases. It does not have to progress to a crisis state. Also keep in mind that it is not the career that is producing the burnout, but rather the difficulty in coping with the stresses the career is producing. Although it may not be possible to change the requirements of the profession significantly, it is possible to learn how to cope more effectively with stress.

Manage Stress and Time

Although there are many schools of thought about stress- and time-management techniques, several common threads run through many of these theories. These views include setting personal goals, identifying problems, and using strategies for problem-solving.

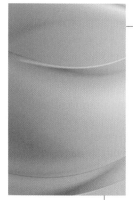

Issues Now

Exercise Myths: True or False

1. Exercise can turn fat into muscle. False.

Muscle and fat are two completely different types of tissue. Exercise can increase the mass of muscle tissue and decrease the size of fat cells by burning fat as energy.

2. If you're gaining weight, it always means you're getting fatter. False.

An increasing amount of fat will make the scale numbers go up, but it's not the only cause. If you are exercising and building muscle, it has a much higher density than fat (i.e., a pound of muscle takes up less space than a pound of fat). It is possible to become leaner and healthier while at the same time gaining weight. The scale can be your friend or enemy!

3. I'm a woman and I'll bulk up if I lift weights. False.

The bulging, bulky muscles that men get when they pyramid train (overwork muscles) is due primarily to testosterone. Also, that type of training requires weight lifting for 6 to 8 hours a day every day. Weight training will help muscle definition in women and help tone muscles, which in turn increases metabolism and reduces weight.

4. Running outside on a track is worse for the joints than running on a treadmill. False.

Running is running and it stresses the joints no matter where it's done. There are some very expensive high-end treadmills that have extra shock-absorbing features, but even those do not completely eliminate the stress on the joints.

5. Any type of aerobic exercise will burn fat. True.

However, the harder you exercise, the more fat you burn. It is important to build up a progressive exercise tolerance before attempting to reach the maximum level of an aerobic exercise.

6. I can eat anything I want as long as I exercise every day. False.

This is a myth that gets some people into a real bind. Any given exercise will burn a certain amount of calories per session. For example, if you weigh 155 pounds and run 1 mile in 12 minutes, you will burn about 560 calories. Or if you ride a stationary bike for 1 hour at a moderate speed, you will burn 439 calories. (For a complete table of exercises and calories, go to http://www.nutristrategy.com/activitylist3.htm.) The key here is not to eat more calories than you burn off when you exercise. So if you stop and get a 1100 calorie super-sized chocolate milkshake after you run your mile, you are going to be 440 calories in the hole! You need to go back and run another mile!

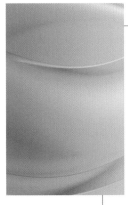

Issues Now continued

7. Using free weights causes more injuries than using weight machines. It depends.

Free weights are very adaptable to all body types and can be adjusted easily to accommodate a person's exercise progression. The danger with free weights arises when people do not know their limits and try to overdo the weights. Also, they tend to pay less attention to good body alignment and configuration when they use free weights. With machines, you are less likely to drop a weight on your toe. They also tend to force the person into the proper body position for the particular exercise. The problem is that machines are based on an "average-sized" person, and if you are very large or very small, it may not be appropriate for you.

8. When you sweat a lot, it means you are achieving the maximum workout. False.

As warm-blooded creatures, humans sweat to keep their internal body temperature in an acceptable range (homeostasis). It may or may not be related to increasing the heart rate or burning fat. Some people have a higher metabolic rate and tend to sweat a lot even with minimal exertion. When exercising on a cold day, a person may sweat little or not at all.

9. No pain, no gain. False.

The corollary to this myth is "A lot of pain, a lot of gain." Although most people do experience a small amount of discomfort or pain when they exercise vigorously, it is due primarily to the toning and stretching of the muscles. If your muscles are toned, you may not experience any pain at all with regular exercise. If you are having an excessive amount of pain, it's your body's way of telling you to stop what you're doing and take a rest.

10. Stretching after you exercise may be more beneficial than stretching before exercise. True.

After you have exercised, the muscles and connective tissues are "warmed up" and comply more readily to being flexed and lengthened. The stretches should be slow and deliberate and held for 10 to 15 seconds while breathing deeply. Cold stretching before exercise may actually cause injuries because the connective tissues are stiff and less elastic. Many people, especially women, are hyper-flexible and do not need to stretch. Although it is a widely accepted practice, cold stretching may not be needed by everybody.

Sources: Boston G. 10 fitness myths debunked. Wellness. *Washington Post,* 2013. Retrieved June 2013 from http://www.washingtonpost.com/lifestyle/wellness/fitness-myths/2013/05/28/28c04d6a-bf25-11e2-9b09-1638acc3942e_story.html; Bouchez C. Top 9 fitness myths. WebMD. Retrieved June 2013 from http://www.webmd.com/fitness-exercise/features/top-9-fitness-myths-busted; Calories burned during activities, sports and exercise chart. Nutristrategy, 2013. Retrieved June 2013 from http://www.nutristrategy.com/activitylist3.htm; Park M. 10 exercise myths that won't go away. CNN Health, 2013. Retrieved June 2013 from http://www.cnn.com/2011/HEALTH/06/24/exercise.myths.trainers/index.html

Set Personal Goals

Goals and goal setting are an important part of client care. Nursing students—and, by extension, practicing nurses—are highly proficient in the planning stage of the nursing process, in which goal setting is the primary task. Nurses know that a good set of goals should be client centered, time oriented, and measurable and that they should write these goals with every care plan they prepare.

In their personal lives, however, these nurses may rush full tilt into one erratic day after another, subordinating their own needs to the needs of others and working long, hard hours but without accomplishing very much and feeling frustrated about it. What is the problem here? Very simply, nurses can prepare realistic, beneficial goals for their clients, but they seem to be unable to do the same for themselves.

Long-Term Goals

Personal goals should include both long-term and short-term goals. Typically, personal long-term goals look into the future at least 10 years and include a statement about what the nurse wants to achieve during his or her lifetime. Some examples are going back to school to obtain an advanced degree, becoming a director of nursing, or even writing a book about nursing.

Practicing nurses who are caught up in the whirlwind of everyday life find it difficult to formulate statements about the future. One other important characteristic of long-term goals is that they need to be flexible. As life circumstances change, modifications are required.

Short-Term Goals

Short-term goals are those that the nurse expects to accomplish in 6 months to 2 years. These goals should be aimed primarily at making the nurse's professional or personal life more satisfying and fulfilling. Like long-term goals, they do not need to be related to work. Perhaps visiting a foreign country, going on a skiing trip in the mountains, and even learning how to paint a picture or play the piano may be achievable in a relatively short time. In the professional realm, joining a professional organization, becoming a head nurse, or changing an outdated

hospital policy are goals that can be achieved in a short time. The fact that everyone ages over time cannot be altered, but that time can also be used to achieve personal satisfaction in life and increase knowledge and accomplishments.

An End Achieved

Although goal setting is an important first step in dealing with the stress that leads to burnout, any good nurse recognizes that a plan without implementation is useless. As difficult as goal setting may be for nurses, carrying it out may be even more difficult. Although goal achievement requires a degree of hard work and personal sacrifice, when people are working toward something they really want, the effort that it takes to achieve the end actually becomes enjoyable. This process takes a lot of work, but it becomes an exciting adventure in its own right.

> *Health-care employers today are looking for nurses who believe that high-quality performance on the job is more important than just having a job. Professional nurses can apply the nursing process to their own personal development, and the evidence of positive outcomes is placed in the portfolio.*

Identify Underlying Problems

Another important step in dealing with burnout is to identify the problems that are producing the stress. Again, nurses are taught as students that they need to identify client problems so that they can work toward solving them. The same applies to resolving their own setbacks. They cannot be addressed if they are ignored or unknown.

Self-Diagnosis

Formulation of a nursing diagnosis is nothing more than precisely stating a client's problem. One thing nurses realize early in the learning process is that what may appear to be an obvious problem may in reality not be a problem at all. Conversely, something that a client only mentions in passing may turn out to be the real source of the client's nursing needs. Perhaps nurses should look at their own lives and attempt to formulate nursing diagnoses that deal with their stress-related problems (setting the North American Nursing Diagnosis Association list aside).

What Do You Think?

List three tasks that you have put off today. Why did you avoid doing these? How can you get them done sooner?

For example, a new graduate has just completed a shift during which he was assigned to eight complete-care clients. He had to supervise two poorly prepared nurses' aides and put in 55 minutes of overtime (for which he will not be paid) to complete the charting. This nurse is feeling tired, frustrated, and even a little bit guilty because of an inability to provide the type of care that he was taught in nursing school.

What is the problem? A possible nursing diagnosis might be "alterations in personal satisfaction related to excessive workload, evidenced by sore feet, headache, shaky hands, feelings of guilt, frustration, and a small paycheck."

Goals and Interventions

Now that the problem has been identified, goals and interventions can be introduced to solve the problem. The goals may range from organizing time better to refusing to take care of so many complete-care clients. Interventions, depending on the goals, can include activities such as attending a time-management seminar, talking to the head nurse, or changing a policy in the policy and procedure book.

> " *It is important to realize that it is not the career that is producing the burnout, but rather the difficulty in coping with the stresses the career is producing.* "

RESPONDING TO MAJOR STRESSFUL EVENTS

Although nurses often learn how to deal with the stresses routinely found in their daily work, major traumatic events that produce overwhelming stress, such as the devastation of the World Trade Center, Hurricane Katrina, or the massive destruction caused by major tornadoes, may leave nurses with a sense of horror, helplessness, and powerlessness in addition to the normal stress responses of shock, disbelief, anger, and grief. Nurses have several skills that help them deal with traumatic events in their workplace; however, they are not super-people and should not expect that they can handle all stressful events without help. The end result may well be a complex of symptoms similar to burnout syndrome, including physical symptoms, depression, and chronic anxiety.

Crisis Intervention

In response to major tragedies in recent years, the **critical incident stress debriefing** (CISD) process was developed to help health-care providers deal with major acts of violence and traumatic disasters. The American Red Cross has been instrumental in training and providing resources for local CISD teams. These are made up of mental health professionals specially trained in crisis intervention, stress management, and treating post-traumatic stress disorder (PTSD).

To be most effective, the CISD teams need to be on-site within 2 to 3 days after serious events, ranging from the death of coworkers to acts of terrorism and natural disasters. The goal of the team is to encourage the participants to verbalize their feelings and thoughts, identify and develop their coping skills, and generally lower overall grief and anxiety levels. They provide an intensive stress management course compressed into a few hours or few days.

Post-Traumatic Stress Disorder

One of the keys to working with nurses is to help them recognize that they are not expected to be able to handle all situations and can appropriately ask for help. Although nurses study the stress response and grieving process in school, it is sometimes hard for them to apply information about normal stress reactions to themselves. When nurses do not recognize their own problems in responding to traumatic stress, they increase their risk for developing long-term stress reactions. When they do not seek help, they can develop the symptoms of PTSD anywhere from a few days to as long as 6 months after the event.

Warning signs of PTSD include:

1. Recurring nightmares and inability to sleep.
2. Intrusive and vivid flashbacks.
3. Prolonged depression.
4. High levels of anxiety.
5. Maladaptive coping behaviors, such as drug and alcohol abuse.

The CISD session generally requires up to 3 hours. Sessions can be longer or shorter, depending on the nature of the event and number of people affected. Besides having an opportunity to express emotions and feeling, the participants are educated in some ways about reducing anxiety and promoting mental and physical health. This advice includes:

1. Not watching televised replays of the event over and over.
2. Staying with friends as much as possible.
3. Avoiding unhealthy, high-fat diets.
4. Engaging in regular aerobic exercise as much as possible.
5. Avoiding excessive dependence on alcohol and drugs for sleep.
6. Getting back to a comfortable routine as soon as possible.
7. Feeling comfortable seeking professional help when it is needed.

During the CISD sessions, nurses are asked for their input about the process. If the team feels it is necessary, additional referrals for long-term treatment may be recommended.

STRATEGIES FOR PROBLEM-SOLVING

Nurses already know the nursing process as a client problem-solving technique. Why not apply the same knowledge and skills to personal problems? The stress level only increases if problems are left unsolved.

Although specific problems may require specific solutions, several widely accepted methods exist to deal with the general stresses produced by everyday work and personal life. Included in these methods are activities such as recognizing that nurses are only human, improving time-management skills, practicing what is preached, and decompressing.

Time-Management Skills
In modern life there is often not enough time to do everything that needs to be done. The key to time management is setting priorities. In the world of nursing and client care, nurses are often required to do many tasks. Multitasking, the process of doing several tasks at the same time, tends to fragment the nurse's attention and concentration.

Nurses need to recognize that only some nursing activities are essential to the safety and well-being of clients. These include performing thorough assessments and ensuring that the clients get their medications on time, that their comfort needs are met, and that accidental injuries are prevented. Beyond these actions, nurses really have a great deal of

discretion in what they can do when providing care to clients.

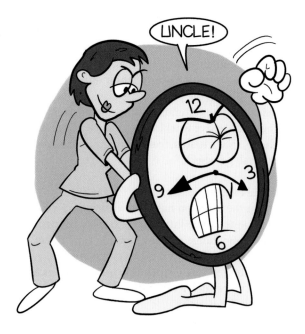

Make Room for Fulfillment
Burnout results mainly from personal and professional dissatisfaction. If nurses feel fulfilled in what they are doing, burnout is much less likely to occur. Activities that may increase nurses' satisfaction include spending time talking with clients, learning new skills, and decreasing the anxiety of families through teaching and listening. After such activities have been identified, time should be set aside for them during the shift. The real secret in using time management to prevent burnout is for the nurse to use the time left for those nursing activities that bring the most professional and personal satisfaction.

Several skills need to be developed to allow time during a shift for these preferred activities. First, the nurse must learn to delegate by letting the licensed practical nurses (LPNs) or aides do those tasks they are able to do. Many nurses graduate from nursing school with the attitude that if you want it done right, you need to do it yourself. After becoming familiar with the LPN's and nurse's aide job descriptions, nurses need to give others a chance to prove themselves.[10]

Overcome Procrastination
Another necessary skill is overcoming procrastination. Most people have a natural tendency toward

procrastination, particularly when unpleasant or difficult tasks are involved. The primary reasons people postpone or delay doing something are that they either do not want to begin or do not know where to begin the task. More time and energy are expended in inventing excuses for putting off tasks than would be taken in doing the tasks.

The Most Distasteful Task

The best way to overcome procrastination is by starting the task, even if it is only a small step. An effective method is to select the most difficult or distasteful task to be done that day and to commit just 5 minutes to it. After 5 minutes are over, you can either set the task aside or continue it. Once you start the task and momentum builds, you will likely carry out the task to completion. If you don't do anything else that day, at least you've completed the most difficult task!

Tasks can be prioritized by listing them in three categories. Category A tasks (e.g., assessments, passing out medications, treatments, and dressing changes) are important and need to be completed on time. Category B tasks (e.g., baths, linen changes, lunch breaks, charting) are important but can be postponed until later in the shift. Category C tasks (e.g., cleaning up, organizing the supply room) are tasks that can either be delegated or wait until the next day.

Problems Don't Solve Themselves

For daily tasks, both pleasant and unpleasant, the best time to do them is immediately. If achievement of the plan requires delegation, it needs to be done at the beginning of the shift, not at the middle or end. Often nurses have a built-in fear of taking chances. As a result, they avoid doing things if there is a chance of failure in the hope that somehow the problem will resolve itself.

Any time an important decision is made, there is a chance that someone will disagree or that the decision will be incorrect. These types of situations need to be viewed as a challenge or an opportunity rather than a life-altering risk to be avoided. Although mistakes in health care do have the potential to be fatal, learning from mistakes is one of the most fundamental ways of increasing knowledge.

Time management, like other skills, requires some practice. Once a nurse masters this skill, his or her life becomes more satisfying.

Practicing What You Preach

Because nursing is oriented toward keeping people healthy as well as curing illness, nurses spend a large amount of their time teaching clients about eating well; getting enough sleep; going for regular dental, eye, and physical examinations; avoiding too much drinking and smoking; and exercising regularly. It might make an interesting student research project to have nurses rank themselves on how well they have incorporated these health maintenance activities in their own lives. The results would probably indicate a low overall score on the "practice what you preach" scale.

Nurses know all about the food pyramid, but they do not translate that knowledge into feeding themselves properly. In reality, there are going to be some busy days when it is impossible to eat right, but it should be possible, on a regular basis, to follow a diet that will promote health and reduce the buildup of fat plaques in the arteries.

"Tension must be released, or it will eventually cause a major explosion or (if turned inward) produce anxiety."

It is important to get enough sleep to avoid chronic fatigue. People can adjust to a state of fatigue, but it tends to decrease the enjoyment that they find in life and make them irritable, careless, and inefficient. Most people need between 5 and 8 hours of good sleep each night. It also probably would not hurt for nurses to take a short nap during the afternoon on their days off.

The Right Kind of Exercise

Many nurses feel they get enough exercise during their busy shifts, and, in truth, the average staff nurse walks between 2 and 5 miles during each 8-hour shift. Unfortunately, this type of walking does not qualify as the type of aerobic exercise recommended for an improved cardiovascular conditioning and stress relief. Exercise, in order to be beneficial, must be done consistently and must raise the heart rate above the normal range for an extended period. The short sprint-type walking involved in client care does not accomplish this goal.

Research studies compared workers' exercise habits with their psychological well-being. The results indicated that the more workers exercised, the less likely they were to experience increases in depression or burnout. Those employees who exercised at least 1.5 hours per week reduced their depression and job burnout tendency by 50 percent over those who never worked out. The group who exercised more than 4 hours per week had the same results as those who exercised 1.5 hours per week.[13]

Further research has shown that exercise actually decreases the production of stress hormones like cortisol and epinephrine while increasing the production of endorphins, the body's natural pain- and anxiety-relief chemicals. Physical activity acts as a strong distraction from problems. Anxiety, anger, and stress can be redirected to physical exercise and may allow a person to achieve a Zen-like state in certain cases. Going to a gym, boxing ring, running trail, biking trail, or a sidewalk in the neighborhood provides a pleasant change of scenery and helps lower stress.[14]

Exercise also helps a person build up an immunity to the stress of the workplace. Studies have shown that people who exercise more tend to be less affected by the daily stress they face. Reasonable exercise also builds up the immune system, making the person less susceptible to common infections; however, excessive exercise may actually deplete the immune system.[15] Exercising with others has the additional benefit of social support. When exercise and physical activity also involves others, the positive effects are doubled by combining stress-relief activity with the enjoyment of friends. Working out with a friend improves motivation, increases happiness, and makes the workout go faster and seem less like work.[14]

Walking 1 to 2 miles a day outside of work is a beneficial, simple exercise that will improve health.

Nurses can also use a wide variety of exercise equipment for those days when walking outside is undesirable. The important requirement is that the exercise be done consistently and frequently. Regular exercise not only improves the cardiovascular system but also helps improve stamina, raise self-image, and promote a general sense of well-being.

Decompression Time

The profession of nursing is stressful, even under ideal circumstances. Nurses are required to deal with other people constantly and to carry out numerous tasks that are potentially dangerous. At the end of any shift, even the most skilled and best-organized nurse has a sense of internal tension. This tension must be released, or it will eventually cause a major explosion or (if turned inward) produce anxiety.

Establish a Daily Decompression Routine

It may take a little time to discover, through trial and error, what works to reduce the tension built up during the shift. Some effective techniques include setting aside approximately 30 minutes of private, quiet time to reflect on the day's activities. Perhaps relaxing in a hot bath or sitting in a favorite recliner might meet the need for decompression. Relaxation activities, such as swimming, shopping, or even going for a drive, can help reduce tension and act as a time for decompression. Of course, stress-management techniques learned at seminars (e.g., self-hypnosis or meditation) can also be used. Finally, meeting with a nurse support group can help the nurse vent feelings and make constructive plans for solving problems.

Conclusion

Although transition shock and burnout are realities of the nursing profession, they can be reduced or even avoided altogether. Nurses should be able to recognize the causes and early symptoms of transition shock and burnout to prevent them from developing into a problem. Therefore, nurses should use techniques to prevent these disorders from becoming insurmountable obstacles. In doing so, nurses will be able to practice their profession proficiently and gain the satisfaction that only nursing can provide.

Critical-Thinking Exercises

- Make a list of the characteristics that would be found in the "perfect nurse." Make a second list of characteristics found in nurses observed in actual practice. Discuss how and why these lists differ.
- Outline a plan for implementing a preceptor clinical experience for the senior class of a nursing program. Make sure to include how many hours of practice are required, criteria for the selection of preceptors, student objectives from the experience, and methods of evaluation.
- Write at least three long-term and five short-term personal or professional goals. Develop a realistic plan and time frame for achieving these goals. Make sure to include what is required to achieve these goals.
- Complete this statement, using as many examples as possible: "I feel most satisfied when I am done with my shift in knowing that . . ." Analyze these answers and discuss how they can be implemented in everyday practice.
- Think of at least three situations in which you were asked to do something that you really did not want to do. How did you handle these situations? How could they be handled in a more assertive manner?

References

1. Fox RL, Abrahamson K. A critical examination of the U.S. nursing shortage: Contributing factors, public policy implications. *Nursing Forum,* 44(4):235–244, 2009.

2. Kydd A. Counting nurses in a nursing shortage: What of the silent attrition? *Reflections on Nursing Leadership,* 36(1): 1–4. 2010.

3. Somers MJ, Finch L, Birnbaum D. Marketing nursing as a profession: Integrated marketing strategies to address the nursing shortage. *Health Marketing Quarterly,* 27(3):291–306, 2010.

4. Plunkett RD, Iwasiw CL, Kerr M. The intention to pursue graduate studies in nursing: A look at BScN students' self-efficacy and value influences. *International Journal of Nursing Education Scholarship,* 7(1):1–13, 2010.

5. Stansfield J, McAleer F. Brought to (Face)book. *Speech & Language Therapy in Practice,* 19:1368–2105, 2010.

6. Olmstead D. A good portfolio puts you ahead of other applicants. *American Society of Respiratory Therapists Scanner,* 42(3):14, 2010.

7. Vallet M. Face(book) the facts. *Massage Therapy Journal,* 49(2):56–61, 2010.

8. Frandsen BM. Burnout or compassion fatigue? *Long-Term Living: For the Continuing Care Professional,* 59(5):50–52, 2010.

9. Laschinger HKS, Finegan J, Wilk P. New graduate burnout: The impact of professional practice environment, workplace civility, and empowerment. *Nursing Economic$,* 27(6):377–383, 2009.

10. Cimiotti JP, Aiken LH, Sloane DM, Wu ES. Nurse staffing, burnout, and health care–associated infection. *American Journal of Infection Control,* 2013. Retried June 2013 from http://www.nursing.upenn.edu/chopr/Documents/Nurse%20st affing,%20burnout,%20and%20health%20care%20associ-ated%20infection.pdf

11. Wood D. Study links nurse staffing and burnout to hospital infections. NurseZone.com. Retrieved June 2013 from http://www.nursezone.com/Nursing-News-Events/more-news/Study-Links-Nurse-Staffing-and-Burnout-to-Hospital-Infections_40308.aspx

12. Fink, JLW. 5 signs of burnout. NursingLink. Retrieved June 2013 from http://nursinglink.monster.com/benefits/articles/2481-5-signs-of-burnout?page=3

13. Toker S, Biron M. Could exercise lower risk of job-related depression and burnout? *Huffington Post,* 2013. Retrieved June 2013 from http://www.huffingtonpost.com/2012/03/07/exercise-lowers-the-stres_n_1327260.html

14. Scott E. Exercise and stress relief: Using exercise as a stress management tool. *Stress Management,* 2012. Retrieved June 2013 from http://stress.about.com/od/programsandpractices/a/exercise.htm

15. Quinn E. Exercise and immunity. *Sports Medicine,* 2012. Retrieved June 2013 from http://sportsmedicine.about.com/od/injuryprevention/a/Ex_Immunity.htm

16. Doyle A. How to make a resume on line. Retrieved August 2014 from http://jobsearch.about.com/od/onlineresumes/tp/how-to-make-an-online-resume.htm

17. Adichie, CN. Hiding from our past. *The New Yorker,* 2014. Retrieved August 2014 from http://www.newyorker.com/culture/culture-desk/hiding-from-our-past

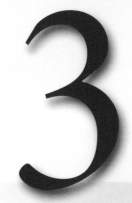

3

Leading and Managing

Leadership, Followership, and Management

11

Joseph T. Catalano

Learning Objectives

After completing this chapter, the reader will be able to:

- Identify and discuss the three major theories used to explain leadership
- Define and distinguish among the three styles of leadership
- Discuss the relationship of transformational and situational theories to leadership style
- Identify the key behaviors and qualities of effective leaders
- Identify the key characteristics of effective followers
- Distinguish the differences between management and leadership
- Identify and discuss the two major theories of management

In today's health-care system, even new graduates who have an "RN" after their name will be placed quickly in positions of leadership and management.

LEADERSHIP

The old saying that "leaders are born, not made" implies that at birth a person either is a leader or is forever relegated to the rank of follower. Not many agree with this statement. Although some people may have an easier time filling the leadership role than others, most experts believe that almost everyone can develop leadership skills.

Many definitions of leadership refer to the ability of an individual to influence the behavior of others. When nurses exert leadership, they inspire other health-care workers to work toward one or more of several goals that include providing high-quality client care, maintaining a safe working environment, developing new policies and procedures, and increasing the power of the profession.

Some leadership theories try to explain why some people are leaders and others are not, but as yet none covers all the possibilities. That may be because leadership requirements differ according to the situation. In the intensive care unit (ICU), for example, where quick decisions are a matter of life and death, the leader is the nurse with highly developed critical-thinking and analytical skills and the confidence to make decisions under pressure. In quality management, where the problems are often long term and complicated, the leader tends to be well organized and can methodically sift through a mountain of information and statistics to develop a policy that covers the widest range of possibilities. Several of the better-known leadership theories are discussed here.

Trait Theory

The trait theory identifies qualities that are common to effective leaders (Box 11.1). Trait theory by itself is limited because it focuses only on the traits of the individual and does not take into account how the person

Box 11.1

Leadership Traits

- High level of intelligence and skill
- Self-motivation and initiative
- Ability to communicate well
- Self-confidence and assertiveness
- Creativity
- Persistence
- Stress tolerance
- Willingness to take risks
- Ability to accept criticism

acts in specific situations. The question left unanswered is why everyone who has these traits is not a leader.[1]

Leadership-Style Theory

One of the best-known theories of leadership looks at three leadership styles:

1. Laissez-faire
2. Democratic
3. Authoritarian

Although these theories are discussed separately, they are a continuum of leadership style that ranges from a mostly passive approach to a highly controlling one (Table 11.1).

The Laissez-Faire Style

The **laissez-faire** (French for "leave it alone") leadership style is also described as permissive, nondirective, or passive. The laissez-faire leader allows the group members to determine their own goals and the methods to achieve them. There is little planning, minimal decision-making, and a lack of involvement by the leader. This style works well in only a few settings, for example, in a research laboratory that is staffed by self-motivated scientists who know what they want to achieve and are familiar with the means of achieving it.

The laissez-faire style works best when the members of the group have the same level of education as the leader and the leader performs the same tasks as the group members. In most situations, however, laissez-faire leadership can leave people feeling lost and frustrated because of the lack of direction by the leader. When they do try to achieve some goal, often the only input from the leader is that they are doing it incorrectly. When faced with a difficult decision, laissez-faire leaders usually avoid making a decision in the hopes that the problem will resolve itself.

The Democratic Style

In the **democratic** (also called *supportive, participative, transformational*) leadership style, all aspects of the process of achieving a goal, from planning and goal setting to implementing and taking credit for the success of the project, are shared by the group. The democratic leadership style is based on four beliefs:

1. Every member of the group needs to participate in all decision-making.
2. Within the limits established by the group, freedom of expression is allowed to maximize creativity.
3. Individuals in the group accept responsibility for themselves and for the welfare of the whole group.
4. Each member must respect all the other members of the group as unique and valuable contributors.

Table 11.1 **Comparison of Authoritarian, Democratic, and Laissez-Faire Theories**

	Authoritarian	Democratic	Laissez-Faire
Degree of Freedom	Little freedom	Moderate freedom	Much freedom
Degree of Control	High control	Moderate control	Little control
Decision-making	Leader only	Leader and group	Group or no one
Leader Activity Level	High	High	Minimal
Responsibility	Leader	Leader and group	Abdicated
Quality of Output	High quality	High quality/creative	Variable
Efficiency	Very efficient	Moderately efficient	Variable

Source: Whitehead DK, Weiss SA, Tappen RM. *Essentials of Nursing Leadership and Management* (5th ed.). Philadelphia: F. A. Davis, 2010, p. 6.

The leader using the democratic style provides guidance to the group, and all members share control. This style works best with groups whose members have a relatively equal status and who know each other well because they have worked together for an extended period. In its purist form, democratic leadership can be time-consuming and inefficient in some situations, particularly when group members disagree strongly, but in the end, when a goal is achieved or a decision made, there is a strong sense of ownership and achievement by the whole group. Hallmarks of this style are trust, collaboration, confidence, and autonomy. Followers of this system have a high level of commitment to the institution, resulting in a strong work ethic and innovative ideas in practice.[2]

Many leaders are uncomfortable with this style of leadership because of the minimal control they have over the group. Participative leadership allows the leader more control over the final decision. After considering all the opinions of the group members, the leader makes the final decision based on what is best to achieve the goal.

The Authoritarian Style

The leader with an **authoritarian** (also called *controlling, directive,* or *autocratic*) style maintains strong control over all aspects of the group and its activities. Authoritarian leaders provide direction by giving orders that the group is expected to carry out without

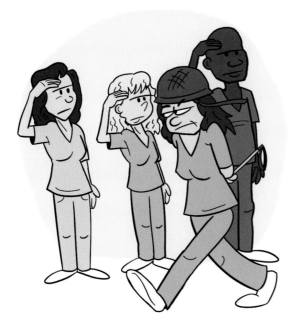

question. The final decision-making authority rests with the leader alone, although input from the group may be considered. The authority consists of micro managers who closely monitor everything that the group members do and often make on-the-spot changes when they believe they know a better way to achieve a task or goal. People who work under this style of leadership usually harbor hostile feelings that they are fearful to express, use passive-aggressive techniques to try to even the playing field, and feel oppressed and unable to use their full potential as a worker.

An extreme form of the authoritarian leadership style is the dictatorial leadership. A leader using a dictatorial authoritarian style is called a dictator. This leader has no regard for the feelings and needs of the group members. Achieving the goal is the only thing that matters, and the dictator will use any means, including harsh criticism, to do so. A military mission to destroy a terrorist group by a Delta Force assault team is an example of this type of leadership.

What Do You Think?

Have you ever had to be a leader in a group? What type of leadership style did you use? How successful was the outcome of the group work?

Another type of authoritarian leadership style is the benevolent leader. The benevolent authoritarian leader uses a more paternalistic approach to achieving the goal. That leader attempts to include the group's feelings and concerns in the final decision, but ultimately the leader makes all the decision. Some group members may feel that the benevolent leader is condescending and patronizing.

The authoritarian leadership style works best in emergency situations, when clear directions are required to save a life or prevent injury, or in situations in which it is necessary to organize a large group of individuals. Although highly efficient in achieving goals and completing tasks, authoritarian leadership suppresses the creativity of the group members and may reduce the long-term effectiveness of the group. Authoritarian leadership also reduces the motivation levels of the group and may lead to passive-aggressive behavior by the members that will further reduce the effectiveness of the group. Although some people can accept the need for the total control exerted by an authoritarian leader, most people in a long-term work relationship with this type of leader will become frustrated and even rebellious at some point.

In reality, few leaders use only one style. Most leaders use multiple leadership styles, depending on the situation. Many factors may influence what type of leadership style is used at any given time, including external regulations and requirements, the ability of the group members, the work setting, and the problem being solved. For example, a nurse manager on a hospital unit may use a highly democratic style in most of the routine activities of the unit, but when a client goes into cardiac arrest, she may revert to a highly authoritarian style while directing the staff through a code.

What Do You Think?

Think of the best leader you have ever worked with. What traits did that person have? Now think of the worst leader you ever worked with. What traits did that person have?

Relationship–Task Orientation

Another commonly used theory rates leaders on whether they are oriented more toward establishing relationships or achieving assigned tasks and resolving problems. The work setting often dictates whether the leader is more oriented toward building relationships or completing tasks.[3] For instance, in a psychiatric setting, relationships are key to successful treatment of the client, and the tasks of self-realization and coping skills are achieved in the therapeutic relationship setting. And in a post-disaster environment, achieving the tasks of sorting victims into appropriate categories for treatment and keeping them alive takes precedence over strong interpersonal relationships.

High Relationship–Low Task

Leaders with high relationship–low task orientations are usually well liked by their groups because of their acceptance of the group members as individuals, consideration of their feelings, encouragement, and promotion of good feelings among all the group members.

However, this kind of leader often sacrifices the achievement of the task or resolution of a problem when it conflicts with the feelings or good will of the group. This leader often allows the group to make its own decisions without regard to the task at hand and ultimately may not achieve the goals the group was organized for in the first place.

High Task–Low Relationship

The opposite extreme is the leader with a low relationship–high task orientation. This form of leadership is similar to the authoritarian style, where the leader does all the planning with little regard to the input or feelings of the group, gives orders, and expects them to be carried out without question. Various forms of punishment are used by this leader, ranging from verbal put-downs to poor performance evaluations that are used to determine pay raises.

Both Extremes

The worst leader is the person with a low relationship–low task orientation. This leadership style simulates the laissez-faire style, in which the leader is uninvolved, does no planning, has little concern for the group members' feelings, and accomplishes little. On the other hand, the best leader is the one with a high relationship–high task orientation. This leader combines the best of both worlds: He or she is open to input and actively communicates with the group members, provides constructive direction, quickly resolves conflicts, and ultimately achieves creative and effective solutions to problems.

Certainly, perfect leaders are difficult to find. Most use a combination of styles and adjust them to the circumstances surrounding the problem. Again, think of the nurse manager who uses a high relationship–high task orientation for managing the unit in most day-to-day operations. In the cardiac arrest situation, this nurse manager may quickly change her or his orientation to one of low relationship–high task until the crisis is resolved.

RECENT THEORIES OF LEADERSHIP

Although the behavior and trait theories remain popular, researchers have come to the conclusion that leadership is really a more complex process. The

> *" The old saying that 'leaders are born, not made' implies that at birth a person either is a leader or is forever relegated to the rank of follower. "*

situational theory recognizes that no one approach works in all situations. A leader needs to acknowledge this and adjust the leadership style and behavior to the situation, considering the many variables that may be involved. Good leaders seem to do this instinctively. One of the key factors is the type of organization in which the group is located. The environment is always important in exercising leadership.

The transformational theory takes the situational theory one step further. This theory recognizes that multiple intangibles exist whenever people interact. Factors such as sense of meaning, creativity, inspiration, and vision all are involved in creating a sense of mission that exceeds good interpersonal relationships and rewards. Although this is true in most work settings, health care and nursing, in which care of human beings is the primary goal, require that nurses do something positive. In many health-care facilities, nursing leaders are expected to inspire excitement and commitment in nurses, who often must provide care to very ill clients in less than ideal circumstances.[2]

KEY LEADERSHIP BEHAVIORS

Traits are characteristics that an individual possesses. Traits may or may not lead to the actions or behaviors that are required for successful leadership. It is also possible to lack leadership traits, yet be able to carry out successful leadership behaviors.

Establish Trust and Cooperation Among Individuals and Groups. A trusting relationship is key to the success of a leader (or manager) on both individual and group levels. The followers must be able to trust the leader and each other.[3] Building that type of trust usually takes some time and involves individuals recognizing that the leader is honest, motivated, reliable, predictable, and consistent. Also, in the health-care setting, nurses tend to trust the individual who works hard and can perform all the required skills. Building trust and cooperation within the group can be very challenging.

Personality is the sum total of a person's genetic composition and experiences. Because no two people have identical genes or experiences, each one has different needs, feelings, and orientations. Because of the many personalities and backgrounds a group brings to the work setting, they often have an inherent mistrust of those who are different from them. However, if they trust the leader, the leader can use this trust to build stable relationships within the group by recognizing the differences and directing people to their highest level of achievement.

Acknowledge Good Work and Success. By providing rewards for the efforts that individuals make in achieving personal and organizational goals, the leader provides a powerful motivation for the nurse to continue working hard and being successful. These rewards do not have to be expensive or even cost anything at all. Positive verbal reinforcement is often more effective than a prize or gift. Saying, "You really did a good job taking care of that difficult client today," or "I was impressed with how well you managed your time in taking care of those five clients," is often more of a reward than most nurses receive in a month. A birthday card or a thank-you card with a personal note is also very effective. At Christmas time, a little homemade gift and a card thanking them for all they do for the success of the unit is also very effective.

Show Respect for Individuals. Although there are some overlaps with trust and reward, showing respect for others has some key elements that are not always easy to master. Treat other people as you would want to be treated (the Golden Rule). If you want to be included in the group when they go to lunch, then include the other person. By treating others as you would want to be treated, you are acknowledging them and recognizing their needs. Be polite and courteous by saying *please, thank you,* and *you're welcome.* Our society seems to have adopted rudeness as its basic mode of response (see Chapter 17 for more detail). Demonstrating politeness can be contagious and others will begin to return the sentiment. Don't make judgments about people before you really get to know them, which may take some time. Often, as the new person on the unit, they may be defensive and trying

> " *The authoritarian leadership style works best in emergency situations, when clear directions are required to save a life or prevent injury, or in situations in which it is necessary to organize a large group of individuals.* "

to protect themselves until they learn the routine and unwritten rules of the unit. Later, they will be more open and more accepting. Show empathy and promote mutual respect. People who are respected by you will respect you back and respect others. Never insult them or say negative things behind their backs.

Provide a Sense of Direction. Leaders need to demonstrate by their actions that they are working toward achieving goals at the personal, unit, and organizational levels. In providing a sense of direction for the group, the leader must be able to convey a vision of what can be achieved rather than how to just survive. Humans have an inborn drive to look toward the future and are attracted to individuals who have a vision of the next big thing coming down the road. If a leader has an unwavering commitment to a greater purpose and a higher goal, it will attract and inspire followers to work for their goals.

Promote Higher Levels of Performance. There are many factors that go into promoting higher levels of performance, including rewards and motivation. One of the best ways to promote better performance is to provide individuals with more difficult challenges. Often nurses become bored with their client care, not because it isn't busy enough, but because it has become routine. If the leader listens carefully to nurses, often they will discover that the nurses' desire for more challenges in a job is a fairly common concern. By providing the nurse with more challenging projects, the leader can increase that individual's performance. Also, the leader can be excited about a project and show a high level of enthusiasm in its completion. Excitement and enthusiasm are contagious and will motivate other nurses to escalate their performance.

Resolve Conflicts Successfully. The primary goal is to resolve conflicts before they get out of control. The main barrier to conflict resolution is that humans have a tendency to avoid overt confrontation because it makes them feel uncomfortable. The result of avoidance is that the unresolved issues continue to escalate to a point where they may no

longer be able to be resolved. The simple solution for managing the conflict between others is to encourage them to discuss the issue openly and honestly between themselves. They need to remember that everybody involved in the conflict has good intentions and truly believe they have the right answer. Leaders need to let people know up front how they go about conflict resolution. Leaders should never take sides, never try to "solve" the conflict, and should bring the conflicting parties to the realization that it is their conflict and they need to resolve it as professionals. (For more detail about conflict resolution, see Chapter 12.)

Foster Cooperation. The goal is to foster a culture of cooperation and teamwork on the unit and in the facility. However, there is some degree of cooperativeness and competitiveness in every individual; few people are 100 percent cooperative or 100 percent competitive. The environment and culture of the workplace also helps determine how cooperative an individual eventually becomes. If nurses who are usually cooperative finds themselves in a highly competitive working environment, then they are likely to become more competitive and less cooperative just to survive in the workplace. Building a culture of cooperation can be a long and difficult process, particularly when a hostile culture already exists. (See Group Dynamics below.)

> *The old question, 'How do you know when you've arrived if you don't know where you are going?' is a truism that all leaders must address at some point by establishing clear goals and outcomes for the group.*

One key behavior that the leader can promote to move toward a cooperative culture is to spend more time with new employees.[3] Instead of the 10-minute "Hi! Nice to meet you. Here's the 50-cent tour of the unit," sit down and talk with new employees. Ask them about their background, work habits, and competencies. Introduce them to at least six employees on the unit and have them ask their new colleagues about their backgrounds. By making this type of connection with at least six other nurses, they develop a sense of trust and establish essential working relationships. The connection also helps develop a cooperative mind-set and encourages them to seek relationships beyond the initial group of six.

Reinforce Goals. The old question, "How do you know when you've arrived if you don't know where you are going?" is a truism that all leaders must address at some point by establishing clear goals and outcomes for the group. Groups who lack clear goals often feel frustrated and lost. Initially, leaders must clearly identify their goals and then continually reinforce the goals or establish new goals as the old ones are reached. Successful outcomes are a result of clear goal setting and continually reinforcing the goals on the way to their achievement.

Develop Staff Strengths. The rapid changes and advancements in health care require nurses to continually learn and develop new skills. Through observation, a good leader can get to know what the strengths and areas for improvement are for each of the nurses on the unit. The leader can then make it known that there are learning opportunities available for those who are interested. If a nurse has a particular talent, ability, or a desire to learn a new skill, the leader will support and nurture it. Another way of developing staff strengths is by cross training a staff member with a particular strength with another staff member who may have a different strength. For example, a nurse in the intensive care unit may be very strong in reading and interpreting electrocardiograms (ECG) of clients but has difficulty with arterial blood gas interpretation. If paired with a nurse who can easily interpret blood gas results but is weak in ECG reading, they will both be able to mentor each other and improve their individual strengths. Actually, the mentoring process is very effective in developing strengths and overcoming weaknesses. The mentor can be another nurse or the nurse leader.

Lifelong learning is a goal that effective leaders seek not only for those whom they are leading, but also for themselves. Leaders can function as teachers in certain settings, but a more effective means of encouraging others to continue to learn is to set a good example. It is important to recognize that learning takes place not only in a formal school-like setting but also in all those encounters and situations that affect attitudes, beliefs, and behavior.

Motivating Personnel. The ability to motivate is an essential behavior for all levels of leadership. Unmotivated nurses merely go through the motions of nursing, producing low-quality care and dissatisfied clients. Motivating staff actually involves many of the behaviors discussed above, including rewarding a job well done, showing respect, establishing reachable goals, and establishing a culture of trust and cooperation. In addition, nurse leaders can become examples of motivation by cheerfully and successfully completing their own duties and avoiding complaining and negative attitudes. Fostering pride in the achievements of the unit and the hospital as a whole can be an effective motivator. Some facilities have a "Unit of the Month" award system that rewards units that achieve high scores on client satisfaction evaluations. Effective leaders also know that constantly berating or correcting other nurses for everything they do that isn't perfect quickly kills motivation and morale.[2] An overall atmosphere of encouragement and reward is a very powerful element in increased motivation.

KEY LEADERSHIP QUALITIES

No matter what style a leader favors, successful leaders have common qualities (Box 11.2):

Critical Thinker. The ability to think critically is a multistep process similar to the nursing process. Critical thinkers must be able to analyze data,

---

Box 11.2

Keys to Leadership

Key Qualities
- Critical thinker
- Problem solver
- Integrity
- Active listener
- Skillful communicator
- Courage
- Initiative
- Energy
- Optimism
- Perseverance
- Well-roundedness
- Coping skills
- Self-knowledge

Source: Adapted from Tappen RM, et al. *Essentials of Nursing Leadership and Management* (5th ed.). Philadelphia: F. A. Davis, 2010, p. 8.

organize and plan, and use creativity in the resolution of problems. Leaders must often make important decisions on the basis of incomplete data.

Problem Solver. Being able to use the problem-solving process effectively is essential to successful leadership. Leaders in the health-care setting face problems that arise from many sources, including staffing and personnel, scheduling, and administrative, budget, and client demands.

Integrity. For many years, nursing has been ranked as the most trusted and respected profession in the annual Gallup Poll of professions. One of the keys to this trust and respect is the integrity of the profession as it is perceived by clients and their families. The public expects nurses, as a group, to be honest, trustworthy, ethical, moral, and professional. The American Nurses Association (ANA) Code of Ethics for Nurses (see Chapter 6 for more detail on the Code) is directed toward promoting and maintaining the integrity of the profession. If a group observes less than complete integrity in their leader, that person's ability to lead is markedly diminished.

Active Listener. To be effective, leaders must be able to hear the words the person is saying and observe the body language and its underlying emotions and meaning. The experts tell us that only 7 percent of communication is verbal; 93 percent is all the other nonverbal content. Leaders often fail in their leadership roles when they do not listen to the full message of the individuals they are attempting to lead.

Skillful Communicator. Communication is a complex process that involves an exchange of information and feedback (see Chapter 12 for more detail on communication). Mistakes happen on both sides when the information being shared is incomplete or confusing. Providing frequent and positive feedback is one of the best methods for leaders to determine how well they are communicating and how open the communication channels remain. It also can boost morale and improve the working environment. Effective leaders should also be able to give and use negative feedback to improve performance. If negative feedback is given in a nonthreatening and encouraging manner, the person receiving it will often appreciate the chance to improve his or her skills.

Courage. Although all leaders must have the courage to maintain their convictions in the face of adversity, certain leadership positions may require a higher degree of courage. Nurses in middle management positions, such as unit managers, house supervisors, or quality control coordinators, often find themselves caught in a no-man's-land between two opposing worlds. Oftentimes staff nurses have the perception that nurse managers work for the administration.[3] For example, higher management may be attempting to implement a plan or procedure that the staff nurses strongly object to, or the staff nurses may be complaining about some issue, such as staffing, that the middle manager has little control over. The leader in this situation may need to risk offending one or the other of the groups to resolve a difficult problem.

Initiative. Effective leadership demands that the leader be a "self-starter" and have the ability to start projects without pressure from above. Often the group relies on the leader to begin the process of completing a task or resolving a problem.

Energy. *Energy* refers to the ability to do work and to display that energy in the form of enthusiasm for the work. Energy and enthusiasm are contagious. Charismatic leaders are the ones who are the most energetic and enthusiastic. The group needs to see that the leader is willing to work as hard as they are being asked to work. However, energy has to be rationed carefully to maintain the optimum levels. It is easy for a leader to burn out, particularly when the expenditure of energy seems to produce little or no tangible result.

Optimism. A positive attitude is also contagious. Conversely, so is a negative attitude, which often leads to discouragement and failure (Table 11.2). A leader who has an overall positive attitude and views new problems as opportunities for success will be much more successful than the leader who constantly complains about each new crisis.[3]

Perseverance. Leaders need to be able to continue to work through difficult problems in difficult circumstances, even when others feel like quitting. Again, if the leader sets the example for the group with a "there's more than one way to skin a cat" attitude, the group will be encouraged to find new and creative solutions.

Well-Roundedness. Leaders, as well as those they are leading, live multifaceted lives. It is important to develop and foster nonwork relationships

Table 11.2 Winner or Whiner—Which One Are You?

A Winner Says . . .	A Whiner Says . . .
We have a real challenge here.	This is a big problem.
I'll do my best.	Do I have to do this?
That's great!	That's nice, I guess.
We can do it.	It can't be done; it's impossible.
Yes.	Maybe, when I have some time.

Source: Whitehead DK, Weiss SA, Tappen RM. *Essentials of Nursing Leadership and Management* (5th ed.). Philadelphia: F. A. Davis, 2010, p. 8.

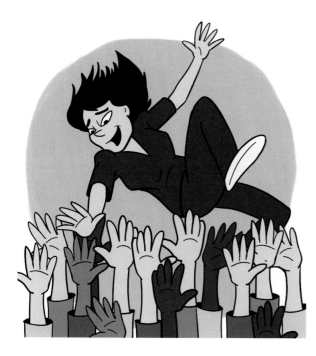

with friends and family. Time at work should be balanced with recreational, spiritual, social, and cultural activities that complete the person and round out the personality. Time must also be invested in maintaining good health through proper nutrition and regular exercise, which will help prevent burnout (see Chapter 10 for more detail).

Coping Skills. All jobs have some degree of stress, although people in leadership positions often experience higher levels. Stress can be handled in two ways: unconsciously, through defense mechanisms, or consciously, by bringing learned coping skills into play. A more productive way to deal with stress is to use coping skills developed in dealing with past stressors to promote a positive and healthy resolution to the stress. Some people learn how to use the stress they experience to motivate them and to tap into the energy it generates to achieve a higher level of functioning.

Self-Knowledge. Leaders who do not know and understand themselves are less able to understand those who are working for them. Self-awareness is the beginning of self-acceptance as a thinking,[1] feeling person who interacts with other thinking, feeling persons. Unless leaders understand and accept their motivations, biases, and perceptions, they will not be able to understand why they feel and react in certain ways to certain individuals and situations.

FOLLOWERSHIP

It is obvious that a leader cannot practice leadership if he or she does not have any followers. Followers, much like leaders, exist in almost all social settings, both formal and informal, and not just in an organizational setting.

Followers

A follower can be viewed as a person who believes in the traditional social hierarchy of leaders and followers and then identifies as a follower in the structure. The concept of subordinate is similar except that it includes the idea of the follower having a title and a formal role in an organizational setting who reports to a supervisor or manager. Almost all leaders are also followers and subordinates at some point in their careers, often simultaneously. And many times followers and subordinates can be leaders.

Individuals who follow are those who think, criticize, and question leaders. They are not always obedient and compliant. When leaders fail to evaluate and know who they are attempting to lead, they also fail to recognize the powerful impact their followers have on their success in achieving organizational goals. Followers have a right to decide which leader they wish to follow and when they will follow. The trait approach discussed above for leaders is also valid when considering followers[4] (see Table 11.3).

Table 11.3 **Types of Followers and Their Traits**

Follower Type	Traits
Effective or Independent	Think for themselves, are active, positive energy, independent problem solvers, challenge the leader
Implementer	Get the job done; do not question authority
Partner or participant	Supports leader but also questions leader on key points
Die hard or activist	Deeply devoted to leaders or are ready to remove them from their position, willing to take risks
Survivors, pragmatics, detached, withdrawn, sheep, bystander, or passive	Wait-and-see strategy, adapt to change but do the minimum necessary to survive, don't know anything about their leaders, don't really care what the leader does, no trust in the leader or organization, doesn't participate
Yes-man or yes-woman	Positive about leader; depends on leader for inspiration; thinking, directions, and project vision; is highly supportive of leader.
Individualist or alienated	Use negative energy to block leader, voice their views but do not necessarily support the leader, don't fit into the group
Impulsive	Constantly challenge authority and authority figures through rebellion, hates the status quo

Source: Kean S, Haycock-Stuart E, Baggaley S, Carson M. Followers and the co-construction of leadership. *Journal of Nursing Management,* 19(4):507–516, 2011, p. 3.

Individuals Versus Groups

Leadership viewed from the mind of the follower links the leader to the followers' perceptions of what a good leader should be and how and when to follow the directions of the leader. This perception varies from each individual and group.

When individuals look at the leader, they bring all of their experiences with past leaders into the evaluation. They base their perceptions on how well the current leader measures up to the "good leader" they experienced in the past, how he or she is managing the current situation, and what differentiates this leader from other leaders. A group brings a collection of past experiences and knowledge when considering a leader's abilities. They share their beliefs about leadership with each other and eventually negotiate a more or less unified perception of the leader's abilities.[4] If the group is cohesive in their belief that the leader is effective and has the qualities required to lead effectively, it is likely that the leader will have a high degree of success, even if one or two individuals in the group do not totally agree with the assessment. On the other hand, if the group decides the leader is not effective, the level of success will be greatly diminished.

Motivating followers is a major undertaking for any leader and is often the key to success. One method leaders can use is to understand how followers view themselves in the organizational structure. By evaluating how followers view the leader's abilities and skills and where they fit into the organization, the leader can better understand his or her own effectiveness. As the leader understands this, he or she can influence followers to improve their self-image with the end result of increasing their motivation levels and their productivity.[4] If the followers believe they are important to the organization and their input is considered in making decisions, they will feel better about themselves and the work they are doing. As a result, they will tend to be more accepting of directions from the leader.

Although the term *follower* may have negative connotations such as inferiority, passivity, submissiveness, or laziness, in reality, followers have a great deal of power and influence over a leader's success. For followers to successfully exercise their followership role in an organization, they must avoid reinforcing the negative stereotypes associated with the term. Rather, they must take a constructive approach and view their roles as ones of co-leaders, partners, and equal participants.[5] The leader–follower relationship is an active and interpersonal process that challenges both sides to participate in better understanding their relationship to each other with an end goal of producing the best possible health-care outcomes.

MANAGEMENT

Nurses who continue employment at a facility for any length of time will likely assume a management position at some point in their careers. These positions can range from middle management such as charge nurse or unit manager to higher level positions such as shift supervisor or chief nursing officer. Although leadership skills are highly useful in these positions, the move to manager involves a new set of skills and behaviors that the nurse must master.[6]

Unlike the development of leadership theory, which primarily focused on the leader, the early study of management was aimed toward influencing employees to be as productive as was humanly possible. Two schools of thought address and define management.

Time–Motion Theory

Time–motion theory developed out of the early industrial age, in which theorists concentrated on ways to complete a task most easily and efficiently. Often their efforts resulted in increased productivity but decreased employee satisfaction. From this viewpoint, management can be defined as planning, organizing, commanding, coordinating, and controlling the work of any particular group of employees. In the time–motion approach, providing the right incentives, primarily money, is expected to increase employee productivity. Although the weaknesses of this approach make it less desirable in today's society, variations of it served as the harbingers of many of the business techniques currently in use.

Human Interaction Theory

Early in the study of management, the limits of the time–motion approach became evident. Researchers observed that some lower-paid employee groups had higher levels of productivity than others with higher pay who were doing the same jobs. It appeared that factors such as employees' attitudes, fears, hopes, personal problems, social status in the group, and visions strongly influenced how they worked.[7] From this perspective, management can be defined as the ability to elicit from employees their commitment, loyalty, creativity, productivity, and continuous improvement.

Issues in Practice

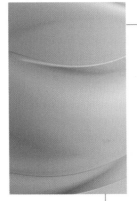

Leadership/Management Case Study

Resolving Staffing Issues

On a busy medical-surgical unit, a group of staff nurses were concerned about the process of making assignments. They believed that the usual practice of assigning nurses to a different group of clients each day eliminated any continuity of care, decreasing the quality of care and lowering morale among the staff. They agreed to meet with the nurse manager as a group to discuss ways of resolving the issues.

The meeting soon became confrontational. The staff nurses expressed a feeling of having very little autonomy in the selection of assignments. The nurse manager expressed the opinion that the nurses were being uncooperative and didn't understand the problems involved in making client assignments. She stated that her primary responsibility was to ensure provision of the best nursing care possible to all clients. The staff nurses countered that the current system wasn't doing that.

The staff nurses proposed a solution: After shift report, they would be allowed to select the clients they felt most qualified to care for, with the same clients reassigned to them on subsequent days until the clients were discharged. The initial response by the nurse manager was that it would be impossible to use this method in a fair and equitable manner. She also wondered what would happen if no one wanted to care for a very difficult client, and how continuity would be maintained on the nurses' days off.

Questions for Thought

1. How would a nurse manager who used an authoritarian system of management resolve this issue?

2. How would a nurse manager who used a laissez-faire system resolve this issue?

3. How would a nurse manager who used a participative system resolve this issue?

4. What initial mistake did the nurse manager make in dealing with this problem?

(Answers are found at the end of the chapter.)

Managers who favored the human interaction theory were required to develop a different set of management skills, including understanding human behavior, counseling effectively, boosting motivation, using efficient leadership skills, and maintaining productive communication. Just being a "nice guy" was not enough to guarantee employee cooperation and commitment. To be successful, management needed to be able to recognize and respond to employee concerns and needs, gain acceptance, and alleviate the pressures impending from higher administration.

It is also important to keep in mind that different management forms are necessary for different work settings. A predominantly time–motion approach may still work best in an area such as manufacturing of automobiles or washing machines. Using the same approach would be inappropriate and probably ineffective for managing a group of registered nurses (RNs) working in an ICU of a busy city hospital.

KEY BEHAVIORS OF THE NURSE MANAGER

Nurse managers often find themselves located on the organizational chart between employees and upper-level management. The functions and duties of nurse managers depend to a great degree on how the institution defines the role. One of the first activities of a new nurse manager is to make sure he or she understands the job description, responsibilities, and level of authority the position has in the institution. Some of the key behaviors that have been identified as being a regular part of a nurse manager's position are listed in Figure 11.1.

In today's health-care system, nurse managers continue to move away from close supervision of the staff nurses' work to helping them complete their work safely and effectively.[8] As this role continues to evolve, the emphasis will shift from traditional management functions to highly supportive functions, such as are seen in the leadership role.[9]

LEADERSHIP VERSUS MANAGEMENT

Several questions arise when people speak about leadership and management.

> *Charismatic leaders are the ones who are the most energetic and enthusiastic. The group needs to see that the leader is willing to work as hard as they are being asked to work.*

Are They the Same Thing?

Leadership can be exerted either formally or informally. Often the most effective leaders in a group are not the ones who are officially designated as the leaders. On the other hand, managers are given the title by some higher authority and have formally designated authority to supervise a group of employees in the achievement of a task. Similarly, managers can be held formally responsible for the quality, quantity, and cost of the work that the supervised employees produce.[10]

Do Managers Need Good Leadership Skills?

The most effective managers will have highly developed leadership skills. However, by virtue of their title and position, even managers with poor leadership skills are still the official authority, although their effectiveness is reduced. Often, in groups in which the manager is not a good leader, unofficial leaders emerge and exert either a strong positive or a negative influence on the group. If the unofficial leader is generally supportive of the manager's and administration's goals, the work group can be highly productive, and the organization's goals will be achieved. Conversely, if the unofficial leader's goals are opposed to those of the manager and administration, productivity may decrease to a point at which higher-level management asks the manager to leave the position. Followership is as important for managers as it is for leaders.[10]

Are Leaders Always Good Managers?

A person who has leadership ability may not have good management skills. This phenomenon is often seen in the nursing profession when a highly effective and skilled staff nurse who functions as the unofficial unit leader is taken out of that role and promoted to an official management position. Some do well; others may require additional training in management principles and skills. Some never quite master the skills needed for management.

Management and leadership skills complement each other.[7] As with all skills, they can be learned and require practice and experience to be developed fully. Even new graduate nurses can be effective leaders within their new nursing roles. As

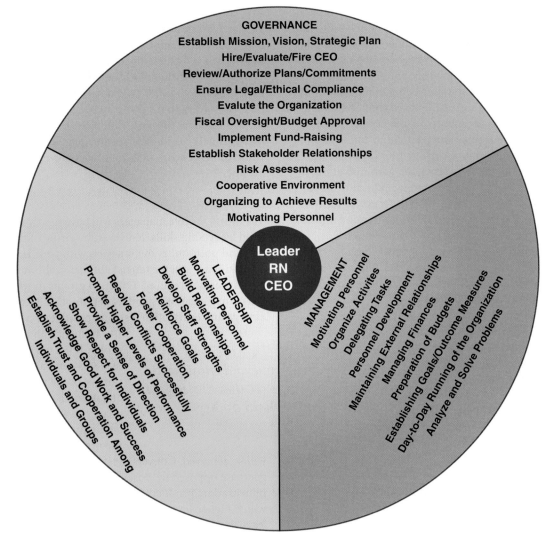

GOVERNANCE
Establish Mission, Vision, Strategic Plan
Hire/Evaluate/Fire CEO
Review/Authorize Plans/Commitments
Ensure Legal/Ethical Compliance
Evalute the Organization
Fiscal Oversight/Budget Approval
Implement Fund-Raising
Establish Stakeholder Relationships
Risk Assessment
Cooperative Environment
Organizing to Achieve Results
Motivating Personnel

Leader
RN
CEO

LEADERSHIP
Motivating Personnel
Build Relationships
Develop Staff Strengths
Reinforce Goals
Foster Cooperation
Resolve Conflicts Successfully
Promote Higher Levels of Performance
Provide a Sense of Direction
Show Respect for Individuals
Acknowledge Good Work and Success
Establish Trust and Cooperation Among
Individuals and Groups

MANAGEMENT
Motivating Personnel
Organize Activites
Delegating Tasks
Personnel Development
Maintaining External Relationships
Managing Finances
Preparation of Budgets
Establishing Goals/Outcome Measures
Day-to-Day Running of the Organization
Analyze and Solve Problems

Figure 11.1 Key behaviors associated with governance, management, and leadership.

they gain experience and develop new skills, their ability and opportunities to provide leadership will also increase. Learning and improving skills in one area will increase the ability in the other.

GOVERNANCE IN THE HEALTH-CARE SETTING

Although nurses are usually not involved in high-level governance activities, there is a considerable amount of overlap among the behaviors involved in governance, management, and leadership. Governance will be mentioned here briefly, although a more thorough discussion can be found in Davis*Plus* Bonus Chapter 2.

As with most complex concepts, there are several definitions of *governance* that often depend on the setting. Governance in the political setting has a different direction and set of expectations than governance in a nursing organization. Governance in large organizations is usually conducted by a board of directors; however, in smaller organizations, the governance role may fall to the chief executive officer (CEO) or president of the organization.[9] In the health-care delivery setting, *governance* can be defined as the process of decision-making at the top levels of an organization that ensures that the organization achieves its goals and produces high-quality outcomes by defining expectations, delegating power to key personnel, and overseeing the administrative process.

Governance is a broader concept than management that involves making decisions at a higher level that:

• Determine expectations.
• Grant power to individuals.
• Establish performance standards.
• Maintain consistent management.
• Set cohesive policies and processes.
• Provide organizational guidance.

Similar to leadership and management, there are a set of key behaviors that are associated with the exercise of governance. Figure 11.1 demonstrates the relationship of the key behaviors associated with governance, management, and leadership. As the behaviors move toward the middle of the wheel, they become more similar and have more overlap. A nurse who is an informal leader on a nursing unit may also engage in management and governance behaviors without knowing it. The circle of responsibility is a flexible structure, much like an elastic band, that can expand, contract, and move in any direction. For the nurse manager, the circle of responsibility completely surrounds the behaviors listed for management and many of the behaviors for leadership, but it also includes some of the governance behaviors. It is important to note that motivation is a key behavior for all three levels because if followers are not motivated, many of the other key behaviors become difficult, if not impossible, to achieve.

TWO KEY TASKS OF MANAGERS

The day to day running of the unit is one of the important tasks with which managers are charged. In addition to activities such as solving problems, developing personnel, and delegating tasks, managers need to master the skills of budget preparation and planning for staffing of the unit.

> *Often, in groups in which the manager is not a good leader, unofficial leaders emerge and exert either a strong positive or a negative influence on the group.*

Budget Preparation

One of the tasks assigned to most nurse managers is creating budgets for their units, usually with a yearly budget that is then broken down into monthly budgets to better monitor the cash flow. The concept of a budget is rather simple. There are two key elements: income and expenses. The goal of creating a budget is to pay all the expenses while not exceeding the amount of income. For the nurse manager, a budget is a plan that helps control expenses and uses money in the most efficient and effective way possible.[11] Of course, this process becomes more complicated as the number of sources of income and number of expenses increase.

Although there are many different types of budgets, the one the nurse manager develops is generally referred to as an *operational budget.* An operational budget helps the nurse manager manage the unit to produce the highest quality care in the most economical manner possible. It details the expenses for the usual maintenance and activities of the year. It is commonly a line-item budget where activities or items that require funding are listed line by line. Much like the client care plan that all nurses are familiar with, the budget has similar elements: problem identification, use of standards, and projected outcomes. A well-developed budget keeps the individual unit—and by extension, the whole facility—out of financial jeopardy.[12]

Key Elements

In developing a successful budget, the nurse manager must keep in mind some key elements and principles. First, the budget should focus on the goals of the institution but yet remain realistic. Limited resources are a reality of the current world of health care. Each item in a budget should be evaluated to see if it will achieve the objectives of the facility in the most economical manner.

Second, the nurse manager must always work within the historical context of past budgets. A budget serves as a predictor of future expenses since it is developed a year before it is actually implemented. By looking at past budgets, nurse managers can better identify areas where there were problems with expenditures.[13] For example, past budgets may not have predicted the steep rise in costs for the replacement of essential equipment used by a unit when it breaks down. Future budgets must take this into consideration, or the budget will be inadequate for the expenses.

Third, all facilities use a standardized format for budgets. The nurse manager must become familiar with this format to increase the efficiency and quality of planning for the institution. Computer skills are required, as budget forms are all computerized on spread sheets.[14] Oftentimes they will have charts and tables the nurse manager must learn how to manipulate.

Fourth, budgets are not static. Over the course of the time period when they are implemented, they must be evaluated and updated. Quite often institutions will have predetermined time frames such as quarterly or semiannually.[15] The goal is to compare what the budget projected and what is actually occurring. By doing this comparison, adjustments can be made in the budget to produce the best results.

Budget Types

Operational budgets can take several different forms. An incremental or historical budget takes the budget from the previous year and adds or deletes money from the various items listed. Also, new items may be added or old items that are no longer appropriate can be deleted. Most nurse managers work with this type of budget.

Performance-based budgeting is based on the belief that traditional methods of budgeting are too simple to account for all the variations in the process and adjusts to produce the best outcomes. Performance-based budgets are totally outcome oriented and allocate resources to achieve certain organizational goals and objectives. For performance-based budgeting to succeed, there must be well-defined key performance indicators developed prior to the process. Without the ability to measure outcomes, performance-based budgeting cannot succeed. Although this has been tried in some health-care settings, defining performance indicators becomes very complicated and most facilities have dropped this method of budgeting.[15]

> *Unlike the incremental budgets that use past experiences to predict the future, zero-based budgets require the nurse manager to start from the beginning each time a budget is created.*

Another type of budgeting that was popular for a time but is now rarely used is zero-based budgeting. Unlike the incremental budgets that use past experiences to predict the future, zero-based budgets require the nurse manager to start from the beginning each time a budget is created. In zero-based budgeting, there is no baseline sum that is automatically approved.[14] Rather, each expenditure item in the budget must be justified and approved each time the budget process is repeated. The nurse manager must adjust expenditures for each item either up or down, based on the amount of funding available. Because the items in most unit budgets remain consistent over time, nurse managers who were required to use zero-based budgeting found that after the first year of time-consuming development of rationales for each item, they could reuse these in the next year's budget, thereby turning it into an incremental budget with justifications.

It is important to note that each facility has its own particular type of budget requirements and forms. One of the steepest learning curves for nurse managers is the budgeting process.

Required Skills

Although it is well beyond the scope of this text to provide a detailed presentation of the budgeting process, there are some skills that nursing students and nurses can learn to better prepare themselves for the nurse manager role as budget designer. These skills include the following:

- Learning basic budget and financial terminology
- Understanding the key elements of a budget
- Manipulating the data on the computerized budget spreadsheets
- Developing strong working relationships with the finance and billing departments
- Monitoring and analyzing the variables in the unit's budget[12]

Although nurse managers often approach the budget process with fear and dread, budget development is a skill that can be learned much like the clinical skills they already possess. Through mastery of the budget process, nurse managers also develop the skills to be change agents for their organization and leaders to their staffs.

Planning for Staff Coverage

Another area of nursing management where there is a steep learning curve is planning for staffing of the unit. Somewhat like budgeting, the basic concepts behind staffing are deceptively simple: Have enough people to meet the needs of clients and the goals and outcomes of the facility. Almost all nurses have up-close-and-personal experiences with staffing, usually when their units are short staffed or they are asked to work extra shifts because someone called in. New nurse manages soon learn that developing staffing plans is much more complex.

Staffing is also highly dynamic and essential to the overall financial health of an organization. It affects almost every aspect of functioning in health care, including achieving institutional goals, ensuring quality and safety of clients, and delivering care goals.[16] The American Nurses Association (ANA) recognized the importance of staffing a number of years ago. In 2005, they published the *ANA Principles of Staffing* as a guide for nurse managers in determining safe and efficient staffing levels. However, since the document's publication, there has been a tremendous increase in published literature about the effects of staffing on morbidity and mortality, medication and care errors, successful client outcomes, and the effects of different types of staff on client well-being. Although this body of literature has contributed substantially to the evidence-based practice databases, some nagging questions still remain: How do you determine just the right amount of staff? How can it be measured? How do you track staffing on a day-to-day basis?[17] (For more information, go to http://www.nursingworld.org/MainMenuCategories/ThePracticeofProfessionalNursing/NurseStaffing.)

Several factors contribute to staffing issues. There is a steep rise in the number of elderly seeking health care as the baby-boomer generation ages. Clients tend to be sicker yet have shorter hospital stays than in the past. The national nursing shortage is having and will have a profound effect on staffing issues—some experts project there will be between 200,000 and 800,000 vacant nursing positions by 2025.[18] The Affordable Care Act (ACA) is projected to inject some 36 million newly insured clients into the health-care system and, with its emphasis on quality of care, will require even more well-educated RNs.

Is There a Perfect Staffing Ratio?

Mandatory staffing ratios were implemented in several states in an attempt to ensure that there were enough RNs on the floor to adequately care for clients. Subsequent research has demonstrated mixed results for mandated staffing ratios. Although there appears to be minimum ratios in certain settings that increase the quality of care, the research has yet to show what the optimum ratios might be.[19] The Registered Nurse Safe Staffing Act is a federal law that is being written to improve RN staffing levels in hospitals that receive Medicare funds. ANA is working closely with lawmakers to write and pass this bill. The key elements to be considered in staffing are client acuity (how sick the client is and how complicated the care), layout of the unit (how far does the nurse have to travel between clients), and ancillary support (how many lesser trained personnel does the RN have to work with).[20]

> *The other important factor is to remember that these are people who are staffing the unit, not just numbers to be filled in on a table. They have individual personalities, inflated or deflated egos, worries, families, personal problems, health problems, and financial needs.*

What Is a Nurse Manager to Do?

What can new nurse managers do to better prepare themselves for the challenges they must face in attempting to staff their units to deliver save and high-quality care? Much like preparing for the budgeting process, learning the basic terminology, becoming familiar with the spreadsheets and technology, and understanding the principles of staffing will go a long way to prepare the nurse manager. The other important factor is to remember that these are people who are staffing the unit, not just numbers to be filled in on a table. They have individual personalities, inflated or deflated egos, worries, families, personal problems, health problems, and financial needs. A considerable amount of facility resources are dedicated to staff such as human resources, continuing education, lawyers, and multiple layers of management.

Although each facility will have variations in their staffing procedures and spreadsheets, some basic human relations skills will greatly aid the process:

- Demonstrating leadership skills. Make a decision and stick with it unless it is proven to be incorrect. Then admit the mistake and make another, hopefully better, decision and stick with that one. Staff soon lose respect for a weak and indecisive leader and eventually will no longer follow.
- Interacting with staff at work. Managers who are out on the floor observing and helping when an extra hand is needed are much more in tune with their staff's skills and abilities (and shortfalls). Staff tend to do a better job if they know the nurse manager is nearby.
- Not interacting with staff outside the work setting. The nurse manager is the person who makes the hard decisions. Although everyone likes to be liked as a friend, being too friendly with staff decreases the manager's ability to lead. Staff can be very manipulative of BFF managers. Also, there is a tendency to develop a group of favorite nurses, which makes the ones who are not in the group feel left out.
- Unfriending from Facebook. Social media sites are great for sharing personal information with friends; however, if staff can access the manager's accounts, they are privy to image-altering information. Was that the nurse manager at the party dancing on the bar with a lampshade on her head? The image does not engender respect.[17]

Maintaining optimal nurse-to-client ratios is a task that nurse managers must face 24 hours a day, 7 days a week, 365 days a year. It never stops, it never gets easier, and it never goes away. Despite the challenges, nurse managers can master the skills required for safe staffing. They are not alone. The ANA and other organizations are working to develop safe staffing guidelines that nurse managers can use to meet staffing needs. It is essential that they know of these resources and can access them when dealing with facility administrators.

"Hygiene factors are also related to the conditions under which the work is performed and not to the work itself. They only serve as negative motivators—when they are not met, work productivity is reduced."

MOTIVATIONAL THEORY

Motivational theory can be defined as the ability to influence the choices people make among a number of possible choices open to them. For example, what factors would motivate a new graduate nurse to work at one hospital when there are four facilities offering her or him a job? Are the pay and benefits better? Maybe it is closer to home. Perhaps the shifts are better and the facility does not require mandatory overtime.

Several theorists have attempted to explain this phenomenon. Probably the best known is Abraham Maslow, who developed the hierarchy of needs theory. (For more information on Maslow's theory, see Chapter 13.) Although nursing students are taught and use this theory to deal with client needs, the theory also has applications in the realm of leadership and management. Maslow believes that human needs are arranged in a hierarchy from the most basic and essential to the more complex. Most basic are the physiological and safety needs, and until these are met in at least a satisfactory fashion, the person is less likely to deal with the higher needs such as social relationships, self-esteem, and self-actualization.[6]

For example, if a nurse was not being paid a salary that would meet the needs for food, housing, and clothing, those needs would become the nurse's primary concern rather than delivering high-quality client care. Realistically, needs are never fully met, but they have to be accommodated to a degree to which the person feels comfortable enough to move up in the hierarchy.

Motivation–Hygiene Theory

Another theory that has become popular is Herzberg's motivation–hygiene theory. Although there are some similarities between Maslow's and Herzberg's theories, particularly in their applications, Herzberg believes that people have two different categories of needs that are fundamentally different from each other.[6]

Hygiene Factors

The first category is referred to as *needs dissatisfiers,* or hygiene factors. According to Herzberg, if these needs are not met, the person feels dissatisfied with his or her job and focuses more on the environment than the work that is supposed to be performed. Hygiene factors are related to the work environment and include, for example, salary and benefits, job security, status in the organization, work conditions, policies, and relationships with coworkers.[7]

Hygiene factors are also related to the conditions under which the work is performed and not to the work itself. They only serve as negative motivators—when they are not met, work productivity is reduced. However, if they are satisfied, there is no guarantee that increased productivity and higher-quality performance will result.

Needs Motivators

The second category of needs, according to Herzberg, is called *satisfiers,* or needs motivators. Unlike the hygiene factors, satisfiers focus primarily on the work. Some of the more important satisfiers that have been identified include elements that expand the work challenges and scope, such as career advancement, increased responsibility, recognition for achievements, and opportunities for professional growth. The satisfiers can have both a positive and a negative motivational impact. If they are satisfied, they can encourage workers to increase their productivity and deliver higher-quality work. If they are not satisfied, they often have the opposite effect.

Motivation in the Hospital Setting

Herzberg concludes that employers must satisfy the hygiene factors as a minimum requirement before there can be any increase in productivity. Programs to promote job enrichment will be effective in upgrading the achievement, roles, and satisfaction of employees. In the hospital setting, career or clinical ladder programs provide nurses with the recognition for achievement and opportunity for advancement, along with financial rewards (hygiene factor), and allow them to remain in direct client care.

It is important for the RN leaders to understand and be able to use incentive techniques, even if they are not in a designated management role. The ability to motivate is one of the keys to success in delegation at any level, and the success of RNs is often assessed by the job performance of people on the health-care team they are supervising. Successful motivation is the door to successful leadership because these are the people who can make things happen in an organization.

> *The ability to motivate is one of the keys to success in delegation at any level, and the success of RNs is often assessed by how well people on the health-care team they are supervising perform their jobs.*

MAKING CHANGES SUCCESSFULLY

The goal of education and growth is always to produce change in the individual. Motivating people to change is one of the most challenging and most important functions of leadership. Simply stated, change is the process of transforming, altering, or becoming different from what was before.[8] Although change is a constant in health care and nursing, it is surprising how resistant nurses can be to even minor changes in their work environment.

Change can produce many emotions, ranging from excitement and anticipation to stress, fear, and anxiety. How people deal with change can affect how they respond to the environment and communicate with others.

At minimum, change makes most people feel uncomfortable. Any change can be simultaneously positive and negative. During the process of learning new skills, treatments, or techniques, most people feel a sense of accomplishment at the same time that they feel afraid of making mistakes, being judged by others, or being labeled as "slow learners."

Fear of the Unknown

Imagine a new graduate nurse starting his or her first day at work, very excited about the new experience and the potential for career development. However, at the same time the nurse is worried about being accepted into the group, being able to practice what was learned in nursing school, and being able to learn the new skills required by the unit. Almost everyone has a sense of dread when moving away from activities with which they have become comfortable. Setting realistic personal goals and time lines for learning new information helps reduce fear and stress when making major changes.

The Need to Take Risks

Change can have both positive and negative effects. Often staff will initially resist a change and fight to prevent it, but once they go through the process, they would never go back to the old way of doing things. All change involves some risk taking, and some people are better at risk taking than are others. Consider the following case study:

> After analyzing the needs of the clients and the nursing workload of a busy medical unit, the unit manager decided to change the work shift times. In addition to the standard 7 a.m. to 3 p.m., 3 p.m. to 11 p.m., and 11 p.m. to 7 a.m. shifts, she decided to add a 5 a.m. to 1 p.m. shift to increase coverage during the busiest period of the shift. The RN assigned to the new shift recognized the benefits to the unit and to clients; thus, she accepted and supported the change with few objections. Also, the change in shift times allowed her to alter her personal schedule so that she could take extra courses toward her master's degree at a local college. For the RN, the change in shifts was a positive experience.
>
> However, the licensed practical nurse (LPN) assigned to this new shift was upset with the change. She was a "late sleeper" and did not want to come in so early. She liked the shifts the way they were and did not see any advantages to changing things needlessly.
>
> After the new shift was initiated, the LPN was usually 15 to 30 minutes late, called in sick frequently, and was "grumpy" and hard to talk to when she did come in to work. For this LPN, the change was negative and unacceptable.

Internal or External Forces?

Two primary forces bring about change: external forces that originate from outside the person or organization and internal forces that start from within the individual or organization. A primary example of external change is what happens when government agencies pass down new rules and regulations, such as the ACA, that affect the delivery of health care. An example of internal change would be a hospital increasing salaries or requiring mandatory overtime from the work action of a group of nurses.

Planned or Unplanned?

Change can be planned or unplanned. Planned change is more productive and occurs when there is a directed and designed implementation of some element within the organization. Change can affect all aspects of an organization, including policies, goals, organizational philosophy, work environment, and even structure. Planned change can be used for all sorts of projects, ranging from the minor to the most complex.

Unplanned change, sometimes called *reactive change*, occurs when a problem forces a person or organization into a situation in which it must respond. These changes are often minor but sometimes can involve projects that are large in scope and complexity.[8] Examples include changes in staffing because of nurses who call in sick, clients who experience cardiac arrest, major disasters, or even equipment failures, such as when the electricity fails or a water main breaks.

> *Planned change is more productive and occurs when there is a directed and designed implementation of some element within the organization.*

A Driving Force for Change

Nurses often take on the role of the change agent—that is, the one who brings about the change (Box 11.3). All change requires the ability to overcome resistance to change (called *restraining forces*) by a driving force that pushes toward change. When the driving and restraining forces are equal, no change occurs, and the status quo is maintained.

Change can occur only when the driving force is greater than the restraining force.[9] Those who want to change have a tendency to push, but those who are being asked to change tend to push back to maintain things as they are. It is important when attempting to implement change to identify the restraining forces and ways to overcome them. Habit, comfort, and inertia are the three most common restraining forces.

Planned change works best when it is well organized, proceeds at a steady pace, and has a definite date for achievement. There is a level of excitement that raises energy levels when a change is near

Box 11.3

Characteristics of an Effective Change Agent

- Is well organized
- Identifies restraining forces
- Is able to motivate
- Demonstrates and maintains commitment to change
- Develops trusting relationships
- Responds to feedback and negotiation
- Is goal directed
- Communicates well
- Maintains optimistic attitude

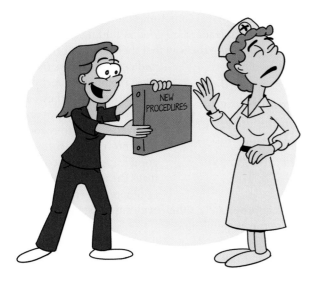

completion, but postponing the date for the change can drain that energy and lead to disappointment.

GROUP DYNAMICS

All successful leaders and managers understand and are able to use the principles of group dynamics. A group exists when three or more people interact and are held together by a common bond or interests.

The power of the group over an individual's behavior should never be underestimated. Groups establish and exert their power through a set of unique behaviors or norms that their members are expected to follow.[21] These norms may be formal or informal, written or unwritten, promulgated or merely understood. Unfortunately, in most nursing units, the norms are often not clearly expressed, yet they may be used as judgment tools or standards for evaluating work behaviors. When new nurses begin work on a particular unit, they must quickly learn the unwritten unit norms and identify the informal leaders to function effectively.

A Common Goal

Groups are open systems that interact with the environment to achieve a goal. The individuals who make up the group are its subsystems and interact with each other and with the environment. Group dynamics provide the principles that underlie team building, which is essential to the success of nursing units. Establishing and sharing common goals is the starting point for successful team building.

When the common goal is to help one another, effective team building results. Members of the team respond most positively when they feel included in the decision-making and when they realize that their input is valued by the other team members.[21] It is important that the leader always ask team members for their ideas about the goal that the team is working toward. A strong team spirit is crucial to the success of the team.

Unwritten Rules

As with most elements in leading successfully, group dynamics may be positive or negative. Nurses who do not learn and fail to display the expected group behaviors may be ostracized from the group, thus making the work environment psychologically uncomfortable and perhaps even physically difficult. For example, nonconforming nurses may find that there is no one around when they need help ambulating an unsteady client. A particular nursing unit staff may have a strong team approach. If the new nurse is highly independent and prefers to work alone, he or she may not "fit in" and may experience hostility or sarcasm from the other nurses on the unit.

Going Against the Group

Consider the following scenario demonstrating group dynamics:

The ICU is responsible for on-call coverage in the recovery room for unscheduled postoperative clients on the evening shifts, night shifts, and all of the weekend shifts. There is no formal written policy, but coverage has traditionally been handled on a voluntary, rotating basis.

Because coverage is "voluntary," one of the ICU nurses has decided that he does not want to be on call anymore. He is the only member of the ICU staff who does not take call. Soon after he announces his decision, he begins to sense anger and experience alienation from his peers. He is very knowledgeable, has highly developed nursing skills, and provides consistently high-quality care to assigned clients on his regular shifts. However, on his semiannual peer evaluation, he receives low ratings from his coworkers on the basis of the informal call coverage standard and expectations. The unit nurses feel that he is no longer a team player.

The nurse becomes angry because he feels that the use of unclear, unwritten standards is an unfair way to evaluate his ability as a nurse. He soon finds that the other ICU nurses accidentally "forget" to invite him to group functions. He also seems to be assigned the most difficult and largest number of clients during any given shift, seemingly to compensate for not taking call.

> *Nurses who do not learn and fail to display the expected group behaviors may be ostracized from the group, thus making the work environment psychologically uncomfortable and perhaps even physically difficult.*

Group dynamics involve many factors, including methods of communication, professional behaviors, professional growth, flexibility, problem-solving, participation, and competition.[22] The ability to understand and use the elements of group dynamics has a direct relationship to the behaviors, cooperation, and effectiveness of the team. Often, when a team labels an individual member as "difficult," it most likely means that the individual is not following one or more of the informal, unwritten group norms. (For more information on difficult behavior, see Chapter 13.)

A Common Understanding

It is evident that the team will only function smoothly when the members understand their roles and the roles of the other members. Their roles identify their places on the team and establish what is expected from each member. To be successful, the leader must establish the belief that all the roles are of equal importance in achieving the goals or purposes of the group.

Mutual Support

Team members need to realize they are not merely responsible for their own roles but also must support the roles of the other members. Although the leader establishes the goals to be achieved, it is important that the team members be allowed to achieve their tasks in ways that are most appropriate for them, particularly in the case of self-motivated professionals such as nurses.[21]

Reward for Achievement

Ongoing or complicated projects require a long-term commitment that is sometimes difficult to maintain. Effective team leaders are good at finding accomplishments along the way that the team can celebrate and enjoy. It allows the team members to feel good about what they have achieved to this point and motivates them to accomplish more in the future. A good leader also recognizes the accomplishments of others and rewards them appropriately. Often even simple statements of praise can be applicable.

Identity and Trust

Finally, establishing a sense of team identity and trust completes the group dynamic and team-building process. Some degree of creativity may be required for establishing team identity, ranging from similar uniforms to buttons or pins. Trust allows the team members to be more open to communications from other members and more willing to take risks. Trust empowers the members, allowing them to make independent decisions and promoting the smooth functioning of the team (Table 11.3).

COMPETITION

Competition can be a very powerful element in group dynamics. Depending on how it is channeled, expressed, and used, competition can be a positive or negative force within the group.[22] The various forms of competition can be individual, team, or unit focused.

Peer Evaluation

A common expression of competition in the group setting is peer evaluations. For peer evaluations to be a positive form of competition, the unit must decide ahead of time on the norms and expectations that they value and then design an objective measurement tool to evaluate whether the individual is meeting the norms. Each individual being evaluated must be aware of the criteria before the evaluation is conducted. The evaluation team must be educated on evaluation techniques and must be as objective and professional as possible.

In the health-care setting, it is important for all professionals, unit groups, and management to promote competition in a positive, progressive, and supportive environment. When competition is channeled positively, it leads to new and creative ideas, better programs, increased growth, more productive interactions, and higher-quality client care (Table 11.4).[23] When the competition is negative, it often produces failures, depression, sabotage, unit turf conflicts, decreased productivity, and lower-quality care. Consider the following case:

> *The ability to understand and use the elements of group dynamics has a direct relationship on the behaviors, cooperation, and effectiveness of the team.*

> The competition on a nursing unit turned negative: The nurses on the 7 a.m. to 3 p.m. shift began competing with the nurses on the 3 p.m. to 11 p.m. shift in order to appear more knowledgeable about client care to the nurse manager. To "look better," the nurses on the 7 a.m. to 3 p.m. shift intentionally withheld selected client laboratory test results during shift report.
>
> As a result of this action, several tests scheduled for the 3 p.m. to 11 p.m. shift were not done, angering the physicians, potentially threatening the safety of the clients, and making the nurses on the 3 p.m. to 11 p.m. shift appear incompetent. In addition, the nurses on that shift had to complete several incident reports on the errors that occurred on their shift.
>
> One informal component the unit manager uses to evaluate the staff nurses' performance is the number of incident reports that a nurse must file. The more incident reports, the poorer will be the nurse's performance evaluation. To the unit manager, the nurses on the 7 a.m. to 3 p.m. shift seemed to be more competent because of the seemingly poor care on the 3 p.m. to 11 p.m. shift, indicated by a large number of incident reports that were being given. However, when the nurses on the 3 p.m. to 11 p.m. shift discovered what had really happened, they devised several ways to "get even" with the nurses on the 7 a.m. to 3 p.m. shift.

CARE DELIVERY MODELS

Nowhere are the elements of group dynamics reflected better than in the nursing units of a hospital or health-care facility. The organizational structure found in the nursing units of a facility reflects how the nursing department interacts with coworkers and participates in the delivery of client care. Various models may be used in the delivery of nursing care. Many health-care facilities have made a transition from one model to another and may even incorporate several different models at the same time.[24] The nurse must recognize which model is being used as well as its strengths and weaknesses. These models include functional nursing, team nursing, primary care nursing, and modular nursing (Table 11.5).

Functional Nursing

Functional nursing has as its foundation a task-oriented philosophy: Each person performs a specific job that is narrowly defined according to the needs of the unit. The medication nurse, for example, focuses on administering and documenting medications for the assigned group of clients.

In this organizational unit, the nurse manager is called the *charge nurse,* whose main responsibility is to oversee the various workers. Charge nurses are also appointed for each shift to manage the care during that time. This model relies on ancillary health workers, such as nurses' aides and orderlies. Some believe this model fragments care too much. Because

Table 11.4 **Do's and Don'ts of Effective Change Agents**

Do's	Don'ts
Do develop a sense of trust.	Don't have a hidden agenda.
Do establish common goals.	Don't be unpredictable.
Do facilitate effective communication.	Don't miss or reschedule meetings frequently.
Do establish a strong team identity.	Don't use threats or bluffs to manipulate members.
Do contribute as much as possible.	Don't volunteer to be the record keeper.
Do find reasons to celebrate and recognize accomplishments.	Don't follow the rest of the crowd.

Table 11.5 **Comparison of Common Client-Care Models**

Model	Nurses Are Called	Description	Where Model Is Used
Functional	Charge nurse Medical nurse Treatment nurse	Nurses are assigned to specific tasks rather than specific clients.	Hospitals Nursing homes Nurse consultants Operating rooms
Team	Team leader Team member	Nursing staff members are divided into small groups responsible for the total care of a given number of clients.	Hospitals Nursing homes Home care Hospice
Primary care	Primary nurse Associate nurse	Nurses are designated either as the primary nurse responsible for clients' care or as the associate nurse who assists in carrying out the care.	Hospitals Specialty units Dialysis Home care
Modular	Care pair	Nurses are paired with less-trained caregivers. Generally involves cross-training of personnel.	Hospitals Home health care Transport teams

many people have specific tasks, coordination can be difficult, and the holistic perspective may be lost.[10]

Team Nursing

Team nursing has a more unified approach to client care, with team members functioning together to achieve client goals. The team leader functions as the person ultimately responsible for the clients' well-being. More cohesiveness is present among the members of the team than is found in the functional model. Rather than having a narrow task to accomplish, team members focus on team goals under the coordination of the team leader. The team conference provides for effective communication and follow-up among team members and is the key to successful team nursing.

Primary Care Nursing

The primary care nursing model gives nurses the opportunity to focus on the whole person. The **primary care nurse** provides and is responsible for all of the client's nursing needs. The nurse manager in this model becomes a facilitator for the primary care nurses. Primary care nurses are self-directed and concerned with consistency of care. The primary care model is similar to the case management model, which has one nurse providing total care for one or more clients. Many home health-care agencies use this method of assigning an RN to work with an individual or family for the duration of the services rendered.[25]

Modular Nursing

Modular nursing, also called *client-focused care,* is one model that was developed in response to professional nursing personnel shortages and to the downsizing of professional nursing staffs. This model is based on a decentralized organizational system that emphasizes close interdisciplinary collaboration. Redesigning the method of nursing care delivery takes much planning and input from the various departments involved, such as nursing, respiratory therapy, physical therapy, radiology, laboratory, and dietary.

> *Leadership can be exerted either formally or informally. Often the most effective leaders in a group are not the ones who are officially designated as the leaders.*

Important aspects of modular nursing include relying on unlicensed assistive personnel (UAPs), also called *unit service assistants,* for the provision of direct care; grouping clients with similar needs; developing relative intensity measures; and emphasizing team concepts in small groups that remain constant.

Strong, Explicit Leadership

Cross-training of personnel is another important aspect of modular nursing. For example, using this system, respiratory therapists provide respiratory treatments but also help clients to the bathroom and turn bedridden clients. Nurse managers in this system are responsible for providing explicit job descriptions, maintaining the work group's cohesiveness, carefully monitoring each staff person's abilities, delegating tasks as appropriate, and evaluating the effectiveness of care.[24]

The role of UAPs is one area of the client-focused care model that needs more definition, particularly in relation to the RN's accountability and responsibilities in supervising these workers. State boards of nursing across the country are considering possible changes in nurse practice acts necessitated by the use of UAPs.

Benefits of this care delivery model include decreased staffing cost and greater autonomy of cross-trained personnel. The nurse manager must be a strong leader for this model of care delivery to succeed. Consistent collaboration between the nurse manager and physician is of utmost importance in planning client care.

Conclusion

Over the years, there has been one constant in the changing health-care system: The registered nurse is still expected to provide leadership and management skills to direct and ensure the highest quality of health care given to clients. Both leadership and management require a set of skills that can be learned. Nurses who learn these skills will become successful managers and the leaders of the health-care system in the future.

Successful leaders and managers understand and often combine the best aspects of the many theories that deal with leadership and management. Knowledge of one's strengths and weaknesses provides the basis for confident and productive leadership. Developing effective leadership and management skills is a lifelong process. Learning from books and articles, as well as from other successful nurse managers, presents an opportunity for professional and personal growth.

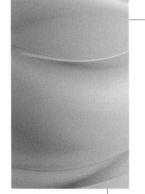

Issues in Practice

Jill, a registered nurse, was recently appointed as the evening charge nurse on a busy postsurgical unit. She has been an active participant in the hospital's quality assurance committee for the past 2 years since her graduation. One of the issues the committee identified as a problem was the higher-than-average surgical wound infection rate on Jill's unit. After some research, Jill determined that a major component of the high infection rate was the procedures that were used when changing postoperative dressings.

After obtaining permission from the unit manager and hospital education director, Jill developed a new procedure for dressing changes, incorporating the most current research. She presented the changes in a short in-service program to the unit personnel and explained the changes several times to each of the three shifts to make sure that all the nurses and staff on the unit were familiar with the new changes. The expectation was that there would be a 25 percent reduction in wound infections after the new procedures had been used for 1 month.

At the end of the first month of using the new dressing change procedures, the postoperative wound infection rate showed no improvement over the previous month's rate. At the monthly staff meeting, Jill discovered that the LPNs on the unit were refusing to use the new procedures because they "took too much time" and had reverted to the procedures they had always used before.

Questions for Thought

1. What was the style of leadership and management that Jill used when attempting to initiate the dressing procedure change?

2. Other than the stated reason, why do you think the LPNs did not want to use the new procedures?

3. How can Jill increase the level of compliance by the LPNs on the unit?

4. What is the role of the unit manager in initiating the new dressing change procedures?

Critical Thinking Exercises

- Look at the list of key qualities of a leader in Figure 11.1. Make a list of the qualities that you believe you already have and the qualities that you need to develop.
- In Table 11.3, there is a list of the types of followers and their characteristics. What type of follower are you? Can you improve your followership skills? How?
- Have you ever been in a management position? Identify some of the issues you faced. Are they similar to the issues listed in the book? How did you resolve them?
- Develop a practice budget for yourself and for your family.
- Are you a Winner or a Whiner? (See Table 11.2.) Be honest!

Answers to Questions in Chapter 11

Issues Now: Leadership/Management Case Study (page 268)

1. A nurse manager who uses the authoritarian system would maintain her position that the proposed plan was unworkable. Relying on her position of authority, she would insist that the nurses continue to use the established system of assignment. Any staff nurse who felt she or he could not work under this system could seek reassignment to another unit.

2. A nurse manager using the laissez-faire system would allow the nurses to try out the proposed system as they wanted. If any problems resulted from it, they would have to figure out how to resolve the problems themselves.

3. A nurse manager using the participative system would recognize that there is always some common ground between herself and the staff nurses. It is important to identify the common points and then work toward resolving the areas of disagreement. For example, the nurse manager could work with the staff nurses to develop a set of criteria for assignments that would be agreeable to all parties and ensure the quality of client care. The nurse manager would then retain the ability to assign clients but would be using criteria that were developed by the staff. In the end, staff cooperation and morale would increase, as would the continuity and quality of care being provided by the unit.

4. The initial mistake the nurse manager made was meeting with the staff nurses as a group. The staff nurses would have done better to select one or two representatives to bring their issues to the nurse manager. Using this approach eliminates the "mob mentality" that sometimes develops with large groups. It also forces the staff nurses to identify the specific issues they want to resolve.

Source: Whitehead DK, Weiss SA, Tappen RM. *Essentials of Nursing Leadership and Management,* (4th ed.). Philadelphia: F. A. Davis, 2006.

R e f e r e n c e s

1. MacPhee M, Skelton-Green J, Bouthillette F, Suryaprakash N. An empowerment framework for nursing leadership development: Supporting evidence. *Journal of Advanced Nursing,* 68(1):159–169, 2012.

2. Casida J, Parker J. Staff nurse perceptions of nurse manager leadership styles and outcomes. *Journal of Nursing Management,* 19(4):478–486, 2011.

3. Azaare J, Gross J. The nature of leadership style in nursing management. *British Journal of Nursing,* 7:20(11):672–680, 2011.

4. Kean S, Haycock-Stuart E, Baggaley S, Carson M. Followers and the co-construction of leadership. *Journal of Nursing Management,* 19(4):507–516, 2011.

5. Bligh MC, Kohles JC. From radical to mainstream? How followercentric approaches inform leadership. *Journal of Psychology,* 220(4),205–209, 2012.

6. De Santis JP, Florom-Smith A, Vermeesch A, Barroso S, DeLeon, Diego A. Motivation, management, and mastery: A theory of resilience in the context of HIV infection. *Journal of the American Psychiatric Nurses Association,* 19(1):36–46, 2013.

7. Ellis P, Abbott J. Leadership and management skills in health care. *British Journal of Cardiac Nursing,* 5(4):200–203, 2010.

8. Shirey MR. Strategic leadership for organizational change. Lewin's theory of planned change as a strategic resource. *Journal of Nursing Administration,* 43(2):69–72, 2013.

9. Tappen RM. *Essentials of Nursing Leadership and Management* (5th ed.). Philadelphia: F.A. Davis, 2009.

10. Ramsay A, Fulop N, Edwards N. The evidence base for vertical integration in health care. *Journal of Integrated Care,* 17(2): 3–12, 2009.

11. Ruger JP. Health capability: Conceptualization and operationalization. *American Journal of Public Health,* 100(1): 41–49, 2010.

12. Kovner CT, Lusk EL. The sustainability budgeting model: Multiple-mode flexible budgeting using sustainability as the synthesizing criterion. *Nursing Economic$,* 28(6):377–385, 2010.

13. Sullivan MT. Nursing budget: Friend or Foe. *Nursing News,* 33(4):13, 2009.

14. Danna, D. Essential business skills for nurse managers. *Strategies for Nurse Managers,* 2013. Retrieved April 2013 from http://www.strategiesfornursemanagers.com/ce_detail/204441.cfm

15. Budgets and Budgeting. Reference for Business: Encyclopedia of Business, 2nd ed., 2013, Retrieved April 2013 from http://www.referenceforbusiness.com/small/Bo-Co/Budgets-and-Budgeting.html

16. Douglas K, Kerfoot KM. Forging the future of staffing based on evidence. *Nursing Economic$,* 29(4):161–167, 2011.

17. Earnhart SW. Have staffing issues? Use common sense. *Same-Day Surgery,* 36(8):86–87, 2012.

18. Knudson L. Nurse staffing levels linked to patient outcomes, nurse retention. *Association of Operating Room Nurses Journal,* 97(1):1, 8–9, 2013.

19. Anderson T. Editorial: Understanding nurse staffing beyond the numbers. *Nebraska Nurse,* 45(1):8, 2012.

20. Cesta T. The importance of adequate staffing. *Hospital Case Management,* 20(3):39–40, 2012.

21. Schimmel CJ, Jacobs E. When leaders are challenged: Dealing with involuntary members in groups. *Journal for Specialists in Group Work,* 36(2):144–158, 2011.

22. What is group work? Retrieved August 2013 from http://infed.org/mobi/group-work/

23. Trukah T. Is competition among coworkers a good thing? Retrieved August 2013 from http://money.usnews.com/money/blogs/outside-voices-careers/2012/05/01/is-competition-among-co-workers-a-good-thing

24. New care delivery models in health system reform. ANA Issues Brief. Retrieved August 2012 from http://www.nursingworld.org/MainMenuCategories/Policy-Advocacy/Positions-and-Resolutions/Issue-Briefs/Care-Delivery-Models.pdf

25. Beattie L. New health care delivery models are redefining the role of nurses. Retrieved August 2013 from http://www.nursezone.com/nursing-news-events/more-features/New-Health-Care-Delivery-Models-are-Redefining-the-Role-of-Nurses_29442.aspx

Communication, Negotiation, and Conflict Resolution

12

Joseph T. Catalano

Learning Objectives

After completing this chapter, the reader will be able to:

- Explain the importance of understanding human behaviors
- Describe conflict resolution and relationship tools
- Identify communication styles
- List the key elements of negotiation and explain each
- Compare and contrast arbitration and mediation
- Analyze and apply problem-solving and conflict-resolution tools
- Discuss the use of the nursing process in conflict resolution

THE NURSE AS COMMUNICATOR

Good communication skills are often advertised as the answer to many of the problems encountered in everyday life. Television personalities, instructors, and psychologists promote improved communication skills as the answer to parental, marital, financial, and work-related problems. The nursing profession recognizes communication as one of the cornerstones of its practice. Nurses must be able to communicate with clients, family members, physicians, peers, and associates in an effective and constructive manner to achieve their goals of high-quality care. Good communication is essential for good leadership and management.[1]

In today's rapidly evolving health-care system, registered nurses (RNs) are called on to supervise a growing number of assistive and unlicensed personnel. One of the keys to good supervision is the ability to communicate to people what they must do to provide the required care and, often, how the care should be given. It is not always easy. Many of the people whom nurses supervise have limited training, lack the theoretical and technical knowledge base of the nurse, and may display attitudes that make them resistant to direction. However, nurse supervisors can be and often are held legally responsible for the actions of those individuals who work under their direction.

UNDERSTANDING COMMUNICATION

Communication is an interactive sharing of information. It requires a sender, a message, and a receiver. After the sender sends the message, the receiver has a responsibility to listen to, process, and understand (encode) the information and then to respond to the sender by giving feedback (decoding). The encoding process occurs when the receiver thinks about the information, understands it, and forms an idea based on the message.

Several factors can interfere with the encoding process. On the sender's side, these can be factors such as unclear speech, convoluted and confused message, monotone voice, poor sentence structure, inappropriate use of terminology or jargon, or lack of knowledge about the topic. On the receiver's side, factors that may interfere with encoding include lack of attention, prejudice and bias, preoccupation with another problem, or even physical factors such as pain, drowsiness, or impairment of the senses.

For example, a staff nurse is in a mandatory meeting where the unit manager is discussing a new policy that will be starting the following month. However, the nurse is thinking about an important heart medication that her client is to receive in 5 minutes. The nurse's primary concern is to get out of the meeting in time to give the medication. After the meeting, the nurse has only a minimal recollection of what was said because she did not encode the information well. The following month, when the new policy is started, the staff nurse is confused about what she should do and makes several errors in relation to the policy.

Effective communication requires understanding that the perceptions, emotions, and participation of both parties are interactive and have an effect on the transmission of the message. Nurses often encounter situations that require clarification of the information for accuracy and encoding.[2] The following is an example of client teaching that requires a return demonstration:

A nurse gave a teaching session to a client who was being sent home with a T-tube after surgical removal of gallstones from the common bile duct. After the nurse finished her instructions, she asked the client whether he understood how to empty the drainage bottle and measure the drainage. The client looked very confused, but mumbled, "Yes," while shaking his head. The nurse recognized that although the verbal response was positive, the nonverbal responses

indicated that he really did not understand. The nurse surmised that further explanation or demonstration was required for this client to encode the message properly. (For more detail on client teaching, see Davis*Plus* Bonus Chapter 3).

Nurses should recognize the many barriers to clear communication and the benefits of clear communication. These are different from communication blockers discussed below. Once the barriers to communication are identified, they can be overcome, and the benefits of clear communication will follow. These barriers and the benefits that result when they are overcome are outlined in Box 12.1.

COMMUNICATION STYLES

There are three predominant styles of communication: assertive, nonassertive, and aggressive. Individuals develop their communication styles over the course of their lives in response to many personal factors. Although most people have one predominant style of communication, they can and often do switch or combine styles, depending on the situation in which they find themselves.[3] For example, a unit manager who uses an assertive communication style when supervising the staff on her unit may revert to a submissive style when called into the nursing director's office for her annual evaluation. Recognizing which communication style a person is using at any given time, as well as one's own style, is important in making communication clear and effective.

Assertive Communication
Assertive communication is the preferred style in most settings. It involves interpersonal behaviors that permit people to defend and maintain their legitimate rights in a respectful manner that does not violate the rights of others. Assertive communication is honest and direct and accurately expresses the person's feelings, beliefs, ideas, and opinions. Respect for self and others constitutes both the basis for and the result of assertive communication. It encourages trust and teamwork by communicating to others that they have the right to and are

> *The encoding process occurs when the receiver thinks about the information, understands it, and forms an idea based on the message.*

B o x   1 2 . 1

Barriers to and Benefits of Clear Communication

Barriers	Benefits
• Unclear or unexpressed expectations	• Clear expectations
• Confusion	• Understanding
• Retaliation	• Forgiveness
• Desire for power	• Recognized leadership
• Control of others	• Companionship
• Negative reputation	• Respect
• Manipulation	• Independence
• Low self-esteem	• Realistic self-image
• Biased perceptions	• Acceptance
• Inattention	• Clear direction
• Mistrust	• Trusting relations
• Anger	• Self-control
• Fear or anxiety	• Comfort
• Stress	• Motivation or energy
• Insecurity	• Security
• Prejudice	• Increased tolerance
• Interruptions	• Increased knowledge
• Preoccupation	• Concentration

encouraged to express their opinions in an open and respectful atmosphere. Disagreement and discussion are considered to be a healthy part of the communication process, and negotiation is the positive mechanism for problem-solving, learning, and personal growth.[3]

Assertive communication always implies that the individual has the choice to voice an opinion, sometimes forcefully, and to not say anything at all. One of the keys to assertive communication is that the individual is in control of the communication and is not merely reacting to another's emotions.[4]

Assessing Self-Assertiveness

Answer the following questions to determine your self-assertiveness:

• Who am I and what do I want?
• Do I believe I have the right to want it?
• How do I get it?
• Do I believe I can get it?

• Have I tried to be assertive with a person I am having difficulty communicating with?
• Am I letting my fears and perceptions cloud my interactions?
• What is the worst that can happen if we communicate?
• Can I live with the worst?
• Will communications have a long-term effect?
• How does it feel to be in constant fear of alienation or rejection?

Rules for Assertiveness

Anyone can learn to use an assertive communication style and develop assertiveness. When first developing this skill, people often feel frightened and overwhelmed. However, once individuals become comfortable with assertiveness, it helps reinforce their self-concepts and becomes an effective tool for communication. There are a few rules to keep in mind while developing assertiveness along with an assertive communication style:

• It is a learned skill.
• It takes practice.
• It requires a desire and motivation to change.
• It requires a willingness to take risks.
• It requires a willingness to make mistakes and try again.
• It requires an understanding that not every outcome sought will be obtained.
• It requires strong self-esteem.
• Self-reward for change and a positive outcome is essential.
• Listening to self is necessary for identifying needs.
• Constant reexamination of outcomes helps assess progress.
• Role-playing with a friend before the interaction builds skill and confidence.
• Goals for assertiveness growth need to be established beforehand.
• Assertiveness requires recognition that change is a gradual process.
• Others should be allowed to make mistakes.

Personal Risks of Assertive Communication

There are always personal risks involved in learning any new skills or in attempting to change behavior. Learning assertive communication is no exception. People often fear that they may not choose the "perfect" assertive response. However, even seasoned assertive communicators may err from time to time because every encounter is unique, involving different people and situations. The person who is new to assertive communication needs to recognize that it is a skill that takes practice.

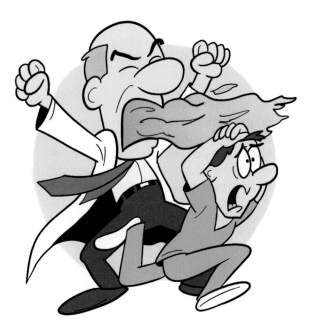

I Win, You Win

Assertiveness does not mean that a person will always get his or her way in every situation, and it is likely the individual will handle some situations better than others. Remember that the goal of assertive communication is to prevent an "I win, you lose" situation and to encourage an "I win, you win" outcome.[4] A win-win goal is achieved when both parties have the ability and willingness to negotiate even though they do not get all they want. However, there may be situations when personal goals are not achieved. Some questions to consider when this occurs are:

- How do I feel about losing?
- Did I express my opinion clearly? Why not? How could I make it clearer?
- Did I do the best I could do? How could I have done better?
- Was I in control when responding to the situation? When did I lose control? What should I have done to regain control?
- Did I stay focused on the issues? What side issues distracted me? How could I have avoided distractions?

- Did I allow the situation to get personal? Did the other person initiate the personal attack? How could I have redirected it away from the personal?
- Was what I asked for under my control? If not, why did I ask for it? What would have been more realistic?

Reviewing these questions and analyzing the answers will help when you attempt to be assertive in future communications. For example, if the answer to the second-to-last question was yes, then during the next communication, a special effort can be focused on avoiding personal attacks during the encounter. Learning to communicate assertively is a process of continual improvement.

Impact of Assertive Communication

Another risk factor that quickly becomes evident when changing to an assertive communication style is the impact that it has on those who know the person best. Sometimes family, friends, peers, and coworkers become barriers to change. Change always produces some degree of stress. Those individuals who are closest to the person trying to initiate changes may feel uncomfortable because they have become accustomed to the old communication styles and behaviors over a long period of time. They can no longer anticipate and depend on the person's responding and reacting in the usual way.[5] In addition, they will have to develop new communication patterns of their own to match the changes caused by assertive communication.

Sometimes family, friends, peers, and coworkers become so uncomfortable that they may try to sabotage the person's attempts at assertive communication. It is important to recognize why and when these sabotage efforts occur and to remember that assertiveness is an internal, personal process. Everyone has a right to change, and it must be respectfully communicated to others that their support for these changes is important.

It is also important to know and periodically review the rights and responsibilities of assertiveness to help reinforce the assertive communication process. The rights and responsibilities of assertiveness are listed in Box 12.2.

Practice and reinforcement of assertiveness skills may be required, especially when preparing for an anticipated conflict negotiation or a confrontational meeting with another. Although a confrontational situation always produces anxiety, rather than

Box 12.2

Rights and Responsibilities of Assertiveness

- To act in a way that promotes your dignity and self-respect
- To be treated with respect
- To experience and express your thoughts and feelings
- To slow down and make conscious decisions before you act
- To ask for what you want
- To say no
- To change your mind
- To make mistakes
- To not be perfect
- To feel important and good about yourself
- To be treated as an individual with special values, skills, and needs
- To be unique
- To have your own feelings and opinions
- To say "I don't know"
- To feel angry, hurt, and frustrated
- To make decisions regarding your life
- To recognize that your needs are as important as others'

being feared, it should be recognized as having the potential to be highly productive. Box 12.3 lists several behaviors that, if practiced and used, will help increase confidence and assertiveness skills during anticipated confrontational meetings.

You can use the checklist in Box 12.4 to determine your own degree of assertiveness.

Nonassertive Communication

Nonassertive communication is also referred to as *submissive communication.*

Submissive Communication

When people display submissive behavior or use a submissive communication style, they allow their rights to be violated by others. Their requests and demands are surrendered to others without regard to their own feelings and needs. Many experts believe that submissive behavior and communication patterns are a protective mechanism that helps insecure people maintain their self-esteem by avoiding negative criticism and disagreement from others. In other situations, it may be a means of manipulation by way of passive-aggressive behavior.

Box 12.3

Assertiveness Self-Assessment

Statement	Communication Behavior
1. I didn't say what I really wanted to say at the last staff meeting.	_____
2. I always express my opinion because it is better than everyone else's.	_____
3. I have the courage to speak up almost all the time.	_____
4. I wish someone else would speak up at the meetings besides me.	_____
5. I am not intimidated by the high-pressure tactics of supervisors, physicians, and/or teachers.	_____
6. I have trouble stating my true feelings to those in authority.	_____
7. I really put that know-it-all aide in her place last shift.	_____
8. After the last meeting with my unit director, I felt hopeless, resentful, and angry.	_____
9. I speak up in meetings without feeling defensive.	_____
10. When I need to confront someone, I avoid the problem because it will usually resolve itself.	_____
11. When I need to confront individuals, I address them directly.	_____
12. When I confront individuals, I let them know in no uncertain terms that they are wrong and need to change their behavior.	_____
13. When I'm reprimanded, I keep silent even though I'm seething inside.	_____
14. The last time I was asked to stay over for another shift, I said no and didn't feel guilty.	_____

B o x 1 2 . 4

Conflict Resolution Tips

In nursing practice, good communication and conflict management skills are essential. The following tips may help resolve communication problems:

Improve Your Conflict Management Skills
- Seminars
- Books
- Mentors

Change Your Paradigm
- Focus on the positive, not the negative.
- Realize that appropriate confrontation is a risk-taking activity.

Achieve Better Communication
- Improved relationships
- Improved teamwork
- Mentoring

Understand Your Values
- Focus on a win-win.
- Be willing to negotiate and compromise.
- Be direct and honest.
- Focus on the issues.
- Do not attack the person.
- Do not make judgments.
- Do not become the third person; encourage peers to go direct.
- Do not spread rumors.

Set Personal Guidelines
- Confront in private, never in front of anyone else.
- Confront the individual; do not report him or her to the supervisor first.
- Do not confront when you are angry.
- Start with an "I" message.
- Express your feelings and opinions.
- Allow the other person to talk without interruptions.
- Listen attentively.
- Set goals and future plans of action.
- Let it go.
- Keep it private and confidential.

What Do You Think?

Recall a recent exchange with someone (e.g., friend, instructor, parent, physician) in which you felt you "lost" the exchange. How did you feel? How did you respond? How could using an assertive communication style have helped?

B o x 1 2 . 5

Assertive Communication Suggestions

- Maintain eye contact.
- Convey empathy; stating your feelings does not mean sympathy or agreement.
- Keep your body position erect, shoulders and back straight.
- Speak clearly and audibly; be direct and descriptive.
- Be comfortable with silence.
- Use gestures and facial expressions for emphasis.
- Use appropriate location.
- Use appropriate timing.
- Focus on behaviors and issues; do not attack the person.

Because of their great fear of displeasing others, personal rejection, or future retaliation, submissive communicators dismiss their own feelings as being unimportant. However, at a deeper level, submissive behavior and communication merely reinforce negative feelings of powerlessness, helplessness, and decreased self-worth. Rather than being in control of the communication or relationship, the person is trading his or her ability to choose what is best for the avoidance of conflict. Every communication by a submissive person becomes an "I lose, you win" situation. However, subconsciously it is more of "You may think you win, but I really am winning because I'm getting what I want or need."

Aggressive Communication

Sometimes there is only a very fine line separating assertiveness from aggressive behavior and communication.[4] Whereas assertive communication permits individuals to honestly express their ideas and opinions while respecting the other's rights, ideas, and opinions, aggressive communication strongly asserts the speaker's legitimate rights and opinions with little regard or respect for the rights and opinions of others. It easily becomes a communication blocker (see below).

Aggressive communication—used to humiliate, dominate, control, or embarrass the other person or lower that person's self-esteem—creates an "I win, you lose" situation. The other person may perceive aggressive behavior or communication as a personal attack. Aggressive behavior and communication are viewed by some psychologists as a protective mechanism that compensates for a person's own insecurities, and others view it as a form of bullying. By demeaning someone else, aggressive behavior allows the person to feel superior and helps inflate his or her self-esteem.

Aggressive communication can take several different forms, including screaming, sarcasm, rudeness, belittling jokes, and even direct personal insults. It is an expression of the negative feelings of power, domination, and low self-esteem. Although aggressive people may seem outwardly to be in control, in reality they are merely reacting to the situation to protect their self-esteem.

Using appropriate methods of communication in conjunction with an assertive communication style enhances the communication and understanding by both parties. Developing an assertive communication style is important in using communication builders. (For more information, go to http://www .ncbi.nlm.nih.gov/ pubmed/21248553).

Verbal, Paraverbal, or Nonverbal Communication

There are three primary methods of communication: verbal, paraverbal, and nonverbal. **Verbal** communication is either written or spoken and constitutes only about 7 percent of the communicated message. **Nonverbal** communication makes up the other 55 percent of communication and includes body language, facial expressions, gestures, physical appearance, touch, and spatial territory (personal space). **Paraverbal** is the tone, pitch, volume, and diction used when delivering a verbal message. How people say something is often more important than what they are saying. A sentence can have a completely different meaning by placing emphasis on different words. Paraverbal communication makes up about 38 percent of the total message and is often considered part of nonverbal communication.[6] When the verbal, paraverbal, and nonverbal messages are congruent, the message is more easily encoded and clearly understood. If the verbal, paraverbal, and nonverbal messages are conflicting, the paraverbal and nonverbal messages are the most reliable. It is relatively easy for people to lie with words, but

> *Through active participation, workers have an opportunity to have an impact on and direct the changes that are being made. Some people mistakenly believe that if they do not become involved, the changes will not happen.*

paraverbal and nonverbal communication tends to be unconscious and more difficult to control.

For example, the nurse suspects that the mother of a newborn infant may be experiencing postpartum depression. The nurse asks the mother how she feels about her new baby. The mother responds in a quiet, very slow monotone (paraverbal message), "I'm so happy I have this baby" (verbal message), while looking down at her feet in a slouched-over posture with her arms folded (nonverbal message). The message from the mother is conflicting. The words are saying she is happy, but all the paraverbal and nonverbal signs indicate that she is sad and depressed. The observant nurse concludes that more assessment for depression is required.

FACTORS THAT AFFECT COMMUNICATION

People are always communicating something, in either a verbal, paraverbal, or nonverbal manner. There often is a degree of overlap among the three styles. Some of the things people do and say help build communication, but other actions or words break communication down. Anything done or said that interferes with communication is called a *communication blocker*. Actions and speech that encourage and build communication are called *communication builders* and are often referred to as *therapeutic communication techniques* Other factors, such as the environment the communication is taking place in, stress levels of the parties communicating, grief and change experiences, and people feeling angry can also block effective communication.

Nonverbal Communication Builders

Eye contact. In general, in North American culture, using eye contact while communicating is a sign of interest in the person and says, "What you are saying is important to me." However, there is a need to be cautious using it. It can turn into a staring contest and says, "I'm trying to dominate you." Also, eye contact has other meanings in other cultures. Some tribes of American Indians believe that direct eye contact is an attempt to take the

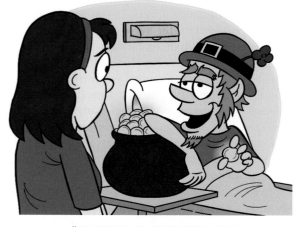

"IF YE LET ME SKIP THIS TEST,
YE CAN HAVE ME POT O'GOLD!"

other person's spirit. In some Hispanic groups, direct eye contact is a sign of hostility and aggression.

Stop what you're doing. This indicates that the other person is more important than the task that is being worked on and encourages more communication.

Nod the head. Nodding while the other person is speaking indicates you are listening closely to what is said and that you either agree with them or accept what they are saying. Shaking the head can also be used as a communication builder if it is used when the person is describing a difficult situation they have experienced.

Positive facial expressions. Smiling or looking surprised at appropriate times while the other person is speaking indicates that what the other person is saying is being accepted. The eyes are often the most expressive part of the face, indicating joy, approval, or excitement.

Sitting or standing in close proximity. Being relatively close to the person speaking shows that they have your full attention and actually makes speaking easier. Leaning toward the speaker also achieves this purpose. This technique also has to be used with some caution. Violating a person's personal space (about 18 to 24 inches in America) may make the person feel uncomfortable. If they back away, then the distance is too close. Personal space also has a cultural component. People from the southwest United States tend to require a larger personal space as compared with persons from

large cities or countries like India or the Middle East, where people experience close proximity in their everyday lives and tend to require much less personal space.

Open posture, directly facing. An open posture, which means arms and legs are uncrossed while directly facing the speaker, says, "I am open to what you are saying—your thoughts are important to me."

Listening empathically. Pay attention to the message so that when the person finishes, he or she can say, "Wow, you really got what I said."

Light touch. Touching the other person's shoulder, arm, or hand, particularly if they are communicating sadness, distress, or grief, can send a message of reassurance; however, there are major cautions with using touch as a communication technique based on cultural and personal preferences. Many Americans dislike being touched by others, especially by people they do not know well, although certain cultural groups within U.S. society such as Italians, Hispanics, and Russians are very open in expressing emotion through touching. **Being aware of the speaker's nonverbal and paraverbal communication.** The messages delivered though facial expressions, gestures, body position, and special distance is as important as the verbal message be spoken.

Paraverbal Communication Builders

Silence. It might seem to be a contradiction to the concept of communication, but silence can be a highly effective communication builder. It is said that "nature abhors a vacuum and will try to fill it with something." Silence is a communication vacuum, and most people abhor it and will not let it go on for more than a few seconds. Waiting for the other person to speak can be very uncomfortable for both parties; however, it provides the speaker with a chance to think about what they said and are going to say. How long is too long? There really is no hard or pat answer to that question, but using a verbal prod such as "Tell me what you are thinking about?" can open up the lines of communication again.

Tone. A calm, soothing tone, particularly when communicating with agitated or hostile individuals who are speaking loudly or aggressively, can ease the situation. It is important not to respond in kind. A calm, even tone conveys the message that the speaker is in control of the situation and that the person who is upset also needs to gain control of their emotions. An assertive tone expresses urgency and a need to respond, particularly in emergency situations. An aggressive or hostile tone usually indicates anger and frustration.

Verbal Communication Builders

Encouraging words. Short responses or interjections such as, "Okay," "Right," "Mmm-hmm" or "Tell me more" says to them, "I'm paying attention," and encourages them to keep talking.

Asking open-ended questions. These are questions that cannot be answered by one or two words and force the person to continue speaking. This type of question includes "Tell me about what made you angry," "Describe the situation that put you in that position," or "What is this person doing that makes you feel inferior?"

Use "I" rather than "you" messages. People are less likely to perceive a communication as a personal attack when the conversation begins with an explanation of a personal view of the situation or even how feelings were affected. Statements such as "I thought it was done this way," or "I heard something the other day," or even "I feel hurt when people judge me" are more productive ways to begin an exchange of ideas and information.

Asking clarification questions. This type of question seeks more information and will keep the speaker talking. Questions such as "Could you explain that a little more? I didn't quite get what you were saying," or "I'm a little confused about your last statement," are nonconfrontational and make the person feel comfortable speaking.

Reflecting feelings and emotions. Sometimes called *paraphrasing*, this response should be used when there is a mismatch between what the person is saying and what their body language is saying. Always believe the body language; it can't lie. These include questions such as "How did you feel about that?" "Why did that make you depressed?" "You seem to be angry (sad, anxious, afraid, etc.). Can you talk about that more?"

Repeating what was just said. This communication builder is called *restating* and helps clarify what the person is saying. Lead into the statement with "Let me know if I heard you correctly. You just said . . ." Restating indicates good listening skills and helps keep the conversation going.

Never, never interrupt. There is always a tendency to identify with the speaker's recounting of an incident and interject something like "I had something similar happen to me." They don't want to hear about your problems. Just let them continue speaking.

Reviewing what was said. This is different from repeating because rather than just repeating one thing that the person said, it requires analysis and synthesis of the key points, usually emotions, of the discussion, which is then summarized. Statements like "Okay, we've been talking for a while, and it seems like you have said that you are anxious because so-and-so keeps saying to you . . ." "Is that a correct summary?"

Acknowledging what was said. Sometimes called *validating*, this communication builder is a combination of reviewing and identifying emotions. It makes the speaker feel that what he or she is saying has value and that someone cares about their issues. Using statements such as "I understand what you are saying," or "I can appreciate your feelings about the situation," validates the speaker.

> " *People are less likely to perceive a communication as a personal attack when the conversation begins with an explanation of a personal view of the situation or even how feelings were affected.* "

Environmental Communication Builders

Calm, nonthreatening environment. A quiet room with subdued lighting is the ideal location to help build communication. However, in the real world, a busy, noisy hospital room or hallway is more likely to be the environment for communication about important issues such as home medications and dressing changes. Nurses, as always, are required to do the best they can with what they have.

Nonverbal Communication Blockers

Eye rolling. When people roll their eyes, they are sending a message of not caring about what the other person is saying. Teens are notorious for this behavior, but adults also use it at times, particularly if it has become habitual.

Arm and leg folding. This generally is interpreted as an indication of disapproval or boredom. The person listening is closed to the speaker's ideas, which are not considered very important. It sometimes can be a sign that the other person is feeling attacked and is trying to defend themselves.

Slouching, hunching, turning away. These nonverbal communication blockers indicate that the listener is just not interested in what is being said. It says to the speaker, "Are we done yet? I'd rather be on the other side of the room."

Fidgeting. This includes picking at fingernails, drumming the fingers, playing with buttons or jewelry, frequent shifting in the chair, rolling and unrolling hair, taking off and putting on glasses frequently, doodling extensively on a pad of paper, frequent checking of cell phone, picking at shoe laces, and so on. It delivers the message that the listener is experiencing extreme boredom and can't wait to leave.

Deep, loud sighs. This message tells the other person that they are boring and should end the conversation quickly. What they have to say is not worth the time it takes to say it, and there are other more productive things to be done with the time.

Multiple watch or clock checks. Similar to deep sighs in that what the person is saying is not very important and the listener is about to die from boredom.

Continuing with an activity while the other person is talking. The message is "I'm ignoring you because you are not that important. What I'm doing is more important."

Failure to make eye contact. This nonverbal technique can be used as a way to show disapproval but is often used when a person is hurt by another and is trying to hurt the person back. On the other hand, an excessively long unblinking stare is a communication blocker that shows aggression and hostility.

Tuning out or failing to pay attention. Another way of saying, "I'm not listening—what you are saying isn't important." (For more information, go to http://www.ncbi.nlm.nih.gov/pubmed/24138223.)

> *An excessively long unblinking stare is a communication blocker that shows aggression and hostility.*

Verbal Communication Blockers

Automatic defensiveness. This communication blocker occurs when one person feels so threatened by the other that the first thing he or she says is of a defensive nature. For example, "It wasn't my fault; the thing just broke," "I really didn't want to do it, but Alexis made me," or "If you didn't push me so hard to speak, I never would have said it."

Asking closed-ended questions. These are questions that a person can answer in one or two words. For example, "How are you feeling today?" Answer: "Fine." "Did you practice your responses like we discussed?" Answer: "Yes."

Accusing or blaming. This is a type of confrontational speech and sends the message that the other person is wrong even before given a chance to provide his or her side of the story. For example, "If you knew how to read a map, we wouldn't be lost in the middle of nowhere."

Using sarcasm. This sends the message that the other person is not respected and is untrustworthy. The statements are often said in a taunting tone with vocal over-emphasis. For example: A co-worker is playing a DVD very loudly in the break room. You comment: "Why don't you turn it up a little? I don't think they can hear it in Toronto!"

Constant interruptions. Over the years, some people have developed a habit of interrupting without any sort of malice or intent to hurt. However, the message is the same whether it is intentional or not—the person interrupting feels that what he or she has to say is more important than the person who is talking.

Judging, name calling, and diagnosing. This communication blocker uses "you messages," indicating that there is something wrong with the other person. These also send the message that the person making the judgment or diagnosis is more intelligent and has a better understanding than the person with the problem. It denotes an air of superiority. It includes statements such as, "You're such a perfectionist—no wonder you don't have any friends," "You don't seem to understand that we need to finish the project on time," "You know what your problem is?" "You really don't care if this issue gets resolved," "You made a mistake," "You said this about me," or "You always do this."

Stating opinions as proven facts. This communication blocker prevents the other person from expressing their opinions and discounts the importance of what they have to say. For example, "Everybody knows that the Affordable Care Act (ACA) allows death panels to decide who is going to get care and who will live or die."

Making generalizations, being patronizing, and offering vague reassurances. Statements such as "You always leave the break room in a mess," "Don't worry, everything is going to be all right," or "It always works out for the best, doesn't it?" makes the other person feel that what they have to say is not important. It also categorizes them in a box that they may not want to be in.

Telling people how they should feel. This invalidates the other person's feelings and shows a high degree of disrespect. This types of statements include "Don't feel like that," "Don't let that bother you," or "Getting upset is very childish."

Changing the subject. Another indicator that what the person is saying is not important and not worth the time.

Expecting mind reading. Sometimes other people expect you to know what they are thinking or to anticipate what they need or are going to say. People who have been very close for a long period of time sometimes get to a point in their relationship where they know the other person well enough to "mind read" (actually anticipate) what they are going to say. However, for the vast majority of communication, telling them what you are thinking, feeling, or wishing them to do is the best approach.

Shaking or pointing a finger while speaking. This combines both verbal and nonverbal blockers. Much like yelling and getting in someone's face, it is an exercise of power over the other person. The message is "You really are stupid and inferior."

Walking away. This is the ultimate communication blocker. If there is no one to talk to, there is no communication.

> *When people say, "I couldn't get a word in edgewise!" it means that the other person totally dominated the conversation. Often the speaker is attempting to avoid confrontation, stress, intimacy, uncomfortable thoughts or feelings, or a difficult situation.*

Paraverbal Communication Blockers

Threatening, ordering, or getting in someone's face. The message here is "I'm angry and I don't care what you think." People often use "clenched teeth speech" or yelling when being confrontational. It threatens other people and makes them keep their distance. People who use these blockers are often deeply insecure, and these techniques push other people away. They also use them to make themselves feel better about themselves. It takes away the need to understand the other person.

Yelling, calling names, or hurling insults. This is a type of negative aggressive behavior that is immature and degrading. It shows a lack of respect for the other person and often creates deep emotional wounds. Yelling and name-calling can quickly rise to the level of physical violence such as pushing or even hitting.

Nonstop, rapid talking. When people say, "I couldn't get a word in edgewise!" it means that the other person totally dominated the conversation. Often the speaker is attempting to avoid confrontation, stress, intimacy, uncomfortable thoughts or feelings, or a difficult situation. In some people, it can become a habit over time and shows disrespect to other people. It may also be an attempt for the speaker to hide feelings of inferiority by showing how intelligent or dominant they are.

Environmental Communication Blockers

Experiencing change. Change can be a communication blocker in various ways. People may be afraid to ask questions about new procedures or policies because they fear that they might appear "stupid" in front of their colleagues. Fear of being criticized closes individuals off to positive suggestions and new ideas.[7] Others may hesitate in sharing ideas because they are afraid of being labeled as confrontational. Nurses also need to keep in mind that the communication abilities of clients experiencing change will be blocked in much the same way as those of nurses experiencing change.

For example, a nurse is reassigned from the medical-surgical unit to the intensive care unit (ICU). This nurse will initially be somewhat fearful in the new environment with the highly trained and assertive expert unit nurses who always seem to be in control. A more positive approach would be for the new nurse to take advantage of the unit nurses' experience and learn from their examples. The new nurse needs to remember that everyone on that unit was a novice at one time. In the current health-care system, almost everyone is fearful much of the time of making mistakes and of not being able to meet the high standards of the profession.

Grief experiences. Most clients who have surgical procedures that result in major body function alterations go through the stages of the grief process: denial, anger, guilt, depression, and resolution. Communication with a client in the anger stage who is hostile, critical of his care, and verbally abusive will be very different from communication with a client in the depression stage, who is withdrawn, reticent, and sleeps most of the time. Recognition of the communication blocking mechanisms of each grief stage is essential to understanding why clients are acting in a particular way. A decision must then be made regarding the most effective communication technique to use when providing care (see below for a more detailed discussion).

> *Most clients who have surgical procedures that result in major body function alterations go through the stages of the grief process: denial, anger, guilt, depression, and resolution.*

Stressful situations. Stress is an environmental blocker that is produced by many factors and always affects an individual's ability to communicate. Some common causes of stress for health-care workers include institutional restructuring, group interaction and dynamics, unilateral management decisions, and personal issues and experiences. Regardless of the source, stress usually decreases people's ability to interact and communicate and increases the demands on their coping mechanisms.[7]

Policy change. Health-care reform is raising many questions about the health-care system and the delivery of care.[8] The changes produced by these transitions will create a high degree of stress at all levels of the health-care system. Change and stress are major barriers to effective communication.[9]

Some techniques to alleviate the stress of change include:
- Active participation of the whole team in planning and implementing change
- Open and interactive lines of communication
- Avoiding rumors, outbursts, feelings of insecurity and fear

Tension and anxiety. When people are unable to successfully cope with a stressful situation, they may experience an increased state of tension or anxiety. They are even more difficult to communicate with than people with stress. They may develop physiological symptoms, such as nausea, stomach cramps, diarrhea, or palpitations; in extreme cases, they may even become paranoid or psychotic. Uncontrolled high levels of stress on a nursing unit may lead to competition among the nurses that affects their teamwork, productivity, and the quality of the care given.

Physicians who are stressed by worry about a severely ill client or threats to their autonomy, practice, and income from changes in reimbursement policies may become tense and highly critical of or even verbally abusive toward nurses. The hospital management may also experience increased stress owing to the escalating responsibility of maintaining high-quality services with ever-shrinking revenues. Management often deals with its stress by becoming more autocratic, making increased demands on the nursing staff while reducing the control that nurses have over their practice and becoming closed off to input from nurses and physicians.

What Do You Think?

List four factors or situations that have produced high levels of stress for you in the hospital or health-care setting. Why did these incidents produce stress? How did you deal with the stress?

Stress is a major contributing factor to a variety of disorders, ranging from high blood pressure to ulcers and anxiety. In the health-care environment, stress is not just experienced by health-care providers. Stress for clients starts when they first come into contact with the health-care system; peaks when they have to undergo physical examinations, surgery, or invasive treatments; and continues throughout the recovery period. The fear that a nurse may not respond to clients' needs increases clients' stress levels, and they sometimes become more demanding of care, which in turn increases the nurse's stress levels.[10] If the nursing staff is experiencing high stress levels, clients often sense this subconsciously, and as a result, clients' stress levels also increase.

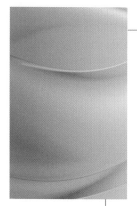

Issues in Practice

Managing Change

The busy nonacute outpatient unit at a large hospital had become disorganized. It consistently received evaluations of "poor" when clients were asked about the care being provided. They often complained about the long waits to be evaluated and treated. The staff also recognized the problems with the care they were providing but didn't have any solutions.

In an attempt to improve the evaluations, the administration replaced the current director with a new director from an even larger facility across town. She was charged with the task of improving client care and was promised that she would have whatever resources she needed.

Within 6 months, the new director completely reorganized the staffing patterns and modernized all the information systems using the latest software. She replaced old equipment with new models and bought additional equipment that the unit had never used before. She also managed to expand and brighten up the unit by remodeling extensively and by securing unused space from the radiology department, which occupied adjacent rooms. She increased the salaries of the nursing staff, hired new nurses, and expanded the hours of service. She implemented a "management by objectives" model for evaluation that allowed the staff nurses increased input into their working conditions and evaluations.

Client surveys indicated an increase in overall satisfaction with the care being provided; the wait time had been decreased to a point at which there were hardly any complaints. However, approximately half the experienced nurses on the unit resigned, and the rest of the nurses began the process of organizing into a collective bargaining unit for the first time in the history of the nonacute outpatient unit.

Questions for Thought

1. What was the underlying issue that led to the nurses' responses to the changes?

2. What could the director have done to increase the staff's acceptance of change?

(Answers are found at the end of the chapter.)

Techniques to Reduce Stress

Several techniques can be used to reduce clients' stress levels so that they can better communicate and become more receptive to teaching. Stress-reduction techniques range from very simple measures that everyone can use, such as distraction with music or simple activities, exercise, or reduction in stimuli, to more advanced techniques such as meditation, **biofeedback**, and even antianxiety medications.

Eliminate the Situation

Nurses need to be able to identify situations that produce stress, recognize the symptoms shown by someone in a stressful situation, know how to reduce stress, and be able to use appropriate communication techniques with someone under stress. Of course, if possible, the best way to reduce stress is to eliminate the stressful situation. Consider the following case:

The hospital management has just sent a memo to all the hospital units that a new client assessment form they have developed is to be implemented next week. This new form is in addition to the ones that the nurses already fill out each day. It is to be completed by RNs only and must be done each shift on every client and then sent to the house supervisor so that management can track acuity. Because of recent facility restructuring and changes in staffing patterns, often there is only one RN on the 3 p.m. to 11 p.m. and 11 p.m. to 7 a.m. shifts to cover a 42-bed unit. This extra, time-consuming, and seemingly redundant paperwork increases the stress of the staff RNs to an unacceptable level.

They meet as a group with management and propose that the assessment forms they are already using be modified to include the data that management wants on the new forms. Photocopies of the revised form could then be made by the unit clerk for each shift and given to the supervisors, thus eliminating the new form. Management notes the high stress levels of the RNs, recognizes that increased stress lowers the quality of care, and decides to follow the RNs' proposal, thus eliminating the primary source of the RNs' stress.

Although all sources of stress cannot be eliminated completely, in most situations they can be reduced to a manageable level. However, high stress levels should never be used as an excuse for destructive anger and behaviors, failure of communication, or abuse of individuals.

Anger

People who are angry almost always find it difficult, if not impossible, to successfully communicate, and as such, it is one of the environmental communication blockers, much like stress. However, because anger is also key in understanding and dealing with difficult people, is one of the stages of the grief process, and is a symptom of personal frustration, lack of control, fear of change, or feelings of hopelessness, it is discussed here in more length than other communication blockers.

Anger is one of the strong primitive natural emotions that help individuals protect themselves against a variety of external threats.[11] Many animals, including humans, that express anger by making loud sounds (yelling or growling), puffing themselves up to appear physically larger, baring and gritting their teeth and staring intently are warning other possible aggressors to stop their threatening behavior. Physical violence between two people rarely occurs without a warning expression of anger by at least one of the parties. Although everyone experiences anger, how it is expressed often depends on a person's family and ethnic background, life experiences, and personal values. In some cultures, loud and physically expressive outbursts are the norm for the expression of anger, whereas in other cultures, anger is internalized and expressed only as a "controlled rage."

Positive or Negative Expression

As with most of the other factors that affect communication, anger can be either positive or negative. When anger is used in a positive, productive manner, it can promote change and release tension. Anger can

> " *At some point, one group's stress always affects the stress level of another group, whose stress in turn increases another group's stress. The process becomes a destructive circle of cause-and-effect responses that increase the stress levels for everyone in the facility.* "

be used positively to increase others' attention, initiate communication, problem-solve, and energize the change process. Sensitivity to internal anger can warn individuals that something is wrong either within themselves or with someone or something in the external environment.

Many individuals have difficulty expressing and using their anger in a positive manner. Anger that is used negatively is very destructive. It hinders communication, makes coworkers fearful, and erodes relationships with others. Anger expressed by abusive behaviors, such as pounding on nursing station counters, throwing charts or surgical instruments, verbal outbursts, or even violent physical contact, is never acceptable and may lead to civil or criminal action against the perpetrator.

The negative expression of anger may cause the person who is the object of the anger to retaliate or seek revenge, but probably the most destructive form that negative anger can take is when it is internalized and suppressed. Long-term suppressed anger has been associated with a number of physiological and psychological problems, ranging from gastric ulcers and hypertension to myocardial infarctions, strokes, and even psychotic rage episodes.[11]

> *Many animals, including humans, that express anger by making loud sounds (yelling or growling), puffing themselves up to appear physically larger, baring and gritting their teeth and staring intently are warning other possible aggressors to stop their threatening behavior.*

What Sets People Off

Nurses who understand what makes themselves and others angry are better able to either avoid anger-producing situations or cope effectively with their own anger or with that of others. For example, even new graduate nurses soon learn that some situations will almost always evoke an angry response from hospitalized clients. These include serving meals that are cold or poorly cooked, not answering call lights in a timely manner, waking up soundly sleeping clients at midnight to give them a sleeping pill, or taking 10 attempts to start an intravenous (IV) line. (See below for more detail on angry clients).

Similarly, unit managers and hospital administrators quickly learn that some of the things they do will almost always produce angry responses from the staff. These actions include unilateral changes in the work schedule, additional paperwork, reduction in staffing levels, or refusal of requests for vacation or time off.[11]

It is important that nurses understand that anger is a normal human emotion. Once it is recognized, it should be dealt with and then let go. Sometimes situations are not going to change, no matter how angry the person becomes, and sometimes no amount of anger will prevent changes from occurring.

What Do You Think?

Consider the health-care providers with whom you have worked in the recent past. What were their communication styles? How did those styles affect the way you communicated with them?

PROBLEM-SOLVING

Problem-solving is a process that everyone uses frequently. For example, on the way to work, a tire goes flat on a person's car. That is a problem. How the person solves the problem depends partially on critical-thinking skills, partially on past experiences, and partially on physical abilities. If the person with the flat tire is a 250-lb, 33-year-old male construction worker in good health, he most likely has changed tires before and will probably be physically able to remove the flat tire and put on the spare without difficulty. However, if the person with the flat tire is a 90-lb, 67-year-old female church organist, her solution to the problem will likely be different. She will probably call her emergency roadside service and have someone come and change the flat for her.

One of the primary activities for nurses in the work setting is problem-solving using the nursing process. It really does not matter whether the problem is client centered, management oriented, or an interpersonal issue; the nursing process is an excellent framework for problem resolution. It focuses on the goals of mutual interaction and communication to establish trust and respect. Using the process of assessment, analysis, planning, implementation, and evaluation helps the nurse organize and structure interpersonal interactions in a way that will produce an "I win, you win" situation.[12]

The basic problem-solving steps of the nursing process form the framework for successful conflict management. Nurses who are good problem-solvers using the nursing process also tend to be good at conflict resolution, and nurses who are good at conflict resolution tend to be excellent problem-solvers. Rather than being avoided in the work setting, conflict should be considered an opportunity to practice and grow in the use of problem-solving skills.

CONFLICT RESOLUTION

Everyone experiences conflict at one time or another as a part of daily life. Often people feel more comfortable addressing the conflict that arises in their personal lives than conflicts that arise in the professional setting. Problem-solving is often perceived as less emotional and more structured, whereas conflict management is considered to be more emotionally charged, with the potential to produce hostility. However, the steps of conflict management and problem-solving are almost identical to those of the nursing process. The one additional element that must be included in conflict resolution is the ability to use assertive behaviors and communication when discussing the issues.

> *Everyone experiences conflict at one time or another as a part of daily life. Often people feel more comfortable addressing the conflict that arises in their personal lives than the professional conflicts that arise in the job setting.*

Contributing Factors to Conflict

There are many things in life and the environment that contribute to conflicts. These can range from a difference of opinion about how a job should be done to major underlying beliefs such as culture, religion, and politics. The focus here is on resolving conflicts that affect the work environment, primarily emotional issues, insecurity, lack of skills, and diversity issues. Understanding the underlying elements of all types of conflict is a key in preventing and resolving many of the issues.[13]

Understanding what motivates a person's behavior permits the individual to better appreciate the full scope of the conflict.[14] Conflict is often a symptom of some deeper problem, and the conflict really never gets resolved without dealing with the underlying issues. When individuals are able to separate themselves from the conflict, they are less likely to take things personally and more likely to begin to focus on the underlying issues causing the problems than on the other person's behavior. The interaction becomes less judgmental and threatening to the other person. However, understanding the other person's motives never excuses unacceptable behaviors such as sarcasm, angry outbursts, and abusive language. Rather, it allows for direct confrontation of the behavior in a more controlled and less emotional way.

Emotions

Emotions and feelings are a primary contributing factor to the development of conflicts. Many people are very sensitive to what others say to them or by threats to their perceived security and react aggressively to demonstrate their hurt feelings.[15]

A common situation that causes conflict is the nurse's feeling of being overworked or overwhelmed by assignments. The overloaded nurse might say something like "I have a huge amount of work today. Why isn't anyone helping me?" rather than asking a particular individual for help. Believing another person is, or should be, a mind reader rarely produces the results the person desires. When the person who is expected to help fails to comply with the implied request, the overworked nurse becomes angry and resentful. The other person may not understand where this anger is coming from and often avoids addressing the angry person for fear of making him or her angrier.[15] This type of poor communication and lack of direct, respectful conflict resolution produces tension among workers, deterioration of working relationships, decreased efficiency, and, ultimately, lower-quality client care.

Insecurity and Lack of Skills

Conflicts sometimes arise because people do not know how to deal with them or feel threatened by the thought of confronting another person. Some of the reasons people give for not resolving conflicts before they get out of hand include the following:

- Fear of retaliation
- Fear of ridicule
- Fear of alienating others
- Mistaken belief that they are unable to handle the conflict situation
- Feeling that they do not have the right to speak up
- Past negative experiences with conflict situations
- Family background and experiences
- Lack of education and skills in conflict resolution[16]

Diversity

Diversity simply means that people are different from each other. It is a multifaceted issue that involves many areas of people's lives, including culture, values, life experiences, instinctual responses, learned behaviors, personal strengths and weaknesses, and native abilities or skills.[17] Each time two people interact, they bring the sum total of all these elements into their communication. To communicate effectively, both parties need to first recognize that the other person is different, then understand how these differences affect the communication, and finally accept and build on these differences. (Cultural diversity is discussed in more detail in Chapter 21.)

> *When the person who is expected to help fails to comply with the implied request, the overworked nurse becomes angry and resentful.*

Diversity Recognition

Conflicts based on diversity issues can be resolved by recognizing the diversity and then using it to promote teamwork, improve communication, and increase productivity. Recognizing diversity helps people better understand each other as well as themselves.[18] The ultimate goal of diversity recognition is to use each individual's strengths, rather than emphasizing the weaknesses, to build a stronger, more self-confident, and productive environment. For example, consider the following scenario:

> Anne B, RN, is a nurse in your unit who has a reputation for being a "nitpicker." She is constantly judging her peers and criticizing their actions on the basis of her own personal standards. Her judgments of others are not well accepted by her coworkers, who try to avoid her as much as possible.

Betty A, RN, another nurse on the unit, always seems to be coming up with ideas for changing things in the unit but then avoids joining the committees that are formed to put the ideas into practice. When she does join a committee, she quickly gets bored and does not follow through on her responsibilities. The other committee members become angry and frustrated by Betty's behavior. They feel that because it was her idea in the first place, she should work as hard as everyone else to make the change.

You have been selected as the chairperson for a committee that has been formed to design a new client care documentation tool. Both Anne and Betty are on the committee. The other committee members are upset because Anne and Betty are on the committee. Everyone knows about Anne's and Betty's personality quirks. As chairperson of the team, you need to draw on everyone's strengths while recognizing their diversities to develop a new, comprehensive, yet easy-to-use form. If you perform well in your chairmanship role, each team member's self-esteem should be enhanced, and the morale of the group should improve.

At first glance, these may not seem like diversity issues. However, Anne is a detail-oriented person, whereas Betty is a visionary. Although their interests and abilities are very diverse, neither one is right or wrong. People who are preoccupied with details are left-brain dominant; creative, visionary individuals are usually right-brain dominant.

Two primary tasks are required to complete the project:

Task 1. Conduct brainstorming sessions with staff members, physicians, and ancillary personnel to develop a general concept of what the documentation should include and how the form should look.

Task 2. Work with the print shop to design the specific layout and content of the final form.

Plan

Task 1. It would be most appropriate to include Betty in the group that directs the brainstorming efforts and collects different ideas. She probably had no preconceived form in mind before starting the process and will feel comfortable investigating and researching a variety of different possibilities. Anne would have difficulty with this task. The lack of structure of the brainstorming process would make her feel out of control and would probably frustrate her urge to consider all the details of the project. Anne would most likely already have a good idea of the form she wanted.

Task 2. Anne would be much better at this task because of her orientation to structure and detail. Working with the print shop, she could focus her attention on each item on the form and decide where it should be placed, how much room it should be given, and how it flows in the document. She would make sure the form met all the standards and regulatory requirements of the Joint Commission and would ensure it was error free. Betty, on the other hand, would very quickly become bored with this aspect of the project. To her, all the attention given to the details would seem like a waste of time, and she would probably start recommending changes in other unit forms.

> *Rather than being divisive, diversity, when recognized and used correctly, can promote teamwork, improve communication, and increase productivity.*

Placing people in the working environments that correspond with their strengths will ensure success for the project. The project will be a successful experience for the nurses and will promote positive changes in peer relationships.

Resolving Conflicts

Several different strategies can be used to resolve workplace conflicts. Depending on a person's communication style and personality traits, different outcomes may occur. People who use an assertive style of communication and incorporate the communication builders have much greater success in the positive resolution of conflicts.[19] Below are listed some strategies for conflict resolution.

Strategy 1: Ignore the Conflict

- Submissive personality: Person avoids bringing the issue to the other through fear of retaliation or ridicule if he or she confronts and expresses honest feelings or opinions.

- Assertive personality: Ignoring the conflict is never an option. They will almost always use strategy 2.
- Aggressive personality: Person has decided not to pursue the conflict because the other person is "too stupid to understand" or it would just be a "waste of my time."

Strategy 2: Confront the Conflict

- Submissive personality: Person does not handle the situation directly but refers the problem to a supervisor or to another person for resolution.
- Assertive personality: Person sets up a time and place for a one-on-one meeting. At the meeting, the two parties focus on the issues that caused the conflict and negotiate to define goals and problem-solve. If conflict is more severe, the parties may resort to negotiation or mediation (see below).
- Aggressive personality: Person confronts the other loudly, in front of an audience, and attacks the other's personality rather than the issue. Person either walks away before the other can speak or keeps talking without stopping and does not allow the other person to respond. The communication is strictly one-sided and very negative.

Strategy 3: Postpone the Conflict

- Submissive personality: Person keeps track of the issues until they reach a critical point, then dumps all the issues at one time on the offender in a highly aggressive manner. The other person generally has no idea why he or she is being attacked and may respond with anger or submission.
- Assertive personality: Hardly ever uses this method except to allow the other person to "cool down" and become more receptive to what others have to say.
- Aggressive personality: Person waits until he or she can either use the incident as a threat or blackmail or express the conflict in front of an audience.

Professional nurses need to be assertive and feel comfortable when handling conflict and confronting others. The conflict situations that nurses may encounter range from uncooperative clients and lazy coworkers to hostile, insecure, but influential physicians and administrators. Practicing assertiveness skills during confrontational situations helps increase the nurse's confidence in handling daily work-related conflicts and allows the honest but respectful expression of opinion and ideas. Keep in mind that unresolved conflicts never really go away. Ignoring a conflict situation may postpone it, sometimes for a long time, but it will not resolve the issue. Unresolved conflicts often fester until they either reach the boiling point or are manifested in negative behaviors or feelings.[19] Some of the feelings and behaviors that are symptoms of unresolved conflicts include the following:

• Tension and anxiety manifested as sudden angry outbursts
• Generalized distrust among the staff members
• Gossiping and rumor spreading
• Intentional work sabotage
• Backstabbing and lack of cooperation
• Isolation of certain staff members
• Division and polarization of the staff
• Low-rated peer evaluation reports[20]

Improved Communication Skills

Often, when conflict is handled appropriately, it produces much less anxiety than was initially anticipated. An individual who prepares for a confrontational meeting by expecting the worst-case scenario may be pleasantly surprised when the meeting and discussion take place. Many conflicts turn out to be merely errors in perception, simple misunderstandings, or misquotes of something that was said. If a situation is cleared up at an early stage, this prevents the development of the symptoms of unresolved conflict (listed earlier) and improves staff relationships. Individuals feel more confident and have better self-esteem when they resolve the conflicts in an adult and productive manner.

Another advantage of good conflict management is the improvement in communication skills. As with any skills, the more these skills are practiced, the

> *Keep in mind that unresolved conflicts never really go away. Ignoring a conflict situation may postpone it, sometimes for a long time, but it will not resolve the issue.*

> *The conflict situations that nurses may encounter range from uncooperative clients and lazy coworkers to hostile, insecure, but influential physicians and administrators.*

easier they will become to use. A conflict situation is illustrated in the second Issues in Practice box at the end of the chapter.

A Focus on Strength

For many people, resolving conflicts based on diversity issues can be difficult, especially when individuals feel insecure about their skills or abilities. When people feel insecure, they may revert to submissive or aggressive behavior or communication styles to hide their weaknesses or differences.

Because assertive people recognize that everyone, including themselves, has both strengths and weaknesses, they feel comfortable with diversity and are more likely to accept and support others by recognizing and using their strengths. Focusing on strengths provides them with positive feedback and helps them grow personally and professionally.[20] Focusing on weaknesses and differences tears down an individual's self-esteem, creates an uncomfortable work atmosphere, and makes people defensive and sometimes hostile. (For more information, go to http://www .ncbi.nlm.nih.gov/pmc/ articles/PMC1291328/.)

NEGOTIATION

There is an old saying that "everything is negotiable." Negotiation is a common method to manage conflicts. Negotiation can be between nurse and client, nurse and nurse, nurse manager and staff, or nurse manager and administration. Negotiation is the process of give and take between individuals or groups with the goal of reaching an agreement acceptable to both sides.[21] It is a specialized two-way communication skill in which individuals or groups with differing needs or ideas settle on a middle ground result that may not completely please either party. Negotiations may be formal or informal, hostile or friendly.[22] A cooperative atmosphere fostered by both sides that recognizes the similarity of each side's demands will be the most productive in reaching a satisfactory solution.

Bargaining is a special type of negotiation that is used most often when money-related issues are being discussed. Collective bargaining is a formal process that is used by groups of workers represented by a union or a negotiating body to solve workplace issues such as salaries, health-care benefits, safe work environment, and hiring practices. Formal contract negotiation is a key element in collective bargaining and requires that the two sides designate negotiating teams that are selected by both management and employee groups. (See DavisPlus Bonus Chapter 2 for more detail.)

Less formal negotiations found at the unit level may still have some of the elements of a formal bargaining effort. For example, if a nurse manager is negotiating with a group of staff, he or she may want just one or two individuals from the group to negotiate the problem. These individuals are designated as spokespersons who will be the primary representatives for the group. A formal written list of issues may be drawn up, but most likely the exchange will be informal in nature during a face-to-face meeting.[23] Informal negotiations between individual nurses can be used to resolve conflicts that if left to fester will eventually cause disharmony and lower morale among the staff.

> *Focusing on weaknesses and differences tears down an individual's self-esteem, creates an uncomfortable work atmosphere, and makes people defensive and sometimes hostile.*

> *Negotiation is the process of give and take between individuals or groups with the goal of reaching an agreement acceptable to both sides.*

Conflicting Powers

In formal contract negotiation, there is an obvious power control conflict. Each side is reluctant to give up power or relinquish any control of key factors such as money or rights. The employees' group tries to gain some power from management and improve benefits for its members. The power tug-of-war also factors into less formal negotiations.[22] Staff negotiating with nurse managers for more staff, different length shifts, longer breaks, or fewer weekend shifts may be perceived by the nurse manager as attempting to usurp some of his or her power. Individual nurses negotiating a conflict may also interpret the negotiation as an attempt to reduce the other person's power.

Learn the Skills

The underlying purpose of all negotiation is to achieve a goal or objective. Negotiation is a skill that nurse managers must learn and with which all nurses should familiarize themselves. Some keys to successful negotiation include the following:

1. Do some research, particularly if negotiating with management or administration. Focusing on issues such as quality of care and client safety will be received more positively than just listing the wants or wishes of nurses.
2. Clearly identify the objectives and goals of the negotiation. The old saying "If you don't know where you are going, how will you know when you get there?" is never so true as in negotiations.
3. If criticized by the other person or side during the discussions, avoid taking it personally. Especially avoid becoming angry and hostile. This will shut the negotiation down immediately.
4. Avoid making personal attacks on the other person or group. It will cause anger and hostility and shut down the negations.
5. Negotiate in good faith. Effective negotiations always require give and take and a willingness to meet in the middle. Digging in one's heels and refusing to give in on any element under consideration is not negotiating in good faith.
6. Respect the other side's goals and objectives. Unless proven otherwise, assume that they are also negotiating in good faith. Trust on both sides is a key element of successful negotiation.
7. Pre-plan the elements of the negotiation list that can be sacrificed in order to obtain concessions from the other side.
8. Attend workshops or seminars on negotiation and bargaining. Nurse leaders in particular need to master the techniques of the negotiation process. Facilities should provide staff-development in negotiating techniques for all nurses so that they can use these skills in all aspects of their professional lives.[22,23]

Mediation or Arbitration?

When the sides are unable to reach a resolution to their differences, they may resort to mediation. Mediation is a form of alternative dispute resolution that can be either formal or informal. In a formal negotiation setting such as a contract dispute, the disagreements are sometimes resolved through formal mediation, in which a neutral third party provided by the Federal Mediation and Conciliation Service meets with each side.[24] The appointed mediator works with both sides to reach an agreement; however, the agreement is nonbinding and either side can reject the settlement.

A less formal mediation process can be used to reach an agreement between two individuals who disagree.[25] Some health-care facilities select volunteers to receive training in mediation techniques. These individuals use the skills they learned to settle conflict situations between employees and colleagues. At the training sessions, the mediators learn skills such as how to identify what situations would be most appropriate for mediation, communication techniques that allow both parties to speak freely and identify their key issues, and methods of reaching a mutually acceptable resolution. The parties involved in the mediation process do so voluntarily and will not be forced to participate by management. All communications during the mediation are confidential.[26] Much like the formal mediation process, agreements developed during the informal process are also nonbinding.

"Trust on both sides is a key element of successful negotiation."

Arbitration is another form of alternative dispute resolution and usually the last step before the dispute is taken to court for litigation. It can be either nonbinding or binding, in which case both parties agree ahead of time to comply with whatever decision is reached by the arbitrator. In a formal setting such as a contract negotiation or settlement for a malpractice suit, an arbitrator with binding power is appointed. This person is a neutral third party who, like the mediator, investigates the conflict, meets with both sides, and makes a recommendation for settlement.[24] Binding arbitration, by its very nature, is not appropriate for informal negotiations. Although the formal process of negotiation and arbitration are usually applied to more formal settings and situations, the skills that are involved in their practice are useful in a number of other settings and situations. (For more information, go to http://www.ncbi.nlm.nih.gov/pubmed/23513710.)

Conclusion

A person's professional and personal lives are influenced by communication styles and behavioral patterns. The ability to analyze personal strengths, weaknesses, and communication behaviors is important in everyday communication but is particularly important in negotiation and conflict resolution.

Certain specific communication qualities and skills are essential for interacting with coworkers and clients. Of primary importance is the skill of assertive communication, which allows people to express themselves openly and honestly while respecting other people's opinions and ideas. Being able to identify submissive and aggressive behavior is also essential in trying to resolve problems, as is recognizing issues of diversity, which underlie many problems in communication. Disagreements with others are ultimately resolved through the practice of conflict management. Because it is an outgrowth and extension of the problem-solving method, nurses should be able to quickly grasp its structure and master its use.

Issues in Practice

Julie H, RN, has been working the 7 p.m. to 7 a.m. shift in a busy, 32-bed surgical unit of a large university hospital since her graduation from a small bachelor of science in nursing (BSN) program 6 months ago. Although Julie was told by the unit director when she was hired that she would have at least a full year of training before she had to work as charge nurse, tonight the other two RNs who usually work the shift called in sick, and Julie was left in charge. The 7 p.m. to 7 a.m. shift is always busy because the unit has to discharge clients who are ready to go home after surgery and admit clients who are coming in for surgery the next day. Hospital policy requires that the RN make and sign both the discharge and admission assessments.

Although Julie is nervous about this new role as charge nurse, she feels that she can handle the responsibility if she has some additional help. Normal staffing for the unit on this shift is three RNs, three licensed practical nurse (LPNs), and three unlicensed assistive personnel (UAPs). Julie calls the house supervisor to see if she can get some help. The only place in the hospital that is not busy that night is the obstetrics (OB) unit, so the supervisor sends two of the OB unit's UAPs to the surgical unit to help Julie.

It was not the help Julie really wanted, but she feels that she can handle the responsibility. However, when Julie begins to make assignments, the older of the OB unit UAPs, Hanna J, informs Julie that for the past 15 years she has worked only in the newborn nursery and does not know anything about the care of adult clients who have had surgery. In addition, Hanna states that she has a bad back and cannot lift or turn adult clients. She is also afraid that she might catch some disease from the adults that she would take back to the babies. Julie asks Hanna, "What do you feel you are qualified to do on the surgical unit?" In response, Hanna crosses her legs, folds her arms across her chest, puts her head down, and mumbles under her breath, "A lot more than a new know-it-all RN like you."

Questions for Thought

1. What messages, both verbal and nonverbal, are being communicated? How should Julie respond to this comment? What should she do to rectify the situation?

2. Using what you learned in this chapter, identify the personality type of each of the persons involved in the situation.

3. How can the RN best communicate with this UAP? What were some of the communication mistakes the RN made?

4. What background, cultural, and diversity factors played a part in this situation? Develop a strategy for resolution of this conflict.

Critical-Thinking Exercises

- Make a list of your values and where they came from. Describe how each value affects your work ethic and communication style.
- List your communication strengths and weaknesses. Rank them on a scale of 1 to 10 (10 being the highest). Determine which weaknesses you want to change and create an improvement plan.
- Identify your primary communication style and character type.
- What methods do you use to resolve conflicts? Do these methods work for you? Identify better methods for resolving conflict situations.

Answers to Questions in Chapter 12

Issues in Practice: Managing Change (page 298)

1. The underlying problem was that there was too much change too quickly. Even though the staff recognized that change was needed, there is always a built-in resistance to change. Sudden, unpredictable change creates the most anxiety and therefore the most resistance. It also can produce a great deal of cohesion among those being asked to change when it is viewed as a threat. This last point is borne out by the nurses seeking to organize into a collective bargaining unit.

2. The director of the unit could have decreased resistance by having the staff "buy into" the changes, allowing them to participate in decision-making from the beginning. Also, the whole process of change could have been slowed down—perhaps spread over 1 year to 18 months. A slower process would have given the nurses a chance to adjust to one change before another was implemented.

Sources: Whitehead DK, Weiss SA, Tappen RM. *Essentials of Nursing Leadership and Management* (5th ed.). Philadelphia: F. A. Davis, 2010; Yu M. Employees' perception of organizational change: The mediating effects of stress management strategies. *Public Personnel Management,* 38(1):17–32, 2009.

References

1. Salmon P, Young B. Creativity in clinical communication: From communication skills to skilled communication. *Medical Education,* 45(3):217–226, 2011.

2. Kinoshita M, Yano E, Ishikawa H, Hashimoto H. Can nonverbal communication skills be taught? *Medical Teacher,* 32(10):860–863, 2010.

3. Gifford R. The dragons of inaction: Psychological barriers that limit climate change mitigation and adaptation. *American Psychologist,* 66(4):290–302, 2011.

4. Kriet K. Management forum. Enhancing and using negotiation skills. *Dermatology Nursing,* 20(2):140, 2008.

5. Hyde J. Learning the art of give and take is an essential nursing skill. *Nursing Standard,* 6–12;26(40):63, 2012.

6. Pichler CB. Effective patient communication: Enhancing learning styles and language yields better outcomes. *American Speech-Language Hearing Association Leader,* 6;15(4):5–6, 2010.

7. Nørgaard B, Ammentorp J, Ohm Kyvik K, Kofoed PE. Communication skills training increases self-efficacy of health care professionals. *Journal of Continuing Education in the Health Professions,* 32(2):90–97, 2012.

8. Gage W. Using service improvement methodology to change practice. *Nursing Standard,* 6;27(23):51–57, 2013.

9. Brass L. Can you cope? How to hang in there—no matter what comes your way. *Vibrant Life,* 29(1):30–33, 2013.

10. Sargeant J, MacLeod T, Murray A. An interprofessional approach to teaching communication skills. *Journal of Continuing Education in the Health Professions,* 31(4):265–267, 2011.

11. Clarke N. Anger, rage & relationship—an empathic approach to anger management. *Counselling and Psychotherapy Research,* 10(1):77–79, 2010.

12. McLaughlin S, Pearce R, Trenoweth S. Reducing conflict on wards by improving team communication. *Mental Health Practice,* 16(5):29–31, 2013.

13. Schimmel CJ, Jacobs E. When leaders are challenged: Dealing with involuntary members in groups. *Journal for Specialists in Group Work,* 36(2):144–158, 2011.

14. Lightman D. Dealing with difficult people by managing hot buttons. *Medical-Surgical Matters,* 21(1):14–15, 2012.

15. Soutschek A, Schubert T. Domain-specific control mechanisms for emotional and nonemotional conflict processing. *Cognition,* 126(2):234–245, 2013.

16. Cortese CG, Colombo L, Ghislieri C. Determinants of nurses' job satisfaction: The role of work-family conflict, job demand, emotional charge and social support. *Journal of Nursing Management,* 18(1):35–43, 2010.

17. Guillaume YRF, Dawson JF, Woods SA, Sacramento CA, West MA. Getting diversity at work to work: What we know and what we still don't know. *Journal of Occupational and Organizational Psychology,* 86(2):123–141, 2013.

18. Singh B, Winkel DE, Selvarajan TT. Managing diversity at work: Does psychological safety hold the key to racial differences in employee performance? *Journal of Occupational and Organizational Psychology,* 86(2):242–263, 2013.

19. Ramscar M, Dye M, Gustafson JW, Klein J. Dual routes to cognitive flexibility: Learning and response-conflict resolution in the dimensional change card sort task. *Child Development,* 84(4):1308–1323, 2013.

20. Beunza JJ. Conflict resolution techniques applied to interprofessional collaborative practice. *Journal of Interprofessional Care,* 27(2):110–112, 2013.

21. Dygert CT, Parang E. Honing your negotiation skills. *Serials Librarian,* 64(1–4):105–110, 2013.

22. Zuma SM. Leadership in negotiation. *Nursing Update,* 32(3):44–45, 2008.

23. Tian X, Jing Z. Feelings and comparisons in negotiation: One subjective outcome, two different mechanisms. *Public Personnel Management,* 41(5):21–33, 2012.

24. Four steps to making arbitration policy valid. *Healthcare Risk Management,* 34(7):79–80, 2012.

25. Mediation process. Financial Industry Regulatory Agency. Retrieved August 2013 from http://www.finra.org/Arbitration AndMediation/Mediation/Process/

26. Oxtoby K. Speaking openly via mediation. *Nursing Standard,* 6; 27 (27):62–63, 2013.

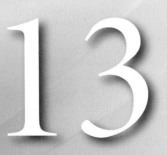

13 Understanding and Dealing Successfully With Difficult Behavior

Joseph T. Catalano

Learning Objectives

After completing this chapter, the reader will be able to:

- Discuss the underlying issues that cause individual to display difficult behaviors
- Develop successful strategies for communicating with persons displaying difficult behaviors.
- Respond effectively to the underlying emotions that persons with difficult behaviors are communicating.
- Successfully resolve problems associated with difficult behavior in both colleagues and clients.
- Formulate coping strategies to adapt successfully to people with difficult behaviors.

UNDERSTANDING DIFFICULT BEHAVIOR

Let's say this up front: There are no difficult people; there are, however, people who display difficult behaviors. It is important to keep in mind that behavior is a form of communication. The term *difficult people* is so often used that it has become a widely accepted way to categorize people. Labeling people as difficult is really stereotyping, which may or may not accurately reflect reality. In dealing with the group labeled as difficult, our goals are to change *our* response to the behaviors and attempt to change the behaviors they are displaying.[1] It is virtually impossible to change an individual's basic personality; however, brain injuries, extreme traumatic events, and potentially lethal illnesses or injuries have been shown to significantly alter a person's personality.

The term *personality* is often misused to mean that an individual is outgoing, humorous, and generally friendly to other people. When you hear people say, "Joe has a great personality," they are usually talking about the fact that he is pleasant to be around, outgoing, and readily engages in conversations. On the other hand, you might hear someone say, "Terry has no personality at all," when they actually are talking about the fact that Terry is quiet, somewhat withdrawn, and doesn't easily engage in conversations.

The truth is that everyone has a personality, and although defined differently by different schools of psychology, an individual's personality is generally recognized as all those elements, both genetic and learned, that go into making them who they are at present.[1] A personality includes strongly held beliefs, attitudes, emotions, and behaviors. Most people have identifiable personality traits soon after birth. Just ask nurses who regularly work with newborn babies. There are some babies who are mostly quiet and seem content except when they are hungry or need to be changed, and there are others who cry all the time and never seem to be content.

All children are genetically stamped in the womb with innate emotions that help them survive in a world that they really don't understand and is very frightening to them.[1] Feelings of anger, jealousy, selfishness, and self-centeredness, along with their behavioral expressions, help children manipulate adults, particularly the parents, and cope with what is to them a big and hostile environment. One of the primary goals parents have in raising their children is to teach them adult coping skills to deal with problems and help them outgrow the immature and childish coping mechanisms of manipulation and exploitation of others. It is evident that this outcome is not always achieved.

Some people go through their whole lives using childlike coping mechanisms and behaviors to deal with the adult world.[1] These mechanisms don't work very well, and often they get labeled as difficult people. For whatever reason, they never learned or accepted adult coping mechanisms. For example, being able to forgive is a learned adult behavior that counteracts the self-centeredness that children use as a survival mechanism. People who have never learned to forgive others, forget about insults, or let go of much of anything are sometimes afflicted, as adults, with conditions such as chronic fatigue and depression. And it's no wonder they act in these ways; they are carrying around a heavy burden of emotional baggage from a lifetime of perceived or actual events in their lives, and every day they are alive, they add another bag to the pile.

You can observe this type of behavior in a 60-year-old woman who seeks to get revenge for the way she was treated by a relative 30 years before at a wedding. She has been carrying that baggage for a long time. Often this behavior manifests itself in activities such as hoarding. They don't have to be extreme hoarders such as seen on the TV show *Hoarders*, but they tend to collect a lot of junk and pile it around the house. If you ask them, "Why don't we throw out these 10-year-old magazines? Everything is online now," they will likely respond, "No,

> *Labeling people as difficult is really stereotyping, which may or may not accurately reflect reality. In dealing with the group labeled as difficult, our goals are to change our response to the behaviors and attempt to change the behaviors they are displaying.*

there might be something in one of them that I'll need someday." If you look at many of the difficult behaviors discussed below from the viewpoint of what a child does to get his or her way, you will see a great deal of similarity between the two.

People who display difficult behaviors are everywhere. They are found at home, at work, and in the health-care setting. It is pretty obvious that communicating with them requires a special set of communication skills. Because communication is such a major part of quality health care, it is an essential requirement that nurses be able to understand why a client is using difficult behaviors and learn the skills that will allow him or her to communicate effectively.[2] The skills learned in resolving conflicts or negotiating often are used when dealing with difficult people. Of course, difficult people are not limited to just clients in the health-care settings. They may also be the family of the client, nurses, physicians, and other health-care workers. Pretty much anyone can become a difficult person under the right set of circumstances. Who knows, you might even be a difficult person.

Identifying People With Difficult Behaviors

What exactly is a person with difficult behaviors, or in common language, a difficult person? To some extent, a difficult person is one of those "you'll know them when you see them" individuals. Also, it is important to recognize that identifying someone as "difficult" is a matter of perception. One individual's difficult person is another's "Oh, old Uncle Freddy acts that way any time there are people around."

Generally, when a person is displaying difficult behavior, they are hard to communicate with or their behavior is such that it makes it very difficult to work with them to achieve a goal or finish a task. Difficult peoples' personalities have been described as "prickly" because if they are touched verbally, they sting back with sharp vocal barbs.[1] They often use many of the communication blockers discussed in Chapter 12 to achieve their goals. Identifying what goals difficult people are trying to achieve, whether they are a client or a coworker, is one of the keys to understanding them and communicating with them effectively.

In the health-care setting specifically, there are two primary groups of difficult people: coworkers and clients. Although the techniques in interacting with either group overlap to some degree, there are important differences between the two groups that need to be considered, particularly the cause for being difficult and the outcomes they are attempting to achieve. Also, although difficult coworkers can make life on the unit uncomfortable, there is no ethical or legal requirement to interact with them. However, heath-care providers' relationships with clients require that nurses do everything they can to establish and maintain effective communication with them, no matter how difficult they are, to achieve the goals of quality care (Box 13.1).

Improved Understanding

All nurses recognize that obtaining a thorough history and understanding the underlying disease processes better prepare them for the physical care of their clients. Similarly, in working with difficult people, a knowledge of their backgrounds and understanding of their needs and goals better prepares the nurse to communicate in a positive way. It would seem that nurses should be adept at handling conflict and difficult people because a large part of their education includes an understanding of the cause and effect and the intricacies of human nature. These are skills that nurses use daily in the care of clients.

Shifting the communication paradigm from instinctual or "knee-jerk" responses to one that uses the communication building techniques discussed in Chapter 12 in combination with the nurse's relationship skills should make interacting successfully with difficult people a less imposing task. The behavior displayed by a difficult person is really a symptom of a deeper underlying problem, just as an assessment of shortness of breath is a symptom of a respiratory disease. Identifying the cause of the problem and the outcomes the client is attempting to achieve permits the nurse to treat the disease rather than just the symptoms.[3] The problem is never cured by merely ignoring it or dealing only with the symptoms. In the long term, the "leave it alone" approach usually only amplifies the difficult behavior. (For more information, go to http://www.oscehome.com/Communication-Skills.html.)

Basic Principles

There are several basic principles to remember when attempting to work with a person displaying difficult behavior:

1. **No change.** Keep in mind that it is highly unlikely that a difficult person will change his or her behavior very much, particularly if that person is a coworker. However, one of our goals in teaching and caring for clients is to change behavior even if they are displaying difficult behaviors. The key to remember here is that we need to change our own perceptions and the way we approach a difficult person.[2] Difficult people tend to make us anxious, frustrated, and angry, but we cannot show them these feelings.

2. **No reinforcement.** It is a basic tenant in psychology that reinforcing a behavior will cause the behavior to be repeated (e.g., Pavlov's dogs). It is interesting that the reinforcement can be either positive or negative. Providing punishment for something someone is doing is often the payoff the difficult person is looking for, and he or she will repeat the behavior to get additional payoffs. The most powerful reinforcement is intermittent reward or punishment. This is where the behavior is rewarded or punished one time and then ignored the next. It keeps the behavior going because the person is wondering when the next reinforcement will come.

> *All children are genetically stamped in the womb with innate emotions that help them survive in a world that they really don't understand and is very frightening to them.*

B o x 1 3 . 1

Seven Principles of Communication

1. Information giving is not communication.
2. The sender is responsible for clarity.
3. Use simple and exact language.
4. Feedback should be encouraged.
5. The sender must have credibility.
6. Acknowledgment of others is essential.
7. Direct channels of communication are best.

Source: Adapted from Whitehead DK, Weiss SA, Tappen RM. *Essentials of Nursing Leadership and Management* (4th ed.). Philadelphia: F. A. Davis, 2006.

3. **No action.** There is an old saying that "doing nothing is doing something!" This means that when dealing with difficult people, if we do nothing, we are in reality reinforcing their behavior.

4. **No anonymity.** Identify the particular behaviors they are displaying as difficult and call the behaviors by name. "Letting it go" actually reinforces the behavior (see #3).

5. **No ashes.** Another old saying is "Fight fire with fire"; however, the result of this approach is scorched earth and ashes. Again, this may be the outcome that the difficult person is seeking. He or she wins when nothing is left but ashes!

6. **No condemnation.** The difficult person had probably developed this type of behavior over a long period of time and is doing the best they can. Although it may not seem so, they usually are not malicious or hateful, and condemning them as such really misses the point.[3] Difficult people lack the basic communication skills to interact successfully with others and are constantly seeking to fulfill a need or achieve an outcome by their behavior.

7. **No robbery.** You must believe that you are 100 percent responsible for your own happiness, because you are. Happiness comes from within yourself, and it is not up to others to make you happy. Similarly, it is up to us to control our unhappiness. Sometimes it is the goal of some difficult people to rob us of our happiness because they are unhappy (misery loves company). Don't let them do it! Find happy people to hang out with! Find some fulfilling activity outside of the work setting.

Remembering Maslow

Maslow's hierarchy of needs is often one of the first important theories that is taught in nursing programs. It is typically introduced in the first nursing course and then reinforced in psychology courses. The primary reason it is taught is because it is one of the most effective ways of prioritizing client care (Fig. 13.1). The needs on the bottom of the triangle, particularly the physiological and safety needs, are necessary for the client's survival and maintenance

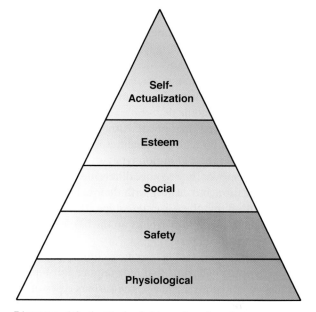

Figure 13.1 Maslow's hierarchy of need

Because communication is such a major part of quality health care, it is an essential requirement that nurses be able to understand why a client is using difficult behaviors and learn the skills that will allow him or her to communicate effectively.

of life. These needs must always be met first. The higher needs, such as love and belonging, self-esteem, and self-actualization, cannot be met if the person is not able to fulfill the basic needs to stay alive and remain safe.[4]

Maslow's hierarchy can also be used in understanding and interacting with people in the health-care setting who are displaying difficult behaviors. Understanding what causes people to behave in a difficult manner is directly related to the hierarchy of needs and differentiates the causality between difficult coworkers and difficult clients. Because the causes are different for each of these groups, interacting successfully with them also requires a different approach.

It is pretty safe to believe that physicians, nurses, pharmacists, and other health-care workers are having their basic physiological and safety needs met. The needs that are producing coworkers' difficult behaviors are generally related to the higher level needs of love and belonging, self-esteem, and self-actualization. In the cases of difficult clients, their illnesses, injuries, or surgeries often threaten their basic needs for merely surviving physically.

Difficult Coworkers

Anyone who has been employed in or even associated with the health-care setting for any length of time soon becomes aware of a variety of personality types among the staff members. These personality types can be identified by their predominant behaviors. The behaviors vary to some degree based on how they are attempting to meet their needs. Although there are several types of difficult personalities in the work setting, the two most common types are the persecutor and the sneak. They require different strategies for communication and dealing with their behaviors. Keep in mind that these are stereotypes that tend to batch individuals into groups on the basis of predetermined behaviors.[5]

In reality, people may have combinations of or overlapping behaviors that may require combining strategies for communication. The various types of stereotypes are all interrelated and based on individual behaviors and communication styles. An increased awareness of the various identifying characteristics and communication strategies will help develop the coping skills and communication techniques necessary for communicating with difficult people.

> *The most powerful reinforcement is intermittent reward or punishment. This is where the behavior is rewarded or punished one time and then ignored the next. It keeps the behavior going because the person is wondering when the next reinforcement will come.*

Also, it is possible for individuals to have true personality disorders, which are diagnosed psychological conditions. Some of these disorders, such as a narcissistic personality or the avoidant personality, may present with the same types of behaviors as seen with difficult people but are more pronounced and extreme.[1] If a person has a true personality disorder, it is likely beyond the floor nurse's skill set to interact with these individuals successfully, unless the nurse specializes in psychiatric practice. These clients are best left to the mental health professionals. However, one of the characteristics of these types of disorders is that the person does not believe there are any problems and rarely seeks help for them.

The Persecutor

Also called the *dictator*, these people generally display an attitude of being superior to others and being in control. They attempt to humiliate, intimidate, threaten, or demean other individuals or groups with the goals of overcoming their own lack of confidence, feeling more powerful, and inflating their low self-esteem. This behavior is probably habitual, being repeated over and over for a long period of time, and becomes the person's primary mode of communication. The persecutor has self-esteem needs that are not being met and may also have love and belonging issues. The goal of their behavior is usually to coerce or intimidate another person into doing something they do not want to do. However, sometimes the goal is to merely humiliate a person or group due to some perceived difference or weakness because it makes them feel better about themselves.[5]

Persecutor Tactics

Persecutors attempt to maintain control by putting others down and ruling from a command post. They often have minions working for them who are fearful of getting on their "bad side" and will help persecutors when they engage a new target. Persecutors have learned over time that being inconsistent (i.e., easy to deal with one day and demanding the next) keeps people off balance and helps them maintain power to achieve their goals. They usually will be unable to accept ideas that are different from theirs and often may use loud speech and treats to keep the other person from expressing a new idea. Persecutors may attempt to provoke the other person into an angry defensive outburst and enjoy the flare-up because they've achieved one of their goals. These are some of the messages they are attempting to convey by their behavior: "If you don't do what I want, I'll make your life miserable," "If you do what I want, I'll stop harassing you," and "If you give into my wants, you can become one of my minions and help me demean others."

What Do You Think?

Recall a recent exchange with someone (e.g., friend, instructor, parent, and physician) in which you felt you "lost" the exchange. How did you feel? How did you respond? What could you have done differently?

If the dictator is in a superior position such as a charge nurse or supervisor, this type of behavior is called *vertical violence*. When the dictator is a fellow employee at the same authority level, the behavior is referred to as *lateral* or *horizontal violence*. (See Chapter 16 for more detail.) It is important to remember that the persecutor's self-image is fragile, and attempting to destroy it will be ineffective. In actuality, it will make them more defensive and will escalate their behavior.

Taming the Persecutor

Using the basic principles discussed above is essential in taming the behaviors of the persecutor. Communication skills can also be coping skills in interacting with these individuals. Everyone develops coping skills as they mature and use them when confronted with complex situations. These coping skills can be used to resolve crisis situations, deal with anxiety, and resolve difficult issues of communication. This basic set of coping skills can be used as the foundation for adding to or building new coping skills to deal with difficult people.[5] Just as developing communication skills requires a willingness to change and a lot of practice, so does the development of coping skills

Also, remember that perception is a significant part of dealing with the difficult behavior of people.[6] However, a lot of people really don't understand what their own perceptions are or how they affect their actions and thoughts when confronting a persecutor. When confronting a persecutor or any difficult person, it is essential to understand one's own motives, preferences, beliefs, and biases.

Dealing with difficult people requires a high level of personal confidence and inner strength: They have learned how to quickly identify weaknesses in others and to use those weaknesses in their attempt to maintain control. Success in dealing with persecutors in particular also requires high degrees of self-awareness and emotional self-control. The only way to develop emotions strong enough to resist the attacks of the persecutor is through self-knowledge. Some of the particular actions that can be used in taming the persecutor include the following:

1. **Set the stage for communication.** This is an environmental communication builder. After a decision is made to deal with a difficult issue or person, it is important to set the stage for a positive experience. The location for the exchange should be private. The format of the meeting needs to be established ahead of time, including an explanation to the other person that both parties will take turns expressing their opinions and feelings without interruption.

2. **Listen to what is really being communicated,** including body language and paraverbal clues. Often persecutors will reveal hidden messages or indications of what their real goals or needs are nonverbally while giving a much different verbal message.[5] You can use the nonverbal communication builders when interacting with persecutors, but be sincere. Persecutors have learned how to quickly detect dishonesty. In some situations, merely allowing a person to vent emotions by using active listening reduces the levels of anger and animosity and sometimes even solves the conflict. Also, when intelligent people are allowed to speak openly and freely, they may be able to develop a new solution to the problem that they had not considered previously.

> *The persecutor has self-esteem needs that are not being met and may also have love and belonging issues.*

3. **Use assertive but not aggressive communication.** If the persecutor is in a highly animated state and speaking rapidly and loudly, your message will not penetrate the tirade. Never yell back or argue with them. Rather, say to them, "You are upset now; we can discuss this issue later." Then walk away.

4. **Use a line of discussion that will get their attention** and not make them defensive or lower their self-esteem. A statement like, "Joanne, this project you have been working on shows what a hard worker you are; however, I am assigned to it also, and we need to figure out how to work together to make it the best possible." "Liz, our relationship feels strained. I would like a good working relationship with you. What can we do to improve it?" "Alexis, I noticed that you excluded me from meetings and communications. I feel left out. Can we talk about this?" Using the person's name eliminates a chance of misunderstanding to whom the statement was directed.

5. **Remember persecutors are acting the way they do because of something they lack in their lives** or because of internal feelings of low self-esteem,[1] so don't take what they are saying personally. They

probably say it to everyone. Also, never react emotionally in front of them by crying or sulking. It shows vulnerability and that is an outcome they are seeking because it makes them feel better about themselves.

6. **Avoid doing nothing.** Persecutors want people to leave them alone so that they can continue their behavior without confrontation. After you've walked away, walk back when they calm down. Identifying their behavior to them calmly and directly is the first step in dealing with the behavior. Their behavior is not likely to change very much, but they will know that you know what they are doing. They probably will take you off their target list and seek a new target.

7. **Avoid personal attacks.** Separate the person from the behavior by focusing on the issues without attacking their personality. Having the facts about the specific behavior to be addressed makes people much more receptive to resolution of the problem than attacking their personality.[5] Remember, persecutors have fragile egos and attacking them will only invite a more vicious counterattack. When situations are made into personal attacks, people feel defensive, responsible, or persecuted, and communication is either blocked or closed off completely. Avoid becoming personally or verbally abusive.[6]

> *Dealing with difficult people requires a high level of personal confidence and inner strength: they have learned how to quickly identify weaknesses in others and to use those weaknesses in their attempt to maintain control.*

For example:

During shift report on a particular client, the 11:00 p.m. to 7:00 a.m. nurse forgot to tell the 7:00 a.m. to 3:00 p.m. charge nurse, Gail L, RN, that the client had fallen out of bed during the night shift. Later in the day, the client's physician and family confronted Gail to find out what had happened and why the client was not placed on "fall protocols." Later, when Gail confronts the night nurse about the omission, she has two options for initiating the discussion of the incident with the responsible night nurse. Which approach would the night nurse probably take as a personal attack?

Option 1. Gail: "I was taken off guard and was ill-equipped when the family and physician asked me about this client's fall, and I felt unprepared to explain the problem or provide a solution to them. My lack of knowledge about the fall really made me feel incompetent."

Option 2. Gail: "You failed to tell me about his fall last night. Because of you, I was not aware of the incident and was not prepared to answer questions. You always make me look like a fool!"

8. **Avoid judging what a person is doing** or what they should have done by your own standards. This type of statement becomes an arbitrary judgment call. Instead, ask the person for his or her ideas on how the situation could have been handled differently or what other options were available.

9. **Ask clarifying questions** that validate the person's concerns, feelings, and perceptions. Validating will help ensure that the responses address the real issues. Also, avoid reflex-type reactions to hostile or aggressive statements. It is a human instinct to become defensive when attacked and to attack back. However, this behavior only escalates the anger and tension and blocks effective communication.

10. **Ignore trivia.** Always make a conscious decision about the importance of the issue that needs to be discussed and stick with it. It is a very human tendency to become preoccupied with trivial and unimportant issues. If people spend large portions of their energy dealing with trivia, they will have little energy left to deal with major issues when they come along. Identifying the causes and needs of people displaying difficult behavior can sometimes be complicated and time-consuming. Often they will try to direct the conversation away from issues they believe are painful and toward topics that are more comfortable.[7] They do not accept criticism well, even constructive criticism. By having a clear idea of the outcomes you wish to achieve, you can redirect the conversation when the person attempts to lead it in another direction.

The Sneak

Another type of coworker with difficult behavior is called the *sneak* because of the devious, underhanded, and often malicious attacks they use to fulfill their self-esteem needs and achieve their goal to be in control. They are also called *double-crossers* or *backstabbers*. Unlike the persecutor, who enjoys direct confrontation and watching others feel uncomfortable under their attacks, the sneak will attack when you aren't looking and gets his or her reward by watching your discomfort and confusion in not knowing where the attack came from. Although they really don't have minions like the persecutor, they often will elicit the help of others who are afraid of them and gang up on a person as a group behind his or her back. This process is called *gossip*, and it is a primary source of recreation and entertainment on many nursing units that should be eliminated.

The methods sneaks use are really forms of manipulation, which demonstrates that they are insecure and unsure of where they belong in the work setting. Interestingly, their behavior has the same underlying causes as the persecutor—a need to feel in control, low self-esteem, and love and belonging issues; however, they use different methods to build up their self-esteem and sense of control.[5]

> *Shifting the communication paradigm from one of instinctual 'knee-jerk' responses to one that uses the nurse's relationship skills should make dealing with difficult people a much less difficult task.*

What Do You Think?

Have you ever been in a situation in which others have intentionally sabotaged your work? What was the situation? How did you feel? How did you deal with it? Did you try to retaliate?

Sneaks often have very few true friends and are generally fearful of close friendships because they don't want others to know what they are really like. Often sneaks subconsciously feel they lack the talent, intelligence, or skills to be successful and use covert manipulative behavior to gain promotions and advance their position. They often will behave in a way to gain attention from a superior and feel a strong sense of jealousy when the superior gives the attention or promotion they want to another person. They will work hard to bring that person down. They are very sensitive to criticism and often feel slighted and angry at people who may have unintentionally said something that hurt their feelings.

Sneak Tactics

Methods commonly used by the sneak to achieve his or her goals include personal digs, rumors, accusations, allegations, finger-pointing, and innuendoes. Sneaks often appear very friendly when they are communicating face-to-face with you, but they do not have your best interests in mind and are looking for a weakness they can exploit to lower your esteem. They will use any underhanded means to discredit a person, and by making that person appear inferior, they feel superior. They also go out of their way to avoid confrontation.

Sneaks like to keep the workplace in a state of uncertainty, tension, and disorder. One of their favorite tactics to achieve this goal is to divide and conquer. For example, the sneak knows that Bill and Cindy have a strong work alliance and friendship and rely on each other to provide high-quality care on the unit. The sneak will try to break up this alliance by first going to Bill, on Cindy's day off, and saying, "Don't repeat this, but did you hear what Cindy said about you? She said you were incompetent and shouldn't be working as an RN." Then when Bill isn't around, the sneak would go to Cindy and say, "Don't repeat this, but did you hear what Bill is saying about you? He said you were too fat to be working on such a busy unit and provided really poor care." And the pot gets stirred!

One of the most powerful tools they use is a mixed rumor, which contains just enough truth to make it completely believable.[7] For example, Aleshia is an RN on the unit who was selected by the hospital to attend an expenses-paid workshop in another state because of her interest in geriatric nursing. Anne, who is an infamous sneak, started a rumor while Aleshia was away by saying, "You know that Aleshia went to that workshop paid by the hospital? Well, I heard that she skipped most of the breakout sessions and spent her time in the bar drinking with strange men!" The truth is that Aleshia did go to the workshop; the rumor is what she did there. There is just enough truth in the rumor to make it credible.

Some of the messages that sneaks send out by their behavior are that no one should confront or tangle with them because, when you are out of earshot, they will put you in your place. Also, because of the covert nature of their attacks, they believe that they are unstoppable and that they are the only ones honest enough to tell the truth about other workers.

Unveiling the Sneak

Using the basic principles discussed above in conjunction with some of the techniques for dealing with the persecutor will work, up to a point, with the sneak; however, there are several different techniques that must also be used to be successful. As with the persecutor, perception and self-knowledge are significant elements in dealing with the sneak's behavior. You need to understand how and why you react the way you do when suffering the aftermath of a sneak's attack. Your reaction is a behavior that you can and need to change. It's unlikely the sneak will change his or her behaviors to any great degree. Understanding your own motives, preferences, beliefs, and biases can help in softening the devastation you feel after the attack.[5] Methods for showing up sneaks for who they really are include the following:

1. **Make the decision to talk to them about their behavior.** They won't change on their own and may not change anyway, but it's worth a try. Talking to them takes a high degree of courage and resolve because the exchange is going to be difficult. Do this only after you have settled down from the effects of the attack and are calm and certain of what you want to do. If you display excessive emotions while talking with them, the sneak wins. They are highly manipulative and will try to make you feel bad about yourself and sorry for them.

2. **Let them know that you know.** Catching them in the act is the best way to let them know you know, but this is often difficult to accomplish. They are sneaky, after all. Pretending that you didn't hear them and doing nothing is what they want you to do. You can say something like, "Anne, you were the only one who knew that I went to that workshop. How come everyone else is talking about what I supposedly did there?" It is important that you talk with others to confirm what you heard. Make sure you have your facts straight when you do talk with the

> *It is a very human tendency to become preoccupied with trivial and unimportant issues. If people spend large portions of their energy dealing with trivia, they will have little energy left to deal with major issues when they come along.*

sneak or he or she sneak will pick apart what you are trying to say and turn the attack on you.

3. **Let the group know that you heard what the sneak said.** Using a statement like, "Did everybody hear what Anne said about me?" will gain you support among your peers.

4. **Don't show your hostility toward the sneak in front of a group.** Avoid being rude and aggressive. Like the persecutor, sneaks do have fragile egos and low self-esteem. Unlike persecutors, who will immediately attack back when confronted, sneaks will use the incident to make themselves seem like the "victim," which is another type of manipulative behavior. They revel in the "poor me" role because it garners sympathy from the other staff members and gives them more ammunition against you. "Did you see how mean Sarah was to me?"

5. **Stay on point when you finally speak with them.** They will try to turn the subject back on you to break your train of thought. Just keep saying, "We're not talking about me; we're talking about your behavior," and then continue with your train of thought. They are expert distracters, so you might want to make a list of things you want to say and take that along. Also, don't laugh at them, don't agree with them, and don't let them gain control of the conversation nor let it go.

6. **Try to treat them with empathy and understanding,** not resentment and anger. Like the persecutor, they have developed this type of behavior in response to something that is missing in their early lives. This has become the only way sneaks can gain attention or exercise any control in their lives. They never developed adult communication skills, and it is likely they've been using these manipulative behaviors for many years in all aspects of their lives. That is probably one of the reasons why they have few friends. Sneaks tend to be negative all the time, and most people steer clear of negativity. Many people already probably have enough negativity in their lives and don't need any more from a coworker.

7. **Listen carefully to their response.** If you are able to complete your thoughts and finish what you are saying without them walking away, it is important

to listen to how they respond. It is important to remain open-minded and to be prepared to understand what motivated them to use the behaviors they use. You might discover that you did or said something unintentionally that they took as a personal insult that triggered their behavior. Sneaks often display paranoid tendencies. You might actually need to apologize to them. Even though you did nothing to deserve their negative behavior, be prepared to listen to what they have to say. They probably need someone to talk to, someone to confide in, and in some peculiar way, you might just be the person who is their first real friend in many years. You might be the first person who has been prepared to really listen to them and not just turn you back on them or try to get revenge.

8. **Plan for future interactions.** After you've listened carefully to them and provided responses to questions or further explained your feelings, set the direction for your future relationship. Make them believe that their behavior must change or you will take whatever actions are required to guarantee that they will never undermine you again. If it becomes clear that the relationship will not work, let them know that you will treat them in a civil and professional manner but the relationship will go no further.

9. **Forewarned is forearmed.** Now that you know what types of behaviors can be expected from the sneak, you can be more cautious about leaving yourself open to future attacks. You are much less vulnerable when you can keep a close eye on the individual and head off covert attacks before they happen.[5]

Clients With Difficult Behaviors

Clients displaying difficult behaviors are in some ways similar to coworkers with difficult behaviors, but in other ways very different. The nurse is legally and ethically bound to provide the best care possible for all clients, even those who are displaying behavior that makes communication or care difficult. Although some clients may actually be persecutors or sneaks in their everyday lives or even have undiagnosed personality disorders, the majority of clients displaying difficult behaviors are acting that way as a response to their illnesses or injuries. Their needs and goals are different from persecutors or sneaks.

Above we discussed the effects of grief on individuals. Although we usually think of grief as being associated with a loss such as the death of a loved one, clients who are severely ill, severely injured, or who have had major surgeries, amputations, or loss of internal body parts or who may be facing death also often go through the stages of grief: denial, anger, guilt, depression, and resolution. The traditional five stages of grief were first presented by Dr. Kübler-Ross, who had investigated grief and suffering for many years before developing her theory on grief. Some more recent theorists believe that Ross's five-stage theory is too simplistic and have added several additional stages to the process and changed their names.[8] However, Ross's five stages remain the gold standard and is the theory that is most often taught to nursing students.

> *They are also called double-crossers or backstabbers. Unlike the persecutor, who enjoys direct confrontation and watching others feel uncomfortable under their attacks, the sneak will attack when you aren't looking and gets his or her reward by watching your discomfort and confusion in not knowing where the attack came from.*

The nurse has two primary goals in caring for clients who are working through the grief stages: (1) to provide the best care possible so that they will survive and recover from their illness (meet their physiological and safety needs) and (2) to help these clients work their way through the stages of grief until they reach resolution.[9] The ideal is to achieve both goals simultaneously, but that is not always possible. Goal 1 will always have the highest priority.

How each client experiences grief is highly individual, and there is no right way to resolve grief. Some clients move rapidly through the stages, some skip stages, and some are unable to move on from the stage they are in. They also don't always go through them in order. The stages of grief are really guides to help determine where the client is in the grieving and mourning process. The key to understanding this is to observe their behavior. It is also important to consider the effects of medications and pain on the client's behavior. Unfortunately, our health system of today often sends people home well before they have had a chance to complete the grief stages. However, if the nurse is able to start the process and move it even one stage, the other stages will progress more easily at home.

Earlier we saw that coworkers with difficult behaviors had need-fulfillment issues at the upper levels of Maslow's hierarchy of needs. However, severely ill clients are often attempting to meet the needs of the lower levels of the triangle—physiological survival and safety. Maslow believed that if the lower level needs are not met, the person is unable to move to the higher level needs fulfillment. Severely ill clients, in some ways, are starting over in their needs development.[3] It is a key responsibility of nurses to aid clients in maintaining their physiological and safety needs so that they can move back up to their prior levels of adjustment.

Even more so than working with a difficult coworker, perception on the part of the nurse plays an important part in understanding and adapting to client behaviors. Quickly stereotyping a client by saying something like "Oh, he's just an old grouch," "She's a real whiner and complainer," or "He doesn't like nurses. He won't do anything I want him to do" completely disregards the underlying issues that are causing the client to behave the way they are behaving. Often, once a client is labeled, the care provided to him or her is based on that label and the client's real issues are never addressed or resolved.

> *It is important to remain open-minded and to be prepared to understand what motivated them to use the behaviors they use.*

Establishing Trust

Establishing trust is key to any successful relationship. In the nurse-client relationship, it is the foundation upon which all nursing care is built and is particularly important when dealing with difficult behavior. In most relationships, it takes a considerable amount of time to develop trust between two people; however, in the health-care setting, time is limited and trust has to be built quickly. Nurses have a head start in trusting relationships with clients. The annual Gallup Poll surveys the nation's population asking which profession they trust most. For the past 10 years, that profession has been nursing.

Respect

Trust can be established by a show of respect for the other person's opinions and ideas and letting them know you accept their behavior even though you do not agree with it. Always be honest with the client even when it isn't pleasant to do so.[10] If clients find out that you have been less than honest with them, it is almost impossible to regain their trust again. We sometimes are tempted to be less than 100 percent truthful because we don't want to hurt their feelings, make them angry, or upset them. By focusing on what is going well with the client rather than criticizing them or pointing out the problems in their behavior, you can soften the impact of a negative statement and show them that you are not being judgmental about them or their condition.

Consistency

Another important element in building trust is being consistent in what you do and say. The client will be able to relax if he or she knows what is coming next. Being reliable and doing what you say you will do, even in small things, acts as a foundation for trust. If you tell the client you will be back to check on them in 30 minutes, make sure you come back on time. If they can trust you in the small things, they will trust you with the more critical things. Generally nurses should not make promises to clients. Health care and health-care outcomes have too many variables to be certain about much of anything; however, if you do make a promise to a client, make sure you keep it. Even promises about small issues like promising to get the client some juice after finishing the client next door can have a huge impact on a person whose world is currently limited to a hospital room.

Confidentiality

In order to trust you, the client needs to know that you will keep his or her confidence. Nurses are bound ethically and legally to maintain confidentiality of client information, but nurse-client communication is NOT considered privileged communication as exists between priest and penitent or lawyer and client or physician and client. (See Chapter 8 for more detail.) Personal secrets that do not affect the client's health care are easier to keep and should remain secret. Information that is important to their treatment or recovery should be revealed to the physician. If a client tells you something in confidence—for example, "Don't tell anybody, but I have seizures from time to time"—and it isn't on their medical record, you need to inform them that the information is important to their treatment and you are going to pass it on to the physician. Sometimes clients will ask you, "I want to tell you something that I don't want anyone else to know about. Can you keep it secret?" A good response is to say, "I can keep secrets, but if what you are about to tell me is important to your care or recovery, I'll have to let the physician know. However, the information won't go any further than that."

Loyalty

Nurses can also foster trust in clients by showing how loyal they are to the client and to the principles of nursing, being proficient in their health-care knowledge and nursing skills, and showing that they are ethically and morally strong. Additionally, demonstrating the use of good judgment in decision-making, being fair, maintaining objectivity in difficult situations, and taking responsibility for your actions also reinforce an atmosphere of trust. Once two people begin to trust each other, even if they disagree about some of the issues, they are much more likely to come to a satisfactory resolution of the problem.

Stages of Grief

The discussion below of managing difficult client behaviors is organized around the stages of grief and prioritized by the levels of Maslow's hierarchy. The behaviors most commonly associated with each grief stage will be presented along with methods to respond to the behaviors. Some of the methods discussed above for managing coworkers with difficult behaviors also work with clients, although, because of their different needs, additional methods are also required.

Denial

Denial, also sometimes called the "I'm Fine Syndrome," is used as a coping mechanism to give people time to adjust to sudden traumatic situations. For some people it becomes a way of life, particularly if they have addiction issues. It is an unconscious process that protects the individual from feeling vulnerable or losing control. Because it is an unconscious process, clients often are unable to accept obvious facts or they greatly minimize the consequences of their condition.

> *It is a key responsibility of nurses to aid clients in maintaining their physiological and safety needs so that they can move back up to their prior levels of adjustment.*

This stage is often very short and may take place even before the client arrives at the hospital. Statements such as "This can't be happening!" "I don't believe what you are telling me!," "Are you sure about that diagnosis?" or "This treatment (surgery, medication, etc.) is a waste of time. There's nothing wrong with me." are all expressions of denial. Some clients, however, get locked into a state of denial and are unable to move from it. They may spend 2 weeks in the hospital being treated for a severe heart attack, including open heart surgery, and the day they go home, they say, "I'm glad there really wasn't anything wrong with me."

Goals

Clients in a persistent denial stage use behaviors that achieve the goal of maintaining their denial. The denial protects them from accepting the reality of their condition, which may significantly alter their body image and prevents the need for them to make lifestyle changes, eat a restricted diet, or limit their activities after discharge.[11] There are different degrees of denial ranging from mild, which is relatively easy to overcome, to impenetrable denial, which is resistant to all rational reasoning. Common denial behaviors include refusing to take medications, refusing to go for diagnostic tests, pulling off monitor electrodes, or not following directions about activity if they decide they are not necessary because they believe they are not really sick. They might even decide to sign themselves out of the hospital against medical advice (AMA).

Autonomy

One of the important considerations in working with clients in denial is consideration of their autonomy or right to self-determination. (See Chapter 6 for more detail.) From a strictly legal and ethical point of view, they have a legal and ethical right to do or not do whatever they want. However, some of their autonomous actions can come into direct conflict with the nurse's obligation for beneficence, to do good for the client.

Clients in denial pose significant challenges for nurses. Physicians sometimes will ask a nurse, "Did Ms. Hart take her antibiotic this morning?" The nurse answers, "No, she refused to take it because she says she doesn't need it." The physician responds loudly, "When did she get her MD? She DOES need it! Get in there and make her take it!" Of course, you really can't force clients to do anything they don't want to do if they are competent. Forcing clients to take medications or undergo treatments they do not want leaves the nurse open to civil suits for assault and battery. So what is the nurse to do?

Approaches

There are several approaches that can be used to achieve the goals of providing quality care and moving the client out of denial:

Walking the tightrope. Approaching clients in denial who are refusing to take their medications or submit to prescribed treatments requires a gentle touch. Providing too much information may overwhelm them, or being too forceful in your approach may result in them stiffening their resolve not to do what you want.[7] On the other hand, diminishing or dismissing the issue will also not accomplish your goals.

Look at the situation from their point of view. Clients have a reason for not taking the medication or going for their treatments. Addressing that reason with compassion and rational arguments about why they should cooperate with you may work if they are in a mild denial state; however, no amount of objective reasoning will penetrate the resolve of the client in persistent denial. You must find another way to motivate them to take their medications. Although it is not ideal and comes very close to violating the "always tell the truth" principle, sometimes you need to use approaches that are somewhat manipulative. Some possible approaches that you can use include:

You can trust me; I'm the nurse. You can use the trust the client has built up for you due to your compassion and knowledge to change behavior. For example, "Ms. Hart, I feel like we've developed a strong relationship over the past few days. You know I have never lied to you and promise I never will. You need to believe me when I tell you that this medication is necessary for your recovery. Please take it."

It can't hurt. Sometimes called the "**humor me**" approach. "Ms. Hart, I know you don't think you

> *Nurses can also foster trust in clients by showing how loyal they are to the client and to the principles of nursing, being proficient in their health care knowledge and nursing skills, and showing that they are ethically and morally strong.*

need this medication, but Dr. Happy wants you to have it. Why don't you take it anyway since it really doesn't hurt anything and if you really do need it, it will actually help." Or "I would really appreciate it if you would take this medication. I want to help you."

Let's try it and see what happens. "Ms. Hart, I know you don't believe you need this medication, but if you look at your incision site, you can see how red and tender it is. Why don't you take this medication and see if it helps with the pain? You'll probably need several doses for it to be effective."

I'll be back. "Ms. Hart, I feel like you have other things on your mind right now. I'll come back in an hour and you can take your medication then."

Don't ask, don't tell. This approach needs to be used cautiously because it can ruin a trusting relationship; however, if you assess that it might work with your client and nothing else has worked, give it a try. Just quietly walk into the room and hand them a glass of water and the medicine cup with the pill. Don't say anything. Sometimes clients have become conditioned to take pills without really thinking about what they are doing. If not, they'll just tell you they're not going to take it.

Tough love (inducing fear as a motivator). (Note: this is to only be used when all else has failed because it is borderline unethical using the Teleological system of ethics. Be careful using this approach, as it has the potential to destroy your relationship with the client.) "Ms. Hart, you have refused all medications and treatments for the last three days. I'm going to get in contact with the people at hospice so that they can make arrangements for your end-of-life care at your home."

These approaches are aimed solely at the physiological needs of the client and do not take into consideration his or her need to work through and get beyond the stage of denial. Below are approaches that can be used in conjunction with the previously discussed approaches in resolving their denial issue. They include:

Establishing a strong trusting relationship. Use the techniques discussed above for trusting relationships. It is particularly important in working with clients in denial.

Being consistent in your message. This approach is similar to the "walk the tightrope" approach, except now it is directed at resolving the issue of denial. You need to move slowly and let the client determine the pace of the discussion. Agree to disagree but do not waver in your message. The client will insist that there is nothing wrong with them, but you need to make it clear that you believe the lab tests, x-rays, and other objective findings that indicate that they are ill; however, do not argue with them or attempt to overwhelm them with facts and data. They will shut down completely.

Use the communication building techniques. The most important ones for the client in denial are:

- Asking open-ended questions and taking the time to really listen to the responses. Try to uncover what they are afraid of losing by accepting the diagnosis: independence? Lifestyle? Life itself? Fear is a powerful motivator.
- Reflecting back emotions that are being expressed. Acknowledge and accept both positive and negative emotions, and remember that crying is a powerful emotional release. "Ms. Bell, although you insist that there is nothing wrong with your leg, I'm getting the sense that you are afraid if the physician treats it, you might not be able to clean your house or care for grandchildren anymore. Am I mistaken?"
- Asking clarifying questions. "Ms. Bell, you said before that you are really okay, but then you just said you were afraid that the pain in your leg might lead to an amputation. I'm a little confused. Can you help me understand what you are saying?"
- Using all the nonverbal and paraverbal techniques. Eye contact, directly facing the client, open posture, quiet tone, head nodding, and light touch.

Encourage family involvement. This one can also be a tightrope act. You need to inform the family members of what is happening, that you need their help and how they can be helpful. For example, "Your dad is denying that he has cancer and is refusing all treatment and medications. We are working to get him to accept his diagnosis. Denial is an unconscious protective mechanism people use to avoid the fear associated with their condition. However, we need to avoid using the 'hard sell' with him. Yelling at him and arguing with him will only make him more resistant. Letting him talk about how he is feeling is a much better approach and more successful. Thank you for your help." Keep in mind that families sometimes go into denial, too, and reinforce the client's denial or have a relationship that involves yelling and arguing as the usual form of communication, which only exacerbates the denial state.[10]

Provide information in small doses. Too much information at one time can overwhelm them and increase their resistance. Leave reading materials in their room that they can consider when they are ready.

> *"The client will insist that there is nothing wrong with them, but you need to make it clear that you believe the lab tests, x-rays, and other objective findings that indicate that they are ill; however, do not argue with them or attempt to overwhelm them with facts and data."*

Anger

Angry behavior between coworkers was discussed above as one of the important communication blockers. Anger expressed by clients is also a significant communication blocker; however, it has different causes and manifestations in clients who are severely ill or injured. As clients move away from the denial stage and the protective veil of refutation and refusal falls away, clients are often not prepared for the flood of intense emotions they are experiencing. They have suddenly become vulnerable and recognize that they have lost most of their control over their lives and their future.[12] When a client accepts that he or she is acutely ill, it means they are literally placing their lives in the hands of the health-care team.

Remember also that mild to severe episodic pain or even mild long-term chronic pain can elicit behaviors that exhibit irritation and antagonism, even though the client is not in any particular grief stage. Assessing the cause of the behavior is extremely important because the techniques used for a client exhibiting grief-stage angry behavior will not be effective. Pain medication and distraction techniques are much more effective. However, sometimes clients displaying grief-stage anger can also be in pain.

Clients' expressions of anger can range from a mild sense of frustration to declarations of injustice or raging destructive behaviors that must be stopped immediately. Clients in the anger stage often use statements that contain a small degree of recognition of their condition. Common statements that can indicate a client is in the anger stage include, "Why is this happening to me?" "This isn't right! I don't deserve this," "What has God got against me?" "If my #%&@$ boss didn't put so much pressure on me, I wouldn't have had this heart attack!"

Other behaviors indicating the anger stage include tightened jaw; clenched fists; aggressive body language and posture; fidgeting; physiological responses such as elevated pulse rate, blood pressure, and respiratory rate; red face; raised voice; making threats; excessive demands for attention; and overt acts that express anger, such as throwing food trays or banging on bedside tables.[9] However, unlike the client in denial, the angry client will comply with most treatments and medications, even if it is done grudgingly, with resentment and with some caustic comments. Most clients who are expressing anger believe their anger is a result of what has happened to them.

Many clients experiencing the anger stage have it come and go quickly while other clients can hang on tightly to their anger stage. Anger can be both a defense mechanism and a form of manipulative behavior. Anger, for those who are unwilling to let go, fulfills their needs for feeling safe and secure and meets the goal of avoiding uncomfortable feelings such as fear, particularly of pain and death, and feelings of helplessness and powerlessness resulting from loss of mobility or independence. Factors that can contribute to the anger stage are feelings of anxiety, frustration with their care, or increased feelings of stress. If they are religious, the anger may also be caused by feelings of abandonment, particularly by God or a higher power.[13] Anger is less of a threat to a client's physical status than the behavior displayed in denial, but anger behaviors have a relatively high potential to affect the client's safety needs, ranging from self-injury to the development of stress-related disorders.

Coping with anger is always difficult, regardless of whether it is our own anger or that being expressed by a client. Some clients express anger easily and openly while other clients have little outward expression of anger and instead suppress and direct it inward. Anger turned inward is hard to assess, is very destructive, and usually is related to feelings of guilt, which itself is also a very destructive emotion. When clients can say, "I'm so angry at (my disease process)," the anger becomes therapeutic and part of the recovery process.

Expressions of anger always need a target, and it is usually a target of convenience and proximity. Nurses are always close by and always around, so expect the angry behavior to be directed toward you. When clients are displaying angry behavior toward you, it is a normal tendency to say, "I've had enough! They don't pay me enough to take this abuse. Put your call light on the next time you want to insult me!" and not go back in the room. This is a knee-jerk reaction and needs to be avoided. By understanding that you really are not the target of the client's anger but that you were merely there when he was expressing his feelings of anger at his situation can lessen the impact of the attack on you, but it still hurts. It is also important to let family members, who are also often targets of a client's anger, know that the client is not really angry at them but is expressing feelings of loss of control and helplessness. Angry retorts from family members toward the client can result in explosive arguments that no one wins.

Because the anger stage has fewer threats to the client's physiological well-being than the denial stage does, the following approaches to working with a client displaying angry behavior are focused more on moving them out of the anger of stage. Many of these approaches are similar to those used for moving a client out of the denial stage. Of course, if the client's anger is being expressed in a self-destructive way, such as punching a glass window or throwing objects around that can bounce back and hurt him, it

> *Other behaviors indicating the anger stage include hostile facial expressions; tightened jaw; clenched fists; aggressive body language and posture; fidgeting; physiological responses such as elevated pulse rate, blood pressure, and respiratory rate; red face; raised voice; making threats; excessive demands for attention; and overt acts that express anger, such as throwing food trays or banging on bedside tables.*

has become an emergency situation and action must be taken quickly to stop the behavior. (For more information, go to http://www.ncbi.nlm.nih.gov/pmc/articles/PMC3208944/.)

Approaches

Release anger safely. Although it is important for the client to "get the anger out," anger should never be taken out on another person. The anger should be redirected to intimate objects or safe activities that hurt neither the client nor others. The ultimate goal is to have the client redirect the anger toward the illness.[7] Throwing small plastic items like cups at a wall, scribbling hard on sheets of paper, tearing sheets of paper into small pieces, breaking pencils or tongue depressors in half, wadding paper into a ball and throwing it hard at a wall or trash can, or punching a pillow are all safe and harmless physical ways of expressing anger. Provide the client with a stress-relief ball that he can squeeze. Be creative!

In the past, "scream therapy" was thought to be an effective way of releasing pent-up anger, but in the health-care setting, loud screaming is considered disruptive in a quiet intensive care unit. However, depending on the unit, the number of clients, and the staffing, it may be possible to allow the client in the anger stage to yell, scream, and stomp the feet, if able, by closing the door to the client's room and other clients' rooms and warning the staff of what is about to happen and why. You can also include the client in deciding on a safe expression of anger. "Mr. Pound, I appreciate how angry you are at your situation; however, yelling at me and the other staff and throwing your urinal when it is full is not appropriate. Is there something that you might want to do to express your anger that is safe and doesn't involve other people?"

> *The statement the angry client made was not a personal attack on you; rather, you just happened to be near when he wanted to express feelings of anger.*

Respond calmly and with respect. Although showing clients respect is an ethical requirement, when responding to angry clients it is usually easier said than done. Clients expressing their anger are insulting, demanding, and in general, very annoying. Outside of the health-care setting, you would likely respond to this behavior by avoiding them, but as a nurse, that is not an option.

A few of the comments heard from clients who are displaying anger behaviors over a 40-year career as an RN include:

"You're not a very good RN, and you're fat too."
"Go get the pretty nurse; at least she knows what she is doing."
"Did you comb your hair with a firecracker this morning?"
"OH NO, NOT YOU AGAIN."
"If even one more person asks me how I'm doing, I'll shoot them!"
"You bring me another tray of this slop you're passing off as food, and I'll throw it at you!" (She did.)
"I want my bed bath now while I'm awake."
"You're supposed to give me my medication at 9:00 a.m.; it's almost 15 after. Where is it?"
"I've had my call light on for 2 hours. Where have you been?" (It was more like 2 minutes.)
"What do you mean you're changing my dressing change procedure? It already hurts enough when you pull the thing off!"
"Take me for my CT scan now! I'm getting hungry."
"The care is so bad here I'm going to call my lawyer and sue you and this torture chamber for every penny it's worth."

The instinctual responses to such statements is to take it personally, fire back with an even sharper verbal bard, or run out of the room crying. None of these responses are therapeutic and do nothing positive for the client or you. As difficult as it might seem, the way to respond to angry behavior and speech is to remain calm, remembering that you are a professional and you are in control.[10] The statement the angry client made was not a personal attack on you; rather, you just happened to be near when he wanted to express feelings of anger. Respond to the underlying message that is in the underlying emotion being expressed using acknowledgment and reflection.

Never respond to the actual statement. Remember the client is trying to achieve the goal of self-protection from the realization of the effects of his illness. However, in your best reassuring, calm, rational, professional, and "I'm in control" voice, while displaying open and accepting body language, respond by saying, "I understand how upsetting all this must be for you and how angry you are. We really need to talk about what is making you feel this way."

Sometimes the client may actually have a legitimate complaint that needs to be addressed. If that is the case, let him or her know that you are doing something to fix the problem so it doesn't happen again. For example, "Ms. Picky, it appears that the food we've been bringing to you is not up to the standards you expect. I called the dietitian and she will be here shortly to see if we can improve the selection and quality of the food you are receiving."

It is also helpful to practice by role-playing with a good friend because many people have never had another person talk to them this way. Have your friend attack you verbally with the statements above or ones that they think up, and analyze how you feel. Practice responding calmly and confidently to the emotion of the statement, not the statement itself.

Keep it cool. If the client is in an agitated state and is hurling a nonstop barrage of insults and demands at you, step back one step, displaying accepting body language (hands off hips and no crossed arms on chest) and wait until he or she finishes. When the barrage is over and the room becomes quiet, speak calmly and softly, addressing the client by his or her name. "Mr. Volatile, I appreciate how scared you are. Everyone here is working hard to help you recover. All I want to do now is to listen to your lung sounds to make sure you are breathing okay." Using a calm, confident approach will help the client relax enough to complete the rest of the physical evaluation. In some cases, the client may even apologize for their outburst. "I'm so sorry I acted that way. I don't know what came over me." This actually may be the opening you need to address his underlying feelings of fear and loss of control.

Defuse a blowup. In response to unpleasant news or some incident involving their care that they perceive as a threat, some clients with anger issues will at times totally lose control, become irrational, and become deaf to anything you have to say. The trigger event or issue doesn't have to be major; clients' worlds get very small in the confines of a hospital room, and small issues can loom as giant monsters to them. The approach to a client who has blown up emotionally is similar to the approach used to defuse the behavior of a toddler having a temper tantrum. Responding by yelling back at the client to "Calm down," "Stop acting like a child," or "This is not acceptable behavior" will only intensify and make the blowup last

longer. In this situation, the client is using the behavior to manipulate the nurse into giving him or her more attention or to get his or her way. Any type of response, either positive or negative, during the blowup just reinforces the behavior, which will be used more and more often in the future.

With toddlers who are having tantrums, the best approach, after making sure they are safe and can't harm themselves, is to walk away. The tantrum usually stops quickly thereafter. The same approach can be used for clients, but a more therapeutic approach is to maintain eye contact with the client in an accepting posture while he or she is exploding and listen actively to the underlying emotions being expressed. Often they will reveal what happened recently in their lives to trigger the outburst. After the client has returned to a relatively rational state and is able to hear you again, acknowledge his or her feelings. If something happened in the course of his or her care that triggered the outburst, let him or her know that you regret the situation and will work to resolve it.

Involving clients in their care in general increases their sense of control and levels of compliance.[9] For clients who have blown up, asking them for their help in resolving the problem is highly effective. Use statements such as, "Tell me what we need to do to resolve this issue," "Give me some suggestions on ways to deal with this," or "If you were in my shoes, how would you go about preventing this from happening again?" Try to reach an agreement with the client on how you and he or she can work together to find an answer. For example, "I hear what you are saying. The night nurses are very noisy and keep you from sleeping. We could approach this by having me talk to the charge nurse on the night shift about keeping the noise down. I will let her know that when you are being kept up by the noise, you will put your call light on and inform your nurse that it is getting noisy. Does that sound like a pretty good approach?" Use short, clear sentences when communicating with this type of client.

Stop, look, and listen. As we saw with clients in denial, it is impossible to push clients off the anger stage of grief or pull them to the next stage. We can, however, facilitate their progress, but they will only move on when they are emotionally ready to do so and see some type of reward for the progress. A strong trusting relationship is essential in making any progress and requires the use of many of the communication builders and time. The goal here is to have the client understand that his or her expressions of anger are really a defense to accepting the realities of their illnesses or injuries.

Set aside at least a half-hour block of time and tell the client that you will be talking with him or her at a predetermined time—that is, make an appointment. Make sure you show up on time and begin the communication by asking them a question like, "Mr. Axelrod, I've been concerned about you for several days now. I really don't know you that well, so could you please tell me something about your background and life?" Then let him talk without interruption. Use body language that shows you are serious about the communication, including nodding, appropriate facial expressions, and eye contact. Turn off your pager or cell phone. Listen attentively to his whole story. For many clients, this may be the first time a health-care provider has shown a real interest in them as a person and not just a disease process. For example, "The amputation in room 234 curses at anyone who comes in the room with medications."

When they stop speaking, allow for a short pause and then begin your response by agreeing with them and showing them that you listened to what they said. "I'm really glad you were willing to share that information with me about yourself. I can see that you have had a difficult life and appreciate the efforts you have made to improve yourself. By getting to know you better, I believe I can take better care of you." However, don't turn your reply into a lengthy monolog. Rather, see it as an opportunity to ask more questions that will help the client attain self-realization of their behavior.

Sometimes gentle confrontation may help the client see the issues more clearly. Statements such as, "You seemed to be upset about something earlier today. Can you tell me about it?" or "You made some angry comments to the orderly who was helping you with your bath. Could you tell me what that was about?" This can open the door to deeper and more meaningful communication; however, be very cautious using any type of confrontation. The answers to these types of questions can lead to additional questions that will direct the course of the discussion.

Other techniques that help reveal the underlying causes of the client's anger include reflection and legitimization.[12] We saw that reflective statements or questions such as, "It appears to me that you became angry because you believed that I didn't think you were in pain. Is that correct?" are aimed at getting the client to talk about their deeper feelings. Legitimization is the acknowledgment of and agreement with the client's perceptions. For example, you can say, "I see now why you became upset. You asked me for pain medication, and I gave you a medication different from the one you usually take without explaining what it was. I'd probably be upset also if I were in your shoes. It seems to bother you to depend on other people to meet your needs when you've been so independent all your life."

Threat of physical harm. Clients who are displaying grief-stage angry behavior usually are not physically aggressive. However, if at any time any client threatens or attempts to harm you physically or you sincerely believe your safety is in jeopardy, contact your coworkers immediately for help and let hospital security know of the situation. Often, after they are alerted to a potential dangerous situation with a client, security will post a guard on the unit but will keep him or her out of the room and out of sight. Some actions by the nurse that may provoke a physical attack and should never happen when working with an angry client, particularly one in an outburst state, include:

> *...if at any time any client threatens or attempts to harm you physically or you sincerely believe your safety is in jeopardy, contact your coworkers immediately for help and let hospital security know of the situation.*

- Interrupting the client during an outburst: "Stop yelling right now!"
- Warning a client not to use insults, cursing, or crude language: "The hospital doesn't allow that type of speech."
- Reciprocating anger back to them when they make a personal insult: "You think I'm fat? Have you looked at yourself lately? You look like a pig in a mud wallow!"
- Challenging the truth of the client's statement: "That's not true and you know it!"
- Criticizing them for their behavior: "You're acting like a 3-year-old having a tantrum!"
- Becoming defensive: "I'm doing the best I can, but you are impossible to please."

- Using touch to try to calm them down.
- Blocking their exit from their room.
- Getting behind the client where they can't see you and talking to them.[12]

Documentation. It's imprinted on all nurses from the first day of nursing school that documentation is a mandatory part of the life of a health-care provider. In working with clients who display angry behaviors, or any of the grief-related difficult behaviors, documenting what was said and done becomes extremely important. Make sure to rate the level of the client's anger, specific actions and statements by the client that indicate anger, interventions you have initiated in response to the client's behavior, and how the client responded to the interventions. Don't hesitate to complete an incident report if the client in any way harms you physically. Good documentation is worth its weight in gold if the client or family decides to initiate a lawsuit.

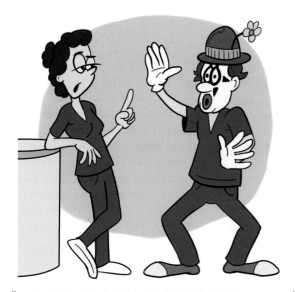

"YOU REALLY NEED TO WORK ON YOUR VERBAL SKILLS."

Bargaining

As the flames of the bonfire of the anger stage are slowly extinguished, reality again comes crashing back in, making the client feel vulnerable. Clients begin seeking other ways to protect themselves from the things that are happening to them. A general definition of bargaining is that it is a form of negotiation in which two parties attempt to reach a deal that is satisfactory to both parties over some item or issue. However, as a

stage of grief, in the bargaining process the client has no one to bargain with except a higher power.

Bargaining is an unconscious coping mechanism that seeks to fulfill the goals of avoiding the bad things that the client anticipates will soon happen to him or her and regaining some degree of control over their lives. It often becomes a type of "magical thinking" that is often seen in young children. Bargaining is also an expression of hope, often unrealistic, on the part of the client, frequently based on irrational beliefs or incomplete information.

There is no set time limit on the bargaining stage: Some clients totally skip it while others find it very comfortable to remain in it almost indefinitely. It can become one of the most difficult stages from which to progress because, rather than having a large physical component that is externally disruptive, bargaining is an almost totally internal mental process.[9] The mind can have a very powerful influence over beliefs and behavior. It can play all kinds of tricks on clients in this stage.

It is interesting that a bargaining stage may actually occur before the official diagnosis, when the client merely suspects something is wrong. It serves as a means of warding off the bad news. The bargaining that occurs after diagnosis serves as a method to negotiate away the changes brought on by their disease process. As with denial and anger, the client is seeking to meet the goals of increasing control over the situation and avoiding pain and suffering.

In all the grief stages, including bargaining, there is a relatively high level of fear and anxiety present. Anxiety is fear of the unknown, and there are many elements of health care that always remain uncertain. Similarly, the feeling of lack of control over the client's own destiny causes him or her to attempt to negotiate with a higher power or someone, something, or anything he or she feels, whether realistically or not, will help them avoid the impending changes. They often make promises to God, hoping that the pain of the illness might not occur or at least be lessened. They look for their lives to go back to how they were before they were given the diagnosis or started the treatment.

Often clients in the bargaining stage are intensely focused on what they could have done differently in the past to prevent what is happening to them now. They also imagine all the things that could have been and how wonderful their lives could be if this bad thing did not happen to them. This type of thinking is actually an improvement over the denial and anger responses to their illness because it moves clients closer to accepting the changes that are occurring in their lives. They are beginning to fully understand and recognize the full impact their condition will have on their lives; however, it is relatively easy for excessive efforts at bargaining to produce high levels of remorse and guilt that will ultimately block their ability to successfully cope with their situation.[10]

Recognizing when clients are in the bargaining stage is fairly easy: There is a unique set of statements they often make. The following are examples of bargaining statements:

"If I do (some action), then you'll (God, nurse, physician) respond by (some action like taking away my disease)."

"I should have done something sooner about this."

"We should have gotten a second opinion from another physician before now."

"If only I had led a better life, this wouldn't have happened."

"I promise to stop smoking, drinking, and cheating on my wife if you (God) make this go away."

"I must have done something terribly wrong in my life to have this happen to me."

"I heard there is a doctor in Mexico who treats this type of cancer without chemotherapy or surgery (or pain)."

"I don't believe that my doctor is as smart as he thinks he is—he didn't even know about that experimental treatment I found on the Internet."

"Go ahead and fix my broken leg, arm, and pelvis. I'm still going to ride my motorcycle when I get out."

"I don't want to start chemotherapy today. Can't we wait until next week when I'm stronger? I promise to do my physical therapy every day."

"I'll give an extra large donation to the church if you can make this go away."

"You're the fifth physician I've seen about this and none of you have given me a good answer."

People in the bargaining stage often hold tightly to irrational or illogical beliefs. However, similar to clients in anger and denial stages, understanding our own perceptions is key to maintaining a balanced approach to clients in this stage. What seems absurd and contradictory to us appears very necessary, logical, and clear to the client. Some beliefs that bargaining clients cling to include:

- There should be no pain involved in this treatment.
- All problems have simple and straightforward solutions.
- Getting better shouldn't involve much time or effort.
- If I continue looking long enough and hard enough, I'll find the cure for my disease.
- Most people work out their own problems; I can too.
- All health-care providers should be smart, kind, gentle, considerate, and able to cure me.
- Health-care providers are totally responsible for solving my problem since I don't know anything about medicine.
- I know that I am the only one who ever had this disease.
- This is my disease; I have to deal with it by myself.
- I can't burden any of my family with treating this illness.
- You must accept any problem that comes your way as a sign of your innate evil; you must accept it as the penance or retribution for your badness.
- If I get help, the problem will go away, and I won't need any more help.[7]

> *The feeling of lack of control over the client's own destiny causes him or her to attempt to negotiate with a higher power or someone, something, or anything he or she feels, whether realistically or not, will help them avoid the impending changes.*

Although there are relatively few immediate threats to a client's physiological health when they are experiencing bargaining, one long-term effect is that they may continue the behavior indefinitely, which prevents them from moving to acceptance. The difficult behavior that nurses may encounter with clients who are in the bargaining stage occur when clients believe that alternative and integrative treatments will work better than the ones they are currently receiving. They may stop the approved treatments and rely on alternative treatments alone or, even more dangerous, combine alternative treatments with approved treatments without notifying the health-care team. (For more detail about integrative therapies, see

Chapter 25.) Also, when bargaining clients attempt to postpone treatments or attempt to seek the perfect physician with the perfect therapeutic plan, they can delay necessary interventions for a significant length of time.

Because there are elements of avoidance and rejection of treatment displayed in the behaviors of clients in the bargaining stage, some of the methods used in the care of the client with denial will also be helpful in the client who is bargaining. However, it is important to take into consideration the differences in what these two groups of clients are attempting to avoid. Clients in denial have the goal of totally avoiding the realization that they are ill or have a severe injury, whereas clients who are bargaining have accepted their diagnosis but are now primarily attempting to avoid the discomfort that is associated with its treatment.

Providing effective care for clients in the bargaining stage requires addressing two issues: (1) the potentially dangerous situations created by their need to postpone treatments and rejecting conventional treatments to seek alternative treatments, and (2) helping them face the issues related to anxiety and fear so they can move toward acceptance. Care for bargaining clients is made more difficult because sometimes they will appear to be cooperative and compliant while in reality they are ignoring your instructions and covertly doing what they want.[6] Resolving the emotional issues involved in bargaining can become a significant challenge. Breaking down a system of false beliefs that a client has developed over time can be as difficult as driving a bicycle through a brick wall.

The other element to keep in mind is that when you finally get through to them and take away their false beliefs, what do they have left? Frequently, even people who are not experiencing a threat to their health and independence have difficulty dealing with the unvarnished truth. Avoid offering clients who are in the bargaining stage false hopes. They may cling to every word, looking for a morsel of something hopeful to hang on to. You need to balance the practical things that you can offer them with their hopes; however, never offer them something that you cannot

> *Clients in denial have the goal of totally avoiding the realization that they are ill or have a severe injury, whereas clients who are bargaining have accepted their diagnosis but are now primarily attempting to avoid the discomfort that is associated with its treatment.*

fulfill. When they are in an active bargaining state, they are often open to your support for change or new ways of believing. If you can use that moment of openness to gain their collaboration in recognizing an illogical belief, you have made a win-win deal.

Approaches

Trust, honesty, and communication approach. Trust again becomes a key to helping the client in the bargaining stage. All the techniques for building trust and establishing open communication are required when working with these clients. They have to trust you enough and feel comfortable enough in talking with you that they will tell you if they are using alternative treatments that you don't know about.

However, if you have a sense that they are using some herbal supplements or other potentially harmful treatments without your knowledge, you may have to ask them about your suspicions. Using a quiet, calm voice, ask nonaccusing and nonconfrontational questions such as, "I noticed you have a printout of an Internet article on herbal supplements for people with cancer on your nightstand. Tell me about the ones you have tried?" "Yesterday you asked me if I knew anything about using a liquid-only diet to cure cystic fibrosis. Tell me how that is supposed to work?" or even a more direct question such as, "Your blood pressure has dropped quite a bit over the last two days. Tell me about what you are doing that is different from before?" This can elicit honest answers if the client trusts you.

What if the client responds, reluctantly, "Well, okay, yes. I've been drinking this liquid that is a traditional cure for most everything. My grandmother, who is 100 percent Creek Indian, makes it. It's made from totally natural herbs and roots and other things she says. I take it when no one is watching. Please don't tell my physician." Now what do you do with that information?

You are now faced with another right to confidentiality versus obligation for beneficence dilemma. Because of the real potential for harm to the client from ingesting unknown chemical substances, you have no option but to inform the physician. The list of substances that American Indians have been using for centuries as home remedies that actually do have physiological effects include minerals such as lithium and selenium, which are found in the ground and in plants such as goat weed, foxglove, willow bark, and cherry bark. Sometimes substances are used such as ashes, which contain mercury and lead, and apple seeds or peach pits, which contain arsenic. The other problem is that the dose or the concentration of the substance is also unknown. Some plants taken in small doses are relatively harmless while larger doses can be lethal. And the interactive effects with other medications are unknown and potentially deadly.

To soften the effect of breaching the client's confidentiality, you can say, "I really appreciate how honest you've been with me, Ms. Crow, in telling me about the potion you are taking. As you know, we have you taking several very powerful medications here in the hospital to combat your disease. The problem is we don't know what is in your grandmother's potion and how it affects the other medications you are taking. There may be something in it that can combine with the medications and make you very sick, or the potion may block the effectiveness of your medication. I am going to have to inform your physician about what you are taking. He will send it to the lab to see exactly what the ingredients are, and the pharmacist will see if any of them affect your medications. However, if they find that there is nothing harmful in your grandmother's medication, the physician may decide that you can continue taking it. Who knows, there might actually be something in it that will help your recovery."

Preempting the postponement approach. Clients in the bargaining stage are more open to logical thinking and rational arguments than clients in the denial or anger stages. Bargaining clients have already accepted that they are sick and need help; they're just trying to find the least painful way of treatment. Conversely, they are also adept at using rational arguments and logic in the attempt to postpone treatments and therapy.

Where a client in the anger stage might say, "Get that #$&@ gurney out of my room; there's no way you're taking me to radiation therapy," bargaining clients would more likely say, "My back really hurts today, so let's hold off starting radiation therapy until it feels better. I don't think I can survive lying on that hard table for 45 minutes," "I've felt too nauseated and weak today to go for another chemotherapy treatment," "I'll take all the pills you want me to take if you'll stop giving me that IV medication," or "I really don't mind starting physical therapy, but I'd like to wait until the new physician I contacted consults with me."

As nurses, we have great compassion for clients we believe are trying to be cooperative and are pleasant to be around. Bargaining clients usually fit that description; however, we have to realize that we must be proactive in dealing with behaviors that may worsen their conditions. When you detect that the client is using bargaining behavior, you need to end the behavior as quickly as possible. However, tying a client to a gurney while he or she is screaming that they do not want to go may leave you open to civil suits for assault and battery.

> *Successful coping with the bargaining stage requires that the client understand the underlying causes of the behavior and acknowledge that they are using bargaining to achieve a goal.*

If you have built up a high level of trust with the client, you may want to gently confront the person, asking her or him to stop by identifying and pointing out the irrational beliefs that underlie the postponing behavior. For example, you can say, "I know the thought of going to radiation therapy is frightening. The machines look very imposing, and you are giving up control of your body to someone you do not know. However, all the radiation technicians are highly trained and have been certified by a national organization, so they're the best. I've seen this type of radiation decrease the size of tumors and decrease the pain it is causing. As far as your back pain goes, I have several medications that you can take to decrease it, and I'm sure the people in radiation therapy can put something on the table to make it softer."

That's a good bargain approach. Successful coping with the bargaining stage requires the client to understand the underlying causes of the behavior and acknowledge that they are using bargaining to achieve a goal. Initially the client needs to recognize that he or she is making bargains and identify what types of bargains they are making. It is essential that the client achieve clarity on what his or her bargain is.[8]

By asking questions that cause the client to consider whether their beliefs are rational or not, you can begin to gradually move them toward a state of reality. Questions that work to achieve this goal include:

"Tell me why you believe that herbal substances are better than the medications we are using in the hospital when you know you have stage four cancer?"

"You've been refusing radiation therapy for almost a week, and your condition has gotten worse. Talk to me about why you feel continuing to refuse therapy will help you?"

"You seem to believe that somewhere there is a physician who can cure you without any discomfort. You've already contacted 25 physicians, and they all basically say the same thing. Does it seem logical that contacting 25 more will be any different?"

"Be honest with me—how is what you are doing now helping you?"

"You have accepted that your leg was amputated in the accident. Is it realistic to believe that nothing will be different in your future life?"

Have clients look at the bargains they have made in the past and evaluate how successful they have been. The underlying reality is not going to change.

Swapping beliefs approach. It is a well-accepted truism that when changing a behavior, we rarely stop one thing without starting something else. If we are eroding the client's unrealistic belief system, we need to be able to replace it with a new system of realistic and rational beliefs or the client will be left with nothing to believe in.[10] The best method to achieve the establishment of the new beliefs is to have the client actively participate in their development. Again, using reflective and thought-provoking questions is the key to the process. For example, "You've told me that seeing 25 more physicians is not going to help. What do you feel would be a better way to approach how you feel about the treatments?" "Identifying that skipping treatments to avoid the discomfort is a major step forward. Talk to me about what you believe the treatments can do for you that is positive," or "Tell me what you think will change if you let go of the illogical beliefs and begin to work with your new set of beliefs."

Practice and repetition approach. Once the client has developed a new set of behaviors to replace bargaining behaviors, these need to be practiced and reinforced.[6] It is very easy for them to slip back into bargaining behaviors, and these behaviors need to be identified immediately. The client will also likely recognize them. For example, "I'll take the medication if you let me finish my lunch first and let it digest." Nurse: "Do you recognize what you just did?" Client: "I guess I'm bargaining again. I know that medication needs to be taken with meals."

Repetition is an essential element in learning. By repeating the nonbargaining behaviors that the client has developed, they will soon become accepted and second nature. However, in letting go of the protective bargaining behavior, the client may begin to experience increased anxiety, anger, and sorrow.

Depression

As the client's stack of bargaining chips continues to dwindle and he or she comes to the full realization of the severity of the illness, the discomfort and length of the treatments, and how the illness is going to affect their future, they may slip into feelings of emptiness and sadness. It is important to keep in mind that grief depression is not a mental illness or clinical condition. Rather, it's a natural response to the loss of independence, control, self-esteem, and, to some degree, hope that the client is experiencing from their illness or injury.

The client must experience the emotions of frustration, sadness, bitterness, self-pity, regret, pain, loss, emptiness, despair, yearning, grief, and sadness that are associated with this type of depression in order to move on to the acceptance stage. It might be helpful to think of it as anger that is being internalized. As they go through the bereavement and mourning process, they may cry frequently and feel emotionally out of control. The client may again experience feelings of guilt and remorse that started in the bargaining stage. They take little or no pleasure in most activities of their day. There is no "normal" time span for the depression stage, but these clients are very close to resolving their grief because they are accepting the reality of their condition.[14] A depressed mood can also be caused by certain medical conditions such as hypothyroidism, or a side effect of some medications such as antihypertensive or certain medical treatments.

Grief-stage depression symptoms can imitate the symptoms of clinical depression at times. The dividing line between the two types of depression is blurry at best, but there are several symptoms that are fairly certain indicators of clinical depression. Clients in a clinically depressed state usually experience a long-term deep state of depression that lasts more than 2 months. The depression interferes significantly with these clients' activities of daily living, and they begin expressing thoughts of suicide, hopelessness, or worthlessness. They can no longer fulfill their daily responsibilities; these clients must be referred quickly to a professional for evaluation.[9]

As with the other stages of grief, there are verbal indicators that the client is experiencing grief depression. These statements include, "I just feel so sad; I don't want to do anything," "I just don't have the energy to get out of bed today," "Why bother? It's not that important," "I'll probably die soon, so what's the point?" "I can't do much of anything I want anymore, so why go on?" and "Just go away; you don't need to be wasting your time on me." The paraverbal indicators include slow, low tone speech and long pauses after you ask them a question before they answer. Nonverbal indicators include apathy, lack of eye contact, slouched posture, and slow body movements.

> " *The client must experience the emotions of frustration, sadness, bitterness, self-pity, regret, pain, loss, emptiness, despair, yearning, grief, and sadness that are associated with this type of depression in order to move on to the acceptance stage.* "

One of the keys in communicating with a client in the stage of depression is to let them talk and not interrupt. Because their thinking is slowed down and they have difficulty making decisions, their speech is often slow and sometimes disjointed with long pauses. There is a tendency for the nurse to jump in and either finish the client's sentences or respond to half of what he or she is trying to say. It takes practice and patience to maintain a conversation with a client displaying depressive behaviors. Active listening for the underlying emotions the client is expressing and reflecting those back or asking about them can help continue the conversation.[1] It is important that clients exhibiting depressed behaviors talk about their feelings as a way of resolving them. For example:

Nurse: "Ms. Daisy, are you awake? It's time for your medication." (Long pause)

Ms. Daisy: "I'm feeling so tired; I don't think I can take it."

Nurse: "It seems like today has been a hard day for you. I'd probably feel tired if I'd been through what you have. What did you find particularly tiring?" (Long pause)

Ms. Daisy: "Going for those radiation treatments always wipes me out. And my family . . ." Nurse: "Your family visited you today?" (Long pause)

Ms. Daisy: "I shouldn't complain; they mean well. But they sit around and yak and yak and yak and then argue about stupid things. They're always messing around with my bed and blankets and trying to get me to drink this awful-tasting water. I don't get a minute of rest. They just don't understand what I'm going through."

Nurse: "It is a lot to deal with—having cancer, being stuck in the hospital, all the uncomfortable treatments. People who haven't been through it never really appreciate how taxing it is."

Ms. Daisy: "I'm beginning to wonder if any of these treatments are really working at all."

Nurse: "When you think of that possibility, what worries you most?"

Ms. Daisy: "I guess I'm most afraid of all the pain I'm going to have to go through if the treatments don't work. And I'm not really happy about the thought of dying and leaving all the things I want to do unfinished."

Nurse: "Tell me how you feel when you think of those things."

Clients in the depression stage of grief do not have as obvious difficult behaviors as the other stages. The primary behaviors that make communicating with clients in the depressed stage difficult are their tendency to withdraw from personal relationships and to avoid interacting with others. They may refuse to see visitors and spend much of the time sleeping, crying, and grieving. These behaviors allow the client to temporarily disconnect from the emotions of love and affection. It is an important time for grieving that must be processed before he or she can move on. These clients often are preoccupied with brooding about their condition and ruminating about what they believe they will lose in the future. They hang on to memories of their past life and daydream about what they might have done differently.

Depressed clients often get labeled as "good clients" because they hardly ever put on their call lights, are not demanding, and tend to be compliant with the nurses' requests. Nurses spend more time with clients who are demanding and have their lights on all the time, and clients in the depression stage are left alone except when it is time for medications or vital signs. Staying away from these clients because they are not asking for anything does not meet their needs, nor is it good nursing care.

There are few serious physiological threats to clients in the depression stage of grief. A decrease in appetite and refusal to eat due to the depression may lead to weight loss, but the nausea often associated with chemotherapy or radiation therapy may also cause weight loss. Because all depression has an anxiety component, they may experience insomnia or restlessness and may pace. Probably the most serious physiological consequence of grief-stage depression is suppression of the immune system, which makes the client more susceptible to any number of infections, such as respiratory infections, wound infections, and urinary tract infections.[6] They have a tendency to remain immobile and can begin to experience skin breakdown. Depression can hurt physically, and it's not unusual for them to experience muscle and joint soreness and pain, particularly if they do not get out of bed or even turn in bed frequently. They may also experience a decrease in their pulse rate and blood pressure.

The three primary goals that we have for clients in this stage are (1) preventing physiological injury of the client, (2) allowing the client to speak about feelings and concerns, and (3) helping the client cope successfully with the reality of the changes brought on by the illness or injury without experiencing the accompanying sadness and grief.

> " *Probably the most serious physiological consequence of grief-stage depression is suppression of the immune system, which makes the client more susceptible to any number of infections, such as respiratory infections, wound infections, and urinary tract infections.* "

Approaches

Observe and encourage. Clients in the depression stage of grief need to be observed closely for refusal to eat and weight loss, signs of infections anywhere, skin breakdown, and extremely low heart rates and blood pressures. Asking the dietician to consult with the client can help with selections of food that the client may prefer to eat. Also, staying with the client and using encouragement during meal time, rather than just dropping the tray off and moving on, is also highly effective.[5] Also, bath time is an excellent time to assess them for skin breakdown and signs of infections. Assess their lungs thoroughly for abnormal or adventitious lung sounds. A real challenge is to keep them mobile. Getting them out of bed into a chair can be a major undertaking; however, keeping them mobile is one of the best ways to prevent respiratory infection and skin breakdown.

Although unlikely with grief depression, if the client expresses any thoughts of suicide, a more direct approach must be used. For example, if the client says, "My life is so worthless—I might as well end it all," the nurse can say, "How long have you thinking about hurting yourself? How would you do it?" If the client provides specific answers to these questions, then it is time for professional psychiatric intervention.

Prompt and suggest. One thing that makes communicating with depressed clients a little different is that they tend to be more receptive to gentle prompting and suggestions than clients in the other stages. They often have some difficulty in making decisions, so offering them choices such as, "Do you want to take your medications now or later?" does not work well for them. However, if you make a suggestion in a quiet, calm, and firm voice, the client is very likely to be receptive to prompting. For example: "Ms. Daisy, it is time to take your medication. Here is a glass of juice and the pills are in this medicine cup. Please take them. Thank you."

What if the client doesn't want to do something? Unless it's a definite refusal, as we saw with the client in the denial or anger stages, using a prompting approach is usually effective with the client in the depressive stage. For example: If the client says, "I really feel miserable today. I don't think I can go through with chemotherapy," the nurse can say, "I can see that you are more upset today than usual and probably want to talk about it. But I also get the feeling that you realize you need the chemotherapy treatment. Let's just have you go today and do the treatment and then when you are done, we can talk about what is bothering you."

Explain and support. Some clients who are in this stage will ask you, "I just feel so sad all the time and cry at the smallest thing. Why can't I seem to be happy anymore?" Although it is pretty obvious to us that the client is in the depression stage, some of them do not realize that it is a normal part of the grief process. This is an excellent opening to do some teaching about why they feel this way and what they can do to move on to acceptance. For example, "I know that you are feeling very confused by your emotions now. You are experiencing some depression because you are beginning to accept that your life may be permanently changed by your illness. It is actually a good sign that you are feeling this way because these feelings you are having now will soon become more manageable. You are a strong person, and I can help you use your inner strengths to feel better."

However, even if the client does not provide an opening for teaching, you need to do it anyway. A lead-in statement you can use is, "You are probably wondering why you cry so much and feel sad. You are experiencing a type of depression that most clients with your illness experience. It is due to . . ."

Life's reality. One thing to keep in mind is that attempting to cheer up these clients or make them happier is probably not going to be successful. Statements like, "Cheer up! It's a great day outside!" or "Stop crying so much; it isn't good for you!" may only worsen the way they feel. They really do not need to interact with cheery, jolly people at this time. Our goal is not to make them laugh, get them to stop crying, or take away their sadness at that moment; the real goal is to have them reconcile what has happened to them with a realistic view of

their future life. To move on from the depression stage, they must adjust their perception from what they have lost of their past lives to what positive things their future holds for them. The important task for you is to allow them to feel your caring presence, concern for them, and willingness to help them deal with their feelings.[7]

Building coping responses. Clients in depression often are unable to summon the energy to build coping strategies on their own. It just requires too much effort for them. Providing them with an opportunity to share their fears and sadness with the nurse makes the client more receptive to teaching and information to help them build their coping skills. Together, the nurse and client will be able to work toward developing an effective repertoire of coping responses. Some techniques that can be effective are slow, deep breathing; visualization exercises (thinking of a place where they feel safe and free from pain); and muscle-relaxation techniques.

The nurse can also help the client to see events and situations from a different perspective or find alternative ways of thinking about them. For example: If the client says, "I know the radiation therapy is frying all my blood cells," the nurse can say, "It's frightening to think that it's killing off all your blood cells, but a different way to think about it is that the radiation is killing off the bad cells and making room for your new blood cells to grow."

> **"** *Depressed clients will often tell you the same thing over and over again, but each time they express these feelings, they are peeling away a layer of grief much as you peel an onion when you cook.* **"**

Peel away the layers. Much like working with clients who are experiencing post-traumatic stress disorder (PTSD), clients in the stage of depression use talking about their feelings to relieve the sadness, anxiety, and stress they are experiencing. They feel a sense of relief in sharing their burden with another. Depressed clients will often tell you the same thing over and over again, but each time they express these feelings, they are peeling away a layer of grief much as you peel an onion when you cook. Eventually, they will get to a point where they can acknowledge how the illness or injury is going to affect their lives without the accompanying feelings of anxiety, sadness, and loss of control.

Medication maybe. The experts on treating depression disagree on whether to use antidepressants for clients with grief-stage depression. Antidepressants do not treat the underlying problems of depression; they only help relieve the symptoms. Some think that the medications may actually postpone the mourning process that the client needs to go through to achieve acceptance.

Selective serotonin reuptake inhibitors (SSRIs) are one of the most widely and commonly used medications to treat mild depression. They work by increasing the serotonin levels in the synapses and have relatively few side effects as compared with the antidepressants used to treat moderate to severe clinical depression. Some clients may have been taking these medications prior to the illness and were taken off of them when they began treatment. Stopping them suddenly can have a rebound effect where they experience more depression than if they had never been on them. They need to restart taking them as soon as they can. Otherwise, generally it is best to avoid antidepressant use in clients with grief-stage depression.[10]

Acceptance

As the layers of depression fall away, the client will gradually move to a mental state where they are willing to accept and to move on with their changed lives. Acceptance does not mean that the client is cured or that they've forgotten about what happened to them. What happened to them will always be a part of their makeup for the rest of their lives, and some days they will feel it more acutely than other days. Being in the acceptance stage means that they are willing to deal with the future and are willing to accommodate the changes wrought by the illness. Acceptance is not a period of happiness and joy but rather a state of calm and peace that comes from coming to terms with the reality they are facing. Often clients will feel a sense of strength in knowing that they have succeeded in getting past their sense of loss of control and loss of self-esteem and can now make sense of how their lives will be.

People in the acceptance stage may use statements such as, "I'm at peace with what is happening to me," "I'm going to fight this disease with everything I've got," "It was a rough few months, but I think I'm going to be okay," or "I guess the world isn't going to end today for me." All of these indicate that they have decided to not let life and its experiences pass them by. Rather they want to participate in life and the decisions that affect them and others.

Non-Grief-Stage Difficult Behaviors

There are some difficult behaviors that are not necessarily related to the stages of grief or Maslow's developmental stages, and they can be expressed by both coworkers and clients.

Inappropriate sexual behavior. Reporting and talking about inappropriate sexual behaviors by celebrities and politicians have become a media spectator sport in recent years. There seems to be no shortage of characters who are willing to display their indiscretions on multiple forms of social media. However, in the health-care setting, inappropriate sexual behavior on the part of either coworkers or clients is harmful to the individuals who are targets of it and decrease the quality of care.

Coworker behavior. Inappropriate sexual behavior or speech on the part of a coworker is really a form of bullying (see Chapter 16 for more detail). Individuals who use it in the workplace are attempting to coerce or influence their coworkers using this behavior. Although it may use sexual content, usually the underlying issues involve elements of controlling others or humiliating others because of feelings of powerlessness, inadequacy, or low self-esteem.[5] The person using sexual harassment has many of the same personality traits as the persecutor discussed earlier.

Workers are now legally protected from sexual harassment, and institutions are required to have written polices about it in their employee manuals. Although the definitions vary slightly from state to state, sexual harassment is generally defined as any unwelcomed sexual advances, requests for favors, or any other verbal or physical behavior of a sexual nature that creates an offensive working environment.[6]

Initially these laws were very strictly enforced, and since the decision of whether or not an offensive work environment existed was determined solely by the perceptions of the person being offended, many individuals had their reputations ruined by inadvertent comments or accidental incidents. It was a backlash to many years of real sexual harassment, particularly on the part of physicians toward female nurses. New graduate nurses often heard, "Oh, that's the way old Dr. Smut usually refers to us. You'll get used to it." It was also frequently used against male professors by female students who disliked the grade they earned.

Recent legal cases of sexual harassment have taken a more common-sense approach to deciding whether statements or actions are creating an offensive work environment. However, if a nurse or anyone employed in a health-care setting really believes that a coworker is displaying sexually inappropriate behavior, he or she should first keep a complete record of the behavior with dates and times and what was done or said, and then contact human resources (HR). It is important to follow the facility's procedures for dealing with alleged sexual misbehavior to the letter; otherwise, the whole case may be invalidated.

Generally these policies start off with confronting the offender with a statement that their behavior is inappropriate and unwanted. For example, "Dr. Smut, I'm a professional nurse and my primary concern is caring for our clients. I feel demeaned and belittled by the way you refer to me and my body parts and do not appreciate the jokes you tell. Please stop doing this around me." However, you need to avoid retaliating with hostile and vengeful jokes that might inflame the situation. For example, "From what I've heard, the newborn babies in the nursery have bigger ones than you!" or "You're not man enough to handle what I've got!"

The second stage in the process is a meeting with the offender, HR, and you. It is always helpful to get support from other nurses who have been harassed. It is likely that the offender has become habitual in this type of behavior and uses it with almost everyone. The third stage usually requires a meeting with the medical or hospital board. If the issue is not resolved satisfactorily by that time, then it is appropriate to seek legal resolution.

Also keep in mind that nurses and other health-care workers in units that experience client tragedies on a regular basis such as the emergency department, intensive care units, and burn units will sometimes use what is called "gallows humor" or "black humor" to reduce the emotional impact of what they are experiencing. It acts as a buffer to painful situations the nurse experiences that otherwise might cause him or her to be unable to continue providing care. In some settings, gallows humor is seen as an expression of resilience that gives the people power over the heartbreaking events they are experiencing.

Newly graduated nurses and nursing students are often shocked when they first experience gallows humor in the clinical setting; however, it has probably been used as a coping mechanism since health care moved from the home to organized institutions. This does not excuse it or make it right, but gallows humor does serve its purpose on busy units where the beds literally do not cool off between clients. Nurses on these units are not afforded the luxury of time to grieve or cry for a client to whom they have become close; rather they must take care of the next seriously ill client coming through the doors. Sometimes the gallows humor contains a sexual component, but unless extreme, it is not considered sexual harassment.

Client behavior. Inappropriate client sexual behavior creates a dilemma for nurses. Nurses must walk a fine line between protecting themselves and providing quality care. However, what most nurses don't know is that federal and some state laws protect them from sexual harassment by clients, and these laws should be reflected, or at least referenced, in the employee manual. Unfortunately, nursing students receive little education on dealing with clients who sexually harass nurses, and there are very few continuing education programs on the topic for the working nurse.

> *What most nurses don't know is that federal and some state laws protect them from sexual harassment by clients, and these laws should be reflected, or at least referenced, in the employee manual.*

Sexual behavior from clients may be related to a stage of grief, particularly anger, but is more typically a form of behavior that is used by clients experiencing anxiety. This behavior is disturbing, increases job-related stress for the nurse, can make the nurse feel humiliated and objectified, and can decrease the quality of care, It can also destroy the nurse-client trust that is essential to quality care.

Clients with mental illnesses or who are diagnosed with dementia or who have brain damage or surgery may not be able to grasp the consequences of their actions or statements and therefore cannot be held legally responsible for them. Medications that have neurological effects may lower client inhibitions, and they will say and do things that they would be horrified doing without the effects of the medications.[9] These conditions create a unique situation for nurses because these clients may not respond to the usual approaches used for dealing with sexual harassment.

Although overt physical sexual assaults are rare from clients, the American Nurses Association (ANA) reports that over 60 percent of nurses have experienced some type of sexual misbehavior from clients, ranging from being called "honey" or "babe" to enduring jokes with sexual content to even unwanted touching.[13] The vast majority of this behavior is against female nurses, although male nurses also occasionally experience unwanted sexual advances.

Nurses tend to avoid these clients, entering their rooms only when absolutely necessary and skipping tasks such as physical assessments, or they may call in sick to avoid providing care for the client. Other nurses will grudgingly provide physical care, but emotional aspects of the care decline. The client will be labeled and his quality of care will decrease. So, how do you effectively approach a client with inappropriate sexual behavior without compromising care?

Approaches

Laugh and deny. Over time, some nurses build up a "resistance" to clients' sexual misbehavior. They often blame it on the client's age, illness, or confused state. They may not even consider the behavior to be sexual harassment. They tend to "laugh it off" as another unpleasant aspect of their profession. However, this is not really the most effective approach. It may work for some nurses, but by ignoring the behavior, they have not taken any positive actions to resolve the issue.

Confront gently. There is always the temptation to respond to these clients with vengeful remarks or jokes. As with the coworker, this is not an effective method in dealing with sexual misbehavior. It is important to speak honestly to the client about what they are doing or saying and how it makes you feel. Sharp retorts such as, "Knock off the jokes," or "It's really inappropriate to display yourself like that when people are around" will usually only exacerbate the behavior. It does not deal with the underlying causes. The behavior may be adaptive for the client and may have developed over a long period of time.

Confronting the client gently but firmly may alter the behavior.[34] If nothing else, it lets the client know you are not pleased with the sexual behavior. For example, you can say, "Mr. Blue, I appreciate the fact that you are not feeling well; however, I feel like you are putting me down and disrespecting me every time you tell one of those jokes or pat my bottom when I'm near the bed. I would really appreciate it if you would stop when I'm in the room." This action by the nurse may make interactions with the client tenser for a while because it creates uncomfortable feelings.

Digging deeper. As mentioned above, the discomfort caused by these clients' behavior often causes nurses to overlook the underlying emotional issues that may be causing the behavior. Rather than ignoring the client or running away when they say something sexually inappropriate, the nurse can use some of the communication builders to help the client recognize why they are behaving this way.[1] The nurse can say, "Mr. Blue, I am very uncomfortable being referred to by that name; however, I realize you are concerned about your heart catheterization tomorrow. When people have high levels of anxiety, they often say things that help them relieve the tension. I'd really like to hear about what you fear most about going for the test tomorrow."

The ANA approach. The ANA has been very emphatic over the years that the work setting be free from sexual harassment from either coworkers or clients. They have developed a four-step approach to dealing with clients who display sexually inappropriate behavior.[13]

Step 1: Confrontation of the offender, which is similar to the "confront gently" approach discussed above; however, the ANA recommends that the nurse leave no room for misinterpretation of what is being said. They insist that the nurse keep the relationship with clients professional at all times by addressing them as Mr., Mrs., or Ms. For example, "Mr. Blue, I respect you as a client who is here to receive care, and I expect that you will treat me as the professional that I am. Please address me as Ms. Locke and not by the foul names you've been using."

In addition, the ANA believes that clients should be aware that there are potential legal consequences for their sexual harassment behaviors. Although not widely known by nurses, there are laws that permit hospitals to transfer a client to another facility if they persist in sexual harassment behaviors. They suggest that the nurse inform the client of the laws associated with sexual harassment. For example, "Mr. Blue, I have asked you nicely several times to stop with the sexual jokes and crude names. The hospital has strict rules about the type of behavior you are displaying, and if you don't stop it immediately, you will be discharged from this facility immediately." Clients in a clinic or outpatient setting are legally required to be given 30 days before they can be dismissed from care.

Step 2: Notify the supervisor of the harassment. This is an important step in the process because when the employer is informed of client sexual harassment of nurses, it becomes their responsibility to do something about it. Employers have become extremely sensitized to sexual harassment issues, and they realize that if nothing is done, they can become involved in a lawsuit from an employee. This often spurs employers to provide more continuing education programs for nurses on sexual harassment from clients and to develop policies and procedures for sexual harassment from clients if they do not already exist.

Step 3: Careful documentation. It is important to keep a record of exactly what the client said and did, what the nurse did in response, and how the client responded to the response. The date and time also need to be documented. This is best done immediately after the incident while it is fresh in the nurse's mind.

Step 4: Involve others. Coworkers on the unit probably have similar experience with the client because the behavior is not targeted to just one person. They can help in developing successful tactics in dealing with the client behavior so that everyone will be consistent in the approach to the client. Inconsistency tends to increase the inappropriate behavior. Having one or two other nurses beside you when you interact with the client may help dampen the inappropriate speech or behavior, and they can serve as witnesses to exchanges. Make sure to include their names in the documentation. The nurse can also seek support from organizations such as the state's nursing organization or even the state board of nursing.[13]

Complaining and Whining Behaviors

One of the most common, if not most annoying, types of difficult person is the constant complainer and whiner. To complain means to verbally express unhappiness or dissatisfaction with a person, place, or thing. The strict definition of "whine" is to make a high-pitched, unpleasant sound that indicates discontent, pain, or unhappiness, often made by infants; in the colloquial usage, it means complaining about something that the person can't or doesn't want to expend the effort to fix, often in a high-pitched voice. The two words *complain* and *whine* are often used in conjunction with each other because they mean basically the same thing.

Everyone knows about the "glass half full and the glass half empty" division of personalities. The glass-half-full people are the optimists who see the positive aspects of life and their situation and attempt to make the best of them. The glass-half-empty people are the pessimists who see the negative aspects of their lives and situations and resign themselves to the idea that they are just going to have to tolerate it. The third type of personality is the "there's nothing at all in the glass" individual, who sees his or her life, work, other people, and the whole world as a black hole of existence. There is nothing good at all, and they are going to let you know about it often and convincingly. They express themselves in chronic complaining and chronic whining.

Causes of Complaining and Whining

The reality is that everyone complains at times as a way to reduce stress, lessen the impact of unpleasant news, and identify areas of concern. These types of complaints are sometimes referred to as *sporadic* because they deal with just one short-term issue or as *constructive complaining* because they are useful in focusing attention on and resolving issues the person is facing.[36] They bring difficult situations to light and allow the person to focus on the resolution of the problem and the opportunity to make right something that is wrong or unfair.

Nurses experience complainers and whiners in the health-care setting as bosses, coworkers, and clients. There are many similarities among the groups, including the reasons why bosses, coworkers, and clients complain and whine to express themselves and the approaches to dealing with them. In the discussion below, the groups are not separated as they were in previous sections because of the similarities. The differences in the care of clients will be pointed out when appropriate. As with other types of difficult behavior, complaining and whining meet some need or achieve some goal that the person has. Often it is used to manipulate others, achieve some type of reward, avoid a troubling situation, or increase their sense of control.

One of the most common underlying reasons that cause people to complain excessively is because their lives have not met the expectations they had for themselves when they were younger. The vision of the things that could have been remains in their memories, but the realities of their present lives are a constant reminder of how short they have fallen. They live in a continual state of disappointment with themselves, their circumstances, and the people around them.[7] They are truly unhappy and use complaining and whining as an expression of their unhappiness with the world.

Many people who excessively complain and whine have a pervading sense that life has not treated them justly. You will often hear from them statements like, "It's so unfair. I work my butt off every day, save every penny I can, and scrape by and have nothing while they sit back and the money rolls in." The underlying emotion leading to these feelings is a lack of control over their lives. This feeling of lack of control is often closely associated with jealousy. Although it is difficult for them to admit, they resent the fact that someone else has something they do not. They might say something like, "How come Betty gets to buy a new car and I don't? She's so selfish; she probably never gives anything to charity." Complaining is a mechanism they can use to gain back some feeling that they are in control again.

A belief and feeling that other people do not appreciate them, understand them, or empathize with them causes some people to complain. Basically they are expressing low self-esteem and "I'm a born loser" self-concept. They might express this feeling by complaining: "You never do anything the right way! You should do it the way I do it because it's much quicker and better than what you are doing now." They believe that others cannot put themselves in their shoes and see things as they see them because they lack empathy for them. No one really understands or appreciates what they are thinking or the other difficulties they have to deal with in their lives. Complaining and whining, they believe, will help others appreciate them more.

> " *One of the most common underlying reasons that cause people to complain excessively is because their lives have not met the expectations they had for themselves when they were younger.* "

They may also complain about feeling left out of important activities or being treated as a second-rate person when someone is selected over them for an important task or position. These complaints usually indicate that they are experiencing a type of anxiety similar to what a child experiences when they are brought to day care for the first time. Complaining makes them feel more dominant or mature when in reality they really feel just the opposite.[9]

People who use complaining to gain power often use the complaining much as the persecutor uses bullying tactics to get what they want. Often these individuals may appear very congenial and cooperative on the outside, but when there is something they really want, like a promotion or to achieve a specific personal goal, they use the complaining and whining to manipulate and harass their targets. They have no regard for how the other person feels and can make the whole work environment toxic to personnel and successful outcomes. They don't accept any excuses for someone getting in their way and often display narcissistic behavior. They are only concerned about achieving their goals and use complaining and whining to torment others until they get what they want.

Effects of Complaining and Whining

Much like the sneak, the chronic complainer loves to keep the pot stirred up and boiling at work. They love to watch the drama and chaos they have created and particularly enjoy observing how their coworkers become irritated and disheartened. Unfortunately, chronic complaining is contagious and chronic complainers may seek out other chronic complainers to commiserate with them. However, at a certain point, complainers and whiners will begin to complain and whine about other complainers and whiners. They seem to recognize the behavior in others as irritating but can't see it in themselves.

Some studies have shown that even after just 30 minutes of listening to someone complain, the neurotransmitter levels in the brain are altered enough to cause memory loss and even permanent brain damage.[10] Even for people who are generally happy, spending too much time around chronic complainers can make it hard to remember all the good that still exists in life. A group of complainers together can make the whole workplace environment toxic.

Chronic complaining destroys relationships and lowers the morale in the workplace. In the health-care setting, it drains the energy out of the staff and decreases the overall quality of care. It creates an intense focus on only the negative issues and even reverses positive aspects of the job. Complaining makes people upset, aggravated, and generally annoyed. People who want to remain positive and provide high-quality care soon become tired of trying to ignore the negativity; it increases their stress levels way beyond what they would normally experience with their daily care activities. Nurses who try to maintain a positive attitude feel very relieved to leave work and go home at the end of the day to get away from the complaining and whining, but because they know what is coming the next day, they dread going back to work.

In facilities where there is a culture of complaining and whining, there also tends to be a higher than average turnover rates of nurses.[5] Nurses would rather quit and move to another facility that has a more positive atmosphere than deal with all the negativity where they are. These optimistic nurses may become depressed because no matter how hard they work, it never seems to be good enough for the chronic complainer. The awful truth is that even one person who continually complains can single-handedly change the atmosphere of a work environment and bring a screeching halt to the productivity of an otherwise highly cohesive nursing unit.

Types of Complaining and Whining Behaviors

Most people can recognize when someone is complaining or whining about something that bothers them, but there are several varieties of this type of behavior. As with the other difficult behaviors, there is considerable overlap between the types of complaining behavior.

Duck-and-cover behavior. Some complainers have become adept at disguising their complaints by intertwining them with real problems so that it is difficult to separate the two. Because they believe they cannot fix the problem themselves, they try to place the responsibility for both the problem and its solution on another person. For example, "It's such a pain to have to document every word we say to these clients. You're the one who suggested it at the last staff meeting, so why don't you do something about it?"

Bulldozer behavior. These complainers want action and to accomplish goals. They use aggressive complaining to manipulate others to achieve their objectives. For example, "No one wants to help me get the stuff ready for the holiday party. I guess I'll just call the whole thing off and chalk it up to your lack of interest in the unit. No wonder we have low morale around here."

Wet blanket behavior. These individuals take negativity to new lows. In their attempts to gain control and manipulate a situation, they will use negative comments and complaints to dampen everyone else's attitudes. They rarely have any good ideas of their own and much prefer to sow seeds of disappointment and failure. At a meeting about a unit project, they would say, "Joe, that's a stupid idea. We tried that in the past, and it was a miserable failure. Why should we waste our time trying it again? Sue, your idea isn't any better. I can name six reasons why it won't work! I can't believe you would even suggest that. I don't think this thing is ever going to get off the ground."

Beyond help behavior. Sometimes when people complain, it can appear that they are seeking help and support with a problem they are facing; however, they immediately reject the helping offer without even considering it. They believe the solution being offered is inappropriate or useless and that their problem is so severe or unique that there is nothing anyone could ever do to fix it.

The goal of their behavior is to gain attention and sympathy from other people, and they really do not want to solve the problem; if it does get solved, they'll find another one.[34] For example, a friend says, "That sounds like a serious problem. Something like that happened to me once and the way I solved it was by talking to my supervisor about it. Why don't you try that as a first step?" Complainer: "Oh, that'll never work. My problem is so much worse than yours and my supervisor is way too aloof to listen to me. I guess it's just another thing in my life that I'll have to live with."

Gossiping behavior. These people use complaining to make themselves look better, cover up their feelings of inadequacy and low self-esteem, and gain recognition or attention. Their tactics include interrupting others, bragging about their accomplishments, and throwing up roadblocks to progress. Some of their most effective behaviors include making unrealistic promises they can't keep and had no intention of keeping, using others as scapegoats, and taking the credit for another nurse's work. For example, "Sorry to interrupt, but, Ellen, you know that error was really your fault, not mine, and if I hadn't straightened it out as quickly and as well as I did, the whole unit would be in trouble now. No one is better dealing with these situations than me."

Needy behavior. By venting and then emotionally and/or physically withdrawing, these chronic complainers are seeking to gain the sympathy of others and develop some type of connection, even if it is dysfunctional. Often they will set up social or work situations where they intentionally fail so that they can become the victim. Being a victim is a role for which they were born and they revel in it.[9] For example, in front of a group they would say, "You have put me down for just about the last time! You couldn't have hurt my feelings more if you had called me a whore! I'm going to the break room and work on my charts and I want to be left alone."

> *By venting and then emotionally and/or physically withdrawing, these chronic complainers are seeking to gain the sympathy of others and develop some type of connection, even if it is dysfunctional.*

Toxic behavior. Although all chronic complaining is destructive to a workplace environment, some complainers are so unhappy with themselves and their lives that they use their behavior to purposely manipulate or poison the environment so everyone else will be as unhappy as them. This can be particularly devastating if the person using this toxic complaining behavior is the boss. They sometimes have secondary goals for their behaviors such as seeking a promotion or recognition rewards. They will attempt to falsely inflate others' perception of their skills and work hard to advance their own agenda. People who use this type of toxic behavior often will retaliate and seek revenge if they are contradicted or challenged. Toxic complaining can deeply torment fellow workers and devastate their emotional state.

Underlying their behaviors may be deep-seated, long-term personality disorders such as narcissism and even antisocial tendencies.[9] Toxic complainers seem to have no conscience or awareness of other peoples' needs or feelings and are totally focused on achieving their own goals. They have developed manipulation into an art form and use it to control situations and people. To your face they can be very supportive of your ideas, charming, and captivating while at the same time they are creating an emotionally lethal work environment.

They may employ any of the other types of complaining discussed above to take the focus off their own unhappiness and lack of knowledge and abilities. For example, while the nurses are still together after receiving shift report and waiting for their assignment, a toxic whiner would say, "Here we go again! Too many clients and not enough nurses. Don't they know we are all working as hard as we possibly can, and by not giving us extra help, they are killing our morale and spirit? I was so tired and my feet hurt so bad yesterday when I went home, I got in the bathtub and fell asleep for 3 hours! It looks like today is going to be a rerun of yesterday. And these clients we have to put up with. They're old, they're grumpy, they smell bad, they can't do anything for themselves, they complain all the time, and their call lights are always on. It's like pulling teeth to get them to do anything. And all the physicians do is bitch at us."

Approaches

One of our goals in approaching chronic complainers is to help them recognize that their behaviors are inappropriate and that expressing their needs by complaining is harmful to themselves and the work environment. Ultimately, we are trying to get them to accept the motto "If you can't say something positive, don't say anything at all!" Of course, once they do internalize this proverb, they may not be saying much of anything for a while.

Another goal is to help them change their perspectives about why they are complaining. Often people complain because they have little capacity for empathy. Primarily we are trying to get them to see from another person's viewpoint. If they can achieve any level of empathy at all and see other persons more positively, they will begin to think differently, have different expectations, and find better ways of handling things in their lives other than complaining.

A goal associated with both changing their perspective and encouraging empathy is to understand themselves better and understand why they have feelings of inadequacy. It is interesting that complainers hardly ever complain about themselves but very frequently compare themselves to others. Because they see the other person as being more intelligent, having better skills, and being more capable than they think they are, complainers are often attempting to bring the other people down to the level where they believe themselves to be.[10] If they can recognize that this is a form of jealously and can understand that they do not have a monopoly on feelings of inadequacy, they will begin to recognize that there are many people who would like to be in their position. They can then focus more on their own lives and what makes them happy.

The chronic complaining behavior observed in clients generally has the same causes and goals as complaining behavior seen in coworkers and responds to the same approaches. However, there are several exceptions when the complainer is a client. It's always important to listen carefully to the complaints of clients, even if they are chronic complainers.

Once a client is labeled as a chronic complainer, the tendency for busy nurses is to dismiss all their complaints as mere indications of an unhappy personality, and indeed, many of them are. However, if the complaints are different from the common complaints such as, "The food is always cold," "The nurses don't talk to me much," or "Why is this room so cold (or hot)," nurses should investigate them more closely. Although all clients' complaints about pain or discomfort need to be assessed, complaints about pain in locations where they haven't complained about pain before need a more thorough assessment. It is possible for a chronic complaining hospitalized client to have a heart attack or develop a kidney stone unexpectedly while they are in the hospital.

One group that requires an approach somewhat different from coworkers is the clients who are in the depression stage of grief. They may express that grief by complaining about almost anything and everything. Using the approaches discussed earlier for interacting with clients in the depression stage of grief will likely be more effective than the approaches listed below, although there are many similarities. Our primary goal for depressed clients is to move them on to the stage of acceptance.

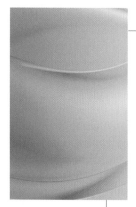

Issues in Practice

The Girl Who Cried Roach!

The incident described here really happened, but the location and some of the names have been changed to protect the innocent.

I had been pulled from the cardiac intensive care unit (ICU) to work on one of the medical-surgical units due to a low census in the ICU. My assignment that day included a 17-year-old girl who, while taking a test at school the day before, felt dizzy, had a "fluttering" in her chest accompanied by a feeling of pressure, and difficulty breathing. The school nurse took her blood pressure and obtained a reading of 72/58 (normally 108/64) with an irregular pulse of 167 (normally 75 and regular). The nurse called the girl's parents and the ambulance. By the time the paramedics arrived, the girl's blood pressure was 104/66 with a regular pulse of 80. After being connected to the cardiac monitor, they observed normal sinus rhythm with no dysrhythmias. However, because of the potential for reoccurring cardiac abnormalities, the girl was taken to the local hospital's emergency department (ED), where she was examined by the ED physician on staff with a consult from a cardiologist. Although she had no more episodes of rapid heart rate, the cardiologist wished to monitor her in the hospital for 24 hours.

Normally, a 17-year-old child would be admitted to the pediatric unit, but that unit was experiencing a highly contagious rotavirus outbreak, and they did not want to expose the girl to the infection. She had a cardiac telemetry unit, which is a portable radio transmitter about the size of a large cell phone, only thicker and heavier, connected by wires to electrodes on her chest that sent her heart pattern wirelessly to a room next to the ICU where monitor technicians watched it 24 hours a day for any irregularities. It allowed her complete mobility, and she was on activities as tolerated, which meant she could do pretty much anything she wanted in the hospital.

I usually was not assigned to female clients, but the charge nurse that day believed that because of my ICU experience, I was the best qualified to handle any emergency situations that might arise with the client. Her fast, irregular heart rate was a type of supraventricular tachycardia (SVT), known as *atrial fibrillation* (A-fib or atrial fib), where the atria of the heart become irritable and take over the pacemaker function from the heart's normal pacemaker, the SA node. Many things can cause this to happen, and it is fairly common and usually transient in teenage girls and young women; however, in elderly clients, it's often chronic and an indication of an underlying cardiac pathology. Causes include increased hormone levels as seen in teenagers, excitement, stress, and use of caffeine, tobacco, alcohol, stimulant street drugs, and a variety of prescription medications.

She was in a semiprivate room in the bed farthest away from the door, by the windows. When I went into the room, she was awake, sitting up and listening to her iPod. I introduced myself: "Good morning, Ms. Bennett. I'm Mr. Catalano and I'm going to be your RN today. How are—"

"Stop right there," she interrupted. "Mrs. Bennett is my mother's name. I'm just Julie."

"Okay, then," I answered. "Good morning, just Julie. I guess you can call me just Joe."

Issues in Practice _{continued}

I saw her start to smile; however, it stopped suddenly when she remembered Rule Number 3 of the Teenager's Handbook on Dealing With Adults: "Never let them know they're funny."

"How are you feeling this morning?" I asked.

"I feel great! When am I getting out of this dump?"

"Well, your cardiologist wanted to monitor you for 24 hours, and if there aren't any more episodes of what you had yesterday, you can go home, probably this afternoon or early evening. The monitor techs tell me everything has been normal since you came in. Have you felt anything like you had at school yesterday?"

"None at all, but these things stuck on my chest are starting to itch, and I kept getting tangled up in these wires last night and pulled them off a couple of times. They won't let me use my cell phone, and this hospital phone with the wire is an antique and doesn't seem to work half the time."

"We can move the electrodes to a different spot on your chest where it isn't itchy. The cell phones send out a signal that blocks the telemetry, so we don't let anyone use them here. I realize those wires are a pain, particularly when you're trying to sleep. How did you sleep last night anyway?"

"You've got to be kidding me, right? Sleep in this place? It was noisier than our band room at break time! It sounded like someone was banging a metal garbage can top against the wall. This one over here"—she pointed to the other client in the room—"snores like a freight train! And then there were the bugs running up and down the curtain all night."

Many teenagers are compulsive chronic complainers and use complaining like an orchestra conductor uses his baton. Complaints are a way to emphasize points, such as not being happy with a situation, and to enhance their expressions of disapproval, particularly of adults. I usually don't pay much attention to them, but when they sound unusual or relate to changes in physiological conditions such as pain or breathing, I tend to become curious. The bugs on the curtain complaint got my attention.

"On which curtain did you see the bugs?" I asked.

"This one here," she answered, pointing to the curtain that separated her bed from the client in the next bed. The curtain was a heavy fabric in pastel-colored stripes and was hung from a roller track on the ceiling so it could be pulled all the way around the bed for privacy. Usually, we just leave them pulled down to the foot of the bed.

"I think they were roaches. We had some under the sink at our new house when we moved in. My mom totally FREAKED OUT! She called the real estate agent who sold us the house and a bug guy was there in 15 minutes! Roaches make kind of a clicking sound when they move around, and I thought I heard that last night."

I assessed that Julie was alert and oriented to person, place, and time and did not appear to be experiencing the side effects of any types of medications that might cause confusion. Actually, she wasn't on any medications at all. So I pulled the curtain all the way open just to be sure and didn't see any bugs of any kind.

"There doesn't appear to be any here now," I observed.

(continued)

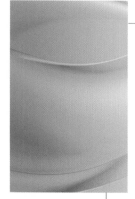

Issues in Practice continued

"Of course not. The lights are on and the sun is out," she noted. "Don't you know anything about roaches?"

"I can't remember any nursing classes covering that topic in nursing school," I inappropriately replied. "And maintenance sprays the whole hospital for bugs about once a month. But hang on a second, I just want to check something out."

I walked around the curtain and saw that the client in the bed by the door was a client I had seen several times in the ICU. It was Mrs. Perry, one of our "frequent fliers" (clients who are admitted to the hospital every month or so), who was 80-something and had difficulty seeing and hearing, but lived alone and was ferociously independent. She vehemently refused any kind of help with her own care or care of her living quarters. Unfortunately for her neighbors in the apartment building where she lived, she had severe self-care deficits and her apartment was known for its cluttered and malodorous condition. I had a strong feeling that some of her admissions were related to her living conditions, because I had heard from my friends who worked in client transport that when they returned her to her apartment after a hospitalization, it was better organized, much less cluttered, and had a lingering sent of Febreze filling the air.

"Hello, Mrs. Perry. How are you feeling today?" I asked her.

"I'm okay. Is that Joey?" (She always called me Joey because she had a son named Joe who was killed in World War II at Midway. I guess I reminded her of him.)

"Yes, Mrs. Perry," I replied. "You remembered me."

"I can't see or hear worth a flip, but my memory is like a steel trap," she replied, and then launched into the story about her Joey.

I let her talk for several minutes; then I interrupted her. "Mrs. Perry, I would like to take a look at your suitcase if you don't mind?" It was one of the old hard side suitcases like Julie Andrews carried in the *Sound of Music* when she left the convent, except Mrs. Perry's was a faded yellow color with travel stickers on it from all over the country. It was on the floor on the curtain side of the room.

"Why would you want to look at that old thing? There's nothing in it. I put all my clothes in the closet over by the sink yesterday when I came in."

"I just want to check something out," I said.

"Well okay, go ahead."

I crouched down next to her suitcase, flipped the two worn brass latches up, and carefully opened the lid about six inches. That's all I needed to see what I was afraid I would see. There were several hundred live and healthy roaches scurrying around in the bottom. I quickly but cautiously closed the lid and latched it. I went over to the sink and got a pair of rubber gloves out of the box and then got a red biohazard plastic bag from under the sink. I carefully slid the suitcase into the bag and double tied it.

"Mrs. Perry, I'm going to need to borrow your suitcase for a little while. Is that okay?" I asked her.

"Sure, Joey, anything you want. But why don't you buy yourself one of those nice new fancy ones with the wheels on it?"

"This one will be just fine, Mrs. Perry. I promise I'll bring it back later." I wasn't sure that was a promise I could keep.

Issues in Practice continued

I gingerly picked it up and carried it at arm's length to the nurses' station. Never having been in this situation before, I wasn't quite sure what to do with it, so I set it down on the edge of the nurses' station counter. Everyone was pretty used to seeing specimens in biohazard bags that needed to be taken to the lab, so they didn't really pay much attention to my little gift. It happened that the unit manager, who was a classmate of mine from nursing school, was in the hall.

"Hi, Joe," she said. "It's good to have you back over here working with us. Did you cure all the clients in the ICU? What's in the red bag there?"

"You're probably not going to believe this," I answered. "I wasn't sure what to do with it because I've never run across this problem before. It's Mrs. Perry's suitcase and it is full of roaches," I said quietly.

I watched the color in her face drain away.

"I'm not sure what to do with it either," she answered. "But we need to get it out of here, now! Fern (the unit clerk), call maintenance and get them up here right now to get rid of this. Tell them it's an emergency!"

Surprisingly, three men from the maintenance department were there within about 5 minutes. We took them to an empty room and explained the situation. They said that their policy and procedure manual actually had a protocol for this. One of them picked up the red bag with the suitcase in it, and all three of them left. I wasn't sure what they were going to do with it. I was thinking incineration, but the suitcase reappeared in Mrs. Perry's room later that afternoon, a little more faded with a distinct chemical odor. I really had no desire to open it again.

"We really need to get the clients out of that room," I said.

"There is an empty private room across the hall where Julie can go, and we can put Mrs. Perry in the isolation room across the hall from the nurses' station," explained the unit manager.

I headed back to Julie's room and found her listening to her music again.

"Julie, we're going to move you to another room. Grab your makeup case and electronics and put on your shoes, okay?"

"What about my clothes?"

"I'll bring them to you later. Actually, it might be better if you call your mother and tell her to bring you some fresh clothes to go home in." We walked across the hall to the private room and got her settled in. I headed back to her old room to help with Mrs. Perry. When I got to the room, Mrs. Perry's nurse had a wheelchair next to the bed, and Mrs. Perry had a death grip with both hands on the bedrail that was still up.

"I like this room. I'm not going to go to another room!" Mrs. Perry shouted.

I walked around to the side of the bed she was facing and said, "Mrs. Perry, is there a problem here?"

"Joey, I'm glad you're back. This nurse here wants me to go to another room and won't tell me why. And she's trying to make me ride in a wheelchair. I'm not a cripple. I CAN WALK BY MYSELF!" she said emphatically.

"Well, Mrs. Perry, it's like this. You've always been such a good client for us when you come in; we wanted to put you in a nicer room. Think of it like an upgrade in a hotel when you used to travel. And you don't have to use the

(continued)

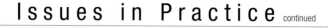

Issues in Practice continued

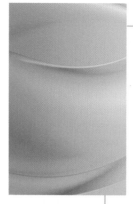

wheelchair. I can walk with you to your new room, you know, like we used to walk together in the ICU?"

"An upgrade? I didn't know hospitals did that. I used to love upgrades when I traveled with my husband. We were in Las Vegas one time and . . . ," she launched into her Vegas story of at least 40 years ago. I actually hadn't heard this one and was kind of interested in what she had to say, but I interrupted her again.

"Mrs. Perry, I really want to hear about Las Vegas, but can I hear the rest of the story after we get you to your new room?"

"Oh sure, let's go!" She was very spry for her age and walked by herself after we got her shoes on. Now, I know you're not supposed to lie to clients because it destroys the trusting relationship. However, if you rationalize it enough, I really wasn't lying, much. The room she was going to was actually better than her old room. She had her own TV, which she couldn't see anyway, and the room had some unique features, like negative airflow and a second big sink by the door. It was larger than her old room and had a full-size rocking recliner where she could sit comfortably. Most importantly, the approach her nurse was using wasn't working at all, and we had to get her out of that room.

A few minutes later, the three maintenance men reappeared. Two of them had Level C hazardous material (hazmat) suits on (see Chapter 25 for more detail) and were carrying a fogger and a 3-gallon spray can. The third man had on his regular blue maintenance department uniform and carried a roll of plastic sheeting and a roll of duct tape. The two with the suits and sprayers went into the room. They bagged up Julie's and Mrs. Perry's clothes in biohazard bags. They also bagged all the linens, towels, and wash clothes that were in the room in biohazard bags. Everything else was thrown away, in biohazard bags of course. A special biohazard laundry cart with a cover was brought to the unit, and all the laundry was sent for washing, no doubt in scalding hot water and undiluted chlorine bleach. I don't think Julie will ever be able to fit into that pair of jeans again.

After they were out of the room, they closed the door and the man without the hazmat suit proceeded to tape the sheet of plastic around the doorjamb. When the other two were finished spraying, they pulled back the plastic just enough so they could duck out and then sealed the room again. A sign was put on the plastic sheet: "Do Not Enter for 48 Hours."

Julie went home later that day and had no more episodes of SVT. The nurse manager called the super at Mrs. Perry's apartment and told him what we had found. When Mrs. Perry went home 2 days later, her apartment had a strong chemical odor and was cleaner than usual.

So what are the lessons to be learned from this incident? I think there are two important ones: First, listen to your clients! When they talk to you, they usually have something to say, although it may be difficult for them to explain it and in may take some time, it's always worth listening. Second, Don't totally disregard chronic complainers. If the complaint sounds strange or is about something physiological, it needs to be investigated more thoroughly.

Under the best circumstances, it is difficult to change complaining behavior. It is behavior that the person likely began using as a young child to gain recognition and attention and manipulate the parents into giving them what they want. Because of the rewards they have received from this behavior, they will be very reluctant to give it up for more adultlike behavior. However, because it is so toxic to the work environment, it must be addressed and dealt with at some point.[5] The approaches listed below can be effective in altering behavior to a degree, but don't get discouraged if the chronic complainer continues to complain at times. At least it is an improvement.

The empathy approach. As it did with several of the approaches for other types of difficult behavior, active listening can also work with the complainer if combined with a response that acknowledges their problems. After they finish talking, say to them, "Wow, that sounds really awful. I can't imagine how you handle all those problems without going crazy. I'm sure I couldn't do it." Make sure you are genuinely sympathetic and not patronizing. Many complainers are looking for someone who understands them as a person, but because of their constant complaining, people tend to avoid them. Quite frequently they will reply, "Yes, but it's not really *that* bad and I'm handling it okay!" For this approach to work, you do need to be sincere and avoid any hint of sarcasm.

Also remember you're not really agreeing with the complainer that their problem is worse than anyone else's or that it is so big it can never be solved. You're just acknowledging the fact that this is a problem for that person, which it is.

Break the vicious cycle approach. This is similar to the first approach, and like the first one it may not completely stop the complainer from complaining. Be patient with the person and respond realistically to their complaints. For example, the complainer says, "You know, this job is really boring. I just do the same thing over and over again and the clients are always the same." You can respond, "Getting bored with a job can be a problem. Why don't you do something about it?" (Long pause and blank look.) Complainer: "You mean there's something I can do?" This will usually stop them from complaining to you at the time you take their unhappiness seriously and offer a practical resolution. You are challenging them to take control of their situation and fix it.

Adjusting the attitude approach. Complainers often do not realize how good they actually have it and how much they can be thankful for. This approach is difficult because it requires the person to shift their perception from one they have been hanging on to for many years. Helping adjust their perception of themselves and what they have and can do will allow them to become more positive and speak of the good things in their lives.[3] They do need some degree of self-awareness, however small, for this to be successful.

This approach can be a slow process, and the key is to get them to acknowledge that they have a negative attitude and that their complaining is not helping them. Continual redirection is needed when they start complaining and being negative again. For example, the complainer say, "This job is so hard. I'm always tired, and I never have any time to do what I want. They're always giving me something else to do, and I can't seem to ever say no because they'll fire me. What's wrong with me? I don't know when my life became so negative." Response: "Why don't you try this. Tell me right now about five things that are good in your life?" Complainer: "Well, I have a great husband who listens to me and encourages me and helps me with the housework. The pay I'm getting here is better than at anyplace else I've ever worked. I live in a nice big house with a big yard. How many is that? I've got some great friends who would do anything for me. And I love my church and the people who are there. That is five." Response: "That's great! Don't you feel better now? You have to keep looking at the positive side of things. Now I'm going to help you with this even though you'll probably get irritated with me at some point. Every time you complain about something, I want you to say something positive also, okay? It'll be hard at first, but if you forget, I'll remind you."

Complaining to the complainer approach. Unlike the first two approaches, the goal of this approach is not to alter the underlying causes of the complaining but to ameliorate the behavior to some degree. Most people who complain all the time have no self-realization of how they come across to other people and how irritating their complaining is.[2] Sometimes by hearing how they sound, they can get a sample of how other people feel about their complaining.

Step 1: Rather than trying to be empathetic and positive in responding to the complainer, complain about everything, including what they are doing and how they are doing it. If they ever do a good job, complain about that. This will be tiring if you're not a born complainer, and others may look at you strangely. At some point, however, the complainer will probably start complaining about your complaining. This is a sign that your plan is working.

Step 2: Keep on complaining and then, when they least expect it, tell them they are doing a great job when they do something well. They'll be surprised at your positive words, and it will likely make them ask you what you are doing. If they ask this, they are showing the first signs of self-awareness and this is your opening to have "the talk."

There are also many things that do not work with complainers. These are listed here so that you don't waste your time on approaches that will only lead to more complaining or nowhere at all.[3] Approaches to avoid:

1. Ignoring or avoiding them. They are seeking attention by complaining, and this will only make them complain more.
2. Having an aggressive confrontation. They will either hide the complaining or play the victim role.
3. Trying to fix their problems. They really don't want their problems fixed; they just want to complain about them.
4. Trying to cheer them up. Saying, "No one can have it that bad," will only make the complainer try to convince you more that, yes, his or her life is *that* bad or even *worse.*
5. Telling them they complain too much. They have no self-awareness of their complaining behavior and will deny it and then complain that you're being mean to them.
6. Commiserating with them. Saying to the complainer, "You know, you're right. This job is awful, and the cafeteria food stinks, and the charge nurse doesn't have a brain in her head," will make you the complainer's best buddy. You can now both face the big bad horrible world, together.
7. Using sarcasm. If you say, "Oh, you poor dear, bless your heart, it sounds like your life is just one big tragedy after another, doesn't it?" they may misinterpret it to mean that you really are acknowledging how big their problems really are, or, if they do get the sarcasm, they will complain about how you are unable to show empathy for them (and the world).[2]

Chronic complaining is bad for the work environment, bad for the people working there, and bad for the chronic complainer. No matter how difficult it is, complaining does need to be stopped somehow. A company in Germany sends employees home when they are having a "complaining day." Many employers are now including complaining behavior as a reason to avoid hiring someone. For chronic complainers, complaining is habitual and they really can't ever hide it, even in an interview. However, because of the nursing shortage, HR personnel in hospitals and other health-care facilities are still using the "warm body" approach to hiring, so there tends to be a much higher number of chronic complainers in hospitals.

There are other types of difficult behavior that people can display that were not discussed here; however, the approaches to changing that behavior are similar to the many approaches talked about earlier. Some additional types of difficult behaviors include the following:

- Procrastination and indecision
- Non-responsiveness and silence
- Yes-men or yes-women

Conclusion

All professional nurses need to develop mechanisms to deal with people who are displaying difficult behavior. The very nature of the profession exposes nurses to a large number of people who are experiencing change, are under stress, and have a wide range of backgrounds and values and varying expectations. By understanding communication, using **behavior modification,** developing **assertiveness,** avoiding submissive and aggressive behaviors, and appreciating diversity, the nurse can develop the coping skills required for problem-solving, handling conflict in the work setting, and confronting the unacceptable behaviors of difficult people.[14]

Dealing with difficult people and resolving conflict are never pleasant undertakings. However, like most skills, the more they are practiced, the more comfortable you will become using the communication techniques discussed both in Chapter 12 and this chapter. The importance of handling problematic situations in a timely, honest, and caring manner is self-evident. The anxiety and fear provoked by confrontation are part of the price that nurses must pay to do their jobs well and provide high-quality client care.

Critical-Thinking Exercises

- Complete this statement, using as many situations or statements as possible: "In a conflict situation, I have difficulty saying _____." Analyze reasons that prevent you from saying it. What would have been the worst thing that could have happened to you if you had said it? Create a phrase that you feel comfortable with that you could use the next time you want to say something difficult to the members of your team.
- Identify the communication and behavior characteristics of your work group or team. List areas of diversity for each member, including yourself. Identify their strengths and weaknesses. Identify methods for using the team members' diversity to enhance the team.
- Identify a person who displays difficult behaviors either at home, in the classroom, or in the clinical setting. Which of the categories discussed in the text does this person fit into? Attempt to communicate with this person using the techniques discussed in the book. Did they work? Why or why not?
- Analyze your own behavior. Are you a difficult person? Most people can have difficult behavior in some situations. What situations trigger a difficult behavior response in you? How does your behavior change when you are angry, depressed, or anxious?

References

1. Berghuis H, Kamphuis JH, Verheul RC. Features of personality disorder: Differentiating general personality dysfunctioning from personality traits. *Journal of Personality Disorders,* 26(5):704–716, 2012.

2. Lightman D. Dealing with difficult people by managing hot buttons. *Medical-Surgical Matters,* 21(1):14–15, 2012.

3. Haas LJ, Leiser JP, Magill MK, Sanyer, ON. Management of the difficult patient. Retrieved August 2013 from http://www.aafp.org/afp/2005/1115/p2063.html

4. Duncan MK, Waibel BA. Maslow's needs hierarchy as a framework for evaluating hospitality houses' resources and services. *Journal of Pediatric Nursing,* 26(4):325–331, 2011.

5. Zanni GR, Wick JY. Dealing with those difficult coworkers. *Consultant Pharmacist,* 26(9):672–678, 2011.

6. Bossheim J. How nurses can fight sexual harassment. Retrieved August 2013 from http://www.nursingcenter.com/lnc/CEArticle?an=00152193-201209000-00015&Journal_ID=54016&Issue_ID=1418247

7. Vroomen-Durning M. Nursing relationship: Five tips for working with a difficult physician. Retrieved August 2013 from http://www.nursetogether.com/nursing-relationship-five-tips-for-working-with-a-difficult-physician#sthash.PxCGclp2.dpuf

8. Michaelsen JJ. Emotional distance to so-called difficult patients. *Scandinavian Journal of Caring Sciences,* 26(1):90–97, 2012.

9. Rich BA. Distinguishing difficult patients from difficult maladies. *American Journal of Bioethics,* 13(4):24–26, 2013.

10. Forrest C. Working with "difficult" patients. *Primary Health Care,* 22(8):20–22, 2012.

11. Brass L. Can you cope? How to hang in there—no matter what comes your way. *Vibrant Life,* 29(1):30–33, 2013.

12. Clarke N. Anger, rage & relationship—an empathic approach to anger management. *Counselling and Psychotherapy Research,* 10(1):77–79, 2010.

13. Powers AD, Oltmanns TF. Personality pathology as a risk factor for negative health perception. *Journal of Personality Disorders,* 27(3):359–370, 2013.

14. Gage W. Using service improvement methodology to change practice. *Nursing Standard,* 6;27(23):51–57, 2013.

Health-Care Delivery Systems

14

Nicole Harder

Joseph T. Catalano

Learning Objectives

After completing this chapter, the reader will be able to:

- Discuss the implications of health-care reform on the profession of nursing
- Analyze the evolution of the health-care delivery system in the United States
- Analyze the evolution of the health-care delivery system in Canada
- Evaluate the factors that influence the evolution of the health-care delivery system
- Synthesize the concerns surrounding the uninsured in the United States
- Analyze industry efforts to manage health-care costs
- Evaluate the efforts being made to ensure high-quality, cost-effective health care
- Describe and list the levels and types of health-care delivery

HEALTH CARE VERSUS HEALTH-CARE DELIVERY

Health care is often defined as the management of the resources of healing. The delivery of health care is the action or activities of supplying or providing services to maintain health, detect illness, and cure those who are ill or injured. In the past, these services were typically delivered in a hospital or clinic setting. A growing awareness of and interest in maintaining optimal health is resulting in a movement toward increasing preventive and primary care as a means of promoting health. This change in focus has produced substantial changes to the ways in which health-care services are delivered and the way health-care professionals interact with these systems. As professionals, nurses need to understand health-care delivery systems. Nursing practice is influenced by political, societal, and cultural realities and needs to adapt to the changing world that affects everyday practice. Today's health-care institutions are heavily affected by the costs of delivery, access to services, and health-care professionals.

It has been long recognized that although individual health-care services in the United States are among the best in the world, the nation's health-care delivery system is mediocre at best. In many key health-care indicators, such as infant mortality and chronic diseases, the United States is well behind other countries, ranking 37th out of 50. One of the goals of health-care reform is to bring the high-quality care experienced by some to those who are less fortunate or do not have employer-based insurance plans.

HEALTH-CARE REFORM

In 2010, passage of the landmark Affordable Care Act (ACA) set the stage for the largest overhaul of the U.S. health-care system in 50 years. Now that the uproar has settled somewhat, nurses must take the lead in implementing ACA to move the U.S. health-care system toward becoming the best in the world for *all* its citizens.

New Provisions for Health Care

Sometimes referred to as health-care reform, Obamacare, or, less frequently, Americare, the primary goal of ACA is to provide affordable health care to U.S. citizens who, before its passage, were unable to pay for or obtain health insurance. Secondary goals include eliminating the insurance industry's stranglehold on the health-care system, addressing inequities in current coverage, and help struggling senior citizens. The legislative process mangled or killed several key provisions of ACA that would have covered the almost 47 million Americans without health insurance. However, it is estimated that some 32 million additional citizens will be added to the rolls of those with health care over the next ten years.[1]

The detractors of ACA remain legion and often cite false or misleading information as their rationale for opposition. The bill does have some limitations, which we discuss later. The provisions of the bill will be phased in over 8 years to be less of a "change shock" to health-care providers and citizens alike. Provisions that took place in 2010 include:

- "Doughnut hole" protection for senior citizens. They will receive a rebate from the government to supplement the $2,700 limit on Medicare drug coverage. However, this fills only 50 percent of the doughnut hole for 2010; 100 percent will be filled by 2020.
- Care for all children by eliminating the pre-existing conditions restrictions found in most policies.
- Access to high-risk pools for all uninsured, even adults with pre-existing conditions.
- Increasing the age to 26 years for young adults to be covered on their parents' plans.
- Ending the insurance companies' ability to drop coverage for someone when he or she gets sick.
- Transparency: Insurance companies must reveal how much money is spent on overhead and administrative costs.

- A customer appeals process to explain to customers how coverage determinations are made and claims are rejected.
- A 10 percent tax on indoor tanning services, with the money being used to fight skin cancer.
- Eliminating health insurance fraud and waste with a new system of inspection and checks.
- Improved quality of information on the Web. A new website makes it easier for consumers and small businesses in any state to find affordable health insurance plans.
- Improved labels of food products for more accurate nutrient content to eliminate the confusing and sometimes fraudulent information provided by manufacturers.
- Less expensive health-care plans offered to early retirees (ages 55–64 years) as part of the benefit package.

Provisions that became effective in 2011:

- Tax credits for small businesses with fewer than 50 employees to cover 50 percent of employee health-care premiums.
- Limited power of insurance companies to exploit small businesses; reduced out-of-pocket expenses for employees.
- A 2-year temporary credit (up to $1 billion) to encourage research into new therapies and procedures.

Provisions that became effective in 2014:

- Eliminating all pre-existing illness limits for adults to obtain health insurance.

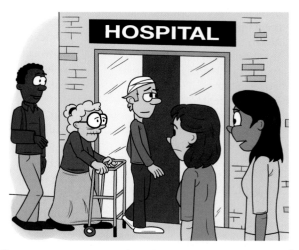

"I GUESS HEALTH-CARE REFORM MEANS JOB SECURITY!"

- Eliminating higher insurance premiums based on a person's gender or health status.
- No lifetime caps on the amount of insurance an individual can receive.
- Expanded Medicare payment to small rural hospitals and other health-care facilities that have a small number of Medicare clients.
- A minimum benefits package defined by the federal government, including certain preventive services at no cost.
- The option of coverage that can be offered through new state-run insurance marketplaces, called *exchanges*. Increased Medicare payroll taxes for high-income earners ($250,000 or more). Unearned income of $250,000 or more, now exempt from the payroll tax, would also be subject to a 3.8 percent levy. (This was postponed until 2016.)

Provisions that become effective in 2018:

- All new insurance plans to cover checkups and other preventive care without copays.

Individuals who have health insurance plans at the time of the Affordable Care Act (ACA) implementation can keep their plans with very little change. The plans will not be increased to match the new policies' increased benefit standards. However, as of summer 2011, no health plans will be able to set annual limits, drop individuals because of illness, drop children from parents' plans until they are 26 years old, or deny children coverage because of pre-existing conditions.[2]

Concerns About Health-Care Reform

Some of the more controversial provisions in health-care reform include the anticipated gradual increase in premiums (up to 13 percent) that will be phased in from 2011 to 2016. However, most individuals and families will qualify for subsidies. These will be a sliding-scale tax break for a family of four making less than $88,000 per year. Federal insurance plans will *not* cover abortions. However, this coverage can be obtained through the state-sponsored exchange programs for an additional premium if the individual exchange plans decide to offer it. States may opt out of the abortion coverage.[3]

Another controversial aspect of ACA is the requirement that most Americans buy health insurance or pay a penalty starting in 2014. The penalty will start out at 1 percent of income in 2014 and rise to 2.5 percent by 2016; however, the total amount will not exceed $2085 per year. Some believe this is an invasion of privacy and limits personal freedom.[4] The underlying idea is that when everyone has insurance, the rates for premiums are lower across the board. Without the requirement, people with insurance would have to pay higher premiums to cover those without insurance. This is what the health-care and insurance industries have been doing for the past 50 years. However, this provision was delayed until at least 2016 and perhaps even later.

A few groups would not be required to purchase health insurance. Most American Indians can receive health care through their tribal health-care systems. Almost all federal government employees are covered by government-sponsored insurance which is very similar to the insurance under the ACA. Also, those who have legitimate religious objections can avoid paying for insurance. Individuals and families with extreme financial hardship would not be penalized for inability to pay if the cheapest plan available would cost more than 8 percent of their income.[5]

Some clinicians fear that the increased number of new clients will overwhelm the health-care system, resulting in long waits at physicians' offices. Another concern is that the Medicare system will be inundated with a flood of new recipients and not have enough funding to cover everyone. New legislation invariably raises issues; these problems are growing pains that can be resolved along with other issues that are sure to arise.[6]

Nursing and Health-Care Reform

Nurses were at the table during the planning of the Affordable Care Act, and nurses will have a key role as the plan moves forward. The influx of some 32 million new clients into the health-care system offers new challenges and opportunities for nurses to expand their profession and practice to the levels for which they were educated.

> "*The influx of some 32 million new clients into the health-care system offers new challenges and opportunities for nurses to expand their profession and practice to the levels for which they were educated.*"

A Goal of Maintaining Health

Sometimes overlooked or discounted in ACA is the increased emphasis on preventive care. All Americans can receive screening procedures such as prostate examinations, mammograms, annual physical examinations, and preventive care such as immunizations at no out-of-pocket costs. Almost all the preventive care measures have been implemented and do not require approval by Congress, like some of the other provisions. This is a major transition in emphasis from illness and disease to prevention and health promotion. One commitment that has always differentiated professional nursing from medicine is this goal of maintaining health and preventing disease.[7]

Opportunities and Challenges for Nurses

The arena where this transition will occur is primary care. During the past decade, physician training for primary care has decreased because of low reimbursement rates from insurance companies and government programs. It is unlikely that the current crop of primary care physicians will be able to handle the increase in clients seeking preventive care. On the other hand, the education of nurse practitioners has increased by some 60 percent during the same decade. In addition, ACA provides about $50 million per year to develop new programs for each of the nurse practitioner roles. Also, public health will find itself on the front lines of the influx of new clients. The opportunity for nurses to lead the cutting edge of health-care reform is ripe with promise.[8]

To fulfill this promise, nurses must continue to do what they have always done, but to do it better. In the past, when demographic swings or governmental programs have created substantive changes in health care, nurses have been the leaders in developing new systems and models to accommodate the changes. Nurses are experts in increasing access to care while maintaining the quality of that care. They must work in the political arena to broaden the ability of advanced practice nurses to provide the services they were educated to provide. They must be at the table to help shape changes in health care.

As evidence-based practice becomes the norm for heath-care practice, nurses need to keep conducting the research and collecting the data that improve care. Without a solid base of research, it will be impossible to demonstrate scientific evidence of the effectiveness of preventive care and improved client outcomes. However, nurses cannot do research in a vacuum. It is essential that they collaborate with all health-care disciplines by understanding and acknowledging the importance of their roles in health-care reform. From collaborating with medical schools to providing training for patient care technicians (PCAs), nurses can establish the trust required to work in concert with others and provided seamless, high-quality care.[9]

Health-care reform can be a double-edged sword for professional nursing. Nurses can lead the reform that will mark the success of health care for decades to come, or they can be overrun by the system and become a footnote to health care. Nurses who educate themselves about the new reforms and find the opportunities will be the leaders health care requires.

> *Although significant strides have been made in treating some acute infectious diseases, many challenges still exist in the management of health concerns such as cancer, heart disease, Alzheimer's disease, diabetes, chronic obstructive pulmonary disease, and HIV.*

THE NEW FACE OF HEALTH CARE

The number of U.S. citizens who were not covered by any type of health-care insurance in 2010 was more than 47 million, about 25 percent of the population. Of the top 25 industrialized countries, the United States is the only one that does not have any type of universal health-care coverage for its citizens.[10] The ACA is a first step to developing a system that will offer all U.S. residents the same type of health care distributed to members of the U.S. Congress. The new law challenges politicians to develop a system that will cover all citizens as they are covered by their governmental health-care plan. Nurses see every day the effect of lack of health care among the most vulnerable population: infants and children.

DEMOGRAPHICS AFFECTING HEALTH-CARE DELIVERY

Age

Between now and the year 2050, the number of persons 65 years or older is expected to double. By 2050, one in five people living in Canada or the United States will be elderly, and their numbers will reach an estimated 80 million.[11] Of this number, many will eventually become more dependent on the health-care delivery system as a result of chronic health problems. (See Chapter 22 for more detail.)

Although an aging population constitutes a sizable number of persons who may require expensive long-term health care, their community activism and powerful influence at the ballot box can provide them with better access to health care than other less vocal and politically savvy groups. Additional at-risk groups consist of persons residing in urban areas with limited incomes and individuals living in remote rural areas where access to care is limited.

Chronicity

Another factor influencing the climate of health-care delivery is the long-term and expensive nature of many health problems. Although significant strides have been made in treating some acute infectious diseases, many challenges still exist in the management of health concerns such as cancer, heart disease, Alzheimer's disease, diabetes, chronic obstructive pulmonary disease (COPD), and HIV. Additional concerns include environmental and occupational safety, drug abuse, and mother and child health care.

HEALTH CARE AS AN INDUSTRY

In most developed countries, health care is one of the largest industries. According to a report produced by the Kaiser Foundation, total expenditures on health accounted for 9.5 percent of the gross domestic product in Canada[12] and 17.9 percent in the United States in 2010 (this is the last year of available statistics), or just under $8,000 per person.[13] Total expenditure was more than $2 *trillion* and is expected to reach $4 trillion by 2015. These numbers alone indicate the significance of health care and health-care spending to the people of these two countries.

In the United States, with the introduction of managed care, the organizations that pay for health care have the capacity to dramatically influence who provides care, how the care is furnished, and who receives compensation. The significance to the economy, along with other factors, is evident.

Health Care in the Global Context

Understanding the approach to health care in comparison with other countries is important in assessing the challenges to and potential of health-care delivery. How and why health-care systems differ is a function of multiple influences. These may include societal values and beliefs, sociocultural climate, the state of the economy, political ideologies, geographic density, international influences, historical realities, established practices and programs, and other factors. For health-care systems to develop, several factors must come into play at different points. This development is consistent throughout the world, as can be seen by examining the contexts in which various health-care systems were developed.

One way to think about system differences is to consider that Western countries provide for health care in several ways, all of which involve variable combinations of private or public funding of services and private or public delivery of services.[13] Table 14.1 shows the degree of public involvement in financing health services and the essential role envisioned for the health-care system.[14]

Type 1 Systems

In the type 1 health-care system, private approaches to health services predominate. Physicians, other caregivers (e.g., midwives), and clients have maximum autonomy. In this plan, individuals who can afford private health insurance, or who simply can pay for their health care, choose their care providers and receive health services. Those who cannot pay do not have choice or benefit.

> *Between now and the year 2050, the number of persons 65 years of age or older is expected to double. By 2050, one in five people living in Canada or the United States will be elderly, and their numbers will reach an estimated 80 million.*

Table 14.1 **Types of Health-Care Systems in the Western World**

	Type 1	Type 2	Type 3	Type 4
System	Private health insurance	National health insurance	National health service	Socialized health system
Primary goal	Preserve autonomy	Egalitarian	Egalitarian	Essential service
Secondary effect	Acceptance of social differences	Preserve autonomy	Public management	Physicians as state employees

In its purest form, the type 1 system would not offer any other option other than to pay for service. In reality, most countries have adopted a mixture of system types. For example, although the United States has a mainly private payment system of health care, some publicly funded programs assist elderly and poor people. Even with these programs, it is estimated that 25 percent of Americans have no health insurance and therefore are limited in their ability to access health care.

Type 4 Systems

On the opposite end of the spectrum from type 1 is type 4. This type of health-care system focuses on keeping the general public healthy so that they can continue to contribute to society and the economy. Health care is considered an essential service or even a right, not necessarily involving compassionate motives. Physicians are considered agents of the state who work to keep others working efficiently.

In Canada, the type 4 structure is seen in such organizations as the military, hockey teams, and other sports teams. Physicians are hired by these organizations to ensure the players stay healthy and can do their part to achieve the goals of the group.

Type 3 Systems

Between the extremes of type 1 and type 4 health-care systems are two types—type 2 and type 3. The type 3 system is funded and operated by the government, as was seen in Great Britain some years ago. With this system, the state-operated and state-funded health services were based on an egalitarian value. Public management of each service was considered key to efficient and effective operation.

Type 2 Systems

The type 2 system is a hybrid of the type 1 and type 3 systems. Egalitarian values are given high priority, but so are practitioner and client autonomy. The type 2 system uses tax dollars to pay for health services through health insurance available from a nonprofit agency (e.g., government).

Each health service is operated more or less autonomously by others, including municipalities, citizen groups, physicians, nurse practitioners, and physiotherapists in private offices, group practices, and other groups. All services rendered to clients are then paid from the central pool of health insurance funds created through taxation. This type of system is used in Canada and embodies the collective sharing of burdens and benefits while allowing a degree of autonomy in delivery.[15]

Third World Alternatives

It is important to note that the four systems described above exclude a group of third world countries that cannot afford the type of health care appreciated in most developed countries. Yet many third world countries have managed to develop primary care systems that are not as institution dependent as the systems found in Canada and the United States. In their systems, primary care includes preventive health care, first point of contact, and continuing care. However, in some countries, the primary and preventive systems have been undermined by the influence of Western countries promoting high technology and institutionalization.

What Do Taxes Cover?

Even in countries that finance health insurance through tax dollars, there are variations in services provided. For example, some fund home care but others do not; some provide coverage for prescription drugs and others do not. Regardless of the type of system, it is important to reflect on the influences that have created it and continue to maintain it.

What Do You Think?

What type of health-care system did you use the last time you accessed health care? Did you use the health-care system for preventive care or illness care?

ADMINISTRATION AND FUNDING OF HEALTH-CARE SYSTEMS

Canada's health-care system is the subject of much political controversy and debate in the United States. Those opposing universal health care question how efficient the Canadian system is at providing timely surgeries, treatments, and access to health care. Regardless of the political debate, Canada does boast one of the highest life expectancies (about 80 years) and lowest infant mortality rates of industrialized countries, which many attribute to Canada's universal health-care system.[16]

Health Care in Canada

Financing and administering health-care systems can be an overwhelming responsibility. In Canada, health-care services are provided under the Canada Health Act. The Canadian federal government collects funds through taxes and gives the responsibility of administering health-care services to the provinces. As in the United States, the cost of financing health-care services has risen tremendously since the first Medical Care Act was introduced in 1967–1968. In Canada, medical insurance premiums became an increasing burden for the federal government as a result of the improved services promised to all Canadians.

Federal Transfer Payments

In an attempt to control the costs to be paid to all provinces, the Canadian government proposed a system of block funding. In 1977, the Federal-Provincial Fiscal Arrangements and Established Programs Financing Act were established after lengthy negotiations with all provinces. The formula for federal transfer payments consisted of four components:

1. Per capita payments were made on the basis of previous expenditures and adjusted regularly in relation to the gross national product.

2. Tax points were transferred by the federal government, allowing provinces to reduce their tax contribution to the government and at the same time increase the portion of tax collected at the provincial level.

3. Equalization of tax points was distributed among poorer provinces.

4. Additional per capita payments were indexed to help pay for nursing home, residential home, and ambulatory care.

This new act changed the funding formulae from a 50-50 cost-sharing arrangement to one that gave taxation points to the provinces in exchange for lower cash transfer payments. The provinces were initially very receptive, as this meant they had more taxation power in an economy that was very healthy. However, with rising costs of health care, owing in part to an aging population and increased technology, some physicians and provinces struggled with health-care coverage. With extra billing or balance billing becoming prevalent, there was a heated public debate, and the new Canada Health Act was passed in 1984.

> *Regardless of the political debate, Canada does boast one of the highest life expectancies (about 80 years) and lowest infant mortality rates of industrialized countries, which many attribute to Canada's universal health-care system.*

The Canada Health Act

Although the Canadian federal government has a limited constitutional basis for making health-care decisions, it has considerable economic clout to develop and shape a national health-care plan. To support their positions on health care, the federal government enacted the Canada Health Act (CHA). The purpose of the CHA is to "establish criteria and conditions in respect of insured health services and extended health-care services provided under provincial law that must be met before a full cash contribution may be made."[16] It was last revised in 2012.

The insured health services defined by the CHA include all medically necessary hospital services and medically required physician services, as well as medically or dentally required surgical-dental services that needed to be performed in a hospital for safety. New criteria, conditions, and provisions were formulated to eliminate extra billing and user charges.

For the provinces to qualify for full cash refunds from the federal government under the Canada

Health and Social Transfer (CHST) agreement, they must meet five basic criteria and conditions. These criteria and conditions must be met for each fiscal year and must include:

1. *Public administration:* The health-care insurance plan must be administered and operated on a non-profit basis by a public authority, responsible to the provincial government, and subject to audit of its accounts and financial transactions.
2. *Comprehensiveness:* The plan must cover all insured health services provided by hospitals, medical practitioners, and dentists and, where permitted, services rendered by other health-care practitioners.
3. *Universality:* One hundred percent of the insured population of a province must be entitled to the insured health services provided for by the plan on uniform terms and conditions.
4. *Portability:* Residents moving to another province must continue to be covered for insured health services by the home province during any minimum waiting period, not to exceed 3 months, imposed by the new province of residence. For insured persons, insured health services must be made available while they are temporarily absent from their own provinces on the following basis:
   - Insured services received out of province but still in Canada are to be paid for by the home province at host province rates unless another arrangement for the payment of costs exists between the provinces. Prior approval may be required for elective services.
   - Out-of-country services received are to be paid, as a minimum, on the basis of the amount that would have been paid by the home province for similar services rendered in the province. Prior approval may be required for elective services.
5. *Accessibility:* The health-care insurance plan of a province must provide for:
   - Insured health services on uniform terms and conditions and reasonable access by insured persons to insured health services not precluded and unimpeded, either directly or indirectly, by charges or other means.
   - Reasonable compensation to physicians and dentists for all insured health services rendered.
   - Payments to hospitals in respect to the cost of insured health services.

Although discussion and debate continue surrounding the federal and provincial responsibilities for health-care funding and the escalating costs associated with health care, the Canada Health Act of 1984 continues to be the operating model for the Canadian health-care system.[16]

Health-Care Systems in the United States

The United States has a far different method of funding and administering health-care services than Canada. According to the World Health Organization, the United States spends more per person on health care than any other country, yet in overall quality its care ranks 37th in the world and last among the 17 leading industrialized nations.[17] Of these 17 countries, the United States has the following:

- The highest rate of death by gun violence, by a huge margin
- The highest rate of death by car accidents
- The highest chance that a child will die before age 5
- The second-highest rate of death by coronary heart disease
- The second-highest rate of death by lung cancer and COPD
- The highest teen pregnancy rate
- The highest rate of women dying due to complications of pregnancy and childbirth[17]

This disparity is attributed in large part to the cost of health-care services, not the quality of the services available.

In an attempt to contain some of these costs, professional standards review organizations (PSROs) were introduced to review the quality, quantity, and cost of hospital care through Medicare. The primary goal of PSROs was to review the care provided by physicians to determine whether the best diagnostic and treatment approaches were being used. Another measure was the introduction of utilization review committees, requiring Medicare-qualified facilities to review admission, diagnostic testing, and treatments with the goal of eliminating overuse or misuse of services.

What Do You Think?

Review the bill from your last hospitalization or the bill of a family member. What do you think about the charges listed? Does the bill seem excessive?

Prospective Payment Systems

Although these measures have assisted with cost containment to some degree, one of the most significant factors that have influenced cost control was the prospective payment system (PPS) established by the U.S. Congress in 1983. This system required facilities providing services to Medicare clients to be reimbursed using a fixed-rate system and included monetary incentives to reduce the length of hospital stays. Medicare clients are classified using a diagnosis-related group (DRG), and the facilities are reimbursed a predetermined amount. Clients may be classified into one of 467 DRGs, and reimbursement occurs regardless of the length of stay. DRGs may be further grouped into major diagnostic categories (MDCs).

If the client is discharged sooner than anticipated, the facility keeps the difference. If the client requires a lengthier hospital stay, the hospital pays the extra cost. Under the PPS, the emphasis is on the efficient delivery of services in the most cost-effective manner.

Capitated Payment Systems

Capitation, or a capitated payment system, was introduced to encourage cost-effectiveness in a growing health-care system. In a capitated payment system, participants pay a flat rate, usually through their employer, to belong to a managed care organization (MCO) for a specified period of time. The health-care providers who serve the participants receive a fixed amount for each participant in the health-care plan.

Controlled Access

The goal of capitation is to have a payment plan for selected diseases or surgical procedures that provides the highest quality of care, including essential diagnostic and treatment procedures, at the lowest cost possible. Any expenses in excess of the capitated rate are the responsibility of the MCO. If the MCO spends less on the care of a client than it is given for delivery costs, it can keep the excess as profit, providing it with a strong incentive to reduce the cost of services.

Another goal of managed care is to enhance the efficiency and effective use of health-care services. A key underlying concept of managed care is to maintain administrative control over access and provision of primary health-care services for the members of the plan. The MCO controls all aspects of care, including delivery, financing, and the purchase of health-care services for clients who are enrolled in the program. Clients are allowed to use only the services of primary care physicians who are approved by the organization. Any referrals to other medical specialists must be approved by the MCO. The MCO contract determines what treatments or procedures will be reimbursed.

A Spending Increase

The effectiveness of the MCO plan rests on the theory that health-care costs can be reduced by decreasing the number of hospitalizations, shortening the length of inpatient stays, providing less expensive home-care services, and keeping people healthy through health promotion and illness-prevention services. It is logical to conclude that if people stay healthy, the cost of health-care services should decline.

Although much debate surrounds managed care and its advantages and disadvantages, the reality is that managed care has *not* reduced health-care costs nationally. Increases in spending are attributed to rising health-care wages, legislation that increased Medicare spending, increasing insurance premiums, technology, and consumer demands for less restrictive plans.

Overview of Health-Care Plans

See Boxes 14.1 through 14.5 to compare the principal features of different health-care models.

QUALITY OF CARE

Although the primary focus of health-care delivery systems is to provide care to as many people as possible, consideration of the quality of care is also a key factor. Delivering low-quality care to large numbers of individuals is not an option. Health-care facilities have implemented several quality improvement measures in an attempt to reduce the large number of injuries and deaths of hospitalized clients. (For more detailed information about quality of care, see Chapter 15.)

> *Under the PPS, the emphasis is on the efficient delivery of services in the most cost-effective manner.*

Box 14.1

Managed Care Organizations (MCOs)

Definition: Provide comprehensive, preventive, and treatment services to a specific group of voluntarily enrolled persons.

Managed Care Structures

Staff model: Physicians are salaried employees of the MCO.

Group model: MCO contracts with single group practice.

Network model: MCO contracts with multiple group practices and/or integrated organizations.

Independent practice association (IPA): MCO contracts with physicians who usually are not members of groups and whose practices include fee-for-service and capitated clients.

Characteristics: Focus on health maintenance and primary care. All care provided by a primary care physician. Referral needed for access to specialists and hospitalization.

Medicare MCO

Definition: Program same as MCO but designated to cover health-care costs of senior citizens.

Characteristics: Premium generally less than supplemental plans.

Box 14.2

Provider Organizations

Preferred Provider Organization (PPO)

Definition: One that limits an enrollee's choice to a list of "preferred" hospitals, physicians, and providers. An enrollee pays more out-of-pocket expenses for using a provider not on the list.

Characteristics: Contractual agreement exists between a set of providers and one or more purchasers (self-insured employers or insurance plans). Comprehensive health services at a discount for companies under contract.

Exclusive Provider Organization (EPO)

Definition: One that limits an enrollee's choice to providers belonging to one organization. Enrollee may or may not be able to use outside providers at additional expense.

Characteristics: Limited contractual agreement; less access to specialists.

Box 14.3

Medicare

Definition: Federally funded national health insurance program in the United States for people older than 65 years. Part A provides basic protection for medical, surgical, and psychiatric care costs based on diagnosis-related groups (DRGs). Part B is a voluntary medical insurance plan that covers physician and certain outpatient services. Part D is an unfunded insurance for medications.

Characteristics: Payment for plan deducted from monthly Social Security check; covers services of nurse practitioners (varies by state); does not pay full costs of certain services; supplemental insurance is encouraged.

Box 14.4

Medicaid

Definition: Federally funded, state-operated medical assistance program for people with low incomes. Individual states determine eligibility and benefits.

Characteristics: Finances a large portion of maternal and child care for the poor; reimburses for nurse midwifery and other advanced practice nursing (varies by state); reimburses long-term care facility funding.

Box 14.5

Private Insurance

Traditional Private Insurance

Definition: Traditional fee-for-service plan. Payment, computed after services are provided, is based on the number of services used.

Characteristics: Policies typically expensive; most policies have deductibles that clients must meet before insurance pays.

Long-Term Care Insurance

Definition: Supplemental insurance for coverage of long-term care services. Policies provide a set number of dollars for an unlimited time or for as little as 2 years.

Characteristics: Very expensive; good policy has a minimum waiting period for eligibility, payment for skilled nursing, intermediate or custodial care, and home care.

HEALTH-CARE LEVELS AND SETTINGS

Even though there are many methods for providing and funding health care, high-quality health-care services remain the highest priority. Consumers who have access to multiple types of health care may not always understand the differences among them.

In the past, health-care services were primarily illness or institution based and focused primarily on treating the ill or injured. The emphasis is now shifting slowly toward prevention and health promotion in the population. It is believed that a focus on wellness and a population living a healthier lifestyle will reduce the number of people who require expensive illness care services.

Levels of Service

Health-care services are frequently categorized according to the complexity or level of the services provided. This complexity relates to the kinds, or levels, of services: primary, secondary, and tertiary.

Primary Care

In nursing, *primary care* refers to health promotion and preventive care, including programs such as immunization campaigns. Primary care focuses on health education and on early detection and treatment. Maintaining and improving optimal health is the overriding goal.

> *It is logical to conclude that if people stay healthy, the cost of health-care services should decline.*

Secondary Care

In the secondary level, the focus shifts toward emergency and acute care. Secondary services are frequently provided in hospitals and other acute care settings, with an emphasis on diagnosis and the treatment of complex disorders.

Tertiary Care

The tertiary level emphasizes rehabilitative services, long-term care, and care of the dying. Nursing services are essential in all three levels of health care, in both the hospital and community settings.

What Do You Think?

Have you ever received care in a "nontraditional" health-care setting? What was it? What role did nurses play in the delivery of care?

Health-Care Settings

While nursing care is provided in traditional settings such as the hospital and the community, nursing services are also delivered in a growing number of nontraditional locations. One growing trend in care is seen in the outpatient departments attached to some hospitals. Outpatient services are used by clients who require a relatively high level of skilled health care but who do not need to stay in a hospital for an extended period of time. An inpatient is a person who enters a setting such as a hospital and remains for at least 24 hours. Whether clients are inpatients or outpatients, they often need assistance from the nurse to identify which services best suit their needs.

Public Health

Public health departments are government agencies that are established at the local, provincial or state, and federal levels to provide health services. The goal of early public health departments was to prevent and control communicable diseases that were rampant in the 18th and 19th centuries, producing epidemics that killed millions of people. Modern day epidemics, such as the Ebola outbreak in western Africa, still remain a threat and Public Health nurses continue their role as the first line of defense against pandemics that can potentially kill thousands of citizens. However, today, the scope of public health, while retaining its contagious disease control and prevention mission, has expanded to areas such as child health, obstetric and pregnancy care, and, more recently, the early detection and treatment of terrorist acts, particularly bioterrorism (see Chapter 26).

Home Health Care

Care of the ill and injured in the home is the oldest of all the health-care modalities. If you were to go back far enough, it might even be called "cave health care." The modern hospital and clinic are relatively new entities in the health-care system, having their origins in the industrial revolution. Before that time, the only place a person could receive care was at home, usually from a female relative.

Care in the Home Setting

Although the interest in and use of home health care have waxed and waned over time, its benefits have received new attention in the era of an aging population and health-care reform. Currently, the number of clients receiving care in the home exceeds 1.4 million, and some of this care is at a high-acuity level.[18] Gone are the days when home health care consisted of a quick visit by a nurse or aide taking vital signs, changing a dressing, and cleaning the house. Home health care now combines the advantages of health care in a safe and familiar setting with the high-tech treatment modalities found in the most advanced hospitals.

The goal of home health care is to make it possible for clients to remain at home rather than use hospital, residential, or long-term care facilities. Most clients prefer the familiar atmosphere of their own home and neighborhood. Clients experience lower stress levels at home and have a more positive outlook, which studies have shown hastens recovery. They are active participants in their own care, increasing their independence and giving them a sense of control over the outcome. Usually the home contains far fewer invasive pathogens than the hospital, so clients have a lower rate of infection with the medication-resistant bacteria commonly found in hospitals and extended care facilities. High-quality home care helps prevent readmissions, which benefits clients and saves money.[19] When nurses and other health-care professionals do visit the home-care client, the client and his or her health needs are the sole focus of the care provided.

> *It is believed that a focus on wellness and a population living a healthier lifestyle will reduce the number of people who require expensive illness care services.*

The majority of home health care remains informal and is mostly provided by relatives and friends. When professionals provide care in the home, nurses are the primary group involved. Other providers include physical therapists, home health-care aides, respiratory and occupational therapists, social workers, and mental health professionals. Professional-level home health-care services can include physical and psychological assessment, wound care, medication and illness education, pain management, physical therapy, speech therapy, and occupational therapy. Assistance with activities of daily living and other daily tasks such as meal preparation, medication reminders, laundry, light housekeeping, errands, shopping, transportation, and companionship is sometimes referred to as *life assistance services.*[18]

The technology long considered the sole domain of the acute care hospital has found its way into the home. Clients who previously could only receive treatment in a hospital can now remain at home and receive the same quality of treatment. A rapidly growing industry of high-tech home care is breaking down the walls between the acute care unit and the bedroom. From the intravenous infusions of antibiotics and total parenteral nutrition to the use of ventilators, hemodialysis machines, and assistive robots, the level of high-tech home treatments continues to grow.[20]

Although it might seem logical that hospitals would resist a trend that reduces the number of clients, the opposite is true. Current funding restrictions for clients who return to the hospital too quickly with the same condition, or who have acquired a hospital-source infection, make earlier client discharge very attractive. More continuity of care is guaranteed when clients are observed in the home. Research shows that home care reduces emergency department visits and unnecessary readmissions to the hospital. Overall, clients report an increased level of satisfaction with the care provided and the improvement of their conditions.

A Need for Skilled Care

Not just anybody can be covered to receive home health care. When a client is referred for home health care by a physician or nurse practitioner, the provider must demonstrate that the client requires skilled needs that can only be provided by a professional nurse or other professional, depending on the client's diagnosis. These skilled needs fall into three categories:

- *Management of care*: for example, injections, intravenous (IV) lines, wound care, diabetes or its complications, urinary catheters, rehabilitation, respiratory therapies
- *Client evaluation*: for example, unstable conditions, pain, response to medications, neurological functioning, environment
- *Client education*: for example, medications, glucose monitoring, disease management, prevention measures, activities of daily living[19]

A Rewarding Practice

Not all nurses are attracted to home health care as a career path. Individuals who thrive on the fast pace and perpetual motion of acute care or intensive care units would find the laid-back pace of home health care boring. Additionally, the mountain of paperwork that accompanies home health-care clients might deter even the most dedicated supernurse. However, many nurses find it a rewarding area of practice. The one-on-one interaction with clients and their families permits a level of care only dreamed of in the acute care setting. The ability to observe a client over an extended period and to watch his or her condition improving makes all the effort seem worthwhile.

However, the nurse who provides care in the home setting must develop a number of important skill sets. Probably most important of all is ethical practice. In the home-care setting, the nurse practices with virtually no supervision. It is up to professionals to maintain their competency and provide a high level of skills. Ethical practice is at the heart of establishing trust with the client and his or her family.

Flexibility is another quality that home health-care nursing requires. Things do not always go as planned. Even though appointments are scheduled well ahead of time, clients often have last-minute condition changes or conflicts that require a reschedule. Even during the visit, the nurse may find that the client is not physically or mentally able to do the required skills or learning. Nurses are visitors in the client's home, and the client sets the pace for the care that is provided. It is sometimes difficult for nurses to let go of the control they had over clients in the acute care setting, but it is one of the keys to success.

Nurses must also increase their skills in cultural competency. Each home has its own unique cultural context. To become **culturally competent,** nurses must develop a high level of cultural sensitivity by respecting and believing that all cultures are equally valid and not attempting to impose values from the nurse's culture. Using a cultural assessment such as is found in Chapter 22 can be a great help in

Today, the scope of public health, while retaining its contagious disease and prevention mission, has expanded to areas such as child health, obstetric and pregnancy care, and, more recently, the early detection and treatment of terrorist acts, particularly bioterrorism.

providing culturally sensitive care. By learning about a client's beliefs, value systems, attitudes, and customs, the nurse can enrich his or her own life.

Often home health-care nurses find that the home is not a very peaceful environment but is filled with tension and conflict. The ability to apply the principles of **conflict management** (see Chapter 12) is a skill that home health-care nurses must master early in their careers. Illness is an automatic stressor, and often the families of ill clients do not know how to deal with the increased levels of stress. Family members may have widely different views of care, and clients themselves may have a variant understanding of what they can and cannot do. It is not unusual for a nurse to hear from family members, "Tell Mama she's too sick to fix supper anymore!"

The most important skill in conflict management is active listening. It is essential for the nurse to listen to clients' fears, concerns, and anger about their condition and their families' reactions and actions. The nurse must also be on the lookout for signs of elder abuse and neglect. It is not uncommon for family caregivers, either intentionally or unintentionally, to harm the client through threats, withholding care and medications, or negative communication.

The future of home health care is full of opportunity. As the population ages, home health care will allow them to stay at home while receiving the same treatments and technology as they would receive in the acute care setting. Health-care reform has placed a brighter spotlight on the areas of quality and cost. Home health care allows for increased continuity of care and enhanced quality of care, while significantly reducing its cost.

School-Based Services

Nurses provide a variety of services within local school systems. These services include screenings, health promotion and illness prevention programs, and treatment of minor health problems. Emphasis is placed on physical, social, and psychological well-being. Concerns relating to self-esteem, stress, drug abuse, and adolescent pregnancy are frequently addressed by the school nurse. In addition, children and adolescents with long-term health problems often attend school, and it is not uncommon for the nurse to be consulted about such issues as seizure management, colostomy care, or gastric tube feedings.

Students who have health concerns are frequently referred to providers within the community, and an important role of the school nurse is that of community liaison. For this reason, the nurse must be knowledgeable about community resources and adept at getting clients into the system in a timely and efficient manner.

Community Health Centers

Community health centers are being more frequently used in many areas. Most centers use a team approach involving physicians, nurse practitioners, and community nurses working together to provide health services. Most centers have diagnostic and treatment facilities that provide medical, nursing, laboratory, and radiological services. Some centers may also provide outpatient minor surgical procedures that allow clients to remain at home while accessing health services as needed.

> *Nurses are visitors in the client's home, and the client sets the pace for the care that is provided. It is sometimes difficult for nurses to let go of the control they had over clients in the acute care setting, but it is one of the keys to success.*

Physicians' Offices and General Clinics

The physician's office continues to be the location where most North Americans access primary health care. The majority of physicians in North America continue to work either in their own offices or with other physicians in a group practice. Services range from routine health screening to illness diagnosis and treatment and even some minor surgical procedures.

The responsibilities of nurses who work in physicians' offices or in general clinics include obtaining personal health information and histories of current illness and preparing the client for examination. Nurses also assist with procedures and obtain specimens for laboratory analysis. Teaching clients basic health information and home management of treatments and medications is also a responsibility of the clinic nurse.

Occupational Health Clinics

Maintaining the health of workers in their workplaces to increase productivity has long been recognized as an important role for nurses. In response to rising health insurance costs, today's employers are increasingly supportive of workplace health promotion, illness prevention, and safety programs. Many companies provide wellness programs and encourage or even require their employees to participate. These services range from providing exercise facilities and fitness programs to health screenings and referrals. Illness prevention focuses on topics such as smoking cessation, stress management, and nutrition. Although some companies may hire health educators to manage their clinics, community health nurses often provide these services.

In Canada, occupational health nurses are registered nurses (RNs) holding a minimum of a diploma or a bachelor of science degree in nursing. Many may also have an occupational health certification or a degree in occupational health and safety from a community college or university. Nurses who are certified in occupational health nursing must meet eligibility requirements, pass a written examination, and be recognized as having achieved a level of competency in occupational health. The certification is granted by the Canadian Nurses Association.

Hospitals

Hospitals, the traditional provider of health-care services, are still an essential part of the health-care system and still provide the majority of nurses with employment. Hospitals range in size from small, rural facilities with as few as 15 to 20 beds to large urban centers that may exceed a bed capacity of several thousand.

Depending on the services they provide, hospitals will have varying classifications. General hospitals offer a variety of services, such as medical, surgical, obstetric, pediatric, and psychiatric care. Other hospitals may offer specialized services, such as pediatric care. Hospitals can be further classified as acute care or chronic care, depending on the length of stay of the client and the services available.

Large hospitals may be designated as specific centers for treatment, such as a trauma or cardiac center, because they can offer specialized services.

Long-Term Care Facilities

The majority of senior citizens in North America continue to live in their own homes. However, a growing group of seniors have health needs that require long-term care or extended care services. Some individuals may require rehabilitation or intermediate care, whereas others require extended, long-term care. These services are provided for both elderly and younger clients who have similar needs, such as clients with spinal cord injuries.

The current trend in extended care facilities is to provide care in a homelike atmosphere and base programs on the needs and abilities of the clients, or residents as they are commonly called, of the facility. Many of these residents require personal services such as bathing and assistance with activities of daily living. Others may require higher-level skilled nursing care such as tube feedings and catheter management or even occasional medical attention. Because of the range of needs of clients, some facilities will admit clients with specific needs to specific areas of the facility where the appropriate services are provided.

In Canada, admission to long-term care facilities must meet specific guidelines. Assessments of client needs and the nursing services available must be completed before the client is admitted to the facility. Frequently, there are waiting lists for admission to extended care facilities.

In the United States, many long-term care facilities are for-profit institutions that rely heavily on Medicaid and Medicare reimbursements.[21] When Medicare coverage is limited, the resident must use private insurance or personal resources to pay the difference in cost.

> *Hospitals, the traditional provider of health-care services, are still an essential part of the health-care system and still provide the majority of nurses with employment.*

Retirement and Assisted Living Centers

As the population continues to age, assisted living centers are increasing in popularity because they allow clients, or residents, to maintain the greatest amount of independence possible in a partially controlled and supervised living environment. These centers consist of separate apartments or condominiums for the residents and provide amenities such as meal preparation and laundry services.

Many centers work closely with home care and other social services to provide the resources required for maintaining a degree of independence. Case coordinators, often nurses, help residents navigate their way through the complex paperwork usually involved in obtaining required services. Some assisted living centers are attached to long-term care facilities. According to the level of care required, residents may be transferred to various facilities as their care needs change. The goal of the Gold Standards Framework program is to ensure that quality of care persists up to the time of death.[22]

Rehabilitation Centers

In many acute care facilities, discharge planning and rehabilitative needs are discussed at the time of admission. Rehabilitation centers or units are similar to some extended care facilities, where the client goal is to restore health and function at an optimum level. Often clients are admitted to rehabilitation units after recuperating from the acute stage of an injury or illness. The rehabilitation unit then provides services to complete the recovery and restore a high degree of independence.

Some common types of rehabilitation units include geriatric, chemical dependency, stroke, and spinal cord injury units. Nurses who work on these units have the responsibility of coordinating health-care services, providing skilled care when required, supervising less qualified personnel, and ensuring client compliance with treatment regimens.

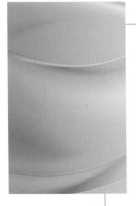

Issues Now

Nursing Home Fall Pays Big

An 82-year-old nursing home resident fell twice within a 6-week period. When she was admitted to the nursing home, the RN assessed that she had an unsteady gait from poor circulation, mild dementia, and at high risk for falls. The family also reported that she had fallen several times at home, and the falls were one of the primary reasons for her admission to the nursing home. The care plan recommended the use of seatbelt restraints and a seat alarm.

The first fall occurred in the dining room when the resident pushed her wheelchair away from the table and attempted to stand. The incident report noted that the wheelchair locks were not engaged. The second fall happened in the recreation room. The client was left alone in her wheelchair and again the wheel locks were not engaged. She attempted to stand by herself and fell again. She did not receive serious injuries from either fall.

The client's lawyer argued that the care plan was not followed and that the staff at the facility had neglected the protocols that called for locking of wheelchair wheels when clients were left unattended. The case was settled out of court by the nursing home's insurance company. The client and her family received $150,000 for the falls.

Source: Cebollero vs. Hebrew Home, 2009 WL 2989743 (Westchester County Court, New York, March 16, 2009).

Day-Care Centers

Day-care centers can be used by any age group. Traditionally, "day-care center" has referred to the care of children; however, during the past 12 years or so, adult day-care centers have become relatively common. Adult day-care centers provide services for elderly adults who cannot be left at home alone but do not require institutionalization.

Services provided by adult day-care centers include health maintenance classes, socialization and exercise programs, physical or occupational therapy, rehabilitative services, and organized recreational activities. Nurses who are employed in adult day-care centers may administer medications, give treatments, provide counseling and teaching, and coordinate services between day care and home care.

Rural Primary Care

Clients living in rural areas face some different health issues than people who live in large cities. Access to health care can be difficult when a client is located in a remote area. They might not be able to get to a hospital quickly in the event of an accident or emergency and have to travel long distances for basic checkups and assessments. Rural areas often have fewer family practice physicians and often no specialists at all. Health problems in rural residents tend to be more serious because of delayed diagnoses. Chronic disease rates are notably higher in clients who live in the rural areas of the United States. (For more information on rural health care, go to http://www.ruralhealthweb.org/.)

A Problem of Distance

Delivering health-care services to the rural areas of North America is a challenge because of the great distances between homes. In many rural towns, it is common to have small hospitals or other health-care facilities available to provide basic health-care services. Most of these facilities have basic laboratory and radiological services available.

In the far north of Canada, aboriginal communities have nursing stations or health centers in the community to provide basic health services. The centers are staffed by nurses. Visiting physicians come in occasionally to provide additional services. The nursing stations also provide emergency services to people who require stabilization before being transferred to a larger facility. For more information, go to http://www.nlm.nih.gov/medlineplus/ruralhealthconcerns.html.

A Problem of Cost

In the United States, paying for health-care services in rural areas is a concern. Many of the residents in rural areas are farmers or employees of small businesses that do not offer health insurance. A type of group insurance called health insurance purchasing cooperatives (HIPCs) is now available to Americans who are self-employed or who do not have health insurance for other reasons. This program was expanded and modified under the ACE to allow larger groups of individuals or employers to band together to purchase health insurance at a reduced cost.

Hospice Services

Hospice care originated in Great Britain and has changed the way end-of-life care is delivered. Disillusioned with health-care services that focused on technology and the preservation of life at all costs, the hospice movement gained momentum in the 1970s. Hospice care emphasizes physiological and psychological support for clients who have terminal diseases. Hospice care provides a variety of services in a caring and supportive environment to terminally ill clients, their families, and other support persons. The central concept of hospice care is not saving life, but improving or maintaining the quality of life until death occurs. With the recent development of the Gold Standards Framework, nurses working with hospice have a defined process to improve the quality of life through communication, collaboration, support, and coordination of care.[22]

Telehealth and E-Health

Telehealth, or telephone health, advice services have experienced major growth in Canada in recent years. These services are generally available 24 hours a day, 7 days a week. Nurses answer the phones, supply answers to health-related questions, and advise callers on how to handle nonurgent health situations.[23]

Although telehealth activities have grown significantly in the past 10 years, their full potential has not yet been reached. The success of telehealth rests on a full and seamless integration of the service as part of the health-care delivery system.[24] Understanding and eliminating barriers to the use of telehealth while capitalizing on the opportunities it presents will eventually improve the acceptance and mainstreaming of telehealth technologies. Telehealth is discussed in detail in Chapter 18.

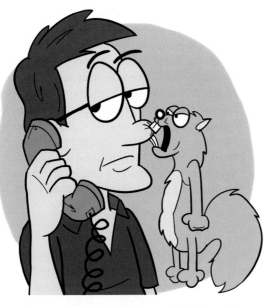

"FOR ANIMAL BITES, PLEASE PRESS 3."

E-health, or electronic health, advice takes the telephone into the computer age. Rather than calling a resource center for information, the client can use a computer, smartphone, or tablet to access any number of sites that provide health-care information. Unfortunately, some of the information available online may not be completely accurate. Persons who use these resources need to evaluate the quality and the accuracy of the information they provide.

Parish Nurses

It is estimated that approximately 2,000 parish nurses throughout the United States are attempting to meet the needs of individuals who are without adequate primary care or who are experiencing escalating health-care costs.[23] Many of these nurses work part-time or are volunteers, and some work in conjunction with community-based programs. Churches engage parish nurses to:

• Serve as health educators and counselors;
• Do health assessments and referrals;
• Organize support groups;
• Visit parishioners who are sick or elderly;
• Serve as client advocates or case managers; and
• Organize and manage parish health clinics.

Parish nurses are in a unique position to exercise their skills as case managers. As nurses, they possess clinical knowledge and skills, understand the health-care delivery system in their communities, and know many of the key health-care providers. As members of their parish, they are intimately familiar with their communities, understand the cultural climate of their clientele, and are familiar with the services that are available. Moreover, as members of the church community they serve, they are likely to be familiar with the spiritual, psychosocial, and financial needs of their clients.[23] However, direct reimbursement is not yet available for most parish nurse services.

Voluntary Health Agencies

Since their inception in 1892, voluntary health agencies have experienced steady growth and now number more than 100,000. The first voluntary health agency was the Anti-Tuberculosis Society of Philadelphia. Some of the more well-known agencies that exist today include the American Cancer Society, American Heart Association, National Foundation for the March of Dimes, National Easter Seal Society for Persons With Disabilities, and Alliance for the Mentally Ill.

These agencies provide many valuable services, including fund-raising in support of cutting-edge research and public education. Some, such as the American Cancer Society, which has a strong emphasis on education and research, also help individuals secure special equipment, such as hospital beds for the home and wigs for chemotherapy clients. The Alliance for the Mentally Ill is politically active and organizes support groups for the mentally ill and their families. These groups are not-for-profit organizations; all revenue in excess of cost goes toward improving services.

Independent Nurse-Run Health Centers

Similar to community health centers, nurse-run health centers tend to focus on health promotion and disease prevention. Historically, they have been service rather than profit oriented and remain so today. Nurses who are interested in autonomous practice often work in these settings.

Several types of nurse-run health centers have been identified. Among these are community health and institutional outreach centers. These facilities may be freestanding or sponsored by a larger institution, such as a university or public health agency. Primary care services are generally offered to the medically underserved, and these centers are typically funded by public and private sources.[25]

Wellness and health-promotion clinics are another type of nurse-run clinic and offer services at work sites, schools, churches, or homeless shelters. Many of these centers are affiliated with schools of nursing, providing health-care services while offering educational experiences for nursing students.

A final type of nursing center includes faculty practice, independent practice, and nurse entrepreneurship models. These facilities are owned and operated by nurses and may be solo or multidisciplinary practices. Services are typically reimbursed through fee-for-service plans, grants, and insurance. The ability of nurses in these centers to secure payments through the newly emergent and complex health-care reimbursement network will largely determine the future financial viability of these types of clinics.

HEALTH-CARE COSTS AND THE NURSING SHORTAGE

Although many efforts have been put forth to solve the nursing shortage over the years, it still remains a major concern for the health-care system. The median age of nurses is 46, and over 50 percent of the nursing workforce is at or over retirement age. The number of people in the over 65 demographic is rapidly increasing and have medical and health needs that will increase the need for qualified RNs. If the ACA is fully implemented, somewhere between 30 and 50 million new clients will gain access to the health-care system. Traditionally, as the economy grows stronger, fewer students seek nursing as a career, further increasing the nursing shortage.

A Cost-Cutting Measure

The origins of the current nursing shortage can be traced directly back to the implementation of managed care in the 1990s as a method of controlling health-care costs. Managed-care companies required many procedures to be performed outside the hospital, leading to clients being sicker when they do enter the hospitals.

An Expensive Mistake

Health-care facilities trying to cut costs hired fewer expensive RNs in favor of less-expensive personnel.

> *Similar to community health centers, nurse-run health centers tend to focus on health promotion and disease prevention.*

Nursing service at most facilities is the largest single budget item, averaging between 50 and 60 percent of the overall operating budget. At first glance, this seemed like a promising way to control health-care costs, but in the long run it turned out to be a very costly mistake. RNs who were employed in acute care settings moved in droves to the home health-care and primary care settings. At the same time, the population was aging, resulting in a need for more nurses who could deliver high-quality specialized care in the acute care facilities.

As a result, the health-care industry has seen a trend of closing hospital units because of a lack of RNs. It is estimated that a closed 20-bed general medical-surgical unit will cost a hospital approximately $3 million in lost revenue per year.

Stress on the Nurse

The nurses who remain are finding working conditions to be less than ideal. Mandatory overtime, short staffing, and increased acuity of client conditions all are adding to the stress these nurses experience. As a result, they call in sick more often or leave for other facilities that have fewer demands. Sick time, recruitment, and orientation costs for many facilities have skyrocketed as a result.

Stress on the Facility

The other area in which health-care institutions feel the cost of the RN shortage is in lawsuits and rising insurance costs. During periods when there is a shortage of RNs, the quality of health care decreases, clients become dissatisfied with the care they are receiving, and serious mistakes are made in care, resulting in injury or death of clients. It takes only a few of these cases with awards in the tens of millions of dollars to reemphasize the correlation between RN care and high-quality care.

Staffing Ratio Laws

One proposed solution to the nursing shortage problem is the passage of mandatory staffing ratio laws. Of course, hospital associations see these as increasing operating costs. However, the presumption is that more RNs will equate with higher quality of care and ultimately reduced long-range health-care costs.[26] For

more information, see http://www.nursingworld.org/
MainMenuCategories/ThePracticeofProfessional-
Nursing/workforce/NursingShortage.

Although laws have been passed in California, Florida, and other states, their implementation
seems to be inconsistent. Hospital association groups
in several states have challenges to the laws that have
effectively blocked their implementation for the time
being. However, nursing groups generally support
these laws and see them as a way to solve staffing
shortages by enticing inactive nurses or nurses who
have sought employment in other health-care areas to
return to the bedside in acute care facilities.

A Lack of Research

Not everyone, including some in the nursing profession, is convinced that enforced staff-to-client ratios
will cure an ailing health-care system. Although there
is an ever-growing body of evidence that shows improved RN-to-client ratios also improve outcome,
more research is required. The increasing amount of
research is a direct result of the Institute of Medicine's identification of a dearth of information about
the quality of care being delivered in the nation's
acute care facilities.

Initially, leaders in the nursing profession
hoped the new staffing ratio laws would help demonstrate the important and critical part nurses play in
providing high-quality care. The American Nurses
Association recognized as early as the 1990s that
there is a direct correlation between the care provided
by RNs and positive client outcomes. The American
Hospital Association (AHA) has formally acknowledged that RNs are critical to ensuring optimal client
care. The AHA still resists the move toward mandatory staffing ratios, characterizing them as an "over-
simplistic" solution to a complex problem. However,
recent research has demonstrated that in hospitals
with low numbers of RNs, clients are more likely to
stay longer, suffer more complications, and die from
complications that would be survivable if they were
identified and treated sooner.[26]

Passing staffing ratio laws was an attempt
to quickly fix an emotional and dramatic concern,
but it does not address a much wider range of
problems hospitalized clients face every day. What
is needed to ultimately cure the industry is a long-
range plan for systemic reform on the basis of
client needs, not the needs of a profit-motivated
insurance industry.[27]

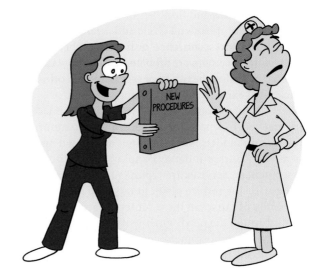

Clients educated to understand what high-
quality care is, and how it can best be achieved, will
ultimately be the most powerful force for attaining
the care they require. When managed care facilities
begin to really listen to the clients they are supposed
to be serving, nurse staffing ratio laws will no longer
be necessary. The facilities will meet the quality expectations by making sure that the needed number of
nurses is there to provide the care the client expects.

Although laws may not be the ultimate solution to a much deeper problem, clients in the states
with staffing ratio laws will be reassured to know they
will have a well-educated, skilled professional nurse
nearby who can act as an advocate for their needs and
monitor the care they are receiving when they are
most vulnerable.

Beyond the Numbers

Some in nursing are concerned that managed care facilities will use the mandated staffing ratio as a ceiling
number rather than the minimum number of nurses
required to provide safe care. There is also a fear that
the facilities will look only at the numbers and not at
the educational, skill, and experience levels of the
nurses they use to meet their quotas. Without consideration of the acuity of client conditions on a unit and
the care needs related to their illnesses, staffing ratios
may actually lower the quality of care and threaten
the safety of the clients. In addition, some fear that facilities in which the staffing ratio laws are unworkable
will close only units where sicker clients are being
treated, thus reducing access to care.[28]

A More Acute Problem

Some farsighted nursing leaders see the passage of staffing ratio laws as an important but short-term solution to a much broader problem. Decreasing nurse-to-client ratios are just a symptom of a much more acute systemic problem in the health-care industry. The underlying problem revolves around an overly aggressive policy of cost cutting by managed care, often at the expense of the very clients who support the system with their insurance premiums.

Conclusion

Health-care delivery systems are complex and multifaceted. Nurses continue to provide the majority of health-care services to North Americans and need to understand the important role they play in the system. Changes in the health-care system are never ending. By understanding the various health-care systems and how they are related to each other, nurses put themselves at the forefront of change and advocate changes that benefit the health of all people.

Nursing is as complex as the health-care system. It occurs in a wide variety of locations, and the role of the nurse will vary just as much as the health-care systems do. How a nurse functions in a hospital is different from how a nurse functions in parish nursing, but the caring and compassion that nurses bring to their roles will not vary. Nurses need to understand and develop their roles, and they will undoubtedly continue to have a significant impact on the further development of the health-care system.

Critical-Thinking Exercises

- Select three clients you are familiar with who have different health-care needs. Describe these clients' medical histories, current problems, and future health-care needs; then determine which health-care setting and which health-care practitioners would be most appropriate for them. Identify any difficulties that might be encountered during their entry into the health-care system. How can the nurse facilitate the process?

- Skilled nursing facilities, subacute care facilities, and assisted living facilities all are forms of long-term, or extended, health care. Identify five specific problems that nurses working in such facilities encounter. What is the best way to resolve these problems?

- Identify cost-cutting measures used at a health-care facility with which you are familiar. Have these measures affected the quality of client care? What other measures to cut costs can be implemented? How have changes within the health-care delivery system altered nursing practice?

- Identify four health-care priorities that may be initiated by the year 2015. How are these likely to affect the profession of nursing?

- Describe the advantages and disadvantages of various health-care reimbursement plans. Which ones will produce the highest-quality care? Which ones are best for the profession of nursing? Are there any payment plans that do both?

- Identify the most important elements in health-care reform. Should nurses support these changes? Why?

References

1. Schwartz RM. Reforming the healthcare delivery system: The impact of the Patient Protection and Affordable Care Act. *Remington Report,* 18(3):5–6, 8–10, 2010.

2. Redwood D. Health reform, prevention and health promotion: Milestone moment on a long journey. *Journal of Alternative & Complementary Medicine,* 16(5):521–523, 2010.

3. Cutler D. Analysis & commentary: How health care reform must bend the cost curve. *Health Affairs,* 29(6):1131–1135, 2010.

4. Doherty RB. The certitudes and uncertainties of health care reform. *Annals of Internal Medicine,* 152(10):679–682, 2010.

5. Chollet DJ. How temporary insurance for high-risk individuals may play out under health reform. *Health Affairs,* 29(6): 1164–1167, 2010.

6. Goodson JD. Patient Protection and Affordable Care Act: Promise and peril for primary care. *Annals of Internal Medicine,* 152(11):742–744, 2010.

7. Ebner AL. What nurses need to know about health care reform. *Nursing Economic$,* 28(3):191–194, 2010.

8. Gardner D. Health policy and politics. Expanding scope of practice: Inter-professional collaboration or conflict? *Nursing Economics,* 28(4):264–266, 2010.

9. Falardeau J. Health care reform and you: The road to implementation paved with speed bumps and potholes. *American Chiropractic Association News,* 6(8):7, 2010.

10. National Health Information Center, U. S. Department of Health and Human Services. *Income Poverty, and Health Insurance Coverage in the United States: 2010.* Washington, DC: Author, 2010.

11. Pew Research Social and Demographic Trends. Retrieved April 2013 from http://www.pewsocialtrends.org/2012/12/14/census-bureau-lowers-u-s-growth-forecast-mainly-due-to-reduced-immigration-and-births/

12. Report: Canadian health care spending unsustainable. Daily Caller New Foundation. Retrieved April 2013 from http://dailycaller.com/2012/07/24/report-canadian-health-care-spending-unsustainable/

13. Health Insurance Cost Statistics. Retrieved April, 2013 from http://www.statisticbrain.com/health-insurance-cost-statistics/, 2012.

14. Statistics Canada. Retrieved April 2013 from http://www.statcan.gc.ca/daily-quotidien/100526/dq100526b-eng.htm

15. Kane J. Health costs: How the U.S. compares with other countries, the rundown, 2012. Retrieved April 2013 from http://www.pbs.org/newshour/rundown/2012/10/health-costs-how-the-us-compares-with-other-countries.html

16. Justice and Laws website, 2013. Retrieved April 2013 from http://laws-lois.justice.gc.ca/eng/acts/C-6/

17. Rubenstein G. New Health Rankings: Of 17 Nations, U.S. Is Dead Last. Retrieved April 2013 from http://www.theatlantic.com/health/archive/2013/01/new-health-rankings-of-17-nations-us-is-dead-last/267045/

18. Storey L, Sherwen E. How to use advanced care planning in a care home. *Nursing Older People,* 25(2):14–18, 2013.

19. Preventing readmissions benefits patients, saves money. *Case Management Advisor,* 24(2):13–15, 2013.

20. Carrera I, Moreno HA, Saltarén R, Pérez C, Puglisi L, Garcia C. ROAD: Domestic assistant and rehabilitation robot. *Medical and Biological Engineering and Computing,* 49(10):1201–1211, 2011.

21. Piamjariyakul U, Ross VM, Yadrich DM, Williams AR, Howard L, Smith CE. Complex home care: Part I. Utilization and costs to families for health care services each year. *Nursing Economics,* 28(4):255–263, 2010.

22. Covington M. End-of-life care: Implementing the Gold Standards Framework. *Nursing and Residential Care,* 15(3):146–149, 2013.

23. Darkins A. Patient safety considerations in developing large telehealth networks. *Clinical Risk,* 18(3):90–94. 2012.

24. Howard H. Compassion in practice nursing. *Primary Health Care,* 22(4):21–33, 2012.

25. Owens D, Eby K, Burson S, Green M, McGoodwin W, Isaac M. Primary Palliative Care Clinic Pilot Project demonstrates benefits of a nurse practitioner-directed clinic providing primary and palliative care. *Journal of the American Academy of Nurse Practitioners,* 24(1):52–58, 2012.

26. Duffin C. Managers reject campaigner's call for mandatory staffing levels. *Nursing Standard,* 6;27(23):7, 2013.

27. Shekelle PG. Nurse-patient ratios as a patient safety strategy: A systematic review. *Annals of Internal Medicine,* 158(5 Pt 2): 404–409, 2013.

28. Johns M. Views from nursing specialists on staffing and nurse ratios. *Lamp,* 67(6):17–19, 2010.

15 Ensuring Quality Care

Viki Saidleman

Learning Objectives

After completing this chapter, the reader will be able to:

- Explain the concept of quality as it relates to client care
- Discuss how safety relates to quality of client care
- Identify three strategies used to improve quality of care
- Describe how the Sigma Six Initiative relates to improved quality of care
- Compare Institute of Medicine (IOM) Competencies, American Association of Colleges for Nursing (AACN) Essentials, and Quality and Safety Education for Nurses (QSEN) Competencies in improving the quality of health care
- Explain how risk reduction relates to quality
- Discuss three factors critical to quality endeavors
- Relate two educational initiatives that promote quality of care and safety

WHAT IS QUALITY OF CARE?

Like most complex concepts, there are several different definitions of quality care. The Institute of Medicine (IOM) defines quality as "the degree to which health services for individuals and populations increase the likelihood of desired health outcomes and are consistent with current professional knowledge."[1] Its three accepted elements are structure, process, and outcome, while care should be safe, effective, client-centered, timely, efficient, and equitable.[2]

98,000 Deaths Per Year

When the Institute of Medicine (IOM) published its first report in 2000, *To Err Is Human: Building a Safer Health System,* it estimated that 98,000 people die per year due to adverse events and medical errors in hospitals.[3] The report focused on faulty systems, processes, and conditions that led to mistakes. It recommended system changes for advocated strategies to reduce the number of errors and improve the quality of health care. The report recommended a four-tiered approach:

1. Establish leadership, research, tools, and protocols to enhance the safety knowledge base.
2. Develop a public mandatory national reporting system and encourage participation in voluntary reporting systems.
3. Use oversight organizations, health-care purchasers, and professional organizations to increase performance standards and expectations for safety improvements.
4. Implement safety systems at the point of care delivery in health-care organizations.

Based on the information from this report, the public became more aware of how frequently medical errors occur. Consumer demand for higher quality care has increased dramatically. Nurses are in a pivotal position to positively influence quality and safety at local, state, and national levels.[1] Nurses can indeed make a difference in ensuring quality of health care.

The IOM's second report in 2001, *Crossing the Quality Chasm,* focused on developing a new health-care system that improved quality of care. It identified six aims for improvement, concluding that care should be:

1. *Safe:* Avoiding injuries to clients from the care that is intended to help them.
2. *Effective:* Providing services based on scientific knowledge to all who could benefit, and refraining from providing services to those not likely to benefit.
3. *Patient-centered:* Providing care that is respectful of and responsive to individual patient preferences, needs, and values, and ensuring that patient values guide all clinical decisions.
4. *Timely:* Reducing waits and sometimes harmful delays for both those who receive and those who give care.
5. *Efficient:* Avoiding waste, including waste of equipment, supplies, ideas, and energy.

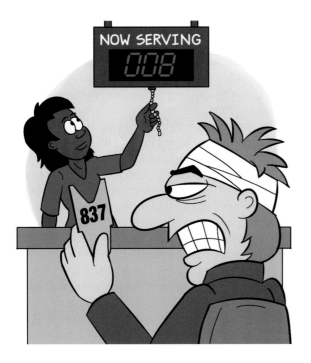

6. *Equitable:* Providing care that does not vary in quality because of personal characteristics such as gender, ethnicity, geographic location, and socioeconomic status.

Redesign elements for health care included evidence-based decision-making, safety, client as source of control, individualized client-centered care, transparency, anticipated needs, decreased waste, interdisciplinary cooperation, collaboration, and communication. Nurses are again positioned to play instrumental roles in enacting the changes necessary to overhaul the health-care system.[2]

What Do You Think?

Are nurses committed to enact the required change? Do they value quality? Do they have the necessary skills to provide safety and high-quality care?

Methods to Measure and Improve Quality

Quality assurance (QA) in health care attempts to guarantee that when an action is performed by a health-care professional, it is performed correctly the first time and each time thereafter. QA requires that actions and activities are continuously measured and compared to a standard of care established by a professional organization and that process of monitoring be in place to provide continuous feedback to prevent errors. Quality control is focused on health-care outcomes.

Quality Assurance

Quality assurance initiatives are essential when efforts are being made to cut costs and, at the same time, maintain high standards of care. To ensure high-quality care, the health-care industry borrowed the philosophy of **continuous quality improvement (CQI)** from the business world. According to the CQI philosophy, there are internal customers and external customers. The external customers are clients and their families; internal customers are individuals working within the health-care setting. The Joint Commission was so impressed with its potential to improve health-care delivery that in 1994 it began requiring hospitals to implement CQI strategies. These strategies target select processes to evaluate and improve.

Exceeding Expectations

Continuous quality improvement, also known as **total quality management (TQM)**, is based on the belief that the organization with higher-quality services will capture a greater share of the market than competitors with lower-quality services. This approach emphasizes customer satisfaction, promotes innovation, and requires employee involvement and commitment. The goal is not only to meet the expectations of the client but also to exceed those expectations. This plan uses a multidisciplinary approach in a systematic manner to design, measure, assess, and improve the performance of an organization. Standards for **benchmarking** are used to classify acceptable levels of performance. These may be written for outcomes, processes, or for structures. Outcome standards focus on results of care given, process standards relate to care delivery, and structure standards relate to the organization, management, or physical environment of the organization. Different tools or indicators are used to measure performance against the set standards. Then actual performance is compared to standards and across institutions. **Dashboards** are electronic tools that act as a scorecard. They can provide retrospective or real-time data to assess quality. These informatics technologies assist the process of quality improvement.

Delivering high-quality services is valued above all else, and the ideal goal is that every constituent be completely satisfied with the services provided.

Client Satisfaction

Client satisfaction is another way to measure quality of care. The Hospital Care Quality Information from the Consumer Perspective (HCAHPS) initiative began in 2008 and provides a standardized survey instrument and data collection method to obtain client satisfaction data on eight key topics: communication with doctors, communication with nurses, responsiveness of hospital staff, pain management, communication about medications, discharge information, cleanliness of environment, and quietness of hospital environment. Three goals directed the survey's development: (1) Produce a method to provide comparison of client satisfaction data, (2) create hospital motivation to improve care quality, and (3) increase hospital transparency in terms of quality of care. This initiative is an example of benchmarking that compares data between similar organizations in an effort to identify areas for growth and areas of strength.[4]

The standardized survey instrument allows health-care organizations to monitor, compare, and improve their performance. It benefits consumers by enhancing the ability to select health-care services based upon the institution's known and shown performance in established key areas.

Leapfrog Group

If you are having problems identifying quality care when you see it, the Leapfrog Group may have a solution. In November 2000, **Leapfrog Group** was officially launched by larger health-care facilities that worked together to improve the quality and safety of health care and make it more affordable. The resulting movement now serves as the gold standard for comparison of hospital performance on national standards of safety, quality, and efficiency, thereby facilitating transparency and easy access to health-care information.[5]

> *Nurses are in a pivotal position to positively influence quality and safety at local, state, and national levels.*

Rewarding Performance and Quality Care

Like many of the quality initiatives, Leapfrog grew out of the 1999 report by the Institute of Medicine concerning preventable medical errors. The group was awed by the finding that up to 98,000 Americans die every year from preventable medical errors made in hospitals alone. In fact, there are more deaths in hospitals each year from preventable medical mistakes than there are from vehicle accidents, breast cancer, and AIDS combined. The report indicated that there was a need for more quality and safety in the provision of health care. Leapfrog's founders realized that they could take "leaps" forward in quality health care for their employees, retirees, and families by rewarding hospitals that implement significant improvements in quality and safety.

Inspired by the Premier/CMS Hospital Quality Incentive Demonstration Project and building on the measures in the Hospital Quality Alliance initiative, the Leapfrog Hospital Rewards Program measures the quality of care and the efficiency with which hospitals use resources in five clinical areas that represent the majority of hospital admissions

Box 15.1

How to Identify Quality Care and Providers

Quality Elements to Identify	YES	NO

Quality Health-Care Plan

Is rated highly by members and on http://reportcard.ncqa.org/plan/external/

People who have the plan maintain their health and recover from illness

Is accredited by a recognized organization

The physicians and hospitals you use are included

Has a list of benefits to choose from that your age and condition require

Is affordable

Quality Physician(s)

Has a certification that is appropriate to your medical requirements

Is rated highly on http://doctorofficereviews.com/index.php?awtil=
    th836452chams9l&aff=gaw2-rating%20doctors

Is focused on prevention as well as treatment

Holds admission privileges at the hospitals you use

Is covered by your health plan

Actually listens to what you have to say and encourages questions

Explains treatments, medications, and instructions so that you understand

Respects you as an individual

Quality Hospital

Is rated highly on http://www.medicare.gov/hospitalcompare/search.html
    or http://www.carechex.com/

Is rated highly by your state's consumer groups

Receives high rating post discharge client evaluations

Has an accreditation by the Joint Commission on Accreditation of
    Healthcare Organizations

Belongs to the Hospital Rewards Program for quality care

Holds Magnet Hospital Recognition

Is included in your health plan and your physician has privileges

Has a comprehensive quality improvement and risk reduction plan

At least 50 percent of the nursing staff are baccalaureate RNs

Has a positive reputation for successfully treating your disease process(es)

Uses a rapid response team to reduce injuries to patients while in the hospital

Bases care on scientific principles and best practices

Provides client-centered care based on respect for the individual

Has a low level of inpatient medication errors

Fosters interprofessional collaboration in all aspects of client care

Has a low number of sentinel and never events

Fosters an environment and culture of safety throughout the facility and expenditures. Hospitals are scored and rewarded separately for each of the five areas and can participate in any of the areas in which they provide care. If they demonstrate sustained excellence or improvement, hospitals are eligible for financial rewards and increased market share.[5]

Hospital scores can become the basis for financial incentives for consumers, such as waived co-pays or deductibles for choosing care at high-performing or improving hospitals. Additionally, these scores can be incorporated into health plans' existing performance-based incentive and reward programs. The program is engineered by Leapfrog, with the input of a vast array of providers and health plans, but it is designed to be implemented by health plans and employers in specific markets.

A key principle of the Leapfrog program is that payers should have a say in what they are purchasing. As a pay-for-performance program for hospitals, Leapfrog makes it easier for health-care purchasers to identify and reward those hospitals that are providing high-quality care for their employees and at the same time helping to gain better value for health-care dollars. Facilities that meet these goals are recognized and rewarded. The Leapfrog Group was launched in 2000 and is supported by the Robert Wood Johnson Foundation, Leapfrog members, and others.

> *Leapfrog's founders realized that they could take 'leaps' forward in quality health care for their employees, retirees, and families by rewarding hospitals that implement significant improvements in quality and safety.*

Leapfrog's Mission and Goal

The Leapfrog Group's mission is to promote giant leaps forward in the safety, quality, and affordability of health care by:

• Supporting informed health-care decisions by those who use and pay for health care
• Promoting high-value health care through incentives and rewards.

There are four concepts that underlie the Leapfrog mission:

1. Health care in the United States is at unacceptably low levels of basic safety, quality, and overall customer value.

2. Major leaps forward in the quality of health care can be achieved if those who purchase health care recognize and reward superior safety and quality.
3. The purchasing power of America's largest employers can be used to encourage other purchasers to join and put additional pressure on health-care providers to improve quality.
4. Guided by specific innovations that present "great leaps" forward in the improvement of safety and quality of care, Leapfrog can increase media involvement and consumer support for the program.[5]

Leapfrog's goal is to promote high-quality health care through incentives and rewards. This is the first ever national private-sector program that responds to the urgent needs of care service purchasers. It provides solutions for escalating health costs and substandard quality. The Hospital Rewards Program builds on incentives for continued improvements in hospital quality and efficiency and enables health plans and purchasers to better provide financially sound rewards for hospitals.

What Do You Think?

Is using rewards a good way to motivate health-care institutions to improve the quality of care? In your experience, do rewards work by themselves as incentives? If not, what other things can be done to increase motivation?

Health benefits are provided to more than 37 million Americans in all 50 states through the Leapfrog Group's consortium of major companies and other large private and public health-care purchasers. The influence that Leapfrog can exert on health-care facilities lies in the tens of billions of dollars the group spends on health care annually. All the Leapfrog members agreed to purchase health care from facilities that encourage and demonstrate quality improvement and consumer involvement. The Leapfrog evaluation is based on four key principles:

1. All evidence-based research shows that these quality and safety leaps will significantly reduce preventable medical mistakes.

2. Implementing the reforms is easily and quickly accomplished by the health industry. Many facilities have already initiated them.

3. Safety and quality improvements will be immediately appreciated by clients.

4. Health plans, purchasers, or consumers will be able to easily determine whether or not the reforms are present or absent in the facilities they are planning to use.

It is estimated that if all U.S. hospitals implemented just the first three of Leapfrog's four "leaps," over 57,000 lives could be saved, more than 3 million medication errors could be avoided, and up to $12 billion could be saved each year. For more information, visit Try: http://www.leapfroggroup.org/, http://www.leapfroggroup.org/news/leapfrog_news/636854, and http://www.leapfroggroup.org/about_leapfrog/eapfrog-factsheet.

Quality Indicators

The Agency for Healthcare Research and Quality (AHRQ) uses **quality indicators** (QIs) as measures of health-care quality from easily accessible inpatient hospital administrative data. Quality indicators include prevention, inpatient, patient safety, and pediatric. The QIs are used to focus efforts on potential quality concerns so they may be addressed by further investigation. QI results are also used to track changes over time.[6]

A Proactive Approach

Continuous quality improvement (CQI) is proactively oriented so that emphasis is placed on anticipating and preventing problems rather than reacting to them after the fact. CQI requires that the service delivery process receive close and constant scrutiny, and everyone is encouraged to generate and test ideas for improving quality. Although CQI encourages change on the basis of systematically documented evidence, it also values standardization of the process so that efficiency is maximized. As an example of the proactive approach, researchers have found that using standardized processes and tools during annual wellness visits for teens with asthma significantly increased

Continuous quality improvement (CQI) is proactively oriented so that emphasis is placed on anticipating and preventing problems rather than reacting to them after the fact.

quality care provision and doubled overall adherence to the medical regime.[7]

Nurses are in an excellent position to implement CQI strategies. On a daily basis, they assess the functioning of the health-care delivery system and the effectiveness of specific treatment approaches. For example, on the basis of evidence that inexpensive saline is as effective as heparin in keeping intravenous catheters patent, nurses at one hospital implemented a new protocol and saved $70,000 within 1 year, while maintaining quality of care.[8]

Case Management Protocols

There is another mechanism for monitoring cost-effective, high-quality care: outcome-based case management protocols, also known as **clinical pathways**. The development of clinical pathways grew out of a need to assess, implement, and monitor cost-effective, high-quality client care in a systematic manner.

Clinical pathways are an outgrowth of nursing care plans but have the advantages of streamlining the charting process, encouraging documentation across multidisciplinary teams, and systematically monitoring variances from prescribed plans of care. The ability to identify how client care and progress vary from a predetermined plan enables more accurate assessment of client-care costs and maintenance of quality-control measures. Integration of clinical pathways into practical use has been enhanced by computerization of client records and online bedside documentation.

Risk Management

Risk management is a component of quality management programs. It focuses on identifying, analyzing, and evaluating risks, and then reducing that risk to decrease harm to clients. When an adverse event does occur, attempts are made to minimize losses. This program is interdisciplinary in nature and includes aspects of detection, education, and intervention. Nursing staff is key to any risk management program. High-risk areas include medication errors, complications from tests and treatments, falls, refusal of treatment or refusal to sign treatment consents, and client/family dissatisfaction. Client records and occurrence/incident reports are used to track and analyze the occurrences. The analysis, often called **root cause analysis**, tracks events leading to error, identifies faulty systems, and processes and develops a plan to prevent further errors.

The Joint Commission sets mandatory National Patient Safety Goals that address particular risks for clients. Hospitals improve quality and safety by making these goals a priority in client care. They include the following:

1. Improve accuracy of client identification
2. Improve effectiveness of communication among caregivers
3. Improve safety of using medications
4. Reduce risk of health-care-associated infections
5. Identify client safety risks inherent in its patient population

> *High-risk areas include medication errors, complications from tests and treatments, falls, refusal of treatment or refusal to sign treatment consents, and client/family dissatisfaction.*

The Joint Commission's central focus is to promote quality evidence-based measures to maximize health benefits.[9]

Issues Now

Healthy People 2020

It seems like the Healthy People 2010 campaign just started, but the 10-year revision is already here. The Healthy People initiative is based on the belief that setting objectives and providing benchmarks promotes tracking and monitoring of progress; these in turn can motivate, guide, and focus actions to increase the quality of health in the United States. The initiative, begun by the U.S. Department of Health and Human Services (HHS), has been renewed each decade since its beginnings in 1980. Starting in 2009, HHS began formulating objectives for the next decade. One of the major changes is that the report produced will be available online and on paper to better deliver the information tailored to the needs of its users. HHS will also be producing a user-friendly disk that will be distributed on request.

Healthy People 2020 envisions the United States becoming a society in which all people live long, healthy lives. The mission of the project is to work through federal and state governmental agencies to strengthen the policies and practices to make people healthier. Some of the strategies include identifying nationwide health improvement priorities, increasing public awareness and understanding of what produces health and what causes disease and disability, developing measurable goals and objectives for all levels of government, and using evidence-based practices to guide actions and focus research to collect data in key areas. Healthy People 2020 rests on four key goals:

- Eliminating preventable disease and death
- Achieving health equity by eliminating disparities and improving the health of all groups
- Creating social and physical environments that promote good health for all citizens
- Promoting healthy habits and behaviors for all ages of the population

The 2020 campaign has increased the number of priority, or focus, areas from 22 in 2000 to 28 in 2020.

Healthy People 2020 is important because it forms a national health agenda that, combined with health-care reform, can be used as a vision and a strategy for the whole nation. Its national-level goals are a road map for where the nation needs to go and how it will get there. Healthy People 2020 will be action oriented and will provide leadership, guidance, and direction for individuals and governmental agencies alike. For more information about the ongoing developments and plans for implementation, go to http://www.healthypeople.gov/hp2020.

Source: http://www.healthypeople.gov/hp2020 (retrieved May 2013).

Sentinel Events

The Joint Commission defines a **sentinel event** as an "unexpected occurrence involving death or serious physical or psychological injury, or the risk thereof. Serious injury includes loss of limb or function."[10] Sentinel events are not the same as errors. Not all sentinel events are due to errors and not all errors cause sentinel events. Sentinel events indicate the need for immediate investigation and response. The Joint Commission reviews organizations' responses to sentinel events in its accreditation process. Its goal is to improve the quality of care and prevent future sentinel event occurrences.

What Do You Think?

Identify an incident that occurred during your time in health-care institutions, either as a student or an employee, that would be considered a high-risk or a sentinel event. How was the incident dealt with? What do you think was learned from the incident?

Six Sigma Quality Improvements

Although Six Sigma was developed and used initially for the manufacturing industry in the early 1980s, it found its way into the health-care system in the mid- to late 1990s. It was seen as a way to identify problems in health-care delivery and find effective solutions.

The Tail of the Curve

Its origins can be traced back to the 1920s and are based on the statistical model of the bell-shaped curve. In the perfect bell curve, there is a mean exactly in the center at the highest point of the curve. Away from the mean, the curve slopes down at a predictable rate on both sides and is divided into standard deviations. Each standard deviation is designated by the Greek letter for a small "s" or "σ" (sigma) and given a number (e.g., plus or minus 1 sigma). Six standard deviations (six sigmas) are so far out in the tails of the bell curve that they are generally considered a total lack of error—in other words, "perfection" (statistically, 3.4 defects per million). Its focus is a quality management program that serves as a measure, a goal, and a system of management to ensure optimal quality results (Fig. 15.1).

The Six Sigma technique was initially used by Motorola to improve the quality of their products and was then adopted by such well-known corporations as

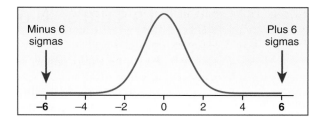

F i g u r e 1 5 . 1 The Six Sigma bell curve.

General Electric and Honeywell. It can be used to reduce the costs of manufacturing items or the steps in manufacturing, making the manufacturing process more "lean."[11]

The traditional Six Sigma process comprises five distinct phases that somewhat parallel the steps of the nursing process:

1. *Define:* The problem is identified. Why are the customers dissatisfied? Why are the costs excessive? Why does it take so long to complete the process?
2. *Measure:* Data are collected to pinpoint the exact issue. The whole process is reviewed in detail and time, or other types of measurement are given numerical values.
3. *Analyze:* The root causes of the problem are identified, and the relationships of external or environmental influences are analyzed. All factors must be considered, no matter how remote.
4. *Improve:* Strategies, based on the previous three phases, are developed to correct the problems. Any number of techniques may be used to make the process error-proof and more efficient. Pilot projects are then established to demonstrate the success of the efforts to correct the problems. Several attempts may be tested before the best one is identified.
5. *Control:* Systems are put in place to continuously monitor the changes in the process. The goal is to detect errors before they affect the whole system. A statistical process may be used to determine the level of correction and as an early warning system for new problems.[11]

Six Sigma in Health Care

How does the health-care system use Six Sigma to improve the quality of care? Traditionally in health care, finding and defining the specific cause of errors have been extremely difficult. Six Sigma provides a wide-reaching and more pragmatic approach to identifying and measuring the problem. By adapting and modifying the traditional Six Sigma methodology, health-care providers can develop more inclusive objectives to increase reliability and quality. The overriding goal of Six Sigma is to develop a fully reliable process or system of care. Such a system will deliver the same quality of care to all clients all the time regardless of who actually delivers the care. Optimal care is provided when it is evidence based.

Black Belts

As a highly structured approach to identifying fundamental problems, the Six Sigma process guides nurses and others through the five-phase process using statistical tools. Specialized training is required to employ Six Sigma, and individuals can become certified as Six Sigma consultants through the Institute of Industrial Engineers or the American Society for Quality. Trained employees of Six Sigma, called Black Belts, serve as well-paid consultants for hospitals and other institutions that believe Six Sigma may be the answer to their problems.[11]

When the Six Sigma process is used to analyze a problem, it looks primarily for two types of statistical anomalies or variations. The primary one, usually at the root of most problems, is called *special* or *assigned variation* and shows a pattern of activity outside the patterns expected to produce high-quality care. Once this variation is detected, the five-step statistical process can be applied. The second type of anomaly is called *common* or *chance variation* and is usually attributed to environmental factors that cannot be controlled. However, in some situations, chance variations can become so significant that they affect the process and have to be addressed.

As a newcomer to health care, the Six Sigma process has been used on a limited basis. The Commonwealth Health Corporation in Kentucky was one of the first to use Six Sigma in 2002. It was used to streamline their radiology department and increase its bottom line by reducing costs. There is only a relatively small body of publications about the successes and problems of using it in the health-care setting. Six Sigma has been used successfully in other hospitals to increase nurse satisfaction and retention by eliminating tedious factors in day-to-day operations, to reduce clients' length of stay, and to speed up the process for transferring clients from outpatient areas to inpatient rooms. In a systematic literature review of 47 articles that met inclusion criteria, studies provided limited data and lacked follow-up. The researchers concluded that Six Sigma can assist in quality improvement, but more evidence base is needed for sustainability of results.[12]

A Hybrid

A hybrid Six Sigma program called Lean Six Sigma focuses on identifying and eliminating waste and therefore improving the flow of processes. A research study has shown that Lean Six Sigma improved the quality of trauma care by reducing inappropriate hospital stays while reducing costs.[13] In a different study, researchers have discovered that the use of Lean Six Sigma improved the collaborative efficiency of meal delivery, radiological testing, and timing of inpatient insulin administration.[14]

There are critics of Six Sigma, and several drawbacks to its use have been identified. Six Sigma is effective in modifying existing processes, but it tends to stifle creative approaches and "thinking outside the box." Although achieving perfection at the statistical 3.4 errors per million level might be adequate for situations such as client satisfaction and nurse retention, it seems to fall short for activities such as administering medications and operating a ventilator. When Six Sigma is implemented in the health-care setting, it is often used as an add-on project not connected with existing quality improvement efforts. Nursing staff tend to resist the strange-sounding jargon and statistical emphasis and may actually attempt to sabotage implementation. Six Sigma has little regard for the interpersonal and institutional culture that is so important in the effectiveness of health-care institutions.

The overall objective of Six Sigma is to increase the reliability of processes by eliminating defects and reducing system variation. Its five-phase structured approach requires high-quality discrete data that are often difficult to obtain in the health-care setting. Its orientation is more industrial than health related: It uses tools such as statistical process control and root-cause analysis to identify anomalies in the processes it is examining. Although yet to be

> " *Trained employees of Six Sigma, called Black Belts, serve as well-paid consultants for hospitals and other institutions that believe Six Sigma may be the answer to their problems.* "

used on a wide scale in the health-care setting, Six Sigma is gradually gaining a following, and its use in health care will probably increase in the future.[15]

EDUCATION AND A COMPETENCY FOCUS

The focus on quality care needs to begin on the first day of a health-care professional's education and continue through the whole education program. Certain initiatives in nursing and medical education focus on developing health-care professionals' competencies critical to

> " *Some nursing leaders believe that by conforming to QSEN-based curricula, they will transform the professional identity of nursing into something other than nursing.* "

providing safe, quality health care. The Competency Outcomes Performance Assessment (COPA) model was started in the 1990s. The American Association of Colleges of Nursing (AACN) has developed program outcomes for baccalaureate curricula that focus on quality. In 2005, the Robert Wood Johnson Foundation introduced the Quality and Safety Education for Nurses (QSEN) project. In 2010, the Institute of Medicine (IOM) issued its report on nursing's future and suggestions for change.

Issues Now

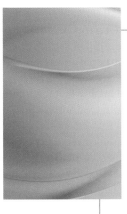

Client Education Is a Quality-of-Care Issue

In the current health-care system, client teaching is not only an expectation but is also an ethical and legal requirement. The enactment of the 2010 Affordable Care Act (ACA) gives nurses new opportunities to provide high-quality care, including preventive teaching. Whether the nurse is providing health promotion, health maintenance, or health rehabilitation, increasing a client's level of knowledge and understanding is required legally and ethically. In recent years, several lawsuits have resulted from the failure of nurses to provide adequate client teaching. Consider the following case:

     The court in *Kyslinger v. United States* (1975) addressed the nurse's liability for client teaching. In this case, a Veterans Administration (VA) hospital sent a hemodialysis client home with an artificial kidney. The client eventually died (apparently while connected to the hemodialysis machine) and his wife sued, alleging that the hospital and its staff failed to teach her or her husband how to properly use and maintain a home hemodialysis unit.

     After examining the evidence, the court ruled against the client's wife as follows: "During those 10 months that plaintiff's decedent underwent biweekly hemodialysis treatment on the units (at the VA hospital), both plaintiff and decedent were instructed as to the operation, maintenance, and supervision of said treatment. The Court can find no basis to conclude that the plaintiff or plaintiff's decedent were not properly informed on the use of the hemodialysis unit." The moral of the story: Always document what was done and what clients and their families were taught. Make sure to include documentation that they did (or did not) understand what was taught.

     Clients are advised to be "smart" and learn as much as possible about their health-care needs. Expert nurses have modeled ways to incorporate client education as a priority in care, and nurse theorists provide worldviews and theories imbued with the primacy of client education. The nation's clients and consumers of health-care services need their most trusted professionals—nurses—to drive substantial initiatives to address health literacy concerns. The ANA's 2010 House of Delegates approved a literacy resolution that addresses the nurse's need to educate. It sets the stage for the ANA to implement the following:

- Promote collaborative nursing initiatives to address health literacy problems
- Use existing research findings to strengthen health literacy knowledge and skills in nursing school curricula and in RNs' workplaces
- Advance nursing research to identify evidence-based practices that promote optimum health literacy

Source: Retrieved May 2013 from http://www.health.gov/communication/literacy/quickguide/resources.htm and http://www.fiercehealthcare.com/story/4-ways-educate-patients-about-affordable-care-act/2012-07-23.

Competency Outcomes Performance Assessment (COPA) Model

The **Competency Outcomes Performance Assessment (COPA) model,** developed in the early 1990s, has been used by medical schools and some schools of nursing to validate the skills and knowledge of their graduates. It is designed to promote competency for clinical practice at all levels. Key components in several of its eight core competencies address quality, safety, and risk reduction, aligning well with the Quality and Safety Education for Nurses (QSEN) competencies. One study explored the COPA model's use in two prelicensure nursing programs and in a graduate nurse internship program. Research has demonstrated the COPA model's benefits for nursing students, nursing graduates, preceptors, employers, and clients. Benefits noted for clients included increased quality and safety.[16]

Quality and Safety Education for Nurses (QSEN)

Driven by community and professional concerns, the Robert Wood Johnson Foundation undertook a three-phase project to improve the quality and safety of client care by focusing nursing education on student competency. The project, QSEN, is built on five competencies initially developed by the IOM:[17]

> *Starting in the fall of 2007, the CMS changed the Medicare payment program to no longer pay for reasonably preventable medical errors that occur in the hospital.*

- Client-centered care
- Teamwork and collaboration
- Evidence-based practice (EBP)
- Quality improvement (QI)[18]
- Safety

A sixth competency, informatics, was later added as the model developed and was revised because of the important role technology now plays in health care. Subsequent research demonstrates that using the QSEN model contributed to the adoption of quality and safety competencies as core practice values.[19] (See Chapter 4 for more detail.)

Essentials of Baccalaureate Education for Professional Nursing Practice

For many years, the AACN document, *Essentials of Baccalaureate Education for Professional Nursing Practice,* has been the gold standard for outcomes for nursing programs. *AACN's Essential II: Basic Organizational and Systems Leadership for Quality Care and Patient Safety* addresses the relationship of safety, quality improvement, and organizational and systems leadership to ensuring quality nursing care. It further outlines skills critical to safety and quality that the nurse must exhibit. Common skills to both QSEN and the *Essentials* include communication and collaboration, decision-making, participation in safety initiatives, quality improvement processes, and cost-effectiveness.[20] Between 2010 and 2011, AACN developed six Web-based learning modules as a free nursing faculty development resource. These focus on QSEN's six core competencies and provide teaching strategies to imbed within the nursing curricula for graduate nursing students. Is there a clear-cut advantage in using the *Essentials* over the QSEN competencies as a curricular model or is the best approach to integrate them?

A Difference in Opinion

Some nursing leaders believe that by conforming to QSEN-based curricula, they will transform the professional identity of nursing into something other than nursing. What about the competencies of caring, integrity, and client advocacy? What about research and scholarship? Where does prevention, a key nursing role since the time of Florence Nightingale, fit in? Those who support QSEN believe that if a nurse is providing high-quality, safe, respectful, and culturally appropriate care, caring and integrity are already included. Others contend that QSEN's inclusion of evidence-based practice as a competency addresses research concerns. QSEN's competency of quality improvement along with its value for updating knowledge and skills also addresses scholarship concerns. Some argue that health promotion and disease prevention are already included in QSEN's model under patient-centered care. Others believe that in order to promote nursing as a unique discipline, a seventh competency, "professional person," should be added to include those aspects of nursing that distinguish it from the medical profession.

The ANA Project

In the fall of 2010, a report by the ANA and the Constituent Member Associations (CMA) moved the discussion to a new level by outlining the key messages from the IOM Report on the Future of Nursing. This report is part of an ongoing project aimed at using evidence-based practice to advance the nursing profession so that nursing can keep pace with health-care reform activities (see Chapter 4 for more information).[21]

Federal Initiatives for Coverage of AHRQ, QIO, and CMS

The Agency for Healthcare Research and Quality (AHRQ) is 1 of 12 Department of Health and Human Services agencies that supports research that improves the quality of health care and helps people make more informed health-care decisions. The agency is charged with developing partnerships that create long-term improvement in American health care. The research goal is to measure those improvements in terms of client outcomes, decreased mortality, improved quality of life, and cost-effective quality care. Its overall focus is in three areas:

- Safety and quality: Risk reduction by promoting quality care
- Effectiveness: Improved health outcomes by using evidence to make informed health-care decisions
- Efficiency: Translating research into practice to increase access and to decrease costs[22]

The Affordable Care Act, Sect. 3501, mandates that the AHRQ work through a Center for Quality Improvement and Patient Safety to conduct research on best quality improvement practice innovations and strategies. The Center's tasks also include identifying, creating, critiquing, sharing, and giving training in these best practices. In addition, the Center must coordinate its activities with the Centers for Medicare and Medicaid Services (CMS) and the Centers for Medicare and Medicaid Innovation (CMI). The Center will award grants to agencies with expertise in providing assistance to health providers in quality improvement activities and to the health-care providers seeking such technical assistance in implementing best practice models.[23]

The Quality Improvement Organization (QIO) is a federal program designed to review medical care, verify its necessity, and assist Medicare and Medicaid beneficiaries with complaints about quality of care. The program is also charged to implement quality of care improvements. According to the Centers for Medicare and Medicaid Services, "by law, the mission of the QIO Program is to improve the effectiveness, efficiency, economy, and quality of services delivered to Medicare beneficiaries."[24] The Centers for Medicare and Medicaid Services identifies three core functions for QIO:

- Improving quality of care for beneficiaries
- Protecting the integrity of the Medicare Trust Fund by ensuring that Medicare pays only for services and goods that are reasonable and necessary and that are provided in the most appropriate setting
- Protecting beneficiaries by expeditiously addressing individual complaints, such as beneficiary complaints; provider-based notice appeals; violations of the Emergency Medical Treatment and Labor Act (EMTALA); and other related responsibilities as articulated in QIO-related law

Researchers linked all-cause 30-day rehospitalization and all-cause hospitalization reductions in Medicare beneficiaries in communities with CQI programs.[25]

What Do You Think?

Have you ever complained about the care you or a loved one received while in a hospital or clinic? If not, why not? If you did, what happened to the complaint? Were there any changes made?

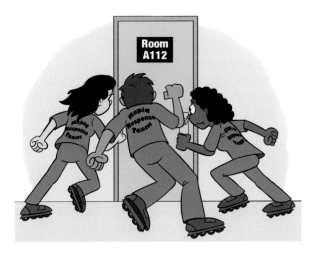

Never Events

Starting in the fall of 2007, the CMS changed the Medicare payment program so that they would no longer pay for reasonably preventable medical errors that occur in the hospital. These events, listed on the CMS website, are referred to as "**never events**."[26] Subsequently, hospitals now have to cover costs for "never events" that do occur. The purpose of this change is to control Medicare costs and improve the quality care; however, quality may come at a heavy price for institutions already financially stressed. This list is likely to be revised substantially as the various elements of the ACA are implemented.

Transforming Care at the Bedside

The Robert Woods Johnson Foundation and the Institute for Healthcare Improvement (IHI) joined forces to create a framework called Transforming Care at the Bedside to institute change on medical surgical nursing units. Their goal was to improve care and staff satisfaction by addressing four main categories:

- Safe and reliable care
- Vitality and teamwork
- Patient-centered care
- Value-added care processes

Ideas for change included use of **rapid response teams** to "rescue" clients whose conditions were deteriorating and prevent their in-hospital deaths, specific communication models to make interdisciplinary communication clearer, a workspace that promotes efficiency and waste reduction, professional support programs, and liberalized diet plans and meal times. These efforts focus on improving the quality of client care on medical-surgical nursing units.[27]

Key Factors to High-Quality Care

IOM, QSEN, and AACN's Essentials of Nursing Education all agree on the importance of scholarship, research, and evidence-based practice in ensuring quality and safety in health care. The developments in technology now make access to this type of information easy and immediate.

Evidence-Based Practice/Research

For this competency, one must "integrate best current evidence with clinical expertise and client/family preferences and values for delivery of optimal health care.[28] Researchers have been finding multiple benefits of evidence-based practice, including cost-effectiveness, increased client safety, improved clinical outcomes, and client and staff satisfaction.[29–31]

Client-Centered Care

According to QSEN, client-centered care occurs when the nurse can "recognize the client or designee as the source of control and full partner in providing compassionate and coordinated care based on respect for patient's preferences, values, and needs.[32] Research about health-care institutions that utilized client and family advisors to promote client-centered care found improved client outcomes in shorter length of stay, higher client satisfaction, and improved levels of reimbursements.[33]

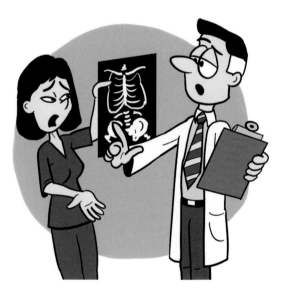

Teamwork and Collaboration

The Institute of Medicine, the Quality and Safety in Nursing Education initiative, and the AACN Essentials of Nursing Education all emphasize the importance of interdisciplinary teamwork, communication, and collaboration in achieving safe, quality health care. This is defined as the ability to "function effectively within nursing and inter-professional teams, fostering open communication, mutual respect, and shared decision-making to achieve quality client care."[17,32] In one study, investigators reviewed the Lewis Blackman case in which a 15-year-old boy died 4 days after surgical repair of a chest deformity. (For more information on this interesting case, go to http://qsen.org/videos/the-lewis-blackman-story/.) Researchers then devised a model to characterize the events leading to the tragic death. They proposed five strategies that nurse educators can use to promote safety and quality in nursing care. These strategies included the following:

- Use "cognitive unmooring questions" in the assessment of clients by students so that they will note subtle changes in the client's condition such as decreased urine output or low blood pressure (i.e., make them think outside the box).
- Incorporate System 1 and System 2 thinking into the curriculum's didactics (i.e., use of both implicit and explicit thinking to solve problems).
- Use case studies during simulation exercises.
- Have an awareness of and strategies for approaching authority gradients (i.e., fear of reporting something to someone in a position of authority) in interdisciplinary collaboration.
- Communication and provision of experiences that recognize client and family as key members of the health-care team.[34]

" *Researchers have been finding multiple benefits of evidence-based practice, including cost-effectiveness, increased client safety, improved clinical outcomes, and client and staff satisfaction.* "

Informatics

IOM, QSEN, and AACN Essentials of Nursing Education all agree on the importance of informatics to ensuring client safety and the quality of health care. Informatics is the "use of information and technology to communicate, manage knowledge, mitigate error, and support decision-making."[32] (For more detail, see Chapter 18.) Canadian nurse experts identified informatics competency as "state of the art communication and technology savvy" and related its linkage to the nurse executive's role as leader to support outcomes of safe, integrated, high-quality care delivery through knowledge-driven care.[35]

Lifelong Learning

Quality and safety in nursing care requires continually updating one's knowledge and skills. Since nursing has multiple levels of entry, formal education must also be viewed as a method for lifelong learning. One research study provided evidence of decreased

client mortality with a higher proportion of baccalaureate-prepared nurses providing care in an acute care setting.[36] The AACN also supports a nursing workforce that is more highly educated.[37] In a review of the literature, researchers have discovered that through increasing nursing education levels, client outcomes and quality of care can be improved.[38]

The Tri-Council for Nursing Issues New Consensus Policy Statement on the Educational Advancement of Registered Nurses declared that healthcare reform requires a workforce "that integrates evidence-based clinical knowledge and research with effective communication and leadership skills. These competencies require increased education at all levels. At this tipping point for the nursing profession, action is needed now to put in place strategies to build a stronger nursing workforce. Without a more educated nursing workforce, the nation's health will be further at risk."[39] Agreeing with this stance is the Joint Statement on Academic Progression for Nursing Students and Graduates' belief "that every nursing student and nurse deserves the opportunity to pursue academic career growth and development."[40]

Environment

Nursing cultures need to make quality and safety a priority rather than focusing on what went wrong after an adverse event happens and trying to blame someone for the error. Other characteristics of blame-free or **just culture** organizations include positive working environments, commitment to safety and quality, transparency, and using errors as learning opportunities. A blameless reporting system assists in reporting errors and near misses voluntarily and anonymously. The just culture holds staff accountable for at-risk or reckless behaviors and does not tolerate them; however, it is prepared to handle human error occurrences. The focus becomes an analysis of the event to identify system improvements that can positively impact quality of care and safety.

In 1983, the American Academy of Nursing (AAN) Task Force on Nursing Practices studied work environments in hospitals that attracted and retained well-qualified nurses who promoted quality client care. Hospitals that demonstrated these qualities were designated as "magnet hospitals."[41] Building upon this study, the ANA board of directors approved a proposal for the Magnet Hospital Recognition Program for Excellence in Nursing Services. The most current Magnet Recognition Model Program has five components:

- Transformational leadership
- Structural empowerment
- Exemplary professional practice
- New knowledge, innovation, and improvements
- Empirical quality results

> *Quality and safety in nursing care requires continually updating one's knowledge and skills. Since nursing has multiple levels of entry, formal education must also be viewed as a method for lifelong learning.*

Several research studies have shown a link between the Magnet hospital experience and increased client satisfaction, decreased mortality rates, decreased pressure ulcers, decreased falls, and improved client safety and quality.[42–45]

Conclusion

Quality can be an elusive goal for the health-care professional, the health-care institution, and the client and family. Quality requires commitment by multidisciplinary team members and health-care institutions to provide, monitor, assess, and evaluate the effectiveness of processes and structures to make improvements and to achieve optimal health-care outcomes. Quality challenges the nurse to be constantly vigilant, to be aware of high-risk situations, and to be dedicated to processes, structures, and policies that ensure quality.

Quality necessitates an informed health-care consumer. It is critical that the consumer is aware and informed of health-care quality and safety issues and utilizes that information to make health-care choices. The benefits of quality include efficiency, cost-effectiveness, timeliness, client and staff satisfaction, safety, and equitable client-centered care. Quality care results in positive client care outcomes. Quality care benefits the client, family, interdisciplinary health team members, and health-care institutions. In this time of health-care change, all stakeholders are poised for the challenge.

Critical-Thinking Exercises

- Identify three quality improvement activities that are being used in the facility where you have clinical.
- Develop a plan for quality improvement using the IOM report recommendations.
- How does the QSEN initiative improve quality and safety in health care?
- Identify provisions in the Affordable Care Act that improve the quality of care.
- How do patient satisfaction survey findings affect quality of care?
- Is there a clear-cut advantage in using the *Essentials* over the QSEN competencies as a curricular model, or is the best approach to integrate them?

References

1. Institute of Medicine (IOM). *To Err Is human: Building a Safer Health System*. Washington, DC: National Academy Press, 2000.
2. Institute of Medicine (IOM). *Crossing the Quality Chasm: A New Health System for the 21st Century*. Washington, DC: National Academy Press, 2001.
3. Bodenheimer T. The American health care system—the movement for improved quality healthcare. *New England Journal of Medicine,* 340(6), 1999.
4. HCAHPS Survey. Centers for Medicare & Medicaid Services, Baltimore, MD. Retrieved March 2013 from http://www.hcahpsonline.org
5. Leapfrog Group. About Leapfrog. Retrieved April 2013 from http://www.leapfroggroup.org
6. AHRQ. Introduction to quality indicators. Retrieved April 2013 from http://www.qualityindicators.ahrq.gov/
7. Weybright D. Standardized processes and tools significantly enhance provision of recommended care to teens with asthma, June 8, 2011. Retrieved March 2013 from http://www.innovations.ahrq.gov
8. Danz MS, Rubenstein LV, Hempel S, et al. Identifying quality improvement intervention evaluations: Is consensus achievable? *Quality and Safety in Health Care,* 19(4):279–283, 2010.
9. The Joint Commission. National Patient Safety Goals 2013. Retrieved March 2013 from http://www.jointcommission.org
10. The Joint Commission: Sentinel events. Retrieved April 2013 from http://www.jointcommission.org
11. Six Sigma project improves documentation of patient status. *Hospital Case Management,* 17(4):55–56, 2009.
12. Glasgow J, Scott-Caziewell J, Kabol P. Guiding inpatient quality improvement: A systematic review of Lean and Six Sigma. *Joint Commission Journal on Quality and Patient Safety,* 36(12):533–540, 2010.
13. Niemeijer GC, Trip A, Ahaus KT, Does RJ, Wendt KW. Quality in trauma care: Improving the discharge procedure of patients by means of Lean Six Sigma. *Journal of Trauma,* 69(3):614–619, 2010.
14. Corn JB. Six Sigma in healthcare. *Radiologic Technology,* 81(1):92–95, 2009.
15. Yamamoto JJ, Lehman A, Juneja R. Facilitating process changes in meal delivery and radiological testing to improve inpatient insulin timing using Six Sigma method. *Quality Management in Health Care,* 19(3):189–200, 2010.
16. Lenburg C, Abdur-Rahman V, Spencer T, Boyer S, Klein C. Implementing the COPA model in nursing education and practice settings: Promoting competence, quality care, and patient safety. *Nursing Education Perspectives,* 32(5):290–296, 2011.
17. Cronenwett L, Sherwood G, Pohl J, et al. Quality and safety education for advanced nursing practice. *Nursing Outlook,* 57(6):338–348, 2009.
18. Barnsterner J, Disch J, Johnson J, McGuinn K, Chappell K, Swartwout E. Diffusing QSEN competencies across schools of nursing. The AACN/RWJF Faculty Development Institute. *Journal of Professional Nursing,* 29(2):68–74, 2013.
19. Armstrong G, Barton A. Fundamentally updating fundamentals. *Journal of Professional Nursing,* 29(2):82–87, 2013.
20. American Association of Colleges of Nursing. Essentials of baccalaureate education for professional nursing practice: Faculty tool kit, 2009. Retrieved March 2013 from http://AACN.nche.edu

21. Nursing Workforce Centers. ANA and CMA activities reflected in the IOM recommendations, 2010. Retrieved March 2013 from http://www.nursingworkforcecenters.org
22. AHRQ at a glance. Retrieved March 2013 from http://www.ahrq.gov
23. Summary of patient protection and Affordable Care Act. Prepared by Health Policy Alternatives, revised 2010. Retrieved March 2013 from http://www.acscan.org
24. Quality improvement organizations. Retrieved March 2013 from http://www.cms.gov
25. Brock J, Mitchell MS, Irby K, et al. Association between quality improvement for care transitions in communities and rehospitalizations among Medicare beneficiaries. *Journal of American Medical Association,* 309(4):381–391, 2013.
26. Department of Health & Human Services Centers for Medicare & Medicaid Services. State Medicaid director letter, 2008. Retrieved March 2013 from http://downloads.cms.gov/cmsgov/archived-downloads/SMDL/downloads/SMD073108.pdf
27. Institute for Healthcare Improvement. Overview: Transforming care at the bedside. Retrieved April 2013 from http://www.ihi.org
28. Houser J, Oman KS. Evidence-Based Practice: *An Implementation Guide for Healthcare Organizations*. Sudbury, MA: Jones and Bartlett, 2010.
29. Hatler C, Mast D, Corderella D. Using evidence and process improvement strategies to enhance healthcare outcomes for the critically ill: A pilot project. *American Journal of Critical Care,* 15:549–555, 2006.
30. Bakke C. Clinical and cost effectiveness of guidelines to prevent intravascular catheter-related infections in patients on hemodialysis. *Nephrology Nursing Journal,* 37(6):601–617, 2010.
31. Bunting B, Lee G, Knowles G. The Hickory Project: Controlling health care costs and improving outcomes for diabetics using the Asheville project model. *American Health and Drug Benefits,* 4(6):343–350, 2011.
32. Institute of Medicine. *Health Professions Education: A Bridge to Quality*. Washington, DC: National Academies Press, 2003.
33. Warren N. Involving patient and family advisors in the patient and family-centered care model. *MedSurg Nursing,* 21(4):233–239, 2012.
34. Acquaviva K, Haskell H, Johnson J. Human cognition and the dynamics of failure to rescue: The Lewis Blackman Case. *Journal of Professional Nursing,* 29(2):95–101, 2013.
35. Remus S, Kennedy MA. Innovation in transformative nursing leadership: Nursing informatics competencies and roles. *Canadian Journal of Nursing Leadership,* 25(4):14–26, 2012.
36. Estabrooks D, Midodzi WK, Cummings GG, Ricker KL, Giovannetti P. The impact of hospital nursing characteristics on 30 day mortality. *Nursing Research,* 52(2):74–84, 2005.
37. American Association of Colleges of Nursing. AACN applauds the new Carnegie foundation report calling for a more highly educated nursing workforce, 2010. Retrieved March 2013 from http://www.aacn.nche.edu/Media/News-Releases/2010/carnegie
38. Lane S, Kohlenberg E. The future of baccalaureate degrees for nurses. *Nursing Forum,* 45(4):218–227, 2010.
39. American Association of Community Colleges. Tri-council for nursing issues new consensus policy statement on the educational advancement of registered nurses, 2010. Retrieved March 2013 from http://www.aacn.nche.edu/education-resources/TricouncilEdStatement.pdf

40. American Association of Colleges of Nursing. Joint statement on academic progression for nursing students and graduates, 2012. Retrieved March 2013 from http://www.aacn.nche.edu/publications/position-statements

41. American Nurses Credentialing Center (ANCC). Magnet program overview. Retrieved March 2013 from http://www.nursecredentialing.org/Magnet/ProgramOverview/WhyBecomeMagnet

42. Cardner JK, Fogg L, Thomas-Hawkins C, Latham CE. The relationships between nurses' perceptions of the hemodialysis work environment and nurse turnover, patient satisfaction, and hospitalization. *Nephrology Nursing Journal,* 34(3): 271–281, 2007.

43. Berquist-Beringer S, Davidson J, Agosto C, et al. Evaluation of the National Database of Nursing Quality indicators (NDNQI) training program on pressure ulcers. *Journal of Continuing Education in Nursing,* 40(60):252–260, 2009.

44. Goode C, Blegen M. The link between nurse staffing and patient outcomes, 2009. National Magnet Conference abstract and presentation at the October 1–3, 2009, Magnet conference; Louisville, KY.

45. Hines PA, Yu KM. The changing in reimbursement landscape: Nurses' role in quality and operational excellence. *Nursing Economics,* 27(1):1–7, 2009.

16 Delegation in Nursing

Joseph T. Catalano

Learning Objectives

After completing this chapter, the reader will be able to:

- Apply the principles of delegation to nursing practice
- Analyze and identify situations in which delegation is used improperly
- Discuss the legal implications of delegation in the current health-care setting
- Distinguish between delegation and assignment

AN ESSENTIAL SKILL

Delegation is an essential component of client care and management of nursing units in today's health-care system. It allows health-care managers to maximize the use of caregivers who are educated at multiple levels in a variety of programs. Delegation, if performed properly, permits nurses to meet the requirements of high-quality care for all clients and is a basic skill that registered nurses (RNs) must learn. However, the skill set required to delegate safely is one of the most complex that nurses must master, requiring the ability to make high-level clinical judgments. The goal of delegation is to meet the increased demands for services as they intersect with the shrinking resources of the health-care system.[1]

Look to All These Things

The concept of delegation has been a part of health care since the time of Florence Nightingale, when she instructed the nurses she educated that "to look to all these things yourself does not mean to do them yourself."[2] As far back as 1991, the American Nurses Association (ANA) initially addressed and defined delegation when it was beginning to become a more widespread practice in health care. They further refined the definition in 1997. The National Council of State Boards of Nursing (NCSBN) also addressed delegation in 1995 and periodically since then. Although some minor revisions have occurred since then, the basic concepts and basic principles of delegation remain essentially unchanged.

DELEGATION OR ASSIGNMENT?

Although delegation and assignment are closely related concepts, they are different. **Delegation** is recognized as designating ancillary personnel for the responsibility of carrying out a specific group of nursing tasks in the care of certain clients. Delegation includes the understanding that the authorized person is acting in the place of the RN and will be carrying out tasks that generally fall under *the RN's scope of practice.* However, the person taking on the RN-level task must be qualified to perform the task within the nurse's state practice act.[3]

Assignment, on the other hand, is designating tasks for ancillary personnel that fall under their *own level of practice* according to facility policies, position descriptions, and, if applicable, state practice act. In the everyday work setting, RNs usually make assignments and delegate tasks, often to the same individuals. It can be puzzling, but clarifying the difference can be helpful in reducing the level of confusion. In either case, the concepts of supervision, authority, responsibility, and accountability are key to successful client care. Supervision is required by the RN in both delegation and assignment.[4]

When nurses delegate nursing tasks to non-nurses, the RNs must always supervise those individuals to ensure that the care given meets the standards of care. However, if the facility, the state board of nursing, or some other official body has a predesignated list of tasks that non-nursing personnel may undertake in the care of clients, the RN is responsible only for supervising them to make sure the tasks are carried out safely.

Legally, the authority or power to delegate is restricted to professionals who are licensed and governed by a statutory practice act. RNs are considered professionals, with state-sanctioned licenses governed by a nurse practice act, and therefore are authorized to delegate independent nursing functions to other personnel. However, not all RN functions can be delegated to assistive personnel because of restrictions in the nurse practice act and institutional policies. For example, performing admission assessments, developing care plans, and making nursing diagnoses are activities generally restricted to RNs only.

RESPONSIBILITY AND ACCOUNTABILITY IN DELEGATING

The ANA defines *delegation* as "the transfer of responsibility for the performance of an activity from one individual to another while retaining accountability for the outcome."[5] The ANA stresses the belief that, even though the leader or manager delegates a task to another employee, he or she remains accountable for the care that is provided.

Nurses often can be heard saying, "If I delegate, then that person is practicing on my license and I don't want the responsibility." This statement implies that responsibility has legal liability attached to it. In reality, it does have liability attached, but only with the performance of duties in the specific role. When they accept a delegated task, assistive personnel accept the responsibility attached to it. Delegatees do not practice on the RN's license. They practice on their own license (licensed practical nurses [LPNs] and licensed vocational nurses [LVNs]) or, if unlicensed, within their own level of education. Assistive personnel, when they agree to accept the delegated task, are responsible for their own actions in performance of the task.[6]

When the RNs accept responsibility for delegating an assignment appropriately, they become accountable for the delegation process. Accountability looks to see if the RN used his or her nursing knowledge, critical thinking, and clinical judgment skills in delegating a task. For example, suppose an RN delegates a task to assistive personnel that is appropriate for the person's educational level and skill set. If the person accepts it, then totally botches the task, leading to the death of the client, the RN has met the requirements of accountability, and the responsibility for the client's death rests on the assistive personnel. On the other hand, if the RN delegates inappropriately to a person who is clearly *not* qualified, and the client dies, the RN and the assistive personnel could both be held liable. So how does the RN make the decision to delegate or not delegate? The steps outlined below are a guide to the decision-making process.

Guidelines for Delegation

The primary goals of staffing decisions are to make sure that optimal staffing patterns are in place and to ensure client safety and high-quality client care. Because health-care facilities and agencies are unable to staff with all RNs, client care today requires the use of health-care workers with a mix of skill levels. It is common for RNs to delegate certain aspects of care to LVNs, LPNs, unlicensed assistive personnel (UAP), monitoring technicians, and other levels of ancillary workers.

Assess the Client

Before delegating any task, RNs should give careful consideration to the condition of the client and the client's health-care needs. Assessing clients is a designated **responsibility** of RNs. Without a thorough assessment, it is likely that critical needs will remain unidentified by less trained personnel, leading to potential errors in care. Clients who are relatively stable and not likely to experience drastic changes in health-care status are the most suitable for delegation. Also, the tasks being delegated must be relatively uncomplicated and routine, must be performed without variation from policy or procedure, and should not require the use of nursing judgment while being performed. For example, the physician has ordered that a client with renal disease have his catheter outputs measured each hour to monitor hydration status. This task requires opening a drainage cap on a special collection device connected to the client's urinary catheter every hour and measuring how much urine is present. It is a low-risk, relatively simple procedure that the RN can easily delegate to an LPN or even UPN. Delegation of repetitive tasks to less educated personnel produces higher efficiency because the time and skills of the RN are used more effectively.

What Do You Think?

Is delegation used in the facility where you have clinical rotations? Who does the delegation on the unit? Does it work well?

Know Staff Availability

The delegating nurse needs to know the availability of staff and the education and competency levels of the personnel to be delegated. These factors must be matched with the level of care required by the client. Key information to obtain is how often the delegatee has performed the required tasks or cared for this type of client, what units he or she has worked on and feels comfortable in, and his or her organizational abilities. It is important to keep the team informed of who is delegated which tasks and when changes are made.

Know the Job Description

One large group of health-care workers to whom RNs delegate is generally called *unlicensed assistive personnel* (UAP). This group includes individuals who have been through some type of training program ranging from a few hours up to several months (Box 16.1). They may receive a certificate of completion, but they do not have any type of licensure and therefore do not have legal status.

The RN needs to know the institution's official position description for the UAP as well as the UAP's abilities. For example, the position description may state that the UAP can care for postoperative clients who have multiple wound drains. However, when the RN assigns a specific UAP to such a postoperative client, the nurse discovers that the UAP has worked only in the newborn nursery for the past 5 years and has no knowledge of how to care for adult postoperative clients.

If the RN delegates this UAP to care for complicated postoperative clients and a major complication develops because of the UAP's lack of competence (even though the position description states that this is an appropriate function for the UAP), the RN will also be held legally liable for the poor outcome. When the RN determines that the client's needs match the skills and abilities of the UAP or LPN, only then should that person be assigned.

Box 16.1

Other Names for Unlicensed Assistive Personnel

Certified nurse assistant (CNA)
Nurse's aide
Home health aide
Registered nurse assistant (RNA)
Nurse technician (NT)
Medication technician (MT)
Nursing assistant
Patient care assistant (PCA)
Orderly
Client attendant
Psychiatric attendant

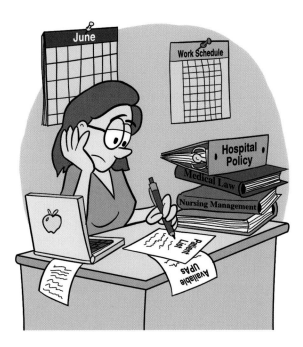

Educate the Staff Member

RNs who delegate are also responsible for educating the UAP about the task to be done. If the UAP is unfamiliar with the task, the RN is required to demonstrate how the task or procedure is performed and then document the training. Education also includes telling the UAP what is expected in the completion of the task and what complications to watch for and

report to the RN. The ANA suggests that the RN watch the UAP perform the designated task at least initially, then make periodic observations throughout the shift to ensure safe and competent care for the client.[7] Furthermore, the RN must always be available to answer questions and help the UAP whenever assistance is required. Consider the following situation:

Elsie Humber, RN, is the evening charge nurse on a busy oncology unit of the county hospital. On one particularly busy evening, she discovers during shift report that one of the scheduled LPNs has called in sick and no other LPNs are available to take her place. Ms. Humber assigns the LPN's duties and clients, including a heat lamp treatment for a decubitus ulcer, to a UAP who has worked on the unit for several months. The UAP protests the assignment, but Ms. Humber rebukes her, saying, "I have no one else. If you don't care for these clients, they won't get any care this shift." In setting up the heat lamp treatment, the UAP knocks the lamp over and burns the client. Because of his suppressed immune system from chemotherapy and generally debilitated condition, the burn does not heal and develops into an infection. The client later sues the hospital for malpractice. The hospital in turn attempts to shift the legal responsibility for the burn to Ms. Humber. Who is legally responsible for the incident? Does the client have grounds for a successful case?

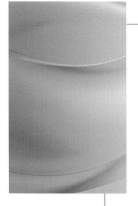

Issues Now

The Professional Nurse Coach—a New Role in Practice

Although RNs coach clients and other nurses informally as a routine part of their practice, the American Holistic Nurses Credentialing Corporation in 2012 recognized it as a formal role and is now offering certification for nurse coaches. Recently, the Interprofessional Education Collaborative Expert Panel in conjunction with the International Coach Federation identified coaching as a key element in the movement toward interprofessional education.

A professional nurse coach must be an RN who is grounded in the holistic concept of nursing care, uses evidence-based nursing theory, and has social and scientific behavioral knowledge to facilitate a process of change and development in clients and other nurses, thereby facilitating their ability to reach their maximum potential. The practice of nurse coach is grounded in the ANA Scope and Standards of Practice, second edition, and the ANA Code of Ethics for Nurses. Nurse coaching is a relationship-based process and necessitates strong interpersonal relationship abilities. The skills required for a nurse coach include the following:

- Being able to identify individuals ready for change in their lives and then establishing a therapeutic relationship with the individual. If clients or nurses are not ready for change, the process cannot go forward.
- Being able to understand and acknowledge where clients are in their movement toward wellness. The client may have issues and concerns that need to be identified to facilitate the coaching process.
- Working collaboratively with the client in identifying goals and outcomes from the coaching process. If the client does not know what he or she wishes to achieve, then the client will not know when he or she achieves it.
- Establishing an agreement with the client, either formally or informally, about how to achieve the goals. This plan should outline what the nurse's and the client's responsibilities are in the process.
- Using communication and dialogue to motivate and help the client work to achieve his or hers goals. In conjunction with the client, actions and activities are selected as interventions. Keeping the client motivated is key in achieving established goals.
- Identifying which goals the client has achieved and which ones remain.

The Affordable Care Act of 2010 began a major movement in the United States away from a disease-based health-care system and toward a health and wellness model of care. The nurse coach will play an important role in the development of the wellness model that is slowly but surely revitalizing the health-care system. Other nonprofessional health-care workers have embraced the coaching role, and some are seeking certification as health-care coaches. RNs, with their education in the behavioral sciences and their familiarity with research and health-care theories, are already well on the way to becoming nurse coaches. By seeking official certification as a professional nurse coach, RNs will gain visibility as leaders in the emerging coach role.

Sources: Hess D, Dossey B, Southhard ME, Luck S, Schaub BG, Bark L. The art and science of nurse coaching. The American Nurses Association, 2012; Professional nurse coach role: Defining scope of practice and competencies, first draft 2012. Retrieved April 2013 from http://ahncc.org/images/AHNCC_WEBSITE_RELEASE_STATEMENT,_MAY_21,_2012-1.pdf

Predictable and Uncomplicated

When a nurse delegates tasks, the outcomes of tasks should be clear and predictable. For example, when a UAP is assigned the task of feeding a client who has suffered a stroke and has hemiplegia, the predicted outcome will be that the client will eat and not choke on the food. The task should not require excessive supervision, complex decision-making, or detailed assessment during its performance. If any of these elements are required, it needs to be reassigned to an RN.

It is important to remember that when nurses delegate nursing tasks, they are *not* delegating nursing. Professional nursing practice is a science, based on a unique body of knowledge, and an art, guided by the nursing process. It is not merely a collection of tasks. Of all health-care workers, professional nurses are the most qualified to provide holistic care of the client by promoting health and treating disease. Nurses' education and experience provide them with the skills and knowledge to coordinate and supervise nursing care and to delegate specific tasks to others.

Although mastering delegation skills can seem like a daunting task, a nurse can take several common-sense steps to attain this skill (Box 16.2). Nursing students often have tasks delegated to them by the RNs on the units where they are having clinical rotations. It is easy to identify the RNs who have developed good delegation skills and those who still need to work on those skills.

Box 16.2

Five "Rights" of Delegation

- Right task: Do the tasks delegated follow written policy guidelines?
- Right person: Does the person have the proper qualifications for the tasks?
- Right direction or communication: Are the instructions and outcomes clearly stated? When should the person report changes?
- Right supervision or feedback: How can the delegation process be improved? Are the client goals for care being achieved?
- Right circumstances: Are the tasks that are being delegated possible without independent nursing judgments?

Sources: Corazzini KN, Anderson RA, Rapp CG, Mueller C, McConnell ES, Lekan D. Delegation in long-term care: Scope of practice or job description? *Online Journal of Issues in Nursing,* 15(2):4, 2010; Vogelsmeier A. Medication administration in nursing homes: RN delegation to unlicensed assistive personnel. *Journal of Nursing Regulation,* 2(3):49–53, 2011; Weydt A. Developing delegation skills. *Online Journal of Issues in Nursing*, 14(2):10, 2010; Whitehead DK, Weiss SA, Tappen RM. *Essentials of Nursing Leadership and Management* (5th ed.). Philadelphia: F. A. Davis, 2010.

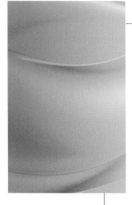

Issues in Practice

Angela is the emergency department (ED) nurse manager in a small rural hospital. Hiring qualified RNs for her staff had become more of a challenge as the nursing shortage worsened. For 8 months, a full-time evening RN position had gone unfilled. During this time, the position was filled by cross-training nurses from other departments, paying bonus shifts and overtime, contracting with agencies, and hiring available nurses from other hospitals. These nurses were excellent, but the continuity of regular staffing was lacking in the ED. Angela believed this lack of continuity was negatively affecting morale and efficiency in the department.

At this hospital, the vice president of nursing services (VPNS) made all the final decisions about hiring new staff after consulting with the nurse managers. The VPNS suggested an employee who was interested in the position but did not have the experience of the nurses usually hired for the ED. Ted, who had been an LPN in a long-term care facility, had gone back to nursing school and received his BS in nursing 6 months earlier. His most recent experience after graduating was working in a physician's office. Although his combined health-care experience was more than 10 years, he had never worked in an acute care setting.

When Angela interviewed Ted, he appeared highly motivated, intelligent, a self-starter, and well groomed. Because of the nursing shortage, it had become fairly common practice to let new graduates work in specialty areas, such as EDs or intensive care units, without the traditional mandatory year of medical-surgical experience. Angela believed that Ted could, over time, learn the ED routines. He would have an experienced RN working with him for at least a year. Also, at this hospital, 90 percent of ED visits were nonurgent, office-type visits. Ted's experience of coordinating and moving clients through a busy office practice would be an asset.

Angela started by giving Ted a thorough and extended orientation to the ED. She consulted with each nurse he would be working with and asked for support in mentoring him. She encouraged the nurses to begin by letting Ted care for the more routine cases and then gradually allow him to care for clients with more acute conditions. During the orientation, Ted seemed to master the assessment and documentation aspects of the job well. Ted was also studying for Advance Cardiac Life Support (ACLS) certification. Obviously, he was unfamiliar with many of the medications routinely used in the ED. Angela encouraged him to ask questions and use the unit's medication reference books.

However, despite all the efforts at orientation, Ted made four serious medication errors during his first 2 months in the ED. Fortunately, they were discovered early enough so that no serious harm came to the clients. Ted was counseled by the hospital's nurse educator, who worked with him on a medication review. He completed the course of study successfully and passed the medication exam.

Angela began receiving feedback from the other ED staff members who had been working with Ted. They expressed insecurity about the quality of the care he was giving, and some believed he was not "carrying his load" during busy times. He would manipulate client assignments and shift work to other nurses. A personality conflict had also arisen between Ted and some of the nurses. They

Issues in Practice continued

had begun watching his every move and documenting what he was doing or not doing. Some observed that he would leave the ED for unscheduled long breaks without notifying anyone. Others remarked that he was not monitoring clients with cardiac problems as closely as they thought he should. Angela noted that Ted seemed to have lost the support of his coworkers and that the overall morale of the unit was deteriorating.

Angela met with Ted and suggested that he attend a certified emergency-room nurse review course to improve his knowledge and skills in emergency nursing. He did attend the course. Angela also met with him several times to develop plans for improving his work. Each time he would complete the requirements of the plan, and the situation would improve for a while. After a week or two, however, he would slip back into his previous behaviors.

As the morale of the unit continued to decline, Angela began feeling depressed and under stress. She sensed that she was losing the credibility and respect of her staff. One day she overheard one of the staff nurses say, "At this hospital, any warm body can have a job," implying that the standards and quality of care were poor. On the other hand, Angela felt responsible for placing Ted in a situation in which he could not succeed.

Questions for Thought

1. Identify the erroneous assumptions used in the initial hiring of Ted.

2. What other measures could Angela have taken to help Ted in his adjustment to the ED?

3. What can Angela do now about the situation?

(Answers are found at the end of the chapter.)

DEVELOPING DELEGATION SKILLS

Clear Communication

In the process of developing delegation skills, students should try to emulate the good delegators. Develop good communication and interpersonal relationship skills. Make eye contact with the other person, be pleasant, and ask for suggestions. However, avoid allowing the person to whom the tasks are being delegated to control the exchange by intimidation or resistance. (See Chapter 12 for more tips on communication.)

After a nurse delegates a task, it's a good idea to make a written list of the responsibilities that are expected from the person, if one does not already exist. The list will help clarify what is expected and head off possible misunderstandings. It is also important to be flexible. Clients' conditions change, new clients may be admitted, and other clients may be discharged. The original assignments may have to be modified in response to changes in the environment.[8]

Simulation Exercises

Both nursing education and nursing service can increase the knowledge and skill required for effective delegation through practice scenarios that reflect daily practice. There is an increasing emphasis on simulation in nursing education, and delegation scenarios can be used alongside clinical practice ones. For students, these scenarios can be an introduction to the type of critical-thinking and decision-making skills required for effective delegation. For practicing RNs, delegation scenarios reinforce earlier learned skills and demonstrate the authority the RN has in the delegation process.

Simulation allows the student or RN to make mistakes and learn from them. Feedback is essential to the educational process and allows participants to self-evaluate their interpersonal, communication, and decision-making skills.[9]

Careful Supervision

Effective delegation, as well as assignment of tasks, requires the RN to master supervision skills. This includes monitoring the delegatees while they are providing care and helping them when they require assistance. Are they doing what they should be doing? Do they understand the responsibilities involved in the client's care? Effective delegation also presumes that the delegator will teach the delegatees who

demonstrate a lack of knowledge. Continual feedback throughout the shift allows both parties an opportunity for ongoing assessment. Most important, at the end of the shift, say, "Thank you. I appreciate the hard work you've done today."

Certain delegation situations may place the RN at an increased risk for liability (Boxes 16.3 and 16.4). When delegating, try to avoid the following:

- Assigning tasks that are highly invasive or have the potential to cause significant physical harm to clients
- Assigning tasks that are designated under the scope of practice or standards of care as belonging exclusively to the RN (i.e., admission assessments, care plan development)
- Assigning tasks that the person is not trained for or lacks the knowledge to complete safely

Box 16.3

Barriers to Effective Delegation

A. Internal barriers (person delegating):
1. Lack of experience delegating
2. Lack of confidence in others
3. Personal insecurity
4. Demanding perfectionism
5. Poor organizational skills
6. Indecision
7. Poor communication skills
8. Lack of confidence in self
9. Fear of not being liked by everyone
10. Micromanaging management style

B. External barriers (circumstances or person being delegated to):
1. Unclear policies about delegation
2. Policies that do not tolerate mistakes
3. Management-by-crisis model for facility
4. Unclear delineation of authority and responsibilities
5. Poor staffing
6. Lack of competence
7. Overdependence on the person delegating
8. Unwillingness to accept responsibility for one's own practice
9. Immersion in trivia and gossip
10. Work overload

Source: Whitehead DK, Weiss SA, Tappen RM. *Essentials of Nursing Leadership and Management* (5th ed.). Philadelphia: F. A. Davis, 2010.

Box 16.4

Delegation Decision Tree

1. Are there laws and rules in place supporting the rules of delegation?
2. Is the task within the scope of practice of the UAP, LPN/LVN, RN, or new graduate?
3. Has there been an assessment of the client's needs?
4. Is the UAP, LPN/LVN, RN, or new graduate competent to accept the delegation?
5. Does the ability of the caregiver match the care needs of the client?
6. Can the task be completed without requiring nursing judgments?
7. Is the result of the task somewhat predictable?
8. Can the task be safely performed according to directions?
9. Can the task be performed without repeated assessment?
10. Is appropriate supervision available?

Source: Whitehead DK, Weiss SA, Tappen RM. *Essentials of Nursing Leadership and Management* (5th ed.). Philadelphia: F. A. Davis, 2010.

- Assigning tasks when there is inadequate time to safely monitor or evaluate the practice of the person performing the tasks[10]

Delegation has the potential to be a powerful tool in improving the quality of client care. The knowledge and judgment of the professional nurse remain essential elements in any health-care system reforms, including clinical integration, case management, outsourcing practices, total quality management (TQM), and continuous quality improvement (CQI).

What Do You Think?

What qualities have you observed in good delegators? What qualities made the poor delegators ineffective?

LEGAL ISSUES IN DELEGATION

One area of fallout from the movement to managed care is the increase in nurses' liability for lawsuits in the area of supervision and delegation. In the search for cost-effective client care, current managed-care strategies attempt to make optimal use of relatively expensive RNs by replacing them with less costly and less educated personnel. As more and more health-care facilities move toward restructuring, the use of UAPs who have minimal education and experience will continue to increase. Although RNs have always been responsible for the delegation of some tasks and the supervision of less qualified health-care providers, delegation is now one of the primary functions of RNs in today's health-care system.

Delegation does have some advantages. It is an RN extender, in that it allows more care to be given to more clients than can be given by one RN. Delegation can free the RN from lower-level, time-consuming tasks so that more time can be spent planning for care and performing those skills that less prepared individuals would be unable to perform. For those to whom tasks are delegated, it can serve as an incentive to learn additional skills, increase knowledge, develop a sense of initiative, and perhaps seek further formal education. Delegation, if performed properly, leaves accountability and decision-making where they belong—with the RN.

WHO CAN DELEGATE—LEGALLY?

As with most activities conducted by RNs, legal and ethical considerations abound. The RN always has to take into consideration the probable effects and outcomes when deciding what task to delegate to which person. It is essential that RNs understand the principles of delegation and know how to delegate effectively to decrease the risk of mistakes that may cause client injuries. (For more information, go to http://www.aacn.org/WD/Practice/Docs/AACNDelegationHandbook.pdf.)

An Ethical Obligation

Most state practice acts do *not* give delegation authority to **dependent practitioners** such as LPNs, LVNs, or UAPs. In addition, professionals who delegate specific tasks retain accountability for the proper and safe completion of those tasks and take responsibility for determining whether the assigned personnel are competent to carry out the task. One exception occurs when the person who is assigned a task also has a license and the tasks fall under that person's scope of practice.[11] Then again, the RN is responsible only for supervision of the other licensed person.

These situations are often seen when LPNs or LVNs are assigned to client care.

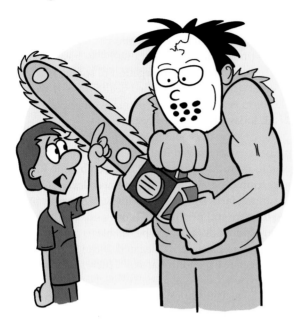

"WHY DON'T I GET SOMEONE ELSE
TO REMOVE MRS. LEMKE'S SUTURES?"

The delegation and supervision responsibilities of RNs have been and continue to be a major concern for the nursing profession, both ethically and legally. The ANA Code of Ethics for Nurses states, "The nurse is responsible and accountable for individual nursing practice and determines the appropriate delegation of tasks consistent with the nurse's obligation to provide optimum patient care" (statement 4).[12] From the ethical viewpoint, RNs have an obligation to refuse assignments that they are not competent to carry out and to refuse to delegate particular nursing tasks to individuals who they believe are unable or unprepared to perform them (Fig. 16.1).

Direct and Indirect Delegation

The legal side of the delegation issue has also been addressed by the ANA in the *ANA Basic Guide to Safe Delegation*. This document makes a distinction between direct delegation, which is a specific decision made by the RN about who can perform what tasks, and indirect delegation, which is a list of tasks that certain health-care personnel can perform that is produced by the health-care facility.[5] (For more information, go to http://www.nursingworld.org/MainMenuCategories/ANAMarketplace/ANAPeriodicals/OJIN/ TableofContents/Vol152010/No2May2010/ Delegation-Skills.html.)

The **consensus** among many experts is that *indirect* delegation is really a form of covert institutional licensure. Lists of activities from the facility that allows non-nursing personnel, who do not have the education of the RN, to carry out professional nursing functions is a de facto permission to practice nursing without a license. Indirect delegation places RNs in a precarious legal position.

Basically, indirect delegation takes away much of the authority of the RN to delegate personnel tasks, yet the RN remains accountable for the safe completion of the tasks under the doctrines of **respondeat superior** and **vicarious liability.** Although some states are beginning to address the UAP and delegation issues in their nurse practice acts, many states either have no official standards for UAP delegation or include UAP standards under the medical practice act.[13]

Delegation and the NCLEX

Because delegation is such an important issue in today's health-care system, and because decisions about delegation require considerable critical-thinking skill, the number of questions about delegation on the NCLEX has been increasing steadily. It is not unusual for 10 to 25 percent of questions to deal with delegation issues. One problem graduates may encounter with these questions is that the NCLEX uses strict parameters for determining delegation. In the real world of health care, LPNs, LVNs, and UAPs often perform functions beyond their legal scope of practice. The following lists may be helpful in answering NCLEX questions about delegation.

Although LPNs and LVNs can do most skills, for the NCLEX they:

- *Cannot* do admission assessments.
- *Cannot* give intravenous (IV) push medications.
- *Cannot* write nursing diagnoses.
- *Cannot* do most teaching.
- *Cannot* do complex skills.
- *Cannot* take care of clients with acute conditions.
- *Cannot* take care of unstable clients.

For questions concerning UAPs, CNAs, and aides on the NCLEX:

- Look for the *lowest level of skill* required for the task.
- Look for the *least complicated* task.
- Look for the *most stable* client.
- Look for the client with the *chronic illness.*

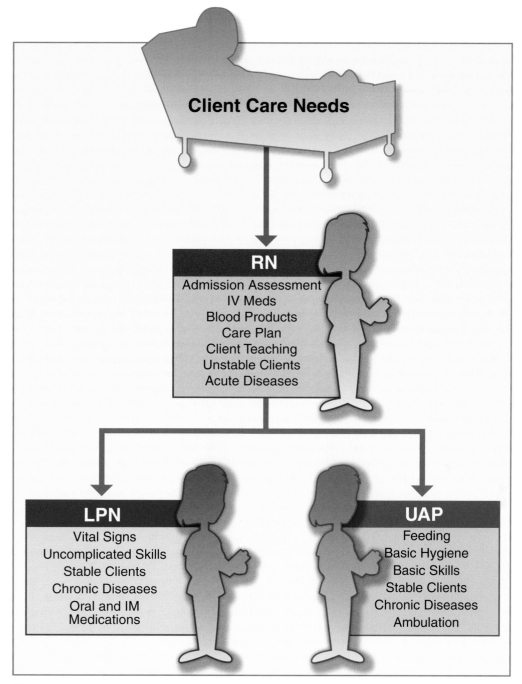

Figure 16.1 Delegation of responsibilities.

Conclusion

With the increased use of less educated and unlicensed personnel in today's health-care system, it is essential that the nurse develop effective delegation and supervision skills. The nurse needs to be mindful that the tasks that can be delegated can change on the basis of work setting, client needs, position descriptions, institutional training of personnel, and the ever-changing requirements of nurse practice acts and professional standards. Nurses also need to know when delegation is inappropriate.

Critical-Thinking Exercises

- Obtain a copy of your state's nurse practice act. Review the section that deals with delegation. Apply those criteria to the case study at the beginning of this chapter.
- As a student, you have had tasks delegated to you. Identify how delegation has changed in regard to your learning and level of skills as you have progressed through your program.
- Obtain a copy of the policy on delegation from at least two of the clinical sites where you have practiced. How do these policies differ? How are they similar? What are the reasons for the similarities and differences?

Answers to Questions in Chapter 16

Issues in Practice: Leadership/Management Case Study (p. 402)

1. The first erroneous assumption was that a nurse with no acute care hospital experience could be taught to provide safe care in a specialty area with only minimal orientation. The second assumption was that the other nurses would be enthusiastic about spending extra time and effort in orienting and teaching a new nurse. This group seemed to resent the imposition. The third assumption was that, because most of the care in the ED was "routine," a person with only limited experience could work there.

2. When Angela first discovered that Ted was having problems adjusting, she could have suggested that he work on a medical-surgical unit and cross-train for the ED. This approach would have given him a range of learning experiences that he could later apply to his work in the ED. After Ted had received 6 to 8 months of medical-surgical experience and cross-training, Angela and the other unit managers would have been able to better evaluate his skills and knowledge.

3. Because of the declining morale and the loss of trust in Angela by the staff, Ted needs to be removed from the ED. If his performance so indicates, he may be terminated. However, in this age of nursing shortages, a better option would be to place him on another unit and evaluate him there. Not everyone is destined to be an ED nurse, and Ted may find another unit with a more relaxed pace to be more suited to his personality and skills.

References

1. Bittner NP, Gravlin G. Critical thinking, delegation, and missed care in nursing practice. *Journal of Nursing Administration,* 39(3):142–146, 2009.
2. Nightingale F. *Notes on Nursing: What It Is and What It Is Not.* London: Harrison and Sons, 1859, p. 17.
3. Potter P, Deshields T, Kuhrik M. Delegation practices between registered nurses and nursing assistive personnel. *Journal of Nursing Management,* 18(2):157–165, 2010.
4. McInnis LA, Parsons LC. Thoughtful nursing practice: Reflections on nurse delegation decision-making. *Nursing Clinics of North America,* 44(4):461–470, 2009.
5. American Nurses Association. Position Statement: Registered Nurse Utilization of Unlicensed Assistive Personnel. Washington, DC: Author, 1997.
6. Resha C. Delegation in the school setting: Is it a safe practice? *Online Journal of Issues in Nursing,* 15(2):1–5, 2010.
7. American Nurses Association. *Registered Professional Nurses and Unlicensed Assistive Personnel* (2nd ed.). Washington, DC: Author, 1996.
8. Anthony MK, Vidal K. Mindful communication: A novel approach to improving delegation and increasing patient safety. *Online Journal of Issues in Nursing,* 15(2):1– 2, 2010.
9. Simones J, Wilcox J, Scott K, et al. Collaborative simulation project to teach scope of practice. *Journal of Nursing Education,* 49(4):190–197, 2010.
10. Vogelsmeier A. Medication administration in nursing homes: RN delegation to unlicensed assistive personnel. *Journal of Nursing Regulation,* 2(3):49–53, 2011.
11. Weydt A. Developing delegation skills. *Online Journal of Issues in Nursing,* 15(2):1, 2010.
12. ANA Code of Ethics for Nurses 2001. Retrieved April 2013 from http://www.ana.org
13. Plawecki LH, Amrhein DW. A question of delegation: Unlicensed assistive personnel and the professional nurse. *Journal of Gerontological Nursing,* 36(8):18–21, 2010.

Incivility: The Antithesis of Caring

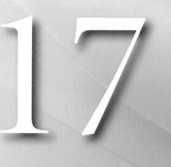

Cheryl Taylor

Sharon Bator

Edna Hull

Jacqueline J. Hill

Wanda Spurlock

Learning Objectives

After completing this chapter, the reader will be able to:

- Define *caring* in the context of civility: the importance of caring relationships
- Define *incivility* and related concepts in academia (among faculty and students) and in the workplace
- Discuss the ethical codes violated by incivility in the profession
- Describe behaviors that are considered uncivil and civil in the academic and clinical settings
- Define and discuss the similarities and differences between bullying and lateral violence

CIVILITY VERSUS INCIVILITY

Many concepts describe a range of actions rather than being all or none. Civility and incivility are these types of concepts, and it can sometimes be difficult to identify when an action is civil or uncivil. For example, if a male employer makes a comment to his female office manager that she looks pretty in her new dress today, most people would consider that a civil comment. However, in today's litigious society, it may also be interpreted as a form of sexual harassment, which is a type of incivility that can lead to a lawsuit.

Current newspaper, television, and Internet reports indicate that incivility is escalating in the world. Some experts believe that the news media's continual reporting of violence between people has desensitized people into accepting this type of behavior as the norm. Incivility in the form of bullying is often exploited in the media on programs that use it for entertainment. Shows such as *The Apprentice, Kitchen Nightmares, American Idol, The Real Housewives,* and *The X Factor* help foster a culture of bullying and intimidation. (For more information, go to http://www.psychologytoday.com/blog/wired-success/201207/the-rise-incivility-and-bullying-in-america.)

What Is Civility?

Although almost everyone has a basic understanding of what civility is and is not, it is more difficult to actually define. The word *civility* is derived from the Latin word for "citizen." It appears that to be a good

Roman citizen, a person had to be polite and helpful to their fellow citizens. In a global context, civility is often thought of as good manners; however, its meaning is much broader. Civility is based on recognizing that all human beings are important. A simple definition of civility is for people to treat others as they would wish to be treated (the Golden Rule). Empathy is key to recognizing how others might want to be treated and what they may perceive as unpleasant actions by others. A more activist view of civility sees it as taking positive actions that fight injustice and oppression while at the same time respecting the rights of others. The Civil Rights Act of 1964 requires that all individuals have equal protection under the law and that human beings matter equally, regardless of race, color, religion, gender, national origin, or disability.[1]

An analysis of existing research shows that even perceived discrimination can produce negative mental and physical health outcomes such as elevated stress levels and self-destructive behaviors. Protection from discrimination can be found in social support, active coping styles, and group identification.[2]

Civility in Nursing

In nursing, civility is one of the underpinnings of caring and can even be considered a moral imperative (i.e., a rule or principle originating in a person's mind that forces the person to act in a certain manner).[3] For most entering the profession, the motivation to be a nurse stems from the moral values of helping and caring coupled with a deep desire to make a positive impact in the lives of individuals.[4]

Civility in the profession enables nurses to make caring the focal point of their practice. Being civil to each other, to students, to colleagues, and to clients promotes emotional health and creates a positive environment for learning and for the promotion of healing. It also develops emotional intelligence and empathy in nurses.[1] Emotional intelligence, which is the ability to be aware of feelings and thoughts of others by using behavioral cues, promotes the nurse's

> " *To learn how to be happy we must learn how to live well with others, and civility is a key to that. Through civility we develop thoughtfulness, foster effective self-expression and communication, and widen the range of our benign responses. Practicing civility means that we are doing more than outwardly manifesting politeness. Being civil is using and developing our emotional intelligence.* "
> —Sophie Sparrow

personal growth. It also transforms negative actions and attitudes into positive responses to health-care issues and is considered critical to the foundation of nursing practice.[4]

Communication and Civility

In Watson's nursing theory (Chapter 3), caring can be demonstrated and practiced through interpersonal interactions (Box 17.1). Similarly, the consideration of others within interpersonal relationships is a fundamental part of being civil.[5] The increase of incivility in nursing today contradicts the primary requirement that nurses be caring professionals. The reason incivility is on the rise can be uncovered by a closer examination of the interpersonal relationships found in toxic work and learning environments.[6,7]

The health and well-being of clients are predicated on excellence in communication and a culture of civility in the workplace. The Institute of Medicine report, *Crossing the Quality Chasm: A New Health System for the 21st Century*, notes that finding new strategies to improve communication is critical in promoting a culture of civility. Furthermore, intimidation, even when subtle, results in harmful outcomes of psychological abuse, horizontal and lateral violence, bullying, relationship aggression, workplace incivility, and mobbing when a group is involved. Ethical codes and values in society affirm civility as the antidote to incivility.[4] (For information, go to http://www.iom.edu/Reports/2001/Crossing-the-Quality-Chasm-A-New-Health-System-for-the-21st-Century.aspx.)

B O X   1 7 . 1

Watson Model of Human Caring

"Caring Science is the starting point for nursing (in) relational ontology that honors the fact that we are all connected and belong to Source."

Source: Watson J. *Nursing: The Philosophy and Science of Caring* (revised ed.). Boulder, CO: University Press of Colorado, 2008.

What Is Incivility?

This conversation between two experienced nurses was recently overheard at a major state nursing conference:

Nurse 1: "I can't believe how impolite people are now. No one ever seems to say *please* or *thank you* or *you're welcome* anymore."

Nurse 2: "I know, I had my arms full of packages when I arrived yesterday, and not even one of the three or four people standing by the door offered to help."

Nurse 1: "I was almost hit in the hotel parking lot by some guy who tried to muscle into a space I was already pulling into!"

Nurse 2: "I guess our society has just gotten a lot more rude over the years."

Society in general and the nursing profession in particular seem to be filled with complaints about "incivility," both in academia and in the workplace. The simplest definition of incivility is the lack of civility. However, it is a very broad term that includes a wide range of what is considered unacceptable behavior in a civilized society. Incivility can be viewed as a continuum of impolite behaviors with a lot of overlap between them. All of the individual stages usually begin with some type of covert, subtle psychological behavior. However, they all can lead to physical violence if taken to their extremes (Fig. 17.1). On the right end of the scale are overt violent actions such as vandalism, physical assault, and battery. On the left end of the scale are more surreptitious and psychologically based behaviors such as discrimination, rudeness, verbal bullying, and psychological abuse. In between the extremes is a range of behaviors that are either more or less overtly violent with a great deal of overlap.

In the academic or classroom setting, incivility is any type of activity that creates an unpleasant or negative learning atmosphere. The end result is that students do not learn and the stress levels of both students and teachers increase. In the health-care work setting, incivility takes on many forms, but they all produce a threatening and polarized work environment that reduces the quality of client care. Subsequently, nurses feel dissatisfied, angry, anxious, and unhappy. Stress levels are unnecessarily high and turnover rates increase.

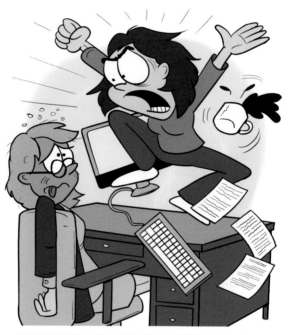

INCIVILITY CAN CREATE A TOXIC CLASSROOM.

Generally, incivility is an enduring human problem in society. Many professional psychologists, educators, and health-care providers agree that civility has declined in society, but they are hopeful that behavior and relationship education will result in more harmonious productivity while elevating expectations in society.[7] People under stress can potentially lose their sense of civility, which can escalate, turning into outright violence if left unchecked.[8]

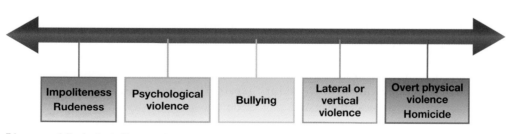

| Impoliteness Rudeness | Psychological violence | Bullying | Lateral or vertical violence | Overt physical violence Homicide |

Figure 17.1 Incivility continuum.

Incivility and intimidation in the academic and workplace environments are not new. However, technological developments have made them even more toxic, widely distributed, and damaging. Research indicates that cyber-harassment, vicious anonymous e-mails, hate text messages, harmful Facebook posts, tweets or other destructive social networking, acts of rudeness, and social rejection are forms of incivility that are on the rise. Often students targeted in this way experience more fear, anxiety, and avoidant behaviors than if they were victims of an actual theft or physical assault.[7]

Incivility in the health-care setting is by no means an original problem. Over the years, it has been called by a number of names: *nurses eating their young*, the *doctor–nurse game*, *assertive versus aggressive*, *passive-aggressive*, *lateral violence*, and *workplace violence*, to mention a few. The ultimate consequence of incivility is that it jeopardizes client safety.[8] Incivility has been linked to increased medical errors and the creation of hostile academic and workplace environments. (For more information, go to http://www.sciencedaily.com/releases/2011/07/110718164024.htm.) Such negative environments can create situations that end in decline of health or even loss of life. For instance, fatal campus violence was seen in 2002 at the University of Arizona, in 2007 at Virginia Tech, and in 2008 at Northern Illinois University. Could it have been prevented by early recognition of the signs of incivility?

> *In the health-care work setting, incivility takes on many forms, but they all produce a threatening and polarized work environment that reduces the quality of client care.*

Bullying

Bullying is a type of incivility that is one step beyond impoliteness. It can be defined as any behavior that could reasonably be considered humiliating, intimidating, threatening, or demeaning to an individual or group of individuals. It can occur anywhere and at times becomes habitual, being repeated over and over.[9] Although almost everyone has experienced some type of bullying during their lives, it is a complex concept that includes a number of elements. In the U.S. legal system, physical abuse, emotional abuse, verbal abuse, or any combination of the three are considered bullying and may be punished by fines in the civil system or jail time in the criminal system (see Chapter 8). The goal of bullying is usually to coerce or intimidate another person or group of people into doing something that they do not want to do. However, sometimes the goal is to merely humiliate a person or group because of some perceived difference or weakness. Hazing and initiation rites are really a form of bullying. Most people who bully others have low self-esteem along with a poor self-image and use bullying to make themselves feel more powerful.[6]

Targets

The victim of bullying, or any level of incivility, is often called the *target*. Elements that may make a person a target include religion, gender, sexual orientation, race, physical characteristics such as weight, physical defects or differences, or a particular skill or ability a person may possess. Bullies perceive targets to be weak or timid. Targets may have a quieter, more self-conscious demeanor, but that is not ultimately why a bully may be pulled to them like a magnet. In actuality, targets have attributes foreign to bullies or bullies hate a characteristic they themselves possess; this is what fuels them to attack—the unfamiliar or a revulsion of themselves. Targets usually feel helpless to stop the bullying and don't know how to defend themselves from it. Although there have been numerous reports of overt bullying posted on social networking sites and other websites, in the workplace or education setting, it usually involves elusive methods of coercion by making intimidating comments on social media (cyberbullying), being ostracized from the group, or being made the butt of practical jokes. One-on-one bullying from peers is sometimes called *peer abuse* or *lateral violence*, but in groups, the primary bully may have co-conspirators that contribute to or prolong the bullying activities. Sometimes a bullying culture can develop in the workplace or educational setting where it is accepted as part of the normal environment. (For more information, go to http://www.education.com/reference/article/who-are-the-targets-of-bullying/ or http://www.workplacebullying.org/individuals/problem/who-gets-targeted/.)

Lateral Violence

Lateral violence, also known as *horizontal violence,* has many of the same characteristics as bullying except that it takes place almost exclusively in the work setting. It has been recognized by the National Institute for Occupational Safety and Health (NIOSH) as one of the leading causes of poor staff morale, excessive sick days, turnover of staff, nurses leaving the profession, poor quality of care, and physical symptoms such as insomnia, hypertension, depression, and gastrointestinal upset. The American Nurses Association has produced many position papers over the past several years that discuss lateral violence as a major problem for practicing nurses (see http://nursingworld.org/workplaceviolence).

Lateral violence can be either covert or overt. Overt lateral violence can include name calling, threatening body language, physical hazing, bickering, fault finding, negative criticism, intimidation, gossip, shouting, blaming, put-downs, raised eyebrows, rolling of the eyes, verbally abusive sarcasm, or physical acts such as pounding on a table, throwing objects, or shoving a chair against a wall. Covert lateral violence is initially more difficult to identify and includes unfair assignments, marginalizing a person, refusing to help someone, ignoring someone, making faces behind someone's back, refusing to work with certain people, whining, sabotage, exclusion, and fabrication.

Lateral violence is a well-known phenomenon in nursing. It has been part of the health-care culture almost since the beginning of the profession. Those experiencing lateral violence also include nursing students, pharmacists, unit secretaries, and others. Oppression theory notes that marginalization is a key contributing factor to lateral violence. Nurses sometimes use horizontal violence to attack one another as a means of venting their frustrations and anger against a supervisor or institution they feel helpless to change. When lateral violence occurs among health-care providers, it leads to decreased communication and, ultimately, poor care and reduced safety of clients.

Vertical Violence

Bullying from a superior, or vertical violence, is a type of harassment that can permeate the entire organization and have a detrimental effect on its effectiveness. The concept of inappropriate use of coercive power becomes a key element in vertical violence. When bullies are in a position of power or are perceived to have power, they can do a lot of damage to the organization and the people who work for them. The people they supervise are in a constant state of fear and work in a defensive mode, avoiding contact with the bully or anything that may bring attention from the bully. They feel anger toward the bully and have a lower self-esteem because they don't know what to do about it. As a result of this type of atmosphere, productivity and innovation decrease, morale suffers, and the best workers seek employment elsewhere.

However, superiors usually forget that vertical violence can move in both directions, and they themselves may become the targets of bottom-up vertical violence. Although subordinates may seem to be powerless in the face of a bullying superior, they actually do have considerable power both as a collective and as an individual (see Chapter 1). The superior's position is often dependent on the productivity of the people being supervised. Some extremely disgruntled employees may devise subtle, passive-aggressive ways to decrease productivity, sabotaging the boss and the organization. When they lower productivity enough, the boss is going to be confronted by his or her superior to see what the problem is and may get fired as a result. In the extreme, bottom-up vertical violence may result in the employee "going postal" and causing physical injury or even death to those he or she holds responsible for their distress. (See "Workplace Violence," below.)

> *Bullying from a superior, or vertical violence, is a type of harassment that can permeate the entire organization and have a detrimental effect on its effectiveness.*

Vicious Circle

Another negative outcome of vertical violence is the "bullying vicious circle" that is perpetuated in the organization. This phenomenon is particularly evident in organizations such as health-care facilities and educational settings where the persons who are bullied when they first start working later are likely to move into supervisory positions themselves. An example is when a new faculty who was bullied when he or she first started now has several years of experience and becomes the bully to newly hired faculty. The same cycle often occurs on nursing units in a hospital where new nurses who were bullied become the charge nurses and bully other new nurses. It becomes part of the culture where it may not even be recognized as bullying. Often there is an attitude of "I went through it, so now it's time for you to pay your dues." (For more information, go to http://www.nursingworld.org/Bullying-Workplace-Violence or http://www.decisionsonevidence.com/2013/03/the-vicious-cycle-of-being-bullied-and-becoming-a-bullier/.)

INCIVILITY IN NURSING EDUCATION

In its broadest sense, academic incivility is any speech or action that disrupts the harmony of the teaching or learning environment.[9] Incivility exists in education as it does in the clinical setting. It takes the form of vertical violence when faculty, students, and staff are demeaning to their peers. Incivility is destructive to the emotional and physical well-being of those affected.[10] Significant financial costs result from a fear-based environment due to missed work, legal fees, rehiring, and decreased work output.[11]

The classroom experience reflects the larger society, with inequities as well as humanitarian qualities such as caring. Academic incivility is an interactive and dynamic process in which individuals or groups make the choice to behave uncivilly. Within nursing education, the three parties or groups who need to take primary responsibility for the disruptive atmosphere are administrators, faculty, and students.[12]

An Escalating Problem

Some nursing faculty are too embarrassed to admit that incivility exists in higher education, particularly in their own classrooms, despite a documented increase in student hostility, insubordination, and even intimidation.[12] Although students are often considered subordinates in the classroom setting, they have a considerable amount of power from their numbers and policies of the institution. They often can exercise this type of bottom-up vertical violence where high levels of student classroom incivility directly relates to the perception of how effective an instructor is in teaching. It often manifests itself in poor teacher evaluations, low levels of attention, inadequate note-taking, and poor grades. Examples of student-to-faculty incivility typically include the following:[5]

- Harassing and threatening behaviors by students toward certain instructors over grades
- Cutting classes because students consider them boring or the instructor stupid
- Cheating on tests and homework assignments to get better grades

- Refusing to participate in class activities
- Being unprepared for classes by not doing reading assignments or written work
- Distracting teachers and other students by asking irrelevant or confrontational questions
- Complaining behind the teacher's back to the teacher's superiors

Examples of student-to-student incivility include the following:

- Obtaining study notes from the previous year's classes and using them as bargaining chips with their classmates
- Ridiculing (bullying) students who are considered outcasts by their classmates because they don't fit the model of the majority in terms of clothing, hairstyle, and disposable income
- Two-faced behavior where students act nice to a classmate's face but are nasty behind his or her back

What Do You Think?

Are any of the above listed behaviors present in any of your classes? What are some other things students do in class to be disruptive?

These behaviors are found throughout higher education. It is critical for nursing faculty to deal constructively with disgruntled students in a timely manner. When students' rude and disruptive behavior is not addressed, it may turn into physical violence. Most nursing students recognize the importance of treating others respectfully, studying diligently, disagreeing gracefully, and listening attentively. However, when stress levels are high, they may struggle to remain civil.[1] Studies show a correlation between increased student stress and student incivility, resulting in some faculty doubting their abilities as educators or even having concerns for their personal safety. The key to effective education lies in the quality of the interpersonal relationship between student and teacher.[13] (For more studies, go to http://digitalcommons.olivet.edu/cgi/viewcontent.cgi?article=1058&context=edd_diss or http://www.nsna.org/portals/0/skins/nsna/pdf/imprint_aprmay08_feat_incivility.pdf or http://www.umfk.edu/pdfs/facultystaff/combatingmisconduct.pdf.)

What can nursing educators do to promote the positive interpersonal relationships that encourage civility? The National League for Nursing (NLN) faculty development program includes strategies to manage incivility and offers a program of co-sponsorship for those interested (go to http://www.nln.org/profdev/PlenarySessionPowerPoint.pdf).

Although many schools of nursing actively engage in curriculum and program improvement measures, few examine the impact of incivility on student learning (Box 17.2). Examples of incivility in nursing education range from minor insults, delivered either electronically or face-to-face, to full-blown acts of physical violence.[14] Regarding the rise of incivility in nursing education, two questions have dominated the literature in recent years: (1) What factors contribute to it? (2) What measures can be taken to minimize its impact on student learning?

Contributing Factors

It is common knowledge that nursing school increases students' stress levels. Identified stressors include juggling multiple roles, such as meeting the demands of work, study, and family responsibilities; financial pressures; time management; lack of family support; demanding faculty; and the student's own emotional issues.[15] As students, they automatically find themselves in a dependent and relatively powerless position as compared to the instructor or institution.

Recent research indicates that the clinical setting is also vulnerable to incivility due to rapid technological changes, staff shortages, and poor staff-to-staff interpersonal communication and relationships. There is a need for ongoing research into the negative consequences of the clinical environment on students and faculty.[16]

One study reported that other contributing factors to incivility included student developmental issues caused by isolation from high-quality professional role models and reduced exposure to the faculty's decision-making process. Other nursing students did not believe in the social hierarchical structure of nursing school but rather that everyone was a peer. For them, the chain of command did not exist, and there were no boundaries in the lines of communication between students and faculty.[9,15]

Colleagues as Targets

On the receiving end, some faculty report being the target of negative remarks, insinuations, and harassment, all of which are counterproductive to their work and their credibility. Some faculty dismiss this type of lateral violence as "part of the job" and look the other way. Others note the rise in incivility and report feelings of anger, disappointment, and embarrassment as the result of colleagues' actions.

Expressed in many different forms, workplace incivility can include a toxic work environment, workplace violence, and bullying. Faculty themselves experience psychological pain as well as anger, fear, anxiety, feelings of being devalued, and decreased self-esteem.[18] These emotions often prompt competent teachers to resign rather than confront the incivility.[19] A famous quote by Martin Luther King is cited in American Association of Critical-Care Nurses' (AACN) Standards for Establishing and Sustaining Healthy Work Environments:[20] "Our lives begin to end the day we become silent about things that matter."

Box 17.2

A Student's Perspective on Bullying

"Wow, I feel as if I'm being kicked to the curb by a faculty member that I trusted. I will know better in the future," came the message from the student. Angry because he had failed a nursing course, he shared his concerns with a nursing administrator and lodged a grievance against the instructor of the course he had failed. Ignoring relationship boundaries, he sent an angry and sarcastic e-mail in retaliation to his instructor from whom he received the "F" because now he was ineligible to advance any further in the program. Many words included in the message fitted the descriptions in the academic literature of uncivil acts committed by students: aggression; anger; and rude, disruptive, violent behaviors. Shocked at the student's approach in managing his academic failure, the administrator began longing for the old days, when, despite the disappointment of a failed course, most students were humble when petitioning for an academic appeal to repeat a course and requesting reinstatement.

Cause and Effect

The increase in incivility in nursing education among faculty has several causes. The academic culture is often controlling and driven by faculty insecurities and competitiveness.[21] It is historically based on a rather inflexible hierarchical management structure. Many nursing faculty, who may have been excellent clinical practitioners, entered the teaching profession with little preparation in the basics of higher education. On-the-job training became the norm as nursing faculty adapted to the academic setting with its triple requirements of teaching, research, and service. Being unprepared, they often found themselves victims of lateral violence through unequal relationships or discrepancies in faculty status and rank.[22]

Normally, nursing faculty work in a highly interactive social system.[23] Most of the day-to-day operations of classes and committees require working closely with other nursing faculty. In some cases, when faculty disagree strongly with policies, procedures, or lines of authority, they may develop feelings of exclusion or alienation. Although nursing educators recognize that challenging the status quo is essential for the growth of the profession, it is still often resisted. Faculty who challenge the system can be silenced and sometimes even shunned by colleagues when they attempt to take a contradictory stance on an important decision.[21] This is most noticeable when a new nurse faculty with many years of experience in the clinical setting, but none in education, is hired and then is expected to blend seamlessly into the academic realm.

Mentoring

High-quality mentoring for new nurses and new faculty helps to build healthy relationships between students and educators. Constructive mentor relationships require respectful listening, focused thinking, maturity, wisdom, and positive energy, all of which help those being mentored correct mistakes and accomplish goals.[22]

It is not enough to just ignore incivility. It doesn't just go away. Disregarding incivility sends the message that uncivil behavior is part of the norm and something to be tolerated. Denial of problems often leads to bigger and more severe problems down the road. It is far better to take precautionary measures to prevent incivility and stop it as soon as it starts. Once incivility becomes a common occurrence, it is almost impossible to stop without radical intervention.[22]

Solutions to Academic Incivility

Once incivility has been identified and acknowledged in the academic and clinical settings, there are effective measures that can be taken to either decrease it or totally eliminate it. All the most effective measures to deal with lateral incivility are based on effective communication skills. Research indicates that in recent years, faculty have become less civil toward one another[17] (Box 17.3).

Don't Eat Your Young

The ritual of "eating your young" is seen both in the classroom and the clinical settings. It really is a form of vertical violence since it is based on an inequality

---

Box 17.3

Civility in the Classroom and Clinical Setting

Dr. Clark's Classroom Norms	Dr. Clark's Clinical Norms
• Practice proper door etiquette. • Assume goodwill. • Listen and respect others. • Be flexible and open-minded. • Keep cell phones on silent and use proper cell phone etiquette. • Use laptop for class work only. • Do not have side conversations. • Give notice of change in advance (faculty). • Be present and on time. • Have fun!	• Assume goodwill. • Respect and celebrate differences. • Communicate respectfully. • Listen carefully. • Come to clinical prepared and on time. • Share work equally among group members. • Resolve conflicts directly and with respect. • Have fun!

of power between the experienced nurse and the new nurse. There has been a long existing practice of having the new members of a profession undergo a rite of initiation. These initiation rites often involve intimidation and belittling of the student or the new nurse to help them "learn their place" in the organizational chain. Common "eating the young" activities include picking on, chewing out, or ridiculing the new nurse for their lack of knowledge. Using caustic humor or setting up the new nurse by placing them in a situation in which they will likely fail also contributes to the demoralization of the new nurse. Although the eating process has diminished to some degree in recent years, it still does exist in many institutions. (For more information, go to http://www.mightynurse.com/dont-eat-the-young/ or http://kdhhealthcomm.wordpress.com/2013/01/22/do-nurses-eat-their-young-whats-wrong-with-communication-in-health-care/.)

As an alternative to on-the-job training in nursing education, universities are now offering master's degrees in nursing education; this teaches students how to teach and explores the political ins and outs of the academic setting. Graduates come into the field of nursing education with an understanding of curriculum development, evaluation, testing, course preparation, and many other aspects of surviving in higher education, such as yearly evaluations, the rank and promotion system, and the need to publish. They are taught to be more assertive and to express their opinions without trepidation. Senior nursing educators are much more sensitive to the needs of new faculty and have a strong incentive to nurture them and help them develop into high-quality educators.[23] They realize that this new generation of instructors will need to replace them as they retire in large numbers over the next few years.

Preceptor and mentoring programs for new graduates have been developed in clinical facilities as a result of the IOM's Report on the Future of Nursing.[23] The chart on page 418 provides examples of classroom and clinical norms for nursing students. These have been co-created with colleagues and clinical setting partners so that everyone is operating with the same behavioral norms.[24]

Alternatives to Incivility

It is a well-known psychological principle that all behavior has meaning. (See Chapter 12 for more detail.) An individual's behavior also expresses his or her intrinsic values, including whether or not he or she treats others with respect and dignity or in a way that disrespects

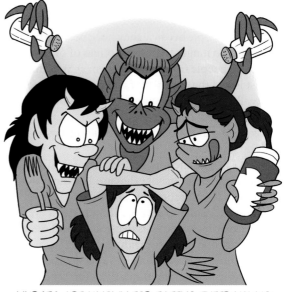

NURSES ARE KNOWN FOR EATING THEIR YOUNG.

them and drags down their self-esteem. An individual who helps in a soup kitchen, provides pro-bono nursing care at a free clinic, or drops a few coins in a street-person's cup is displaying behavior that indicates a fundamental belief that all human beings are valuable and deserve basic respect.[25] As noted below in the discussion of the ANA Code of Ethics and civility, disrespectful and poor treatment of others, whether they be coworkers, clients, family members, or strangers, is inconsistent with the basic tenants of nursing.

Because every action towards others, whether conscious or reflex, either contributes to a culture of civility or incivility, it is essential that every individual be committed to eliminating negative, uncivil thoughts and behaviors. For example, simple negative actions that should be eliminated include groaning out loud when a classmate in the front row asks another a complicated question, gossiping about a classmate during break times, disparaging the instructor's teaching style because it is monotone, making cynical comments about a classmate's presentation, and so forth. Instead, it is much more productive to use positive actions such as saying "good morning," "please," and "thank you" to everyone, even individuals who are not well liked, opening doors for people, putting the personal communication device away when someone is trying to talk to you, complimenting people when they do a good job, asking people if they need help, and so forth. A culture of civility is based on respecting everyone's dignity all the time.[25]

Over time and with the accumulation of life experiences, many people become cynical. Cynicism develops in people because they have been hurt by others and no longer trust the motives of others and try to keep people from hurting them again. This distrust is just the opposite of what is required for civility. Belief in the good intentions of others and the ability to trust in that the intentions of others are positive and good is a key to establishing a culture of civility.

Another method to decrease incivility is to avoid escalating uncivil behavior. It is a natural tendency that when someone is uncivil to us, we respond with similar behavior. This creates a cycle of incivility that just continues to escalate until the cycle is broken by one of the individuals. It seems that it would be much better to break the cycle at the beginning. However, breaking the cycle doesn't mean that others' inappropriate actions need to be ignored. Dealing with conflict and the difficult behavior of individuals is a skill that all nurses must master.[25] For a more detailed discussion of dealing with difficult behavior, see Chapter 13.

A Model for Civility

Administrators have an important role in building a proper workplace environment. This begins with the first interview of the hiring process. Applicants need to be asked specific questions about civility. Some samples of these questions include, "What things about the people you are working with really irk you?" "What do you do when you become angry or irritated with another employee or supervisor?" "On a scale of 1 to 10, with 10 being the best possible, how would you rate your abilities in the areas of collaboration, collegiality, and civility? Explain your answers."[24] The positive or negative attitude of administrators can determine whether stressful situations are addressed or ignored. Unaddressed, the culture of incivility permeates all aspects of the organization, but when constructive problem-solving and respectful encounters are the norm, a culture of civility can prevail. A civil climate enhances both teaching and learning.

A recently developed model allows faculty and students to promote civility in the academic setting. Although the model does not include administrators, their responsibilities, or their perceptions about incivility, it emphasizes the critical importance of the climate and infrastructure established by administrators. It is called the Conceptual Model for Fostering Civility in Nursing Education (Fig. 17.2).[25] The model depicts how, as stress levels increase for both students and faculty, student attitudes of entitlement and faculty attitudes of condescending superiority can lead to incivility.

The Conceptual Model provides a basis for creating a culture of civility by focusing on the levels of stress for nursing faculty and students. Possible research questions include the following:

1. What do you perceive to be the biggest stressors for nursing students?
2. What uncivil behaviors do you see nursing students displaying?
3. What do you perceive to be the biggest stressors for nursing faculty?
4. What uncivil behaviors do you see nursing faculty displaying?
5. What is the role of nursing leadership in addressing incivility?[26]

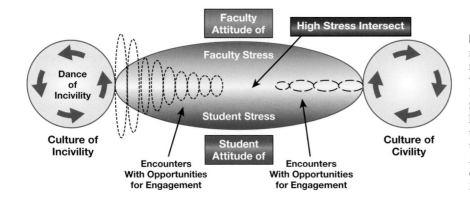

Figure 17.2 Conceptual model for fostering civility in nursing education. (Reprinted with permission from SLACK Incorporated: Clark CM, Springer PJ. Academic nurse leaders' role in fostering a culture of civility in nursing education. *Journal of Nursing Education*, 49[6]:319–325, 2010; doi: 10.3928/01484834-20100224-01. Epub 2010 Jun 3.)

There are some methods faculty can use to overcome academic incivility. Becoming a catalyst and a change agent in one's own nursing program will set an example that others can follow. Make civility and cooperation a key element in the vision, mission statement, and outcomes of the program. Revise the curriculum so that shared values, collegiality, and collaboration are threads that guide students and faculty in the learning process.[24]

ETHICAL PROHIBITIONS TO INCIVILITY

As of now, there are no federal standards to regulate workplace violence; however, several states have attempted to develop laws to control it. In most cases, these laws are confusing and difficult to enforce. To help fill this void, the Joint Commission (TJC) developed new guidelines under their "Leadership" standard to deal with behaviors that are interpreted as lateral violence. These include the following:

- Requiring hospitals and other organizations to develop their own codes of conduct defining behaviors that are considered lateral violence
- Requiring hospital administration to develop and implement a process for managing individuals who are displaying disruptive and inappropriate behaviors
- Requiring additional standards for medical staff to follow for the credentialing process, including demonstrating interpersonal skills and recognizing interprofessionalism.

A Guide for Caring
The Joint Commission notes:

"Intimidating and disruptive behaviors can foster medical errors, contribute to poor patient satisfaction and to preventable adverse outcomes, increase the cost of care, and cause qualified clinicians, administrators, and managers to seek new positions in more professional environments. Safety and quality of patient care is dependent on teamwork, communication, and a collaborative work environment. To assure quality and to promote a culture of safety, health care organizations must address the problem of behaviors that threaten the performance of the health care team."[27]

The American Nurses Association (ANA) Code of Ethics also has principles that support ethical, civil, and caring relationships. (For more information on the Code, see Chapter 6.) It was developed as a guide for carrying out nursing responsibilities in a manner consistent with quality in nursing care and the ethical obligations of the profession. The National League for Nursing (NLN) website gives high priority to the Code of Ethics and to faculty responsibility as a way of dealing with student behavioral problems. The specific parts of the ANA Code of Ethics (2014) that relate to incivility are as follows:

1. "The nurse, in all professional relationships, practices with compassion and respect for the inherent dignity, worth, and uniqueness of every individual. . . ."
1.5 Principles of respect extend to all encounters, including colleagues. "This standard of conduct precludes any and all prejudicial actions, any form of harassment or threatening behavior, or disregard for the effect of one's actions on others."
3.5 "Nurse educators have a responsibility to . . . promote a commitment to professional practice prior to entry of an individual into practice."[27]

> *Make civility and cooperation a key element in the vision, mission statement, and outcomes of the program.*

The Joint Commission, the ANA, and the NLN make it clear that underlying attitudes of caring and respect are essential expectations of those who enter the profession of nursing. It is essential for nurses to learn and internalize these attitudes. A caring attitude is *not* transmitted from generation to generation by genes—it is transmitted by the culture of a society.[3] The ANA has had a Task Force on Workplace Violence for several years (http://nursingworld.org/Search?SearchMode=1&SearchPhrase=workplace+violence). It developed a website that assists nurses in understanding more about this problem.

Professional Standards
Ethical behaviors in nursing school correlate with ethical behaviors in professional practice.[27] The American Association of Colleges of Nursing (AACN) notes the importance of professional

standards, including the development and acquisition of an appropriate set of values and an ethical framework. It stresses that incivility is unethical and notes that nursing faculty have a "moral imperative" to deter incivility.[15] Early identification of incivility in a culture of violence is very important in preventing severe physical harm (see Figure 17.3). The AACN strongly suggests that educators try to determine the presence of incivility before students enter a program.[27]

Codes of Conduct

Some universities and colleges have instituted honor codes. Studies have shown that academic settings with an honor code have less cheating. One type of honor code for students and faculty is called HIRRE, which stands for "honesty, integrity, respect, responsibility, and ethics." In HIRRE, students sign a pledge promising not to cheat or plagiarize.[27] Faculty and students can use a reporting system to identify violations of the honor code. Enforcement by faculty, directors, or the dean can include expulsion for honor code infractions.[9,15]

The Internet Society has an established code of conduct that is used as a guide for responsible behavior of Internet operators. It is important to remember that the Internet relies on the good conduct of those who use it.[12] However, because of recent misuses that have led to teenage suicides, ethical codes are continuing to evolve.

WORKPLACE INCIVILITY

Workplace incivility is a broad term that includes workplace hostility, bullying, lateral violence, horizontal violence, vertical violence, and workplace violence. It is the threat of violence or the actual causing of physical harm to workers either inside or outside of the workplace. Workplace incivility runs along the continuum, ranging from verbal abuse to physical violence and homicide.

Workplace Violence

Over 2 million workers are targets of workplace abuse each year, and it is blamed for the deaths of more than 1,000 people a year in the United States. When the uncivil behavior is directed toward harming someone, it is moved to the far end of the continuum and becomes physical workplace violence. The estimated cost of workplace violence in the United States is $4.2 billion per year.[21] Whether in the form of mere workplace incivility or full-blown workplace violence, these behaviors result in negative outcomes for clients as well as employees and administrators.[21]

Workplace violence in the health-care setting is a growing problem. It is important to be able to recognize characteristics in a person that may indicate escalating cycles of violence, including nurses, physicians, clients, family members, or others. A survey conducted in 2013 of 550 nurses' perceptions of how workplace hostility affected client safety revealed several major concerns. In the survey, a large number of the nurses indicated the following actions could occur in an environment of horizontal hostility leading to the compromise of client safety and quality of care:

> *Once a tipping point is passed, the potential for violence increases dramatically. Interrupting the spiral with positive interventions and communication before that tipping point is important in defusing the anger.*

- Failing to clarify an unreadable order because of fear of the physician
- Lifting or ambulating heavy or debilitated clients without assistance rather than asking for help
- Using an unfamiliar piece of equipment without asking for instructions first
- Carrying out orders that the nurse did not believe were correct[28]

Institutions need a comprehensive plan to deal with violence, including client violence toward health-care workers. Without appropriate interventions, disrespect and unresolved conflict can quickly spiral out of control and eventually lead to physical violence.[14] The Occupational Safety and Health Administration has developed a set of guidelines for limiting workplace violence and stopping it once it gets started (see http://www.osha.gov/OshDoc/data_General_Facts/factsheet-workplace-violence.pdf). This is an appropriate place to start developing an institutional plan. It is comprehensive yet flexible and can be modified to fit almost any workplace environment.

Stop the Spiral

The incivility spiral (Fig. 17.3) depicts uncivil behavior between two people or two groups. The behavior can escalate into violence, or those involved can let go of their resentment and stop the incivility from progressing. The path chosen depends largely on communication, both at the beginning of the conflict and during its progress. Conflict resolution interventions are essential to the process.[9,15]

The higher up the spiral the uncivil behavior advances, the more coercive behavior is displayed and the greater is the desire for violent revenge. The victim of the incivility experiences loss of face, increased anger, and a desire to fight back against the one creating the hostile environment. Once the tipping point is passed (i.e., the point in the spiral where neither party can back down), the potential for physical violence increases dramatically. Interrupting the spiral with positive interventions and communication before the tipping point is reached is essential in defusing the anger.[9,15]

What Do You Think?

How do you think incivility compares with child abuse or elder abuse? Are the measures to overcome child or elder abuse similar to those required to overcome workplace violence?

Solutions to Horizontal Violence in Nursing

Nurses must prevent a situation from reaching the tipping point where incivility turns into violent actions. The importance of providing safety in practice needs to be continually reinforced to prevent negative outcomes from an unsafe work environment. The Quality and Safety Education for Nurse (QSEN) competencies developed by the AACN can be successful in reducing educational and workplace incivility when they are efficiently implemented into a facility or nursing program. The six QSEN areas for prelicensure and graduate nursing programs include client-centered care, teamwork and collaboration, evidence-based practice (EBP), quality improvement (QI), safety, and informatics.[29] Although these areas

Sample Incivility Spiral

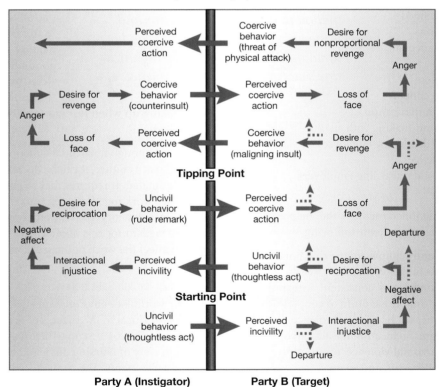

Party A (Instigator)   **Party B (Target)**

Figure 17.3 The incivility spiral. (From Anderson LM, Pearson CM. Tit for tat? The spiraling effect of incivility in the workplace. *Academy of Management Review,* 24(3):453–471, 1999. Retrieved May 2014 from http://www.jstor.org/stable/259136, with permission.)

are being addressed in the clinical setting, there is still a need to promote these competencies in education (see Chapter 4).

Creating a Positive Work Environment

Alertness is essential to defuse incivility in the work setting. Listening to fellow workers' accounts of incivility is a first step and should be followed by reflection and development of an action plan. Ignoring the problem never solves it and often escalates the frequency and intensity of the incivility. To break the cycle, it is necessary to be proactive about incivility incidents and to see them as signs of potentially more dangerous problems.

The Nursing Organizations Alliance recommends eight actions to help build a positive workplace environment and overcome incivility:

1. Building a collaborative culture that includes respectful communication and behavior
2. Establishing a communication-rich culture that emphasizes trust and respect
3. Making accountability central to the culture with clearly defined role expectations
4. Maintaining adequate staffing
5. Training leaders competent in cooperation and communication
6. Sharing decision-making with all those it will affect
7. Continuously developing employee skills and clinical knowledge
8. Recognizing and rewarding employees' contributions[25]

Other identified methods that help reverse horizontal violence include the following:[24]

9. Recognizing and acknowledging that horizontal violence exists in the workplace
10. Adopting a continuous, consistent, integrated approach to promote a culture of cooperation and address instances of horizontal violence
11. Providing regular education for all staff on the subject of horizontal violence; for example, what it is, how to address it, and so on
12. Instituting mechanisms that enable and allow staff members to safely address issues of horizontal violence
13. Talking to all staff members about the phenomenon, breaking the silence

Nurses can break the cycle of incivility by looking at their own acceptance or participation in the negative behavior and using organizational structures and personal influence to change the organization's culture of horizontal violence.[30] Some important actions nurses need to take individually to reduce the effect of lateral violence on their own careers and lives include:

1. Naming the problem—call it *horizontal violence* to refer to the situation.
2. Raising the issue at staff meetings—bring the light of day to the problem.
3. Asking supervisors about developing a process for dealing with incivility in the workplace.
4. Learning from experience—keeping a journal raises self-awareness about personal values, beliefs, attitudes, and behavior, and it is a good source of documentation.
5. Pursuing a path of personal growth—finding those things that create happiness and satisfaction and developing them goes a long way to counteract incivility.
6. Ensuring the nurse is part of the solution, not part of the problem.
7. Maintaining self-care behaviors—peer support, good nutrition, adequate sleep, time-outs, meditation, and exercise.
8. Speaking up when horizontal violence is witnessed.[29]

Although horizontal violence is endemic in the workplace culture, it can be decreased and maybe even eliminated. It requires that all employees of every workplace work together to eliminate oppression and unhealthy behaviors from the environment. Nurses must be vigilant for acts of incivility that are less obvious but affect the work of nurses in all settings.

Leadership for Job Satisfaction

Healthy workplace environments that empower nurses are critical to the success of the profession. At a conference in 2013, Sigma Theta Tau International Honor Society of Nursing discussed healthy workplace environments. The conference identified the key attributes of both healthy and unhealthy workplace environments and interventions for improvement. (See http://www.nursingsociety.org. Read the Posts from CHWE blog by Kathleen Stevens, EdD, RN, ANEF, FAAN, posted on Reflections on Nursing Leadership.)

> " *Nurses can break the cycle of incivility by looking at their own acceptance or participation in the negative behavior and using organizational structures and personal influence to change the organization's culture of horizontal violence.* "

Box 17.4

Thirteen Qualities of Transformational Leaders

1. You hold a vision for the organization that is intellectually rich, stimulating, and rings true.
2. You are honest and empathic. People feel emotionally safe and trust that you have their interests at heart.
3. Your character is well developed, without the prominent dark side of ego power.
4. You set aside your own interests in looking good and getting strokes, instead making others look good and giving others power and credit.
5. You evince a concern for the whole (not just your own organization), reflected in your passionate and ethical voice being heard when necessary.
6. Your natural tendency is to help others engage, deepen their perspectives, and be effective.
7. You can share power with others—you believe sharing power is the best way to tap talent, engage others, and get work done in optimal fashion.
8. You risk, experiment, and learn. Information is never complete.
9. You have a true passion for work and the vision. It shows in your time commitment, attention to detail, and ability to renew your energy.
10. You communicate effectively both in listening and in speaking.
11. You understand and appreciate management and administration. They appreciate that you move toward shared success without sacrifice.
12. You celebrate the now. At meetings or anywhere else, you sincerely acknowledge accomplishment, staying in the moment before moving on.
13. You persist in hard times. That means you have the courage to move ahead when you are tired, conflicted, and getting mixed signals.

Source: Johns C. Becoming a transformational leader through reflection. *Reflections on Nursing Leadership,* 30(2):24–26, 2004.

Healthy workplace environments are supported by the Magnet Hospital Designation (Agency for Healthcare Research and Quality [AHRQ], 2008). It is critical to develop a healthy workplace environment to decrease absenteeism, increase productivity, and dramatically reduce turnover rates.[29] Mentoring has been shown to lower incivility in the workplace. Mentoring partnerships, along with updated educational models, increase cultural competence and enhance job satisfaction for both the new person and the mentor.[30] It eases the new nurse's transition into his or her new role and helps the mentor to better understand the problems the new nurse is having in completing the role transition. It also helps make the new person a genuine member of the group much more quickly than if they were learning on their own by trial and error.

Transformational leadership (TL) is a key element in reversing incivility in the academic or workplace environment. TL acts as a lens through which leaders can see themselves and the workplace inequalities that need to be changed.[31] As an intervention, TL requires an extraordinary capacity for self-restraint, self-reflection, and deep consciousness of the inner sense of responsibility. In addition, TL plays an important role in implementing needed changes in present and future practices.[31] Box 17.4 lists 13 transformational leadership qualities that can work toward increasing civility in the workplace.

Conclusion

Incivility violates trust and undermines the nurse's obligation to care. It creates insecurity and hostility and degrades learning, collaboration, and performance in all institutions where it is found. In all settings, relationships are adversely affected by incivility. Research and active efforts to deal with the problem will help to ensure better client care. TL qualities can transform incivility into civility and caring. TL can stop upward-spiraling incivility and help with spotting, intervening in, and overcoming incivility. Constructive mentor–mentee rather than tormentor–tormentee relationships will promote professional growth in nurses and improve both the academic environment and the health-care setting. Emotional intelligence arising from the practice of civility is essential and basic to the practice of nursing.

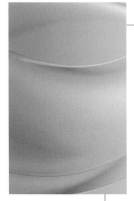

Issues Now

Promoting Civility Through Reflection on Your Personal Qualities

Job satisfaction is important to the attitude brought to the workplace. The likelihood of workplace incivility being present is high. Job satisfaction helps to deal with incivility.

Likewise, the Department of Labor also lists preferred qualities for different career choices (http://www.onetcenter.org/content.html). These are not personality tests, but rather are measures of qualities that meet common core expectations. It is hypothesized that a match between your qualities and those of your chosen career helps job satisfaction.

As you prepare for employment or further professional development, reflect on your own qualities. Identifying them will provide a lens through which to preview your chosen field. Be prepared to have them tested as you progress in your health-care career, reflecting on the assets and competencies that you bring to the world.[32]

Critical-Thinking Exercises

- Obtain the policy and procedure manual for your nursing program. Try to find the policy on lateral violence or bullying. Does it include the elements to stop bullying discussed in this chapter? What things should be added? If your nursing program does not have a policy, ask the dean if you can develop one.
- Obtain the policy and procedure manual for your primary clinical site. Try to find the policy on lateral violence or bullying. Does it include the elements to stop bullying discussed in this chapter? What things should be added? How does it compare to the policy from your nursing program? If your clinical site does not have a policy, ask the CEO if you can develop one.
- Ask your fellow nursing students about their experiences with lateral violence. Take notes and see if there is a common thread that runs through the stories.

References

1. Sparrow S. Practicing civility in the legal writing course: Helping law students learn professionalism. Retrieved December 2013 from http://www.lexisnexis.com/

2. Pascoe E, Richman L. Perceived discrimination and health: A meta-analytic review. *Psychological Bulletin,* 135(4):531–554, 2009.

3. Watson J. Nursing: The philosophy and science of caring, revised edition. Boulder, CO: University Press of Colorado, 2008.

4. Sherwood G, Horton-Deutsch S. Reflective practice: Transforming education and improving outcomes. Indianapolis, IN: Sigma Theta Tau International Honor Society of Nursing, 2012.

5. Dellasega C. Recognizing and overcoming the cycle of bullying: When nurses hurt nurses. Indianapolis, IN: Sigma Theta Tau International, 2011.

6. Townsend T. Breaking the bullying cycle. *American Nurse Today,* 7(1):12–15, 2012.

7. Wilkins K. The civil behavior of students: A survey of school professionals. Retrieved December 2013 from http://cdm15999.contentdm.oclc.org/cdm/ref/collection/IR/id/1454

8. Lamontagne C. Intimidation: A concept analysis. *Nursing Forum,* 45(1):54–65, 2010.

9. Cleary M, Hunt G, Horsfall J. Identifying and addressing bullying in nursing. *Journal in Mental Health Nursing,* 31,331–335, 2012.

10. Fontaine D, Kohl E, Carroll T. Promoting a healthy workplace for nursing faculty and staff. *Nursing Clinics of North America,* 47(4):557–566, 2012.

11. Johnston M, Phanhtharath P, Johnson BS. The bullying aspects of workplace violence in nursing. *JONA'S Healthcare Law, Ethics, and Regulation,* 12(2):36–42, 2010.

12. Internet Society. All about the Internet: Code of Conduct. Retrieved December 2013 from http://www.isoc.org/internet/conduct

13. Poorman S, Mastrovich M, Webb C. Teacher's stories: How faculty help and hinder students at risk. *Nursing Education Perspectives,* 5(29):272–277, 2008.

14. Taylor C, Mpotu F. Embracing mentors and facing tormentors. Imprint. *Journal of the National Student Nurses Association,* Nov/Dec 2010.

15. Clark C, Springer P. Academic nurse leaders' role in fostering a culture of civility in nursing education. *Journal of Nursing Education,* 49(6):319–325, 2010.

16. Hunt C, Marini Z. Incivility in the practice environment: A perspective from clinical nursing teachers. *Nurse Education in Practice,* 11;366–370, 2012.

17. Twale DJ, DeLuca BM. *Faculty Incivility: The Rise of the Academic Bully Culture and What to Do About It.* San Francisco: Jossey Bass, 2008.

18. Purpora C, Blegen MA. Horizontal violence and the quality and safety of patient care: A conceptual model. *Nursing Research and Practice,* 2012. Retrieved May 2013 from doi: 10.1155/2012/306948.

19. Clarke C, Kane D, Rajacich D, Lafreniere K. Bullying in undergraduate clinical nursing education. *Journal of Nursing Education,* 51(5):269–276, 2012.

20. American Association of Critical Care Nurses. *AACN Standards for Establishing and Sustaining Healthy Work Environments.* Aliso Viejo, CA: AACN, 2005, p. 11.

21. Walker, WO, et al. Mentoring for the New Millennium. Retrieved August 2014 from http://www.ianphi.org/documents/pdfs/New%20Millennium.pdf

22. Nursing Organization Alliance Position Paper 2010. Retrieved December 2013 from http://www.nursing-alliance.org

23. Clark C. Faculty and student assessment of and experience with incivility in nursing education. *Journal of Nursing Education,* 47(10):458–465, 2008.

24. Clark C. *Creating and Sustaining Civility in Nursing Education.* Indianapolis, IN: Sigma Theta Tau International Honor Society of Nursing, 2013.

25. Luparell S. Incivility in Nursing Education. Nursing Student National Association, *Imprint.* 2008.

26. Sentinal Event Policy, Office of Quality and Safety in Health Care 2008. Retrieved January 2013 from http://www.safetyandquality.health.wa.gov.au

27. Code of Ethics for Nurses. Retrieved December 2013 from http://www.nursingworld.org/MainMenuCategories/EthicsStandards/CodeofEthicsforNurses/Code-of-Ethics.pdf

28. Wilson BL, Phelps C. Horizontal hostility: A threat to patient safety. *JONA'S Healthcare Law, Ethics and Regulation,* 15(1):51–57, 2013.

29. Dellasega C, Volpe R. *Managing Bullying, Bad Attitudes and Total Turmoil: Toxic Nursing.* Indianapolis, IN: Sigma Theta Tau International, 2013.

30. Hill J. Mentoring African American women leaders in nursing. Unpublished dissertation. Baton Rouge, LA: Louisiana State University, 2003.

31. Johns C. Becoming a transformation leader through refection. *Reflections on Nursing Leadership,* 30(2):24–26, 2009.

32. Pearley M. Lateral violence among nurses. Unpublished manuscript. Baton Rouge, LA: Southern University and A&M College, 2013.

Nursing Informatics

18

Kathleen Mary Young

Joseph T. Catalano

Learning Objectives

After completing this chapter, the reader will be able to:

- Discuss the impact of the information revolution on society in general and on health care specifically
- Define *nursing informatics*
- Explain the importance of nursing informatics to nursing practice
- Analyze the availability of resources and references in the practice site
- Evaluate the importance of human factor engineering concepts on equipment design
- Compare the electronic health record with the paper record system

INFORMATION CHANGES EVERYTHING

The quality, type, and use of information technology continue to evolve at a rapid rate, transforming almost every aspect of life. Since the advent and widespread adoption of technology, society has become more and more dependent on smartphones, tablets, featherlight laptops, and other wireless communication devices. Smart technologies are found in cars, home entertainment devices, house environmental control systems, and all aspects of the workplace. In health care, clients are using their cell phones and handheld devices to look up health-care information, check on the backgrounds of health-care providers, and even assess the quality of hospitals. Health-care providers are also embracing technology, but not always enthusiastically.

These technologies are changing both the way teachers teach and the way learners learn. It is changing the way people work, communicate, and play. Teaching in public schools and colleges now demands fast-moving, entertaining lessons that capture the students' attention because classroom teachers must compete with television, portable electronic games, and the latest free app with which this generation has been raised.

Schoolchildren and college students no longer read as extensively as they once did. Media technology has accustomed many to 30-second "sound bites" of information. Libraries have evolved from repositories of hardbound volumes and journals to providers of Internet access to online journals and books. Many people spend 8 to 10 hours a day in front of a computer or on a handheld device. People who have lost traditional jobs in manufacturing and service industries are finding that, to become marketable in today's workplace, they must have computer skills.

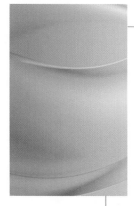

Issues Now

There's an App for . . . Health Care?

Yes! There's an app for that! The popularity and number of health-related apps for wireless devices has doubled since 2011. Many of them deal with exercise, diet, and healthy living, but some apps are specific for medical care. Currently there are over 8,000 heath-care-related apps.

People who are about to undergo surgery often have high anxiety levels due to fear of the unknown. What's going to happen? Is it going to hurt? How long is it going to take? Well, there's an app for that. "Touchsurgery" is an app that allows clients who are preparing for operations to download videos on their mobile devices of their actual surgery or computer-based simulations. Health-care facilities can use these apps to help educate clients about procedures and may also help build trust and confidence in anxious clients. Some of the surgeries that can be viewed include removal of the gallbladder (cholycystectomy), removal of the appendix (appendectomy), and common orthopedic surgeries such as hip and knee replacement and shoulder reconstruction. Because many of these surgeries are done in one-day surgery units, nurses have little time to educate clients about postoperative care. The app also provides clients with instructions about deep breathing exercises, activity limitations, and the use of medications. The app has the potential to increase client satisfaction and improve outcomes.

Feel like you have a lot of stress in your life? If you have an Android phone, an app can monitor that for you! The Android Remote Sensing (AIRS) app monitors your daily stress by using all the sensors built into mobile devices that measure physiological changes. A device built into the phone called an ac-celerometer can measure environmental noise level; social activity, such as the number and frequency of texts and calls; temperature; and even the user's pos-ture. If monitoring wires are attached to the user, it can also track moods and emotions by analyzing pulse and heart-rate data, even when you get a particular e-mail or text. The app can make people more aware of their internal stress levels, which may be helpful for clients with cardiovascular disease or anxiety disorders.

Although not an app, there is a new website where clients can find out if the hospital they are being admitted to has had any violations. By logging on to hospitalin-spections.org, the client can find information about deficiencies cited during complaint inspections at acute care and critical access hospitals throughout the United States since January 1, 2011. The site is run by the Association of Health Care Journalists (AHCJ) in conjunction with the U.S. Centers for Medicare and Medicaid Services (CMS). The goal of the site is to make federal hospital inspections easier to access, search, and analyze. However, inspections of psychiatric or long-term care facilities are not included in the database. Previously, this information could only be accessed in writing and on paper through Freedom of Information Act requests. Because this site is so new, the data is incomplete; however, AHJC is continually updating and fill-ing in missing information. The data should not be used to try to rank hospitals.

Sources: Clark C. CMS Unveils Hospital Violations Database, Health Leaders Media, 2013. Retrieved April 2013 from http://www.healthleadersmedia.com/content/QUA-290217/CMS-Unveils-Hospital-Violations-Database; Glatter R. Worried about your surgery? Skip the Valium and download the app. *Forbes,* 2013. Retrieved April 2013 from http://www.forbes.com/sites/robertglatter/2013/03/31/worried-about- your-surgery-skip-the-valium-and-download-the-app/; Now track your stress level through Android smartphone app. *TelecomTiger,* 2013. Retrieved April 2013 from http://www.telecomtiger.com/Technology_fullstory.aspx?passfrom=topstory&storyid= 17164&section=S210

TECHNOLOGY AND COMMUNICATION

The information revolution has changed both the form and the format of communication. Before the advent of the telephone, people communicated through the written word. Letter writing was an art. Before television and the computer were invented, people gathered together in neighborhoods and developed a sense of community.

Today the whole world is the community, and every corner can be reached from a home computer or wireless device. Senior citizens use their computers to chat and to organize get-togethers and other social activities. Younger people use their cell phones and text-messaging to meet friends and stay connected, even when they are in the bathroom with their pajamas on.

Asymmetrical Information

Not only does technology change the way in which people communicate and work, but it also creates new decision-making processes that affect all aspects of industry and commerce, including health care. Informed decisions produce better outcomes. When people are able to sift through and use the vast amount of information available to them, it gives them a decided advantage in conducting business.

> *Not only does technology change the way in which people communicate and work, but it also creates a new decision-making process that affects all aspects of industry and commerce, including health care.*

The use of multiple data sources in economics and business is called **asymmetrical information.** Many businesses currently work with asymmetrical information: Individuals on one side of the transaction may have much better information than those on the other. Borrowers know more than lenders about their repayment prospects, managers and boards know more than shareholders about the firm's profitability, prospective clients know more than insurance companies about their accident risk, and in some cases, ill clients know more about their disease process than the health-care provider. The fact that the person with more information has an advantage seems like common sense, but a grasp of the impact of asymmetrical information will lead to a better understanding of day-to-day economic activity.

Competitive Health Care

One of the key elements of health-care reform is the increased use of informatics to help drive down the cost of health care. The goal is to have every U.S. citizen's medical record in electronic storage. When the Health Care Reform Act was passed, only 8 percent of the more than 5,000 U.S. hospitals had completely computerized medical records and charting.[1] The American Recovery and Reinvestment Act of 2009 established incentive payments of several billion dollars to encourage electronic health record development through the federal and state medicare programs. Over 77,000 health-care providers have applied for these grants, but the implementation of the systems is lagging behind the goals set by the government.[2]

Competition has long been a driving force in the pricing and marketing of health care. Payment methods that promote competition are encouraged by Medicare and Medicaid prospective payment systems (PPSs), health maintenance organizations (HMOs), preferred provider organizations (PPOs), and managed care. For an organization to offer competitive and high-quality services, information must be available for decision-making. More information is available to decision-makers with information technology.

Technologically driven organizations have a competitive edge through the collection of large amounts of information and its application to decision-making in health care. To stay competitive in national and international health care, the health-care delivery system—specifically nursing—must open itself to new information and ideas.

The health-care information revolution is continuing to progress rapidly. Handheld wireless devices are being used in almost every area of client care today, including assessment of the quality of care, decision-making, management, planning, and medical research.[1]

DEFINING INFORMATICS

Two definitions of informatics are commonly used in health care. The term *medical informatics* was coined in the mid-1970s. Borrowed from the French expression *informatique medicale*, it included all the informational technologies that deal with the medical care of the client, medical resources, and the decision-making process.[3]

Health informatics is a more comprehensive term, defined as the use of information technology with information management concepts and methods to support health-care delivery. Health informatics includes the medical field but also encompasses nursing, dental, and pharmacy informatics as well as all other health-care disciplines. The definition of health informatics focuses attention on the recipient of care rather than on the discipline of the caregiver.

Models for Nursing Informatics

The nursing community has made marked progress toward developing a discipline of informatics that is specific to the delivery of nursing care based on the science of nursing. Nursing has distinct and discrete information needs. The content and application of nursing information are substantively different from those of other disciplines. Data gathered by the nursing profession present unique problems for the use of information in the delivery of nursing care based on critical thinking.[3]

Three Basic Elements

An early model for nursing informatics can be traced back to 1989. Although somewhat simplistic, it primarily combined computer science, information science, and nursing science in a manner that would help the nurse in planning and delivering care. These technologies aid in the collection and analysis of data so that the nurse can make informed and accurate decisions about the type of care clients require.[4]

In this early definition of nursing informatics, computer science was seen primarily as the computer and the institution-wide system to which it was connected. *Information science* refers to the computer software, including how data or tasks are processed, how problems are solved, and where products are produced. Nursing science is all the research data from nursing and other associated disciplines that relate to and support nursing practice.

More Complex Elements

In newer models of nursing informatics, a fourth element, cognitive science, has been added. Cognitive science combines psychology, linguistics, computer science, philosophy, and neuroscience in a way that enhances the delivery of client care. Cognitive science is also concerned with perception, thinking, understanding, and remembering. This model unites information science, computer science, and cognitive science into a framework of nursing science.

It is also believed that wisdom should be added as a component of nursing informatics along with data, information, and knowledge. With wisdom, the nurse is able to know how and when to use the available information in managing clients' problems and meeting their needs.[5]

Data, Information, and Knowledge

In most theories of nursing informatics, *data* are defined as raw and unstructured facts. For example, the numbers 102 and 104 are raw data: By themselves, these numbers have little meaning because they lack interpretation. *Information* consists of data that have been given form and have been interpreted. If the numbers 102 and 104 are given additional descriptors so that they become a 25-year-old man with an oral temperature of 102°F and a heart rate of 104 beats per minute (bpm) taken on admission to the emergency room, they become information that has meaning to the nurse.

Knowledge takes the process one step further because it is a synthesis of data and information. Knowing that an oral temperature of 102°F is higher than normal and a heart rate of 104 bpm is faster than normal for a 25-year-old man, and combining that information with an understanding of human physiology and pharmacology, the nurse is able to decide what treatment should be given.

> *The nursing community has made marked progress toward developing a discipline of informatics that is specific to the delivery of nursing care based on the science of nursing. Nursing has distinct and discrete information needs.*

What Do You Think?

Have you used computerized health-care records? Describe your experience.

This process relies on critical thinking and decision-making and can be used in research to create new knowledge.

The data-to-information-to-knowledge model of informatics is linear, but the process of synthesizing data into information to create knowledge is circular. New knowledge creates new questions and areas of research, which in turn lead to more new knowledge. To answer any research question, new data are required that must be processed into information to create more knowledge. The goal of this process is to provide the most accurate and current information so that nurses can make informed decisions in their daily practice.

Areas of Focus in Informatics

Over the years, the specialty of nursing informatics has evolved through three levels of special interest: technology, concepts of nursing theory, and function.

Technology. The earliest attempts to define nursing informatics focused solely on the use of technology. A commonly used early definition of nursing informatics stated that it existed whenever the nurse used any type of information technology in delivering nursing care or in the process of educating nursing students.[6] Here are some key points in the use of technology or computer systems to store, process, display, retrieve, and communicate health-care information quickly in the health-care setting:

- Administer nursing services and resources
- Manage the delivery of client and nursing care
- Link research resources and findings to nursing practice
- Apply educational resources to nursing education

Informatics is no longer just an elective subject. In today's competitive and rapidly changing health-care delivery system, mastery of informatics is a basic requirement.

Nursing theory. As nursing informatics evolved, it began to combine nursing theory and informatics. Without a well-articulated theoretical basis to guide the gathering of data, nurses soon become overwhelmed with meaningless data and information. Obviously, there is a need for common definitions, a standardized nursing language, and criteria for organization of the data.

Function. An additional step in the evolution of nursing informatics is the inclusion of the concept of function. The function of nursing informatics is to manage and process data to help nurses enter, organize, and retrieve needed information. Technology is then developed to achieve specific purposes related to client-care needs. Although technology forms the foundation of informatics, the nurse's ability to use that technology and make it function to meet clients' needs is the real test of the system's effectiveness.

In reality, nursing informatics includes all three of these areas—technology, nursing theory, and function. However, the field of informatics has become so large that it is difficult for any one person to be an expert in all three areas.

INFORMATICS AS A SPECIALTY

Informatics has been identified as one of the keys to the movement toward quality improvement by all the entities concerned with quality health care. One of the best ways for nurses to incorporate all the new health-care technologies, medications, treatments, and procedures into their daily practices is through the use of informatics. One truth in nursing care is that nothing ever goes away. Nurses are expected to be able to assimilate all the new knowledge while retaining all the things they have learned in the past. Applying that knowledge to client care becomes more manageable with the effective use of technology. (For more information, go to http://www.ahrq.gov/research/findings/factsheets/informatic/informatics/index.html.)

A Broader Definition

A broader definition of nursing informatics is provided by the American Nurses Association (ANA). It defines nursing informatics as:

A specialty that integrates nursing science, computer science, and information science in identifying, collecting, processing, and managing data and information to support nursing practice, administration, education and research; and to expand nursing knowledge. The purpose of nursing informatics is to analyze information requirements; design, implement and evaluate information systems and data structures that support nursing; and identify and apply computer technologies for nursing.[7]

Nursing informatics is now recognized as a nursing specialty for which a registered nurse (RN) can receive certification. The catalogue of the American Nurses Credentialing Center (ANCC) states that the nursing informatics practice:

> . . . encompasses the full range of activities that focus on the methods and technologies of information handling in nursing. It includes the development, support, and evaluation of applications, tools, processes, and structures that assist the practice of nurses with the management of data in direct care of patients/clients. The work of an informatics nurse can involve any and all aspects of information systems, including theory formulation, design, development, marketing, selection, testing, implementation, training, maintenance, evaluation, and enhancement.[8]

Nursing informatics supports all areas of nursing, including practice, education, administration, and research. It facilitates and guides the management of data.

Articulation

Informatics is no longer just an elective subject. In today's competitive and rapidly changing health-care delivery system, mastery of informatics is a basic requirement. The importance of the role of informatics is apparent in the need for the articulation of nursing practice. Articulation is an important way for nursing to demonstrate its accountability and credibility so that it can remain an essential element of the health-care system.

The Need for a Standard

Historically, the nursing profession has had difficulty in locating relevant nursing information quickly because there was no universally accepted nomenclature and taxonomy for either nursing clinical information or management data. In the past, this lack of access to information has presented several seemingly insurmountable challenges for nurse executives, including identifying what the nursing staff actually does, determining the impact nurses have on outcomes, and establishing appropriate reimbursement for nursing activities.

For example, how does a nurse interpret the term *weak grasp* in a client's chart? The meaning of "weak grasp" differs widely depending on the client. If the client is a premature infant, the term has an entirely different meaning than if the client is a 25-year-old professional football player with a head injury or a 60-year-old with a stroke. Imagine the difficulty

that a researcher will have when investigating the phenomenon of weak grasp—there is no standardized definition among the nursing community. Because a standardized nursing language is needed to name and communicate what nurses do, nursing classification schemes, taxonomies, and vocabularies have come to the forefront with the evolution of nursing informatics.

What Do You Think?

Think of four terms, not defined actions, carried out by nurses that have multiple meanings. How could these terms be clarified?

Unified Nursing Language System

The ANA Database Steering Committee was formed in 1991 to develop a common nursing language called the Unified Nursing Language System (UNLS). UNLS maps concepts by identifying common terms from different vocabularies and acknowledging them as synonyms of the same concept.

Twelve classification systems are recognized by the ANA as uniquely developed to documenting nursing care. They are designed to record and track the clinical care process for an entire episode of client care in the acute, home, or ambulatory setting or any combination of these. Standards and scoring guidelines for nursing languages can be found in Box 18.1.

Box 18.1

Standards and Scoring Guidelines for Nursing Languages

1. Terms in data dictionaries and tables are appropriate to the domain of nursing.
2. Terms from ANA-recognized languages for nursing are used as a core for the nursing vocabulary.
3. The system allows for the development and addition of new terms as needed, without duplicating existing terms or disrupting the integrity of existing languages.
4. In "local" languages, terms are mapped to appropriate ANA-recognized nursing languages, which may include reference terminologies.
5. The system accommodates the use of reference terminologies to map nursing languages to other existing standardized data sets, classification systems, or nomenclatures.

Nursing Minimum Data Set

Standardization of the data in a client's record is the first step toward unifying information to make it usable to the bedside nurse. The second step is the development of criteria to determine the necessary elements that must be included in every client record or encounter. The Nursing Minimum Data Set (NMDS), developed in 1985 and accepted by the ANA in 1998, is a list of the data elements necessary in any computerized client record system or national database. The NMDS is considered to be the umbrella for other nursing process schemes. The purpose of the NMDS is to:

1. Describe the nursing care of clients and their families in various settings, both institutional and noninstitutional.
2. Establish comparability of nursing data across clinical populations, settings, geographical areas, and time.
3. Demonstrate or project trends regarding nursing care provided and allocation of nursing resources to clients according to their health problems or nursing diagnoses.
4. Stimulate **nursing research** through linkages of detailed data existing in nursing information systems and in other health-care information systems.
5. Provide data about nursing care to influence health policy and decision-making.[9]

The NMDS focuses on 16 elements divided into three main categories. The three categories are (1) nursing care, such as nursing diagnosis, intervention, outcome, and degree of nursing care; (2) client demographics, such as the client's personal identification, date of birth, gender; and (3) service elements, such as the unique service agency number, the admission and discharge dates, client's condition, and the expected payer.

Accountability

Intuitively, the nursing profession has long known that the presence of RNs improves the quality of care and client outcomes while decreasing the cost of health care. According to the Congressional Office of Technology Assessment, better use of nurse practitioners could result in savings for clients, employers, and society, owing to the cost-effectiveness of both their training and their services. Nurses affect client outcomes positively and contribute measurably to the goals of a competitive health-care delivery system.

This process forms the basis for evidence-based practice (EBP). Although nurses traditionally have not been very good at documenting their worth and effectiveness, a recent surge in research identifying how nurses increase the quality of care is adding to the database for EBP.[10]

To measure effectiveness with accurate information about client care and outcomes, nurses must use standardized language in both practice and documentation. The ability to measure the resources used and the client outcome achieved will help distinguish one health-care provider from another. As nursing practice becomes more efficient and can demonstrate improved client outcomes, the quality of care will increase, and health-care organizations will become more financially stable.

Credibility

The credibility of the nursing profession rests on its ability to document how nursing care improves clients' health and saves money for health-care institutions. Nurses must be able to measure their effectiveness with accurate information about both the care given and the client outcomes achieved. Having control over the process of care, as well as the information and assessments of the quality of care, is an important element in achieving this goal.

Improvements in quality do not occur in isolation. They result from a continual process of assessing care and measuring outcomes that better treatments, change care procedures, and increase the number of support services (see Chapter 15 for information on quality of care).

A standardized language will facilitate the nursing profession's ability to distinguish the costs and benefits of nursing care from the costs and benefits of other health-care providers. If the nursing profession cannot articulate and measure the unique contributions that nurses make to the client's health and well-being, the profession will continue to have difficulty maintaining its higher costs over less educated and less qualified health-care providers.

Accessing Information

Anyone who has been involved in health care for more than a few years realizes that health-care information has increased at an astonishing rate. For example, MEDLINE, a database that contains references to articles in the biomedical literature and is maintained by the National Library of Medicine, added more than 460,000 references between 2011 and 2012. This quantity of new information makes it virtually impossible for nurses to keep up with the latest research upon which to build a strong evidence-based practice. (For more information on the rapid growth in health-care literature, go to http://www.ahrq.gov/research/findings/factsheets/informatic/informatics/index.html.)

An Information Explosion

Health-care journals and textbooks combined form a key element in the information explosion. The amount of health-care information contained in scientific journals has grown to a point where no individual is able to read all of the material. With just a nightly perusal of the latest journals, even the most conscientious practitioners will have difficulty keeping up with all the current research and new developments in their specialty field.

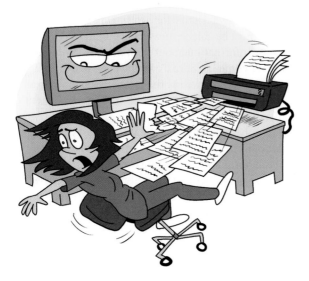

Coping with the volume of biomedical and nursing literature is an enormous task. Since 2010, 35,000 references from 4,000 journals were added each month to the National Library of Medicine MEDLINE database from among the more than 100,000 scientific journals published. More than 612,000 references were added in 2011 alone.[11] In the past 20 years, the number of articles indexed annually in the MEDLINE database has nearly doubled, the number of clinical trials in cardiology has increased five times, and the number of clinical trials in health services has increased 10 times. One new article is added to the medical literature every 26 seconds.[11]

Conflicting Paradigms

Although a large amount of new information is available, only a small portion is read by and incorporated into the practice of many health-care professionals. The traditional paradigm that still seems to guide the decision-making process for many nurses is to:

• Refer back to the knowledge learned in school.
• Confer with a colleague.
• Look up the problem in any textbook or reference book available in the work setting.
• Use previous experiences and "gut" instincts.

This process is useful and has some merit, but it is questionable whether it is adequate for the delivery of high-quality care in today's complex health-care system. For the information age, EBP is more appropriate.[12] This process includes:

• Accessing current literature concerning the latest diagnostic techniques and treatment modalities.
• Conferring with a knowledgeable colleague.
• Evaluating the effectiveness of previous experiences.

Research on the Job

Ironically, even though EBP produces higher-quality care, the nursing profession has only recently embraced its use. With the changes in information technology ushered in by wireless handheld devices and free online nursing databases, nurses are increasingly improving the quality of care by using EBP. Nurses no longer have to leave the practice setting and go to a library to access relevant information. Literature can be searched from the nurses' station or even the client's bedside using available information systems. Nurses find that having access to literature about clinical issues increases their confidence levels in dealing with clients and other health professionals. It also allows them to contribute more fully to the multidisciplinary health-care team.[13]

Nurses must continue to search databases that promote improved client care (Box 18.2). Nurses must have workplaces where they can easily access client information, including research information, to maintain high-quality nursing practice.

THE HUMAN FACTOR

When information tools, machines, and systems are developed, they must include recognition of human factors, including knowledge about human capabilities,

Box 18.2

Principles for Access to Library and Information Services

1. All nurses should have access to a free library service funded by their employer that contains appropriate literature and multimedia resources.
2. Library services should have flexible opening hours and be staffed by qualified librarians.
3. Nurses should have equal rights, similar to those of other health-care professionals, to paid study time to update their practice.
4. Every nurse should have access to training on the Internet and appropriate databases.
5. Every nurse should be educated in electronic systems and services to support evidence-based practice.

Source: Urquhart C, Davis R. The impact of information. *Nursing Standard,* 12(8):23–31, 1997.

limitations, and characteristics that may affect the use of the system. The terms *human factors, human engineering, usability engineering,* and *ergonomics* are often used interchangeably.

Is the System Friendly?

The study of human factors examines how to make the interaction of people and equipment safe, comfortable, and effective. Cognitive science, one of the components of informatics discussed earlier, forms part of the foundation for the study of human factors. Cognitive science includes the human acts of perception, thinking, understanding, and remembering.

In order to manage and process information, especially with an automated system, the individual must be able to understand and remember a great deal of data. The more logically this information is arranged, the easier it is to use the system. "User-friendly" systems are intuitive, self-evident, and logical, even if they are complicated. The best systems will provide the users with on-screen "prompts" or directions to move them on to the next step in the process.

Does the System Make Sense?

Every day in their client care, nurses use complex machinery, including many types of monitors, ventilators, intravenous (IV) pumps, feeding pumps, suction devices, electronic beds and scales, lift equipment, and assistive devices. The directions for using many

of these machines are not self-evident and may be highly complicated. Although hospital equipment producers are becoming better at incorporating the human factor into the design and use of this complicated equipment, consulting with practicing nurses or "field testing" equipment in the workplace before its mass production would make it more user friendly.

Confusing Technology

New computer systems present many learning challenges for health-care providers. Many computer systems are not as user friendly as they might be. Computer system designers are notorious for supplying computers with numerous advanced but obscure functions. These systems often seem to make relatively simple daily tasks much more complicated. Millions of dollars have been wasted on computer systems that are not used or are underused because the user's needs were not considered before the systems were designed.

Individuals encountering complicated computer systems for the first time commonly feel that they are stupid, incompetent, or too old to learn because they cannot quickly master the new technology. However, the fault often lies not with the individual but with the design of the technology.

Nurses, through their education and philosophical orientation, are generally more in tune with the human factor than computer designers, particularly as it relates to client care. Nurses can use their human factor orientation in the process of evaluating new technology before it is purchased. Also, nurses may be able to make suggestions to medical equipment producers to help improve the equipment after it has been used for some time.

Is the System Well Designed?

The lack of well-designed, user-friendly health-care technology is one of the reasons why the health-care industry continues to have high rates of medical errors and poor client outcomes, even after a decade of increased emphasis on client safety.

Poor Design

Poor user design is responsible for thousands of health-care "accidents" each year. Complex medical devices are often used under extremely stressful conditions in which the user's cognitive abilities are not as focused as they might be in a less stressful situation. Often the users are not considered during the design phase because the designers believe they know what is needed. It is no wonder why medical error ranks as the eighth leading cause of death in the United States.[14]

The proliferation of new medications and the increasing complexity of medication therapy have dramatically increased the risk for medication errors and adverse drug events both inside and outside hospitals. Although the information is difficult to obtain, a study in 2013 managed to determine the top 10 categories of health-care errors in U.S. hospitals:

• Improper medication dose and/or method of use
• Technical medical error
• Failure to use indicated tests
• Avoidable delay in treatment
• Failure to take precautions
• Failure to act on test results
• Inadequate monitoring after a procedure
• Inadequate patient preparation before a procedure
• Inadequate follow-up after treatment
• Avoidable delay in diagnosis

(For more information, go to http://www.covermd.com/resources/Medical-Errors-List.aspx.) Also, the increased use of "fast-tracking" medications through the testing process has led to withdrawal of several medications from the market because of long-term complications not seen in the initial shortened testing phase. Well-designed computerized physician-order entry systems can reduce serious prescribing errors by more than 50 percent.[14]

Errors Increase

The inevitable result of poor design in all types of equipment, ranging from laboratory forms to life-support devices, is an increased error rate. Cognitive science studies have shown that the average person's memory can retain only six to eight pieces of information at a time. A well-designed system takes these elements into account (Box 18.3) and should reduce the number of errors. However, a poorly designed system can have the opposite effect and just as easily increase the number of errors. Although bar-code technology in medication administration has reduced errors by as much as 54 percent in some settings, other settings, such as critical care units, found that the number of medication errors remained the same or actually increased after implementing new electronic medication monitoring and delivery systems.[15]

Training Doesn't Compensate

Employees are commonly trained to use an information system to reduce errors. Although training is important, by itself it may not be adequate. In one study, there was no reduction in the number of errors even with an increase in training time. However, well-designed computer-based reminder systems did help clinicians reduce errors significantly. Even after the clinicians received additional training, errors returned to the previous level when the computerized reminder system was removed.[16]

Well-Designed Technology

Designing well-functioning health-care technologies includes both form and function. These technologies need to look good, and they need to do what they are supposed to do. Health-care information technologies attempt to unwind the tangled threads connecting government regulation, confusing insurance policies, and day-to-day care while at the same time attempting to integrate the multiple technologies used to administer medication, assess vital signs, provide clients with oxygen, and other necessary aspects of care.

> *If the nursing profession cannot articulate and measure the unique contributions that nurses make to the client's health and well-being, the profession will continue to have difficulty justifying its higher costs over less educated and less qualified health-care providers.*

When automated and computer systems are made user friendly by incorporating engineering techniques based on human needs, they can make a valuable contribution to monitoring and preventing error in clinical practice. Nursing professionals need to understand that human performance is not perfect and that education and training cannot make it so. Professionals must look for well-designed systems that can reduce and even eliminate errors. (For more information on well-designed health-care technology, go to http://tech.fortune.cnn.com/2013/07/31/can-design-rehabilitate-the-ailing-healthcare-industry/.)

THE ELECTRONIC HEALTH RECORD

Partially due to the provisions in the Affordable Care Act (ACA), the number of hospitals using some form

Box 18.3

Elements of a Good Technology Design

- Intuitive operation with minimal reliance on complicated manuals
- On-screen prompts to the next step
- Easy-to-read displays that are logically arranged
- Controls that are easy to use and reach
- Positive, safe electrical and mechanical connections
- Alarms that sound only when there is a real problem so that they are not turned off because of annoyance
- Long-life reliability with few malfunctions
- Easy, quick repair and maintenance

Box 18.4

Advantages and Disadvantages of the Paper Record

Advantages
- People know how to use it.
- It is fast for current practice.
- It is portable.
- It is unbreakable.
- It accepts multiple data types, such as graphs, photographs, drawings, and text.
- Legal issues and costs are understood.

Disadvantages
- It can be lost.
- It is often illegible and incomplete.
- It has no remote access.
- It can be accessed by only one person at a time.
- It is often disorganized.
- Information is duplicated.
- It is hard to store.
- It is difficult to research, and continuous quality improvement is laborious.
- Same client has separate records at each facility (physician's office, hospital, home care).
- Records are shared only through hard copy.

of electronic health record system has tripled since 2009 and is estimated to be almost 86 percent. However, only 42 percent of hospitals now meet federal standards for collecting electronic health data, and a mere 5 percent also meet federal standards for exchanging that data with other facilities and providers to allow easier access to a client's health records. In the manufacturing and communication industries, experience has shown that it can take up to 10 years after the introduction of a new technology for it to realize its full potential. Hopefully it will progress more quickly in the health-care industry.[14]

A health record serves multiple purposes. It is used primarily to document client care. It also provides communication among health-care team members. It acts as a financial and legal record and is used for lawsuit resolution, research, and continuous quality improvement (CQI). Although the health record can take many forms, the most common form is either paper or electronic. Both forms have advantages and disadvantages (Box 18.4). (For more information, go to http://www.healthit.gov/sites/default/files/oncdatabrief9final.pdf.)

Advantages

Electronic health records (EHRs) have many advantages. Multiple care providers can access them simultaneously from remote sites. They can provide reminders about completing information or carrying out protocols as well as warning of incompatibilities of medications or variances from normal standards.

Redundancy is supposed to be reduced with the EHR. Rather than every health-care worker asking a client for his or her health history, allergies, and current medications, ideally the information is captured once and then transmitted to every record requiring the information. EHRs require less storage space, are more difficult to lose, and are much easier to research. Improved communication, increased completeness of documentation, and reduction in error are the most important advantages of the EHR.

Disadvantages

Electronic health records have some obvious disadvantages. There is a high front-end cost in buying an electronic system and converting from a paper system. Employees may have problems adapting to the new system because of the steep learning curve involved. EHR systems are becoming more portable with the advent of the wireless network; however, they are also subject to all the glitches of electronic systems.

Decisions must be made about who can enter data into the system and when the entries should be made. The Health Insurance Portability and Accountability Act (HIPAA) regulations currently creating so many headaches for health-care providers were written specifically to address the many legal and ethical issues involving privacy and access to client information (for more detail, see Chapters 8 and 9). Some issues still need to be resolved.

The Ideal Record

The ideal EHR would be a lifelong continuous record of all the care the client has received, rather than the episodic, piecemeal data that it now provides. This one record would reflect an individual's current health status and lifetime medical history. It would be unique to the person and not to the institution. This record would reside in multiple data sites and would accept multiple data types (e.g., graphs, pictures, x-rays, text) and be accessible worldwide.

Several Places at Once

The information on the EHR does not physically have to reside in one place, like a paper record. When viewed from a computer workstation, the EHR only appears to be in one place. In reality, particularly with the new cloud technology, the individual records are retrievable from many information systems, such as laboratory, radiology, document imaging, anatomic pathology, anesthesiology, bedside, and accounting.

> *The creation of workplaces in which nurses can easily access client information, including research information, is essential to high-quality nursing practice.*

With proper authorization, this record could be accessed from anywhere in the world, at any time. Many people around the world could look at the same record simultaneously. If an individual became critically ill on a cruise ship or in a foreign country, the local health-care provider would be able to access the medical record to facilitate the client's diagnosis and treatment.

New Forms of Access

Although EHR has been in use in one form or another for a decade, ideal EHR is yet to be designed and implemented. Many of the issues surrounding confidentiality and security have been resolved to some degree. The high cost of starting up the system is still a barrier.

Access to the system would probably require a universal ID code or a unique client identifier. Many organizations may resist a universal ID because they now use either their own client numbering system or Social Security numbers to identify individual records. Neither of these systems is adequate for the global access of the future. Fingerprinting, iris and retinal imaging, face prints, and voiceprints all are identification methods under investigation for use as the universal ID.[17]

Bedside or Point of Care?

Bedside system. Some currently used systems allow nurses to enter information through bedside systems. A bedside system, as the name implies, is a computer terminal installed in each client's room or next to each bed. Portable devices are also now being used in bedside medical records.

Point-of-care system. A point-of-care system has a broader meaning and includes not only the bedside but also many other points of care in the health-care environment and community, including the laboratory, radiology department, outpatient clinics, and even the client's home for home health-care providers. Many facilities currently have a unit system that can be accessed at only one terminal in the client-care area (e.g., the nurses' station).

A Process Redesigned

Taking a paper record and typing or scanning it into a computer does not, in itself, constitute a modern electronic record. Automating the paper record in its present form only automates inefficient practices based on outdated requirements. Modern systems go beyond merely computerizing paper records. These new systems gain control over the generation of information and develop new techniques for using it creatively.

One of the most important characteristics of a bedside or point-of-care system is that client information can be input directly from the terminal. Then the nurse is freed from having to keep notes or chart from memory at the end of the shift. Documenting at the time of care is an important change in workflow for most health-care workers, who are accustomed to documenting at the end of a shift in a workroom with other professionals.

The re-engineering and streamlining of departmental workflow is accomplished by the automatic and continual routing of electronic documents and medical images from one person or department to another throughout the shift. With this system, traditional manual tasks are now automated, increasing the efficiency of management decisions and improving the distribution and evaluation of complex client records and electronic documents by authorized staff. This redesign of the old manual processes provides the real return on investment for implementing the electronic health record.

ETHICS, SECURITY, AND CONFIDENTIALITY

Most people assume that all doctor–client communications are strictly confidential. However, in the new electronic world, confidential information has become a commodity that is bought and sold in the electronic marketplace. Although the HIPAA laws have tried to deal with this issue (see Chapter 8), people who use the Internet or e-mail quickly realize that their personal information is no longer so personal.

Information for Sale

Examples of violations of client confidentiality abound. One of the most egregious occurred in 1996. A convicted child rapist working as a technician in a Boston hospital rifled through 1,000 computerized records looking for potential victims. He was caught when the father of a 9-year-old girl whom the rapist was harassing used caller ID to trace a call back to the hospital.

More recently, in California in 2011, a class-action lawsuit was filed by clients of the University of California–Los Angeles (UCLA) health system. An external hard drive was removed from the home of a former UCLA physician with information pertaining to more than 16,000 clients. Although the hard drive was encrypted, a piece of paper with the password was also taken. In the class-action suit against UCLA, the lawyers were seeking $1,000 for each client as well as attorneys fees and other costs, exceeding the $16-million mark.

In 2010, a family member of a client in the Charleston Area Medical Center discovered how to access the facility's client information database while trying to find information on the Internet about the quality of the hospital. The database contained thousands of clients' names, Social Security numbers,

Estimates of how many people die annually in the United States as a result of medical error range from 44,000 to almost 100,000. On the basis of these numbers, medical error ranks as the eighth leading cause of death in the United States.

medical information, and demographic information. The breach resulted in a lawsuit, *Tabata v. Charleston Area Medical Center,* based on the lack of security for confidentiality of the system. In another case, a banker on Maryland's State Health Commission pulled up a list of clients with cancer from the state's records, cross-checked it against the names of his bank's customers, and revoked the loans of the clients diagnosed with cancer. Additionally, at least one-third of all Fortune 500 companies regularly review health information before making hiring decisions.[18]

A Question of Ownership

One of the key ethical questions is, "Who owns the client's health-care data?" Does the individual's health-care information belong exclusively to the individual? Does it belong to the organization (e.g., insurance company, PPO) that paid for the care, or should it belong to the physician who directed and ordered the care? What about the facility in which the care was given—can they claim some ownership to the information, particularly if it is stored there? Do all these groups and individuals own a part of the information?

Should Society Benefit?

Those who argue the "individual rights" end of the ethical spectrum believe that each individual should have total and exclusive control over the information concerning his or her health and the care rendered. Those on the utilitarian, or "social good," end of the ethical spectrum believe that society as a whole benefits from shared information about disease occurrence and treatment. Therefore, the information should be available to all interested parties. As with most ethical dilemmas, a single definitive answer has not been proposed regarding who owns the data.

However, there have been increasing public policy debates concerning the collection of health-care information for use as aggregate databases to underpin health-care planning. Many consumers are concerned about the status of future physician–client relationships. Driving the development of data collection policy is the public's fear about the damage that may result from excessive and uncontrolled disclosures through automated health-care information systems.

The Implications of Consent

When clients enter the health-care system, they are generally asked to sign consent forms so that other organizations can obtain information about their health status and the care that they received (particularly insurance companies so that bills can be paid). They are usually unaware that this information can be supplied to many other organizations or institutions.

For example, reports are made to the trauma registry about injuries resulting from accidents. The tumor registry collects information about benign and malignant tumors, and infectious disease reports are made to the public health department. Currently, health-care information is shared to develop payment systems, examine access to care, identify cost differences in treatment modalities, research disease trends and epidemiological implications, and expand consumer information.

The Evolution of HIPAA

The HIPAA policies covering the collection, development, and use of client data are based on issues of confidentiality and security. In 1996, the federal government started to develop the guidelines that have become HIPAA. The primary objectives of HIPAA include:

- Ensuring health insurance portability.
- Reducing health-care fraud and abuse.
- Guaranteeing security and privacy of health information.
- Enforcing standards for health information.

In 2000, rules governing the exchange of electronic administrative health-care information were developed and added to HIPAA. The object of these rules was to simplify and standardize the electronic forms required for claims for services rendered. Every organization must now use the same form.

Rules for Disclosure

In 2001, HIPAA was modified by the addition of rules that address the use and disclosure of individually identifiable health information in any form, electronic or paper. Health-care providers and facilities must obtain client consent before using or disclosing client information for treatment, payment, or health-care operations. The full HIPAA was enacted in 2004. It is constantly being updated and revised to include new technologies such as handheld devices and cloud data storage.[19]

What Do You Think?

Who do you think owns health-care information? How does your decision affect health-care policy in the future?

Even with HIPAA regulations, confidential client information can be legally used for a wide range of purposes, including quality assurance, institutional licensing and accreditation, biomedical research, third-party reimbursement, credentialing, litigation, regional and national databases, court-ordered release of information, and managed-care comparisons, to name a few. It is estimated that at least 100 hospital staff have access to a client's medical information as soon as they are admitted to a facility. If that information is used by an outside entity such as an insurance company or the public health department, another 100 gain access to it. Although automated information systems do not cause these types of information uses, electronic records do make acquiring this information much easier.

Threats to Security

Unauthorized Access

Unauthorized sharing of health-care information is generally unethical and now is always illegal. The code of ethics for most health-care professionals

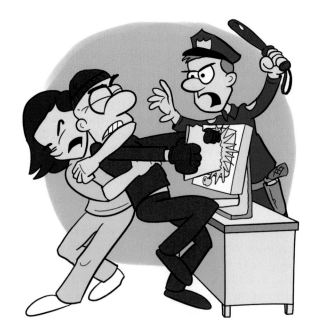

prohibits unauthorized or unnecessary access to client information. In addition, most health-care institutions have policies prohibiting unauthorized access to confidential information. Individuals can lose their jobs because of unauthorized access or sharing of client information and, under HIPAA laws, may be convicted of a crime.

A new wrinkle has been added to unauthorized access to health-care information. Under the policies of a previous administration's Patriot Act, some national governmental agencies, such as the Federal Bureau of Investigation (FBI) and National Security Administration (NSA), now have the authority to wiretap or access, without court approval, any electronic information they believe may be associated with a terrorist threat. This information includes physicians' and nurses' records, laboratory information such as DNA profiles and blood type, and financial information. Although some believe this unrestricted access is necessary to prevent future attacks against the United States, others believe that it is a major violation of U.S. citizens' right to privacy. It certainly seems to violate the regulations set forth in HIPAA.

Unauthorized access or sharing of information is not a new problem associated only with the electronic age. It is just as easy to gain unauthorized access to a paper record as it is to the automated electronic record. The professional codes of ethics that stress confidentiality have always been the primary protector of client information. Still, access to the paper record is available to anyone who picks up the chart.

> *. . . most health-care institutions have policies prohibiting unauthorized access to confidential information. Individuals can lose their jobs because of unauthorized access or sharing of client information and, under recently enacted HIPAA laws, may be convicted of a crime.*

What Do You Think?

Have you witnessed any violations of HIPAA in your clinical practice or in your interaction with the health-care system? How could they be prevented?

In some ways, the automated electronic record provides greater privacy. Access to the automated record is generally restricted to employees who have been issued a password. Also, most organizations have periodic **audits** that can track each person who has accessed a record, and some systems can

even detect unauthorized access at the time of entry into the system.

Accidents

Threats to information security can be either accidental or intentional and can affect both paper and electronic systems. Accidental threats involve naturally occurring events such as floods, fires, earthquakes, electrical surges, and power outages.

The paper record has little security against natural events. Typically, paper records are secured in a locked file cabinet or medical records room. Although current safety regulations require fire detection and suppression systems in these areas, even a small fire can destroy a large number of paper records very quickly. Little can be done to protect paper records against major flooding. Once the charts are destroyed, they cannot be reproduced.

Facilities with automated systems usually have well-developed natural disaster plans built into the system design. These plans include the automatic production and storage of a backup tape at a protected location some distance from the health-care facility. The frequency of data backup varies with the organization's requirements. Most systems automatically save all the data in the system every 24 hours, although this time interval can be shortened or increased to meet the facility's needs.

Although these measures provide a high degree of protection from major natural events such as floods and fires, power surges and outages create problems for electronic systems but leave paper systems unaffected. Anyone who works with computerized equipment recognizes the major disruptions in service and work that occur when the system goes down. Again, some safeguards can be built into the system so that not all the most recent information is lost when the power goes out. Power surges can be controlled with surge protection devices.

Intentional Acts

Intentional threats to the security of information involve the actions of an individual or individuals who wish to damage, destroy, or alter the records. In most cases, it is difficult to protect paper records from intentional tampering. It is a rather simple task for a determined individual to gain access to paper records and erase, add to, or rewrite sections of the chart. These changes are often very difficult to detect. In addition, a person could simply remove the chart and destroy it so that there would be no record left at all. Although automated electronic records are vulnerable to several kinds of intentional threats, they are, overall, more secure than the paper record. All current automated systems have computer virus–checking programs that protect the automated record from both intentional and accidental introduction of destructive computer viruses into the system.

Once data have been entered into the automated system, they are difficult to alter. Modern automated systems are designed with "write once, read many" (WORM) programs. If a legitimate change in the electronic record needs to be made, it must be an addendum. Any changes made in the electronic record are logged by the time and the person who made them and can always be tracked to the point of origin.

Although a determined and gifted hacker can still obtain access to almost any electronic database, electronic security systems are becoming more and more difficult to breach. However, terrorist acts, ranging from detonation of bombs in key locations to development of "superviruses" to destroy electronic records, are difficult to defend against and present an increasing threat.

" Although automated electronic records are vulnerable to several kinds of intentional threats, they are, overall, more secure than the paper record. "

USES OF THE INTERNET

For nursing professionals, the Internet has become a valuable resource for communicating with colleagues and professional organizations, researching clinical information, and educating consumers about health resources and information. Because of the lack of standardization and regulation, it is important that the nurse evaluate each site for accuracy of information, authority, objectivity, currency or timeliness, and coverage.

A Resource for Professionals
Most professional organizations maintain a website containing information about the organization. Many include policy statements and lists of publications. **Continuing education units (CEUs)** can be obtained through the Internet to help nurses remain current and retain licensure. The Nurses Network (http://www.nursesnetwork.com), for example, is a site that lists education courses, position vacancies, conferences, and other pertinent information. News groups, such as those listed at http://www.nursingworld.org, provide professional information and access to experts in specific areas of interest.

Disease-specific websites publish clinical information for both the consumer and the professional. OncoLink (http://www.oncolink.org) is an example of a resource for information about cancer. Often the most recent information about a disease is found on the Internet. Publishing is quicker and easier on the Internet than in a peer-reviewed journal. Web-based support groups disseminate information on both technical and consumer levels. Protocols and policies are shared through websites and news groups.

A Guide for Consumers
Today, consumers are more knowledgeable about health care due to the information available at their fingertips through the Internet. Clients are better informed than they were in the past because they now have easy access to a wide range of health-care information. Preventive and wellness services are available electronically through articles, chat groups, and health risk assessment surveys posted on consumer websites. Clients can now purchase medications over the Web, often at a much lower cost than they can get from their local pharmacies.

Healthfinder (http://www.healthfinder.gov) is one of hundreds of consumer health and human services information websites created and maintained by the federal government. The site links the user with online government publications, clearinghouses, databases, websites, and support and self-help groups, as well as the government agencies and not-for-profit organizations that produce reliable information for the public. The goal of this information source is to help consumers make better choices about health and human services needs for both themselves and their families.

TELEHEALTH

Health Care at a Distance

From its fledgling beginnings more than 40 years ago, clinicians, health services researchers, and others have been investigating the use of telecommunications and information technology to improve health care. Physicians examine and treat clients from distant sites with video cameras, thus saving money by exchanging office visits for online appointments.

The terms *telehealth* and *telemedicine* are often used interchangeably.[20] As defined here, telehealth is the use of electronic information and communications technologies to provide and support health care when distance separates the physician and the client. Telehealth includes a wide range of services and technologies, from "plain old telephone service" (POTS) to highly sophisticated digitized cameras, telemetry, voice systems, and even interactive robots that can be controlled by the practitioner to assess clients. Telemedicine is just one of the services provided by the overall telehealth system that primarily involve consultation with a physician.

Telehealth is being used in emergency departments (EDs) across the United States. The University of Pittsburgh offers neurological consultations to physicians at seven linked hospitals. In Baltimore, providers are using cellular telephone technology to transmit live video and client data back to home base.

Some uses of telehealth, such as emergency calls to 911, are so common that they are often overlooked as part of telehealth systems. Other applications, such as telesurgery, involve advanced technologies and procedures that are being used on a limited basis and are still considered experimental.

Serving Remote Populations

Historically, consumer concerns about access to health care have been the driving force behind the development of many clinical telehealth systems. Early applications focused on remote populations scattered across mountainous areas, islands, open plains, and Arctic regions where medical specialists, and sometimes even primary care practitioners, were not available.

Many telehealth projects from the 1960s through the early 1980s failed because they were expensive, awkward to use, and often not guided by the strategic plans of the facilities using them. However, as the technology has become more common, the costs of many systems have decreased dramatically. With the development of cellular technology, many of the newer systems are tapping into the systems already in place for telephone service.

Renewed interest in telehealth has been spurred by managed-care initiatives seeking to reduce health-care costs while maintaining or increasing quality and access to care. Overall costs have decreased for many of the information and communications technologies used by telehealth systems. In addition, the ever-developing National Information Infrastructure is making these technologies more accessible and user friendly. Medicare reimburses some types of telehealth care, although other third-party payers have been slow to include reimbursement for telehealth services.

Telehealth in an Emergency

Telehealth offers many advantages that will affect the cost of and access to future health care. The telehealth system allows access to centralized specialists who can support primary care providers in outlying areas. Outlying areas can be either rural or urban areas that lack access to the full range of health-care services. Outlying clinics staffed only with nurse practitioners or physician assistants have immediate access to physician referrals through the telehealth system. Many are now using handheld devices for telehealth applications.[20]

University medical centers can offer specialist consulting services to primary care physicians at distant locations, thus reducing unnecessary travel and increased cost to clients. Here is an example of how the telehealth system functions in an emergency situation:

> In 1996, a 72-year-old man with a collapsed lung walked into the ED in a small town in North Dakota. The general practitioner, who usually saw routine emergency cases, immediately called the trauma II medical center in Bismarck and arranged a teleconsult with an ED physician and a thoracic surgeon. The man would have died without a thoracotomy. Following the surgeon's instructions, the physician was able to insert the chest tubes needed to safely transport the client by helicopter to Bismarck.

Telehealth services often save lives and prevent permanent disability, especially when time is a factor in treatment. For example, health-care providers know that if thrombolytic medications are given within 3 hours after the onset of stroke symptoms, the likelihood of death or permanent disability is reduced by 50 percent. Using telehealth technology, neurology specialists can evaluate a client's condition while he or she is still in the ambulance en route to the hospital, thus saving valuable time in deciding about using lifesaving medications. The ED is prepared to administer the medications as soon as the client enters the department, rather than having to wait several hours for all the routine evaluations and consultations to be completed.

Issues Now

Are the Five Rights Enough?

Nursing students have had the five rights of medication administration drilled into their heads all through nursing school. Recent research indicates that five rights may not be enough. Although the majority of medication errors are caused by failures in the systems of obtaining and administering medications, up to 38 percent of errors can be attributed directly to nurse mistakes. When it comes to medications, the nurse serves as the last line of defense between the system and the client. Traditionally the five rights are the following:

1. Right patient
2. Right drug
3. Right route
4. Right time
5. Right dose

However, in today's complex health-care system, many potentially lethal medications are used in all settings. Safe medication administration now seems to demand more than following the basic five rights, a system developed almost a century ago. Research shows that even nurses who meticulously observe the five rights are prone to medication errors. While the nine rights system does not guarantee error-free medication administration, it does increase the safety and quality of client care throughout the process. The four additional rights are the following:

6. Right documentation
7. Right action
8. Right form
9. Right response

Right documentation: It is a major legal requirement that after nurses administer a medication, they must sign the medication sheet or make the appropriate entry in the electronic health record. The signature is legal evidence that the client received the medication. Students are taught to never sign the medication chart before administering the medication. Doing so is illegal and endangers the client, who may refuse the medication; in some cases, the nurse may forget to administer it. More dangerous is failing to sign when a medication has been administered. Another nurse may conclude that it has not been administered, and the client will end up with a double dose. For prn medication, it is essential to document the reason for administering the medication and what effect it had on the client.

Right action: For many years now, the legal defense of, "I was just following the physician's orders" has not been available to nurses. Nurses need to know why the client is receiving a medication and how the medication works. They need to know if the prescribed medication and its dose are appropriate for the client. Administering an antihypergylcemic agent to a client who does not have diabetes but does have an infection is a medication error even if the medication was prescribed. Nurses also need to be aware of laboratory values associated with certain medications. Administering a daily dose of potassium to a client whose morning laboratory work shows a blood potassium of 7 mEq/mL could lead to cardiac arrest.

(continued)

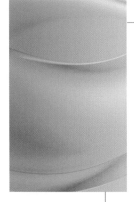

I s s u e s   N o w continued

Right form: This one is similar to right route, although it goes one step further. It is possible to administer various medications by different routes. For example, a licensed practical nurse (LPN) in a long-term acute care facility became confused about how to administer a bag of tube feeding. The nurse on the shift before had mistakenly put IV tubing on the bag of tube feeding and had hung it at the bedside to save the next nurse time in hooking it up. When the LPN on the next shift heard the pump alarm that the bag was empty, he came in and hooked the tube feeding to the IV. The client died about an hour later. In another case, a pharmacist drew up an oral medication in a syringe to obtain a more accurate measurement. The nurse was not familiar with the medication and, because it was in a syringe, gave it by IV.

Right response: This could also be called *right assessment* or *right observation*. After the medication is administered, the nurse must go back to evaluate whether the medication is doing what it is supposed to do. Most nurses know this is mandatory for pain medications and recognize the need to chart whether or not the pain level was reduced. However, it is also important for almost all other medications. If the client was given an antacid for ulcer pain, the nurse needs to note whether or not it helped. Right response is particularly important for dangerous medications such as insulin, anticoagulants, and cardiac medications.

The nurse must respond quickly if a client on anticoagulants begins to have blood in his urine or is oozing blood from the IV site. This may indicate that he is receiving too high a dose of the medication. And of course it is essential to check for allergic reactions to antibiotics and other medications.

The goal, as always, is to make the client's stay as safe and beneficial as possible. Observing the four additional rights can help to achieve this outcome.

Sources: Elliott M, Liu Y. The nine rights of medication administration: An overview. *British Journal of Nursing,* 19(5):300–305, 2010; Health system sets "zero errors" as its goal for patient safety, quality. *Healthcare Benchmarks & Quality Improvement,* 17(4):37–41, 2010.

Issues for the Future

A Boost for Home Care

In the future, home care may benefit the most from telehealth. By investing in telehealth technologies, home care providers should be able to balance cost reductions with increased quality of care.

Clients can be monitored at home using a combination of telephone calls, home visits, video visits, and in-home monitoring using the telehealth system. In-home monitoring devices for conditions ranging from congestive heart failure and diabetes to cancer and cardiac conditions can send information from the client's home to a central base for assessment by professionals.

Future Challenges

System design. Many of the older systems are poorly designed and may be totally incompatible with the systems used in modern health-care facilities. The human factor design and user assessments must be carefully considered in developing any new technologies.

Expense. Although the overall costs of electronic systems continue to decrease gradually, initial expenditures are still a barrier to implementation, especially in smaller facilities. Lack of **third-party payment** for telehealth systems also limits their development and use.

Legal issues. Several legal issues still need to be resolved, including health-care provider licensure when consultations are given across state lines and the liability incurred by providers who examine a client by television rather than in a face-to-face, hands-on encounter. Federal and state policies protecting privacy and confidentiality need to be developed with specific provisions for telehealth systems.

Effects on nursing practice. The telehealth system also affects nursing practice. Nurses are the primary users of telephone triage systems that rely on computerized decision-making trees to suggest appropriate actions when given a set of client symptoms. Nurses who practice in rural and underserved urban areas will have more autonomy and provide higher-quality care when linked electronically with the support services of a large medical center. The use of remote monitoring devices provides nurses with immediate information about changes in their clients' conditions, improves outcomes, reduces complications, and lowers the number of readmissions to the hospital.

> *Nurses who practice in rural and underserved urban areas will have more autonomy and provide higher-quality care when linked electronically with the support services of a large medical center.*

Education and conferencing. The same types of technology used for telehealth can be used for distance and **nontraditional education** applications. Widespread use of **continuing education** is achieved through distance technology. Courses are video-conferenced with two-way interaction. Continuing education credits can be earned through courses on the Internet. Even college credits can be earned through Internet access. Grand rounds are conducted at multiple sites with video-conferencing equipment, and in-services are beamed to multiple locations.

Conclusion

The demand for nurses trained in informatics will continue to grow at a prodigious rate and presents nurses with exciting opportunities. The federal incentive to develop the industry will make it a highly sought after health-care specialty. The information revolution affects every aspect of health care, not only in the United States but also throughout the world. Advanced communications technology and its increased availability worldwide promote ties between people and nations, bridging the gap between isolated rural communities and major metropolitan areas.

The nursing profession needs to be actively involved in developing clinical information systems and the electronic health record, establishing care standards, safeguarding client privacy, using the Internet, and researching better ways of improving access and the quality of care through technology. The nursing profession is transformed, enhanced, and enriched as nurses become active participants in the information revolution.

Critical-Thinking Exercises

- Debate the ethical issues of personal privacy and the greater social good in relation to availability of health-care information.
- Discuss how the design of equipment increases or decreases error rates.
- Discuss uses of telehealth for patient teaching and monitoring of home health clients.
- Write a vision paper describing your view of technology in health care in the year 2030.
- List all the pieces of data you had to give at your last visit to the doctor or hospital. Was all of the information necessary for your care? Who needed the information? How was the information recorded or transmitted?

References

1. Communication Technology and Social Media. Opportunities and implications for healthcare systems. *Online Journal of Issues in Nursing,* 17(3):1, 2012.

2. Conn J. Head of the pack: Early EHR subsidy recipients may have experience. *Modern Healthcare,* 41(32):14–15, 2011.

3. Cipriano PF, Murphy J. Nursing informatics: The future of nursing and health IT: The quality elixir. *Nursing Economic$,* 29(5):286–292, 2011.

4. Nickitas DM, Kerfoot K. Nursing informatics: Why nurse leaders need to stay informed. *Nursing Economic$,* 28(3):141, 158, 2010.

5. Vincent D, Hastings-Tolsma M, Effken J. Data visualization and large nursing datasets. *Online Journal of Nursing Informatics,* 14(2):1–13, 2010.

6. McBride SG, Tietze M, Fenton MV. Developing an applied informatics course for a doctor of nursing practice program. *Nurse Educator,* 38(1):37–42, 2013.

7. American Nurses Association. *Scope and Standards of Nursing Informatics Practice.* Washington, DC: ANA, 2001.

8. *American Nurses Credentialing Center Catalog.* Washington, DC: American Nurses Publishing, 2001.

9. Skiba DJ. WANTED: Informatics resources and learning activities. *Nursing Education Perspectives,* 31(3):183–184, 2010.

10. Dellefield ME, Kelly A, Schnelle JF. Quality assurance and performance improvement in nursing homes: Using evidence-based protocols to observe nursing care processes in real time. *Journal of Nursing Care Quality,* 28(1):43–51, 2013.

11. Koltay T. Information overload, information architecture and digital literacy. *Bulletin of the American Society for Information Science and Technology,* 38(8):33–35, 2012.

12. Bove LA, Finley JJ. ANIA-CARING 2010 Annual Conference. "Re-Evolution in Nursing Informatics." *ANIA-CARING Newsletter,* 25(2):9–11, 2010.

13. Rivett M. Evidenced based practice: Who do we need to convince? *Journal of Family Therapy,* 35(1):1, 2013.

14. Bradley CK, Fischer MA, Walsh KE. Trends in medical error education: Are we failing our residents? *Academic Pediatrics,* 13(1):59–64, 2013.

15. Shadid GW, Shadid J. Compounding and dispensing errors before and after implementing barcode technology in a nuclear pharmacy. *International Journal of Pharmaceutical Compounding,* 16(3):253–256, 2012

16. Bowie P, McKay J, Kelly M. Maximizing harm reduction in early specialty training for general practice: Validation of a safety checklist. *Family Practice,* 13(1):62–71, 2012.

17. Poulton M. Patient confidentiality in sexual health services and electronic patient records. *Sexually Transmitted Infections,* 89(2):90, 2013.

18. Dodson, C. Legal health information exchange, 2012. Retrieved April 2013 from http://www.legalhie.com/lawsuits/

19. Regola N, Chawla NV. Storing and using health data in a virtual private cloud. *Journal of Medical Internet Research,* 15(3):e63, 2013.

20. Brackett C. Telehealth and the role of technology in future patient care. *Caring,* 31(10):14–17, 2012.

19

The Politically Active Nurse

Joseph T. Catalano

Learning Objectives

After completing this chapter, the reader will be able to:

- Explain why it is important for nurses to understand and become involved in the political process
- Discuss how a bill becomes a law
- Identify the major committees at the federal level that influence health policy
- Identify four points at which nurses can influence a bill
- Give examples of how nurses may become politically involved
- List and describe four methods of lobbying

A NUTS-AND-BOLTS APPROACH

Politics, and the consequences of political action, touch people's lives at the national, state, and local government levels. As one of the largest and most trusted professional groups in the country, nurses need to understand how politics work. They have the potential to influence policy decisions that could ensure both optimal health care for clients and ideal work environments for themselves. Subsequently, it is important for nurse to be able to critically analyze proposed policies for any unintended consequences. With their understanding of the health-care system, their understanding of human experiences, and their leadership and negotiation skills, nurses are well prepared to become active in the political system.

This chapter provides a foundation for understanding the political basics with the intention of motivating nurses to become active in the political world. Politics is examined both within the profession of nursing and within society at large. In addition, this chapter discusses the forces that drive politics and the three concepts it comprises: partisanship, self-interest, and ideology.

Almost everyone, ranging from political candidates to academicians, members of the press, and regular citizens, has something to say about politics. People define politics in many ways, but essentially it is the process of influencing public policy. Understanding how it works and what can be influenced is the key to ensuring effective public policy.

Nurses are taking political leadership positions. In the 113th U.S. House Of Representatives, six nurses represent five states. Marilyn Tavenner, who is also a nurse, currently serves as the administrator for the Centers for Medicare & Medicaid Services (CMS).

THE INTERSECTION OF NURSING AND POLITICS

Policy that most influences nursing is instituted at both the state and federal levels while sometimes overlapping. States are responsible for licensure and nurse practice acts, so any legislation that regulates the criteria for licensure and certification or defines what is the scope of practice is determined by individual states. Nurses who aspire to influence their work environment or practice would need to become active at the state level, preferably through state professional organizations.

The American Nurses Association (ANA) has been involved in politics at the federal level for many years and has the ANA Political Action Committee (PAC), which is now the second-largest federal PAC in Washington focused on political activities exclusively at the federal level. The ANA focuses on influencing policy to ensure high standards of nursing practice, promoting the rights of nurses in the workplace, projecting a positive and realistic view of nursing, and lobbying Congress and regulatory agencies on health-care issues affecting nurses and the public.[1] Provision 9 of the ANA Code of Ethics for Nurses calls for nurses to be active in social policy and political involvement (see Chapter 6 for more detail on ethics).

However, there is overlap that sometimes leads to conflict between the federal and state governments about what constitutes a legitimate course of action for the federal government and what constitutes the same for the state government. The 10th Amendment to the Constitution says that any powers not expressly identified as being under federal control should be delegated to the states, unless they are willing to give control to the federal government. This amendment is part of the current debate about whether the states should be responsible for administering certain elements of the Affordable Care Act, particularly where they pertain to Medicaid and Medicare. This becomes an issue because, unlike the federal government, state governments are required by law to balance their budgets. When the federal government passes unfunded mandates onto the states, such as with Medicaid, the governors are left to struggle with funding and possibly administering programs they cannot afford. (For more information, go to http://constitutionus.com/.)

> *Almost everyone, ranging from political candidates to academicians, members of the press, and regular citizens, has something to say about politics.*

Federal Issues

Federal concerns that directly involve nursing include the nursing shortage, burdensome tuition debts, and client safety. Indirectly, passing legislation, such as the Affordable Care Act, significantly affects nursing services, in particular, by potentially expanding the demand for nurse practitioners and the way nurses work within health care under the new legislation.

The Nursing Shortage

According to the U.S. Bureau of Labor Statistics, the latest estimate is that there will be a 26 percent rise in demand for registered nurses (RNs) by 2020 and a 57 percent increase in demand for nurse practitioners by 2025.[2] Shortages vary in different areas of the United States, and both the federal and state governments are searching for solutions. The current U.S. Senate has created a 12-member Senate nursing caucus to provide a forum to address these issues. Nurses can contact members of this caucus to offer suggestions and help work toward effective solutions. In addition, the American Association of Colleges of Nursing (AACN) has a position statement on the nursing shortage and is working with policymakers at both the state and national levels to bring attention to this health-care concern and develop plans to resolve the shortage. (For more information on the AACN efforts, go to http://www.aacn.nche.edu/media-relations/fact-sheets/nursing-shortage.)

Tuition Debt

Not unlike other college students, nursing students often leave college with large amounts of debt. The federal government can assist education costs with programs such as the Nursing Education Loan Repayment Program administered through the Department of Health and Human Services. Title VII and VIII of the Health Resources and Service Administration (HRSA) is a loan repayment plan that awards several different types of loans to nursing students and also has loan repayments in exchange for working with underserved populations and in rural areas. These programs need to be funded biannually by Congress; nurses can contact their representative to ensure they understand the importance of funding these programs. (For more information and loan applications, go to http://www.aamc.org/advocacy/diversity/74120/laborhhs_labor0028.html.)

Client Safety

While nurse-client ratios and whistleblower protections are best left to the states, the federal government can influence these issues via language included in health-care funding legislation and by administrative regulations.

What Do You Think?

What experiences have you encountered, either as a client or as a health-care worker, related to the nursing shortage? How might the political system help solve the shortage? How might the political system worsen the shortage?

States Issues

States regulate licensure and certification, pass nurse practice acts, and regulate hospitals. The states are ultimately responsible for client safety, so they have the capacity to pass any legislation and to set the requirements for who is qualified to practice and how and where they may practice. The mandate for nursing is to help legislators understand how nursing standards are established and then help develop legislation with an achievable agenda for political action by nurses at the state level through the State Boards of Nursing.

The mandate for nursing is to help legislators understand how nursing standards are established and then help develop legislation with an achievable agenda for political action by nurses at the state level through the State Boards of Nursing.

Like the federal government, states are searching for solutions for the nursing shortage. Some states are opting for a short-term solution of recruiting foreign nurses. The National Council of State Boards of Nursing (NCSBN) requires that all nurses who work in the United States must hold a license to practice in the state where they work. The federal government has the authority to provide the required visas to allow them to work in the United States, but states have the authority to ensure that they obtain a license to practice. Many boards require a CGFNS (Commission on Graduates of Foreign Nursing Schools) certificate before they will issue a license (see http://www.cgfns.org). To avoid the delay in allowing foreign nurses to practice, some institutions are attempting to influence legislation to allow them to practice without a license until their license is obtained; this potentially risks client safety. Nurses can contact their state legislators to effectively influence upholding nursing licensure so that the same standards apply to foreign nurses as they do to U.S. citizens.

States also vary on advanced nursing practice. For instance, what nurse practitioners (NP) can do varies among the states. Currently, 18 states have laws that allow NPs to evaluate clients, diagnose, order and interpret diagnostic tests, and initiate and manage treatments, including prescribing medications. This is the model recommended by the NCSBN. In 22 states, NPs must have a collaborative agreement with another health discipline, such as a physician, to provide client care. In the remaining 12 states, providing client care must be done under the supervision, delegation, or team-management of another health discipline.[3] Nurses can work with their professional organizations and directly contact their representatives to help enact legislation to ensure all NPs can practice to the full extent of their education.

Professional Organizations

Professional organizations provide another way to influence policy change and legislation at both the state and federal level. As previously mentioned, the ANA has a large PAC focusing on influencing federal legislations. Additionally, since they establish the standards for nursing, they are able to influence how nurses deliver care.

Magnet Hospitals

In 1980, the American Academy of Nurses conducted a study to identify the elements present in hospitals that attracted and retained nurses. Retaining nurses is cost-effective for hospitals since recruiting and training new staff is very expensive. Several key factors were identified in hospitals that seemed to fulfill the magnet status, including a participative management style, allowing the nurses a relatively high degree of autonomy in practice and decision-making; high-quality leadership at the unit level; a horizontal organizational structure, allowing nurses to practice as full professionals; opportunities for career development; and high-quality client care.

Nurses employed at magnet hospitals have a high degree of job satisfaction and a much lower than average turnover rate than nurses in other hospitals of similar size.[4]

The magnet hospital program has grown markedly since the original study. The ANA has established rather rigorous standards for hospitals to meet and obtain the magnet designation. Most hospitals have found achieving magnet status to be very challenging, and only a small percentage are able to achieve it on the first try.[5] However, hospitals that do acquire magnet status have achieved a well-deserved level of prestige among their peers. Nurses working at these hospitals have more control over their practice, and the end result is that higher-quality care is provided to the clients.[6]

Nursing Education Organizations

In the past, most nursing students entered the profession out of high school, and recruiting sufficient students was not a huge issue. Before the 1960s, nursing was one of the few occupational opportunities for women. Society has changed markedly since that time, and now women have opportunities to pursue more fields that were traditionally male dominated. Recently, however, there has been a trend for students seeking nursing school admission to be in their late 20s and early 30s. Some are associate or baccalaureate graduates looking for a second career, possibly motivated by the well-publicized nursing shortage and the promise of a well-paying career with lots of job security. So far, the effect of recruiting nontraditional students has not reduced the nursing shortage or its projections for the future. Increasing the supply of nurses by any means remains a high priority for heading off the impending nursing shortage.[7]

One cause for the nursing shortage that has been identified is the acute shortage of nursing school faculty, which causes nursing schools to turn away qualified students. Although there has been some movement to resolve this issue, the American Association of Colleges of Nursing reports that 75,587 qualified applicants were still being turned away from nursing programs in 2011, primarily due to a faculty shortage and resource constraints.[8] For those who do choose to enter the nursing profession and manage to get into nursing school, the future looks bright. There are many opportunities, and health-care facilities are beginning to appreciate and reward nurses at the level they deserve. Funding to increase educational resources is essential to help resolve the nursing shortage.[9] The best source would be to contact a federal representative to ensure that funding for nursing education is placed in the federal budget.

POLITICS AND POLITICAL ACTION

Politics can be seen as the complex interaction between public policy and various public and constituent interests. Politics is directly and indirectly influenced by the self-interest of political officials, both elected and appointed. The mass media also have both a direct and indirect impact on the political process through numerous political commentators, commercials, and investigations into the backgrounds of selected political figures.

Political action is a set of activities, methods, tactics, and behaviors that affect or potentially affect governmental and legislative processes and outcomes. Examples of political action include grassroots efforts to change policies or deal with issues such as voters' rights. *Grassroots* refers to political movements that start at the local level by volunteers in the community who give their time to support an issue that is important to them. These are typically spontaneous in nature, unlike the movements that are organized and supported by money from traditional political organizations.

Another example of political action is the activities of lobbyists to change elected officials' opinions or votes and support the give and take of political compromise within legislative bodies. A lobbyist is anyone who talks to a legislator to express his or her opinion about an issue that interests them. Lobbyists provide information about issues that legislators may know little or nothing about. For example, nurses who speak with legislators about health care or nursing issues they wish them to support are acting as lobbyists. Most legislators come from a legal or

> *Nurses employed at magnet hospitals have a high degree of job satisfaction and a much lower than average turnover rate compared with nurses in other hospitals of similar size.*

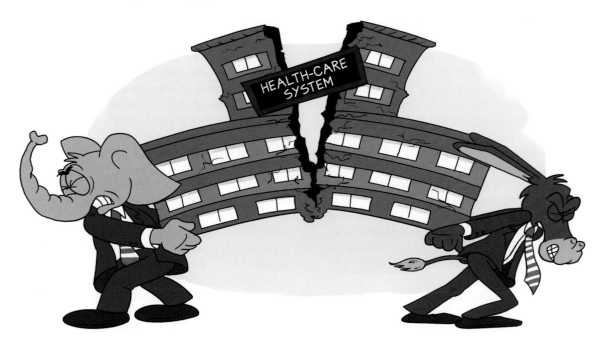

business background and are often very appreciative of health-care information from nurses.

The image of lobbyists has been tainted in recent years because of the excessive amounts of money provided by large corporations and personal interests groups to change legislators' positions on issues. Although there are regulations to control this type of activity, some savvy lobbyists have found loopholes and ways around them. (For more information, go to http://dc.about.com/od/jobs/a/Lobbying.htm.)

A Series of Processes
Government is often thought of as a series of processes used to maintain society. As both an element of and a result of politics, government is also influenced by the forces that drive politics. The three concepts that constitute politics include partisanship, self-interest, and ideology.

Partisanship
Partisanship refers to membership in a political party. Because of its limited scope, this chapter focuses on Democrats (who tend to be progressives or liberals and are considered to be on the "left" side of the political spectrum), Republicans (who tend to be conservatives or Tea Party and are considered to be on the "right" side of the political spectrum), and to

a lesser extent, Independents (who tend to be populists and incorporate positions that are both left and right).

Self-Interest
Self-interest is almost always the most important factor in politics. It dictates the kind of issues that legislators become involved in and present to their constituencies as the key issues. For instance, a congressman who resides in a blue-collar industrialized district that has a majority of constituents who support unionization will most likely be pro-union. The legislative structure in the United States was designed so that elected officials represent the people in their districts rather than having the whole population of the country trying to make policy decisions. If a candidate does not represent the beliefs of the district, it is unlikely that he or she will succeed in that district.

In the larger world of electoral politics, the principle of self-interest often means that an elected official will not make legislative or political decisions that could lead to professional damage, namely loss of an election. There have been exceptions to this rule where elected officials were so ideologically committed to an issue that they defied conventional wisdom and made decisions that went against their self-interest. When the politician's ideology doesn't represent his or her constituents, they are often not reelected.

Generally, to be effective in politics, a person needs to understand and accept the self-interest of his or her constituents and use it as the driving force in political decision-making.

Ideology

Ideology is a broad concept that embodies the beliefs and principles of an individual or group. However, within each group, not every member shares the same opinion on every issue. For instance, persons can be conservative on fiscal issues and liberal on social ones. Conservatives, ultra-conservatives (e.g., Taxed Enough Already [T.E.A.] Party), liberals, populists, libertarians, and radicals represent six examples of ideologies. It is important to understand the underlying principles that influence one's policy decisions. Ultimately, all groups have a vision for an America in which all citizens can prosper. They differ mostly on who should be responsible for ensuring that happens. However, it is important to consider all ideological visions as a right to free speech so that America remains free. These opposing ideologies act as counter points for each other and prevent one ideology from taking over the government and moving the country in just one direction.

> *Most legislators come from a legal or business background and are often very appreciative of health-care information from nurses.*

Conservatives

Traditionally, conservatives support personal responsibility, individual liberty, smaller government, fewer regulations, less federal involvement in everyday life, lower taxes, social programs that support personal growth rather than encourage dependency, and strong national defense. The general characterization of the conservative belief system is "less government equals better government." Many base their ideology on the famous saying of President Ronald Reagan: "Government is not the answer to the problem; it is the problem!" (See http://www.youtube.com/watch?v=6ixNPplo-SU.)

Applied to the current range of issues, conservatives tend to be pro-life and believe in taking personal responsibility for family planning. They are typically pro-gun ownership, pro-personal ownership of property without any limits and property rights, pro-enforcement of immigration laws, pro-death penalty, anti-public education, in support of fewer regulations for business, and against government-controlled health care. They believe that lower taxes, free enterprise, and capitalism are the ways to generate more jobs, increase wages, and improve the overall standard of living for all U.S. citizens, and they believe that the government is not empowered to prevent free exercise of religion in the public domain. Conservatives, as a demographic group, tend to be older, possibly due to life experience. (For more information, go to http://www.c-span.org/video/?318148-11/2014-conservative-political-action-conference-demographics-panel.)

Progressives

Progressives, also known as *liberals*, believe that government has a moral responsibility to do good for society and that government intervention is necessary to achieve equality for all citizens. They believe that only government can alleviate certain social problems because of its size, organizational structure, and virtually unlimited funding ability. Progressives maintain that a big business approach is not workable for taking on problems and taking over systems that produce little or no profit, such as social programs, health care, and education. This ideology traditionally translates into larger government structures, taxes at a level to maintain programs without deficit, and more spending for a wide range of social programs to guarantee that no one is in need.

Progressives are traditionally pro-environment, pro-choice with government funding for women's reproductive issues, pro-gun control, pro-universal health care, pro-voters' rights, pro-public education, and anti-limits on immigration, including providing all their educational and health benefits and supportive of minority groups rights. They believe that government has the right to use eminent domain to seize private property even if it is given to private enterprises to better the community for all. They also believe that religion belongs in places of worship and in the home but never in the public domain.

Populists

Populists are probably the most dominant political force in the United States at a grassroots level. Although populists in general do not like paying high taxes, ideologically they may represent a variety of positions on any particular issue. For instance, one group of populists may be against restrictions on gun ownership, whereas another group of populists may be pro-gun control.

The common bond among all populists is that they have a sense of being burdened by a large, oppressive government structure. Populists constitute the middle ground between liberals and conservatives and are often considered the group that has the most influence in deciding national elections.

Libertarians

As a political partisan group, libertarians used to differ from populists because they often did not take overt political action as much as the populists did. However, in recent years a small but vocal group of libertarians has been elected to national political office and has managed to push the majority of elected conservatives towards their ideology. They believe in strong fiscal conservatism, dislike paying taxes, and have taken up extreme conservative positions on the size and function of government and all social issues. They have become embroiled in ideological battles over gun control, health care, schools, and reproductive rights issues such as abortion. They believe strongly in state rights over the Federal Government and believe that all choices, except over reproductive rights, should remain with the individual rather than with the government.

Radicals

Radicals exist at both ends of the ideological spectrum in both of the major parties. It is important to recognize that, although most voters tend toward the middle of the political spectrum between conservatism and liberalism, radicals attempt to force their parties to the extreme ends of the spectrum. Sometimes a person may be labeled as a radical just because they do not agree with another person's or group's position or belief.

UNDERSTANDING THE PLAYING FIELD

Structure

The three branches of the U.S. government are the executive, judicial, and legislative branches. These branches exist simultaneously at the federal, state, and local government levels.

The Executive Branch

At the federal level, the executive branch consists of the president, vice president, cabinet, and various executive administrative bodies. Only the president and vice president are elected by the people. The others are appointed by the president and accountable to him, not to the constituents. The executive of a state is the governor, who is elected by the people. Boards and commissions can also be construed as part of the executive branch because they are appointees of the chief executive. In county government, one or more elected county commissioners function as executives. Larger cities usually have an elected mayor. Smaller cities and townships sometimes also elect mayors (see Fig. 19.1 and Box 19.1).

> "*Self-interest is almost always the most important factor in politics. It dictates the kind of issues that legislators become involved in and present to their constituencies as the key issues.*"

The Judicial Branch

The judicial branch is the court system. It is important to note the distinction between federal court, state court, and local court; appeals and supreme courts are found at both levels. At the federal level, there is the Supreme Court, federal courts of appeal, and district or circuit courts. At the state level, there are supreme courts, appeals courts, and the lower courts. Many cities and counties also have a local court system. Justices in the federal system, including the Supreme Court justices, court of appeals judges, and district court judges, are nominated by the president and confirmed by the U.S. Senate, as stated in the Constitution. State court judges are selected in a variety of ways; some are elected, some are appointed for a given number of years or for life, and others by a combination of these methods (e.g., appointment followed by election). Local court judges are usually elected.

The judicial branch of government should not be discounted nor perceived as unimportant to nurses. Over the years, both federal and state courts have decided several important issues that have an effect on the practice of nursing. These include the U.S. Supreme Court's decision regarding the right of nurses to organize into collective bargaining units, the requirement of health-care providers to report potentially violent clients to the police, the obligation

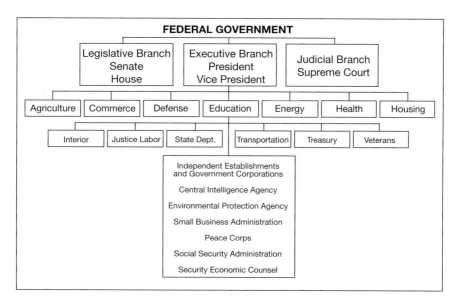

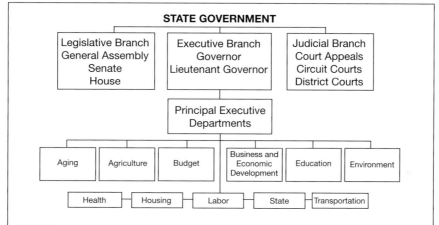

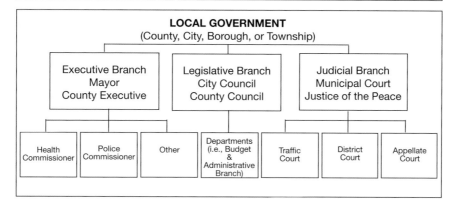

Figure 19.1   The organizational structure of the U.S. government.

B o x   1 9 . 1

Know the Structure to Play the Game

One of the keys to creating power is understanding the organizational structure of the government. The Constitution of the United States establishes three separate branches of the federal government: legislative, judicial, and executive. Unless specifically granted to the federal government by the Constitution, the powers are supposed to go to the individual states. However, since the Constitution was signed, the federal government has taken on more power than was originally intended by the framers. It is the role of the state governments to serve their citizens within these parameters and to delegate discrete areas of activity to local governments.

Beneath the federal and state level of government, there exist five layers of local government identified by the U.S. Census Bureau: county, municipal, township, school district, and special district governments (which include various utility, construction, and facility authorities). The qualifications for the classification of these local government structures are generally determined by the parent state governments. State governments are defined by their individual state constitutions and in turn delineate responsibility for the local governments.

Nurses must understand that there are three levels in each governmental sector: federal, state, and local. These distinctions are important and are the most common source of confusion for nurses.

of nurses to refuse to carry out physician orders they deem dangerous, and criteria permitting nurses to withdraw life-support measures. New test cases that are continually being brought before the U.S. Supreme Court have the potential to dramatically change the way nurses are perceived and what they are permitted to do in the workplace. Because of the influence courts can have on nursing practice, it is important to be aware of judicial decisions and keep them in mind when electing judges to office.

The Legislative Branch

At the federal level, the legislative branch of government consists of the House of Representatives and the Senate. Each state also has a legislative branch of government, and, except for Nebraska, all states have a bicameral legislature with both a house of representatives and a senate. The primary function of the legislative branch of government is the formation of policy by making laws.

Key Players in the Legislative Process

Members of the legislative branch of government have a wide range of ability and influence. It is important to remember that legislators are human and respond to the same forces that all people respond to, including interpersonal dynamics, peer pressure, and both internal and external factors. They are elected by the people to represent their views and, as such, it is essential to ensure that they do that rather than focusing on their own self-interest.

The Majority Leader

The majority leader in the House of Representatives is the person who generally supervises and directs the activities on the House floor. Some consider this to be the most powerful job in politics. The majority leader has control over the legislative calendar, which ultimately determines when many of the House session activities take place and even when, or if, bills are introduced for consideration. The majority leader is also the central figure in crafting the budget, which is the most important activity the legislature performs on an annual basis.

The Majority Whip

The majority whip is responsible for collecting votes when legislators may be leaning toward voting against their party. At the same time the majority leader is supporting a bill, the whip is negotiating on the House floor for the votes necessary to pass the bill. The whip is responsible for collecting support and votes for various issues both during the legislative session and when it is in recess.

The Minority Leader

The minority leader represents the party that does not have a numerical majority in the House and helps organize support against bills introduced by the majority leader. The minority leader presents an alternative point of view. There is an expression in the legislature: "The majority will have their way, and the minority will have their say."

In most cases, the majority party has the capacity to pass almost any bill they support over the objections of the minority. The minority leader usually only has the capacity to speak against it. However, there are some issues that legislators will almost never vote against: "mom," "pop," and "the little guy." When these issues are included in a bill, most legislators will support it even if they must vote against their party. To ensure representatives vote the will of the people, they need to hear the opinions of their constituents.

The Conference Committee

The conference committee attempts to reconcile differences in bills where one is passed by the House and another by the Senate on the same issue. The rules governing the structure, composition, and function of the conference committee vary from state to state. Generally, they consist of an equal number of appointed members from both the House and the Senate. Often a specified combination of votes, such as two votes from the House and two votes from the Senate, is necessary to approve a compromise bill and move it out of committee.

> *It is important to recognize that, although most voters tend toward the middle of the political spectrum between conservatism and liberalism, radicals attempt to force their parties to the extreme ends of the spectrum.*

What Do You Think?

Who do you know in the legislature of your state government? Who is your representative or congressperson? Make a list of the things you would want that person to do for health care and the nursing profession.

Caucuses

Caucuses are formed when the legislature divides into groups consisting of people with mutual interests. These groups operate as a unit, trading on their capacity to bring a block of votes for or against an issue or bill, rather than an individual vote. Examples are the Senate Nursing Caucus, the Women's Caucus, Black Caucus, the Hispanic Caucus, and the Business Community Caucus.

Although caucuses may be bipartisan, many are partisan. For example, the largest caucus groups are the Democratic Caucus and the Republican Caucus. Each caucus develops its own internal governance structure and leadership, including a speaker who leads the caucus and speaks for the group. After a group member achieves a leadership role, he or she must try to balance the wishes of the group against his or her own political survival in the caucus and the political pressures exerted by the larger world.

THE POWER OF THE MEDIA

The media and the voters are external forces that influence policymakers. The media have become a tangible power in government, often driving and shaping public opinion that eventually evolves into a legislative agenda. The public often perceives media personalities as the people who know, write, and speak about important public issues and matters of substance.

When Is It News?

Although they claim to be objective, the major news organizations decide what is and what is not news. They can focus on certain elements of the news, making them more exposed and public, thereby seeming to be more important. For many years, it has been suspected that the major news media outlets tend to focus their stories on those issues important to the ideological principles of liberals. As a counterbalance, other networks were developed to provide the viewpoint reflecting the ideological principles of conservatives.

In recent years, the Internet has become a major source of information for people. Those interested can, and should, view the positions of both sides of the issues and determine which one best fits their views and beliefs without newscasters emphasizing their opinions. And, just as it is when doing research in nursing, it is advisable to locate and read the original sources rather than count on the presentation of an issue presented by news agencies that may only present the positions that support their viewpoint. (For more on website credibility, see Chapter 18.)

Politicians well versed in electronic media have learned to use this media form as a tool to get their message out. Younger voters no longer rely on the national networks' nightly newscasts to get their information about politics and other issues, but use the Internet and the short "sound bites" through which it conveys ideas. Some politicians have learned that the Internet is a practically free and unrestricted way to publicize their positions and slant their information. Keep in mind when viewing these sites the ideological position of the creator. It is always best to also consider the counterargument before making a personal decision. Most legislators now have weekly newsletters and updates by e-mail and wireless media that they will send out to anyone who wishes to sign up for them.

Often, fringe radical groups put rather sophisticated and professional-looking political advertisements on the Internet that attack the other candidate in a personal way or falsely attribute a radical viewpoint to their own candidate. In other cases, unsubstantiated or even blatantly false charges are made against a candidate on the Internet by partisan elements. These ads and charges are then picked up by the network media, and candidates have to spend time and money letting the voting public know that the ads or charges are not true or not from them and that they do not support the position. However, once these stories are out in the media, they often become true whether they are or not and the media may not highlight any corrections.

> *The media have become a tangible power in government, often driving and shaping public opinion that eventually evolves into a legislative agenda.*

Election by Media

Before media campaigns became the norm, with millions of dollars being spent on television and radio advertising, the printed news media used to publish what the candidate said and often printed whole speeches. This approach allowed the public to read the speeches and make up their minds about which issues the candidate supported. Today, the trend is to give a 30-second sound bite of a speech, then have 10 minutes of political analysis by a well-known commentator who tells the public his or her opinion of what the candidate is saying.

Some of the printed media have adopted a similar approach to political issues. In newspapers, it is not unusual to see a lengthy editorial comment positioned next to a statement made by a candidate. Elected officials have a great respect for the power of the media to influence public opinion. The media can

be used by a candidate to give them an advantage for election.

Unfortunately, in recent elections, huge sums of money from foreign countries with business interests in the United States have been funneled through political organizations and PACs in an effort to influence election outcomes. Because the laws that required the tracking of these sources of money have been repealed, no one really knows where the money comes from. The result has been a blizzard of negative political attack ads that can influence the outcome of both state and national elections.

Legislator Beware

Legislators, while recognizing and using the power of the media to promote their messages, have also become wary of it. Statements made by them are at risk of being taken out of context and used to undermine the real intent of their message by news organizations and websites that oppose their views. So, while it is important to use the media to promote their position, it also puts them at risk for potentially unfair criticism. Political organizations that support candidates for election have become highly sensitized to the negative advertisement attacks and generally try to post rebuttal ads within 24 hours of the airing of attack ads. This helps prevent the attack ad from going viral. But it remains important to beware of media presentation of issues without checking with the original source to make sure the presentation or sound bite has not been taken out of context.

A Story With Legs

As an example, suppose a legislator has a large population of senior citizens in his district who have supported him for many years. The legislator publicly supports senior citizen issues and believes that the senior citizen support will always be there. However, during an election campaign, a political opponent's investigation uncovers information that the legislator voted against several bills that would have increased senior citizens' benefits. Keep in mind that amendments are routinely added to unrelated bills. So, the legislator may have not voted for a bill he views as detrimental to his constituents but an amendment that was beneficial to them was added on. So, while he may agree with the amendment, he elected not to vote for the entire bill. Still, an opponent can take that fact out of context and use it to harm the legislator's reputation.

Scandals involving moral issues, such as sexual misconduct, have overshadowed all other issues recently, even those as serious as violations of the U.S. Constitution, such as the erosion of separation of powers and misuse of executive power. If a legislator's opponent finds something that is questionable and posts this information on some obscure website, it can be picked up by the network media, immediately reported on television news programs, and make the front page of the local newspaper.

If the story develops "legs," meaning it takes on a life of its own and continues to grow without further information from the opponent, it will be on other Internet sites, all the television news programs, and in the major national newspapers. Eventually, the major networks will do investigative reporting on the issues. The talk show and television tabloid programs will become interested and begin interviewing people who know or have heard more "dirty little secrets" about the legislator. A normal news cycle is about 24 hours, which means that a story will be reported for one day, then dropped for the next new thing. Stories with legs can stay in the news for days or even weeks and the media often do little to correct a misleading story.

The Internet has contributed to the "legs" phenomenon. Today, almost everything a person in a public position has ever said or done is recorded on tape somewhere, and political websites show these recorded clips. If they are entertaining enough, they are often picked up by the network media and shown over and over again, giving the information a much wider audience than it might otherwise have had. Internet-savvy people are proficient at "data mining" and can obtain private records and information on individuals running for office. This information can become a potent tool in the hands of a political rival. Unfortunately, in some instances the actual story may be untrue but since it gets so much exposure by respected news sources, it becomes true.

At this point, the legislator who is the subject of that story is in political jeopardy. There is little that a politician fears more than being the subject of this type of negative story. Constituents need to be wary of stories such as these. It would be good to consider who may be the beneficiary of the story before accepting it as fact. It is also a good reason to get to know your representative by keeping abreast of the work he or she is doing and how he or she votes. That can help discern whether the information might be true or not or if it seems to represent the positions that representative generally takes.

THE POLITICAL PROCESS

Laws maintain order in a complicated society and regulate the interactions of its citizens. As society becomes more complex, existing laws are analyzed or new ones are passed to ensure they are still relevant for the survival and smooth functioning of the population.

> *Laws maintain order in a complicated society and regulate the interactions of its citizens. As society becomes more complex, existing laws are analyzed or new ones passed to ensure they are still relevant for the survival and smooth functioning of the population.*

Who Introduces Legislation?

Where Laws Begin

Laws are legislative, meaning they are passed by Congress and signed by the president. For example, although computers and electronic communications have increased the quantity of information individuals can process and the speed at which it is transmitted, they have also added to the complexity of the world. Just a few years ago, there were no laws that dealt with hacking, computer fraud, computer theft of bank funds, or online pornography. Today, there is an ever-growing body of law that focuses on computers, and whole sections of police agencies, such as the Federal Bureau of Investigation's Computer Crime Unit, are dedicated to enforcing these laws. Where do ideas for laws and policies come from, and how do these ideas become laws?

Elected Officials

Any elected official, including governors, mayors, county commissioners, and city council members, can propose a program or initiative that requires passage by the legislature. These are called *legislative laws*. This initiative is called a *bill*. The elected official goes to the legislative leadership in the parties and asks them either to submit the bill or to help move the bill through the legislative process.

Lobbyists, the constituency, and advocate groups are a major source of proposed legislation. They represent various interests ranging from public interest groups to corporate lobbyists. Lobbyists frequently craft legislation and then pass it on to a friendly legislator. Consumer groups are often visible at the legislature through demonstrations and lobbying.

Constituency groups are groups of individuals and networks of people who share common interests and concerns with a major organization. They work collaboratively with the primary organization on specific issues to support and develop policies and provide additional voices to influence legislators' opinions. For example, the ANA is composed of individual nurse members who are interested in advancing an agenda that promotes a range of issues based on quality health care and the nursing profession. The state nursing associations and other organizations such as the National Organization of Nurse Practitioner Faculties or the American Association of Critical-Care Nurses (AACN) are constituency groups to the ANA.

Advocacy groups are sometimes known as pressure groups, campaign groups, or special interest groups and are different from constituency groups in that their main focus is to change the way the public views an issue. Advocacy groups can range from very small to very large and freely use the media to increase their power and influence. They can be motivated by a current hot political issue or a long-term issue that affects society. Examples of these groups include organizations such as the AARP, who are concerned about the long-term effects of legislation on the elderly or groups like Prolife America and the House Obamacare Accountability Project (HOAP) that focus on issues that are in the current headlines.

Government Agencies

Legislation is also generated from government agencies. When agencies are seeking fee increases or another type of policy reform, they can introduce legislation. For example, policy reforms in the Internal Revenue Service are a type of agency-initiated legislation. Frequently the employees of the agency draft the legislation and then direct it toward a supportive legislator.

These agencies can also create regulations referred to as administrative law. Bureaucratic agencies, such as the Department of Health and Human Services (DHHS), create the regulations of issues under their authority. These regulations that have the force of law can be problematic, as they are written by unelected administrators, so elected representatives are not accountable for the consequences of imposing these regulations on their constituents. This process is one of the criticisms of the Affordable Care Act (ACA). The bill as passed defines outcome goals and provides the DHHS with wide authority to write the rules. That places the responsibility on unelected administrators and provides some cover for elected officials who then do not need to take responsibility for any problems.[10]

What Drives Legislation?

Funding. Because almost all government agencies depend on legislative funding to sustain their operations, they become actively engaged, overtly or covertly, in seeking the passage of a budget that will sustain their survival.

Public Demand. Legislators are very careful to listen to the demand of their voters and avoid voting against an issue to which the majority of their constituents disagree. A classic example of this process was seen in New Jersey, where a child was sexually molested and murdered by a known convicted sex offender who moved into the child's neighborhood. The tragedy prompted a public outcry: How could this happen? Something needed to be done! Ultimately, the outcry produced the now famous Megan's Law, which requires public disclosure of a known sex offender's residence. The power of individual constituents to demand laws or changes to laws should not be underestimated. Legislators listen and will conform to the will of the people if they hear from enough of them.

Program Issues. These issues recur periodically and require legislative attention. Requests for increases in television cable rates constitute an example of a programmatic issue. The cable industry will be very interested in the outcome of legislation that may affect what they can charge for their services. Both cable and consumer group lobbyists actively seek the opportunity to influence key legislators on these and similar issues.

Constituent-Specific Issues. Groups of voters may have specific interests that can lead to introduction of a bill. For example, in legislative districts where a large population of senior citizens resides, the escalating cost of prescriptions may be an important issue. Legislation specific to that constituency will be introduced at a greater rate than in areas with fewer senior citizens. Issues related to nursing practice regulations fall into this category.

How Bills Become Law

The Tracking Number

Legislators in both the House and the Senate can introduce a bill from any source into their respective chambers. Additional legislators can sign on as the bill's cosponsors. A bill is considered to be strong if it has strong sponsorship, including a number of powerful cosponsors, a high degree of bipartisanship, and the interest of powerful individuals, both political and nonpolitical. After the bill is introduced, it is taken to the chief clerk, who assigns it a number that permits it to be tracked throughout the process.

> *A bill is considered to be strong if it has strong sponsorship, including a number of powerful cosponsors, a high degree of bipartisanship, and the interest of powerful individuals, both political and nonpolitical. After the bill is introduced, it is taken to the chief clerk, who assigns it a number that permits it to be tracked throughout the process.*

What Do You Think?

Visit your state legislature's website and identify two bills that deal with health care. How do you feel about these bills? How should your representative vote on this issue? How can nurses influence these bills to ensure effective health-care policy?

The Committee

After the bill is assigned a number, it is referred to a **committee.** Most congressional committees deal with passing laws. Thousands of bills are proposed in both chambers of Congress, but only a small percentage ever gets considered for passage. A bill that is favored usually goes to a committee that focuses on the issues that the bill would address, but House and Senate leaders decide which committee considers the bill. This decision, greatly influenced by politics, is critical to the survival and ultimate passage of a bill.

In committee, they consider written comments on the measure, hold hearings in which witnesses testify and answer questions, make any needed changes based on the information gathered, and then send the bill to the full chamber for debate. Conference committees, usually composed of standing committee members from the House and Senate who originally considered the legislation, help reconcile one chamber's version of a bill with the other's.

It is no coincidence that most bills die in committee. Invariably, the leadership discusses their expectation for the bill with the committee chairs. If the leadership wants a bill to fail, it is referred to a committee that will never vote on it or will pass it on to the House.

In the U.S. Congress, the committees with greatest jurisdiction over health matters and their subcommittees are the following:

- *House Ways and Means Committee:* Social Security and Medicare (health-care subcommittees)
- *House Commerce Committee:* Health legislation, including Medicaid (Subcommittee on Health and the Environment)
- *Senate Finance Committee:* Medicare and Medicaid (health subcommittees)
- *Senate Labor and Human Resources Committee:* Health legislation in general; also works cooperatively with the Senate Finance Committee in considering issues involving Medicare and Medicaid
- *House and Senate Appropriations Committee:* Authorizes all money necessary to implement action proposed in a bill (subcommittees for labor, education, and health and human services)

The Next Step

As a result of full committee hearings, several things may happen to a bill. It may be:

- Reported out of committee favorably and be scheduled for debate by the full House or Senate.
- Reported out favorably, but with amendments.
- Reported out unfavorably.
- Killed outright.

For example, a bill reforming the way judges are elected ideally would go to the judiciary committee.

However, there is no legal requirement that the Speaker of the House or the Senate president pro tempore send the bill to any particular committee. For political reasons, the speaker may refer the bill to the committee on intergovernmental affairs, where it will languish and die.

Can the Bill Survive?

For a bill to survive, its sponsor must have the knowledge and the political standing to move the bill out of committee. If sponsors are truly committed, they will trade on their political capital. **Political capital** generally refers to some type of favor or action that a politician can exchange for something he or she wants. It is an extremely important element in the legislative process and consists of, but is not limited to, votes, amendments to bills, appointments, and support from constituency groups. Political capital often consists of an "if you vote for my bill, I'll vote for your bill" type of exchange. Legislators can be pushed into considering a bill they would prefer not to if they get feedback from enough of their constituents.

A Scheduled Debate

After a bill has been reported out of a House committee (with the exception of the Ways and Means and appropriations committees), it goes to the rules committee, which schedules bills and determines how much time will be spent on debate and whether or not amendments will be allowed. In the Senate, bills go on the Senate calendar, after which the majority leadership determines when or if a bill will be debated.

After a bill is debated, possibly amended, and passed by one chamber, it is sent to the other chamber, where it goes through the same procedure. If the bill passes both the House and the Senate without any changes, it is sent to the president for signature.

Opposing Versions

However, if the House and Senate pass different versions of a bill, the two bills are sent to a conference committee, which consists of members appointed by both the House and the Senate. This committee seeks to resolve the differences between the two bills; if the differences cannot be resolved, the bill dies in committee. When the conference committee reaches agreement on a bill, it goes back to the House and Senate for passage. At this juncture, the bill must be voted up or down, because no further amendments are accepted.

Passage or Veto?

If the bill is approved in both houses, it then goes to the chief executive—at the federal level, the president, or at the state level, the governor—who makes determinations about the bill. Governors can do one of two things: sign the bill into law or actively **veto** it. At the federal level, the president has the same options, with the addition of the pocket veto. Pocket vetoes, found only at the federal level, occur when the president, rather than actively vetoing a bill, simply does not sign it so that it does not become law. If vetoed, it is sent back to the House and Senate. To override the veto, a two-thirds vote by both chambers is required.

> *. . . there is no legal requirement that the Speaker of the House or the Senate president pro tempore send the bill to any particular committee. For political reasons, the speaker may refer the bill to the committee on intergovernmental affairs, where it will languish and die.*

The Fiscal Note

Clearly, the passage of a law can be a long and difficult process. This is often quite frustrating for action-oriented nurses who are used to seeing immediate outcomes—forming plans and making things happen quickly.

All bills that are passed need a fiscal note attached to them. Therefore, the appropriations committee is operationally very powerful. A piece of legislation that is passed without a fiscal note attached will never become a law. Over the years, many pieces of legislation have been passed by the legislature but have been starved to death financially. These are called *unfunded mandates.*

Housekeeping Bills

Major regulatory change occurs in laws in the form of housekeeping bills. Legislators can use this tactic to move a piece of legislation through the process, especially when the bill is more significant than the leadership acknowledges it to be. Although regulatory reform and change may seem tedious, they are important to the legislative process and have the capacity to benefit the public immensely or do irrevocable harm.

Executive Orders

Executive orders provide the chief executive, the governor or the president, with a means for moving an agenda item forward. Executive orders are in many cases a convenient way to formulate policy with minimal involvement of the legislature. They also allow the executive to make a statement about an issue that can be entered on the public record.

The legislature can leave executive orders uncontested or challenge them by characterizing them as beyond the scope of the executive branch. This may involve turning to the third branch of government, the judiciary.

HOW TO BE POLITICALLY ACTIVE

The first step in becoming politically active is to identify the specific goals that nurses, as a group, want to accomplish.

Why Be Active?

Nurses recognize many important issues in today's health-care system:

> *Once nurses identify exactly what it is that needs to be accomplished and understand what is possible within the political framework, they can use their significant political power to make changes that will benefit both the clients and the profession.*

- Increasingly acute conditions of hospitalized clients, who require higher levels of care and more complex levels of support than ever before
- Increasing responsibilities for nurses in supervision of rising numbers of unlicensed health-care personnel
- Loss of control of the work environment caused by managed care organizations
- Ever-shortening hospitalizations resulting in clients being sent home "quicker and sicker"
- Attempts by non-nursing groups to alter nurse practice acts and change the nature of state boards of nursing

Any one of these issues can become a focal point at which nurses aim their considerable political power.

For example, most nurses are concerned that RNs, who have traditionally been at clients' bedsides, are being replaced by individuals who are less prepared and less able to deal with high-acuity clients. Nurses believe that when they are replaced in large numbers by unlicensed assistive personnel, including nursing assistants, and by personnel who provide specific services, such as technicians who sit in front of cardiac monitors, the quality of client care decreases. Nurses know that these technicians often take on responsibilities for which they have had little training. Rarely are there established national standards that require these assistive personnel to demonstrate their ability to provide a specific level of care, or even standards that protect public safety.[11]

Feeling Powerless

Nurses are usually employees at will and can be fired for any reason. Although some efforts have been made in this direction, whistle-blower protection is generally not available to protect nurses who wish to speak out against unsafe staffing levels or employment practices. Nurses are, at times, torn between their obligations to maintain high standards of safe, ethical care, and their obligations to their families.

Although nurses often feel powerless against a monolithic health-care bureaucracy, in reality they have the potential to be a potent political force. Nationally, with almost 3 million nurses licensed to practice, the nursing profession constitutes the largest single body of health-care providers in the country.[9]

Finding a Voice

Nurses in all health-care settings are saying, "Somebody's got to do something about this situation." The reality of the situation is that nurses themselves are the best group for the job. Once nurses identify exactly what it is that needs to be accomplished and understand what is possible within the political framework, they can use their significant political power to make changes that will benefit both the clients and the profession.

Three Groups of Constituents

Although most nurses understand the problems they face as a profession, not all will be motivated to take the steps to make changes. Some are more comfortable taking leadership roles in political encounters while others prefer to follow and provide needed support. Others may want to get involved but need to weigh family responsibilities and their perception of their ability to make a difference. As situations change, they may choose to become more active. Generally, however, they can be grouped by their state of involvement and beliefs.

Group 1: Have a Little

One problem nurses in this group encounter is the ongoing conflict between the status quo and progress. They want to obtain more power and control, gain more benefits, earn more money, and have more respect as professionals. However, the strong desire to advance is counterbalanced by fear of jeopardizing their current jobs and/or their professional standing. Their motivation to be something more, to do something new, or to believe in something bigger is held back and pulled in another direction by their fear of change or the demands of their personal life. The result of this internal tug-of-war is an attitude of inertia and ambivalence that has prevented nurses from organizing politically and effectively using their numerical power.

Group 2: Want More

Despite the inertia and ambivalence of individuals in the "have a little" category, some of the most notable revolutionaries in history have come from this group, including Thomas Jefferson, Martin Luther King Jr., and Loretta Ford, who founded the nurse practitioner movement. Each of these individuals came from the working middle class with a belief that it could be made better and that they could "want more." Nurses who overcome their fear of change and risk their comfortable status quo position can make great strides in the industry. They can use their actions as examples of what individuals can accomplish to raise their own motivation levels to a point at which they overwhelm their trepidation.

Group 3: Sit Back and Watch

A third group of people, who share the inertia found among the "have a little" and "want more" groups, are the "do-nothings." These individuals can be heard saying things like, "I agree with what you are saying; I just don't agree with your means," or "I'm not going to get involved in this," or "I'm too busy to belong to the organization." The do-nothings tend to watch the activities of others, and if their efforts are successful, then they will join in as beneficiaries because they feel they have supported the effort from an ideological standpoint. However, they avoid any active involvement in

politics. The 18th-century British politician Edmund Burke recognized the danger of the do-nothings. He said, "The only thing necessary for the triumph of evil is for good men [and women] to do nothing" (http://www.goodreads.com/author/quotes/17142.Edmund_Burke).

What Can One Nurse Do?

It is important to remember that politics is a free-market enterprise open to anyone who is willing to become involved and play the game. Success in the political arena is contingent on three elements:

1. Knowledge and understanding of the process
2. The ability to offer something of value to the political figure
3. The capacity to identify what will be necessary to accomplish the objective

Anyone who is interested in becoming politically active must recognize that all candidates and elected officials need three things: resources to run their political operation (money and volunteers), votes, and a means to shape public opinion. Learning about politics through the mentoring process is often a successful strategy for nurses who have had little past political involvement but are interested in advancing a health policy.

Resources
Money

Sufficient resources are essential to running a political campaign. The first and most necessary resource is always money. Would-be candidates soon discover that a lack of money to fund a campaign will inevitably lead to political failure. An unfunded candidate cannot travel, send mailings, produce radio and television commercials, post signs, or organize a telephone bank.

Voters often fail to realize that political candidates are only as available as finances permit. Frequently, promising candidates lose because they fail to garner the financial resources necessary to run an effective campaign. Nurses can gain a candidate's support for issues by donating to his or her campaign chest. Many nurses feel that they are just struggling to make ends meet and do not have a lot of extra money to spend on candidates. The reality is that everybody can afford something, even five or ten dollars. Although the small sum may not seem like much when compared to the millions and millions donated by big business and foreign donors, because of the large numbers of nurses, the small amounts will quickly add up. The nurse's name will show up on the candidates' donor list and he or she will be more likely to consider the nurse's opinion when they call or write about an issue.

Nurses can also contribute to PACs such as ANA or state-level organizations that collectively can have a greater voice than one individual.

Volunteers

A second important resource in an election campaign is volunteers. Volunteers work in campaigns by manning telephone banks, making literature drops, placing signs, conducting voter registration drives, and distributing issues electronically to garner more interest in one's position. Usually political candidates are very glad to have free help for their campaigns, and many movements gain significant traction at the local level.

Although nurses may not be able to make large monetary contributions to a candidate's campaign, they can always volunteer some time. Working closely with a candidate on a volunteer basis allows individuals to discuss important issues and helps candidates who support issues important to nurses. Most candidates need a considerable amount of education on health-related issues because of their lack of knowledge about medical and nursing concerns.

> *Nurses can gain a candidate's support for issues by donating to his or her campaign chest. The reality is that everybody can afford something, even five or ten dollars.*

Votes

Obviously, votes are essential to any candidate. If a candidate does not have votes, he or she will not be elected. One of the most significant activities nurses can become involved in is to join and support a political party and then vote in elections for the candidates who most closely reflect the nurse's value system and fundamental beliefs.

Although the 14th and 15th Amendments emphasize that the right to vote is the most fundamental act in a democracy, some individual states in recent years have enacted restrictions to voting based on the need to save money. Also, in 2014, the Supreme Court repealed several requirements in the Voting Rights Act that prevented certain states from enacting regulations that would restrict minority voting. (For more information, go to http://www.washingtonpost.com/blogs/wonkblog/wp/2014/01/16/the-supreme-court-gutted-the-voting-rights-act-now-a-bipartisan-gang-wants-to-put-it-back-together/.)

The first step in being able to vote is to meet the established requirements for voting. These are established by the individual states but are very similar in many states. They include being a U.S. citizen, establishing residency in a particular location, not being a convicted felon (some states), and being 18 years of age or older. If the person meets these requirements, they next go to a location where they perform voter registration. In some states this can be done by mail or even at the voting poles the same day as people vote. In other states, it is much more restrictive and the locations may be at state offices. Also, some states are now requiring a government-issued photo ID, birth certificate, written proof of residency, or passport.

There are several different types of elections in which people can vote. Local elections are for the election of local officials such as council persons, mayors, and various other local officials. State elections are for the election of state officials such as governors, state senators, and state representatives. General elections are for the election of national officials such as the president and vice president and are held every 4 years on the first Tuesday in November. Sometimes local, state, and general elections all occur at the same time or they may be at different times throughout the year.

Primary elections are for the selection of candidates for the various levels of elections. These are held at times selected by the governors of the individual states. Most states require that the person voting must vote within their own party (i.e., if they are Democrats, they must vote for a Democratic primary candidate; if they are a Republican, they must vote for a Republican primary candidate), but there are several states that have open primary elections where the person voting can vote for any primary candidate regardless of party affiliation.

Keep in mind that there is never a perfect fit with any political party. Almost everyone who belongs to a political party will disagree at some point with some element of the party, usually with the extremist views. However, differing opinions and beliefs should not be a barrier to membership in a political party. The only way to change a view or opinion is by active participation from within the party.

The ultimate political power is the vote. Nurses must be registered to vote and must go to the polls on election day. They can make the difference for a candidate who supports legislation that empowers nurses and who recognizes what is needed for beneficial health-care reform.

Shaping Public Opinion

Candidates need endorsements from their constituents (voters) so they can build their support base. They generally consider endorsements from nurses as one of the most valuable assets to their campaign.

Public Trust in Nurses

Supporting nursing organizations such as the ANA or the American Academy of Nurse Practitioners that lobby for the concerns of nurses is essential because this is exactly the type of organizational endorsement that candidates try to get. By careful selection of candidates who support legislation favorable to nursing and health care, endorsements can give nurses the capacity to shape public opinion, and those organizations have people whose job it is to study the candidate's position of issues important to the profession. Periodic polls conducted by national news magazines, asking readers to rank various professions by how much they are trusted, have consistently shown that the public views nurses very highly, in the same category as police officers, firefighters, and teachers. For the past 10 years, nurses have ranked number one on the Gallup Poll list of the most ethical, honest, and trusted professionals, outranking the second-place finisher, pharmacists, by 12 points. (For more information, go to http://www.gallup.com/poll/1654/honesty-ethics-professions.aspx.)

Why the Governor Matters

Nurses should use endorsements by choosing candidates in campaigns that have an impact on important issues. Often the campaign for governor falls into this category because governors, as chief executives, have a great deal of political power and can appoint people to a number of boards, committees, and other positions. Nurses need to recognize that the members of the board of nursing in their state, as well as other important appointed positions in health departments and other regulatory agencies, may be appointed by the governor and that this board has the final decision on the way that nurses practice.

When nurses establish a working political relationship with the governor either individually or via their state nursing organization, the governor is more likely to look favorably on them as those who have sustained him or her, provided financial support, and given endorsements during the political campaign. They will be the people the governor appoints to a board position.

Targeting endorsements will prevent nurses from making blind political decisions. Candidates should be assessed first on their willingness to support issues that nurses are interested in and then on their capacity to win the election.

> *Another way to become politically involved is to develop a political relationship with an elected official at the state or local level or a political operative who can mentor and guide the nurse in finding a route through the political maze.*

Grassroots Effort

A model for individual political development encourages grassroots involvement in local issues. This model is based on the belief that grassroots efforts may be more fulfilling than involvement in partisan politics.[12] This model is an activity-oriented ladder, including activities at four distinct levels:

- *Rung 1: Civic involvement.* Children's sports, parent-teacher association (PTA), neighborhood improvement group
- *Rung 2: Advocacy.* Writing letters to public officials and newspapers and making organized visits to officials to discuss local issues
- *Rung 3: Organizing.* Independent organizing on local issues, incorporation of single-issue citizens' groups, and networking with similarly situated citizens' groups.
- *Rung 4: Long-term power wielding.* Campaigning for oneself or another, local government planning, and agenda setting.

Sometimes grassroots movements are not so grassroots. How can you tell the difference? The primary key is the funding source, which they often attempt to hide. If the source of money for the movement is from a large corporation, a political party, or other organization that has strong leanings toward one particular position, it is not a true grassroots organization. If large groups of people are bused in for rallies from a great distance away and their signs are professionally printed, this may be a tip-off that they are being funded by a politically motivated enterprise. Large donors tap into a radical wing of the party with high levels of anger and resentment over a particular issue or event. Unfortunately, these types of groups can produce the "arrow shot in the air" effect whereby no one knows exactly where the arrow will land or when it comes down. Unleashing a group of radical ideologues tends to produce considerable backlash and over time can actually cost the party major elections. They can even push the party to take positions that are detrimental to achieving its fundamental goals.

True grassroots movements tend to be more spontaneous and less well organized. They have little funding and come from a locally developed movement. They tend to focus on one particular issue, and the life cycle of their organization is relatively short, lasting a few weeks or months at most, although some may spin off a better-organized group that can have considerable political power.[12]

Nurses in Office

Most nurses prefer not to get involved in running for political office. However, some do and achieve high status in public office. Those congresswomen who are nurses were mentioned earlier.

One way that nurses can become more politically involved is to become knowledgeable about key issues that may have an effect on health care and the profession. Often issues that may not seem at first glance to be associated with health care or nursing, such a reducing taxes, have a very profound influence on how a state can care for those most in need. Almost always, the first items cut from a budget are social and health-care programs such as school nurses.

Another way to become politically involved is to develop a political relationship with an elected official at the state or local level or a political operative who can mentor and guide the nurse in finding a route through the political maze. As discussed earlier, the principle of self-interest is one of the most critical elements in politics, and to establish a relationship with a political figure, nurses must demonstrate that the issues they support have value to both themselves and to the politician.

Making Alliances

There are several ways that a nurse can decide who to support when becoming involved in the political process. A first step is to identify those legislators interested in issues related to health care and nursing. Editorial opinion pieces in newspapers can give legislators a sense of the issues of concern or check the websites of your representatives to determine their positions on issues.

It is a good idea to begin with local legislators and candidates, such as the state representative, state senator, or councilperson serving the neighborhood. Call their offices and find out when and where they are scheduled to speak, then go and listen to the speech to get a sense of who they are and what issues they support. Their speeches and the way they answer questions will reveal their ideology and partisanship. Also, during question-and-answer periods, ask elected officials what they think about issues important to you.

Attending some of the partisan events that occur during an election season or volunteering at election headquarters will help with getting exposure to prominent political figures. An advantageous way to visualize the local political landscape is by observing who is talking to whom at the event. Nurses can make their own assessments of political candidates by observing the candidates in action, calling their

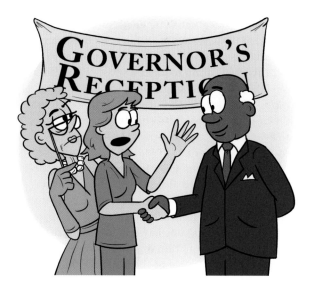

offices for information, reading published literature, checking their positions on their website, and talking to people who know the candidates.

Beginning the process may seem difficult, but once you decide to become politically active, you'll become more confident.

Know the Issues

For nurses to be successful in the political process, they must know and understand the issues. At times an issue may be readily apparent in a nurse's community—for example, an increased number of homeless people. Other issues are easily identified by reading newspapers and a variety of websites that focus on current issues. Issues are generally presented in the editorial section; most newspapers also have a political watch section, which reports the results of any significant votes at the state and federal levels. Keep in mind, however, that most media outlets have a political view that influences the way they present their news and opinions. It is best to research an opposing view to get a full understanding of the issues.

The American Nurses Association (ANA) newspaper, *American Nurse,* is an excellent source of information on issues of concern to the profession. In addition, the *American Journal of Nursing* Newsline feature and *Nursing and Health Care*'s Washington Focus are excellent, easily readable sources of information in journals. *Capitol Update,* the ANA legislative newsletter for nurses, reports on the activities of its nurse lobbyists and on significant issues in Congress and regulatory agencies. This publication requires a subscription but is available in most nursing school and hospital libraries. Most state legislatures now have online access to their proceedings so that bills of interest to nurses can be tracked as they progress through the legislative process.

State nurses' associations and many specialty nursing groups also publish newsletters or legislative bulletins. Many of these are free to members but may be sent only when requested. Most state nurses associations have websites where members can find information on important bills that will affect their practice or the health of their states.

Tracking these bills is very important. The best time to influence a bill that will adversely affect nursing practice or health care is by presenting an opposing view when it is in committee. Writing or calling committee members is key to the success of this tactic. The practice in the past was to have public hearings when a bill is in committee. This allowed for thoughtful discussion about the effects of the bill on the various constituencies. However, in recent years in some state legislatures where one party has an overwhelming majority, some house speakers have adopted the practice of not permitting public debate in committee. They site "streamlining the process" as the reason but use the practice to quickly move their partisan agendas to approval. Constituents often have less than 24 hours to do anything while the bill is in committee.

Action alerts may also be sent by e-mail or phone to inform members of vital issues that come to the table. It is critical that nurses take action and make their position known. Oftentimes, as few as 20 phone calls to a legislator can make a difference in the way he or she votes. Remember a legislator is not a health-care practitioner and probably knows little about the issue. A nurse's opinion provides a valuable level of expertise.

> *Tracking these bills is very important. The best time to influence a bill that will adversely affect nursing practice or health care is by presenting an opposing view when it is in committee.*

Tactics

Tactics, essential tools for those who desire to be politically active, are the conscious and deliberate acts that people use to live and deal with each other and the world around them. In a political sense, *tactics* usually means the use of whatever resources are available to achieve a desired goal.

Nurses, with their long history of accomplishing much with few resources, are natural tacticians. As nurses learn how to organize themselves for political purposes, they can use their well-developed tactical skills to achieve important political goals. Listed below are some easy-to-use tactics for political action.

Engage in Bipartisan Tactics

All nurses need to be politically active to achieve unified goals. Political action across the spectrum of issues and across partisan lines is necessary to pass legislation that is in the best interest of all citizens regardless of party affiliation. Nurses should understand that only by supporting candidates who advocate for nursing, whether Democrat or Republican, can the profession make changes that will advance its agenda. The most important thing, always, is the issue being addressed, not the personality or party of the candidate.

Lobbying

Sometimes communication with legislators takes the form of lobbying. *Lobbying* may be defined as attempting to persuade someone (usually a legislator or legislative aide) of the significance of one's cause or as an attempt to influence legislation. Lobbying methods include letter writing; face-to-face communication or telephone calls; Mailgrams, telegrams, or e-mails; letters to the editor; and written or verbal testimony. In addition, legislators have a place on their websites that invite comment on issues (see Issues in Practice: How to Effectively Lobby Your Legislators).

To lobby effectively, one should be both persuasive and able to negotiate. Lobbying is truly an art of

> *" Nurses need to recognize that the communication skills they use on a daily basis, as when explaining complicated medical jargon to clients, are the same skills they can use in translating health-care issues into language that the public and elected officials can understand. "*

communication, an area in which nurses can become skilled. Before beginning any lobbying effort, it is vital to gather all pertinent facts. If the legislator asks you a question you do not know the answer to, be honest and reply that you will get that information. Then get back to the legislator as soon as you can.

If the plan is to visit the legislator's office, an appointment should be set up in advance. Usually, the meeting will actually be with the legislative aide, particularly at the federal level. This should not be discouraging because this individual is often responsible for assisting in the development of position statements and offering committee amendments for the legislator.

To ensure that legislators and support staff listen to your concerns, it is important not only to be well prepared but also to show that others support your position. When one person speaks, legislators may listen, but when many people voice the same concern, legislators are much more likely to pay attention. Always leave a business card, contact sheet, or both with your personal information so that the legislator can contact you. Send a thank-you note expressing your gratitude for the meeting.

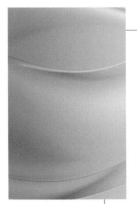

Issues in Practice

How to Effectively Lobby Your Legislators

The first time you communicate with a legislator can be intimidating. The key element to remember is that they are people, just like you. They work for you because you put them in office. The other thing to remember is that they really don't know much about nursing and health care, but you do. You are an excellent source of information for them.

There is a hierarchy of communicating with legislators, listed below in order from the most effective to the least effective:

1. **Personal contact.** This is the best way to make your opinion known, but it's unlikely you will be able to do this very often. During legislative sessions, lawmakers are very busy and have little time for personal interaction with constituents. The next best option is to meet with their staffers. Ask for the one who deals with the specific issue. During times when Congress is not in session, you might reach them when they are home in their districts.

2. **Phone calls.** During legislative sessions, this is a very powerful method of communication. It is timely if you are attempting to influence a vote on a particular bill that is being considered. It is unlikely that you will talk to the legislator directly. Rather, you will get one of their office staff. Make sure you give the number of the bill you are either supporting or opposing and make sure you make it clear as to which position you are taking. What happens is that the staff person has a sheet of paper with the bill number at the top that is divided in half with pros in one column and cons on the other. Your phone call will get a check mark in one or the other of these two columns. This may not sound important, but decisions about how to vote have been decided by as little as 20 phone calls.

3. **Written letters.** These are effective but tend to have a time-lag problem. If a bill is being pushed through a committee in 24 hours, the letter may arrive a day or two too late. If you know the bill is coming up in a week or so for a floor vote, they are more effective. Make sure you identify the bill number and whether you are for or against it in the first paragraph. Keep it short—one page is best—and sign it with your name and address. The legislator will probably not read your letter, but the staff will then place it in one of two piles—a pro pile or a con pile. At the time of the vote, they count the number in each pile.

4. **E-mails.** All of the legislators' websites have a place for constituents to comment on issues.

No matter how you communicate with your legislators, consider following these practical suggestions to maximize the success of your message:

Know your legislators. You will be most effective by getting to know your senator and representative from *your* district on a personal basis. Find out which committees and subcommittees your legislators serve on and their voting record. They have much more influence over legislation within their committees' and subcommittees' jurisdiction. This information is available on your state's legislative website.

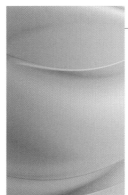

Issues in Practice <small>continued</small>

Know the legislation. Just as your time is very limited, so is a legislator's. Know the bill number and the issues. Have your facts ready when you approach a legislator. State your position clearly and then be available to either answer any questions the legislator may have or offer to find out the answer to any question you don't know. All bills are listed on the legislative website by number and have a reference to the full text.

Know the legislative process. Understand the steps that a bill goes through to become law. Review the steps in this chapter.

Be firm but friendly. Do not try to force a commitment on how your legislator is going to vote. However, when your legislator is aware of the issue and your position, it is then time to begin asking for a position. Remember to be courteous.

Keep in touch throughout the year. Legislators don't like it when the only time you contact them is when you're upset about something. Send them a Christmas card—you'll get one back!

Concentrate on the issue, not the person. Doing your homework and preparing for your conversation with your legislator will allow you to concentrate on the issue. Even though it isn't always possible to remain in harmony with your legislator, remember that with rare exceptions, they are honest, intelligent public servants trying to represent *all* of their constituents.

Lobby like you run your unit/floor/hospital/business. Be cooperative. Be realistic. Be practical. Never break your word. If you tell a legislator that you will do something, keep your promise. Continue to educate yourself regarding the legislative issues that are of concern to you. Bills change during the process. Sometimes you may find yourself supporting a bill and the next week opposing it because it was changed. Know where your bill is and what it looks like at all times. Despite popular opinion, things sometimes happen fast with legislation.

Don't threaten the legislator. Saying things like, "If you don't support this bill, I'm not going to vote for you next election," or "I'm not going to give any more money to your campaign" is counterproductive. Think about how you respond to threats.

Don't try to do it by yourself. Work with your fellow nurses in your community and your state. Work with and through your place of employment, your local chamber of commerce, state chamber of commerce, and of course your state nurses association.

Source: Oklahoma Nurses Association, 2013.

Collaborate With Constituency Groups

Nurses can increase their political power by making alliances with other powerful constituency groups that support similar issues, such as the American Hospital Association or the American Medical Association or other organizations interested in health-care issues, managed care, national health insurance, and the decreased quality of care from the increased use of unlicensed personnel. Nurses who are organized into collective bargaining units can use an alliance with powerful unions. Unions are traditionally concerned with issues such as working conditions, including staffing patterns in hospitals; wages; job security; and benefits. Nurses are concerned about the same issues.

Be a Political Organizer

"Know thy enemy" is one of the most fundamental rules that tacticians must follow, whether in war or politics. Napoleon was successful as a tactician and general because, before he fought any battle, he walked the battlefield. He knew what the terrain was like and where the rocks and crevices were. He knew what to anticipate when he arrived on the battlefield. Nurses who want to be successful in a political battle must first learn the hills, valleys, rocks, and crevices of the primary political battlefield, their own state demographics.

Comparing numbers helps define the political landscape of a state. Important demographics for organizing nurses at the state level include:

- Total population of the state. This provides a demographic overview of the political arena.
- Total number of registered voters.
- Total number of registered voters by political party.
- Total number of likely voters in any given election cycle. To determine this number, the difference between an on-year and an off-year election cycle should be understood. An on-year election cycle occurs when there is a major race in the state, usually during a presidential or gubernatorial race. An off-year cycle occurs when a major race is not being run. Lower levels of political activity are seen in an off-year election cycle.
- Total number of registered nurses. This information can be obtained from the state board of nursing. Comparing the number of actual voters with the number of RNs in a state provides an indication of the potential power of an RN voting block. For example, if there are 800,000 people who regularly vote in a state and there are 100,000 nurses in the state who are organized into a voting block about a particular issue, that group of nurses represents a significant percentage of voters, and candidates running for statewide office will be interested in having nurses' support. Nurses must be encouraged to register and vote to increase the power of the block.[13]

Important Characteristics of an Organizer

Many of the characteristics of an organizer listed in Box 19.2 are the same characteristics that are required of nurses on a daily basis in the practice of their profession. Although these characteristics may have varying degrees of value for the organizer, the one critical element a political organizer has to have is the capacity to communicate in an honest and factual manner. Although nurses usually have a well-developed ability to communicate at the bedside, they may lack the confidence to communicate in the larger public and political arenas. Nurses need to recognize that the communication skills they use on a daily basis, as when explaining complicated medical jargon to clients, are the same skills they can use in translating health-care issues into language that the public and elected officials can understand.

One way to gain the public's interest and elected officials' support is to personalize health-care issues by stressing the fact that nurses are the professionals who provide the bulk of direct care for their mothers, fathers, siblings, and children. Communication of issues that touch people personally is usually the most effective method.

B o x   1 9 . 2

Characteristics of an Organizer

- Curiosity
- Motivation
- Reverence
- Realism
- Flair for the dramatic
- Sense of humor
- Charisma
- Self-confidence
- Communication skills
- Clear vision of the future
- Capacity to change
- Persistence
- Ability to organize
- Imagination

WHAT FOLLOWS ORGANIZATION?

Drafting Legislation and Creating Change

Certain critical questions must be asked. The first question always must be, "Who is the decision-maker?" For example, if an issue needs to be resolved in the state board of nursing, the first step is to identify who makes the decisions at the board. Although the board members make decisions, it is important to remember that the people who sit on the board are appointed. Who appoints them and what is the basis of those appointments? If they are political appointees, they usually have some sort of political benefactor or a political relationship with someone in power.

Understanding these types of relationships makes it easier to determine the appointees' ideological and partisan positions on many issues. For example, if a nursing board is newly appointed by a recently elected Republican governor, there is a chance that most of the board members are Republicans who agree with the governor on many key issues.

The second question to address is, "How accessible is the appointee's benefactor?" Sometimes board members are appointed by the legislative leadership, not the governor. It is important to discover who appointed the board and whether or not individual voters have access to them. Generally, access by individual voters to the power figures who make these types of appointments is very limited. Organized groups, such as the ANA, provide the best avenue of access at the federal level while state nursing organizations focus their efforts on states issues.

Also consider which organizations have opposing views. Understanding their positions provide the opportunity to research data to refute their position.

Questions About Health Care

Other questions that need to be answered include:

- How successful have nurses been in the past in achieving specific goals?
- What positions do nurses hold in government?
- What does the state board look like politically?
- Which legislators have supported nursing issues in the past?
- Which legislators traditionally oppose nursing and health-care issues?
- What is their voting record on similar bills? Do they have a record of support?

Because of the failure to ask and answer these questions, numerous pieces of pro-nursing legislation have died in committee or lacked sponsors to move the bill through the process. In states where nurses are in tune with the political issues and powers, they have more success moving bills through the legislative process so that they become law than in states where nurses are apathetic about the political process.

If a Bill Isn't Filed or Doesn't Pass

Even if a bill favorable for nurses or health care does not pass the first time, the fact that it was brought to a vote is important for several reasons. First, it has brought an issue to the attention of the whole legislature that they might otherwise have dismissed as unimportant. Also, it can expose those entities that support or oppose the issues and provide important information about planning future efforts.

Second, the legislative process brings to light the proponents and opponents of the issue and allows nurses to specifically target legislators who voted against the bill. One of two approaches can be used at this point. Nurses can either communicate with the legislators to explain why the bill is important in hopes of changing their minds, or they can organize as a voting block and attempt to vote the opposing legislators out of office.

Third, after a bill has gone through the process the first time, it becomes much easier to identify the obstacles and sticking points in the language of the bill. Before the bill is reintroduced in a later session of the legislature, it can be modified and amended to eliminate those parts that may have caused ideological problems for specific legislators.

The Nurse as Political Ally

Very few nurses have sought or been elected to governmental positions. However, it is important to realize that not all nurses who hold elected positions are allies for nursing. Currently there are approximately 6 nurses in Congress and 80 nurses in state legislative positions or high administrative positions across the nation. Nurses who are elected to political office should identify with the nursing profession and have the courage to support legislation that promotes health care and the nursing profession; however, after they are elected, for whatever reason, some decide to support legislation that is contrary to the profession's best interests. They need to be reminded by their constituents of the values that make nurses the most trustworthy profession.

Conclusion

There is nothing magical about nurses becoming involved in politics. It is simply a matter of hard work and use of the critical-thinking, decision-making, and persuasion skills that nurses already possess. It is clear, however, that nurses can and do make a difference in the political arena. Nurses must ask how and where they can make a difference and how they can become involved in the process. Not every nurse will choose to run for political office, but each nurse can and should make a contribution. The willingness of nurses to become involved in politics is the key to developing legislative respect for the profession and improving health care.

Issues in Practice

How Do Politics Affect You and Your Family?

Why should nurses be involved in politics? Does it really make a difference who is elected and who makes the laws? Take a minute to go through the questions below and check the items you think may be affected by politics.

Between the time you wake up and the time you leave the house, several things usually happen to you. Do you think any of the following subjects are affected by politics?

- The water with which you wash your face and brush your teeth
- The electricity that lights the room
- The price and quality of food you have for breakfast
- The safety of the products you buy

As the average person's life span grows longer and the retirement age is lowered, these later years become more meaningful. Are any of the following decisions affected by our political systems?

- The age at which you can retire
- The income that you get during retirement
- The quality and cost of health care
- Our life expectancy

We value our leisure time and the chance to get away from it all. Are any of the following areas affected by politics?

- The parks and lakes where vacationers fish and swim
- The air you breathe
- The radio and television programs that entertain you

Take some time to think about these questions. The answers will make you think some more.

Critical-Thinking Exercises

1. Go online and find out who the state and national senators and representatives are for your district. Ask your classmates and professors who their state and national representatives and senators are. Are you surprised by the results?
2. Are you a registered voter? If not, investigate the voter registration process in your state. Was it easy or difficult? If it was difficult, what factors contributed to the difficulty? How can you change the voter registration process?
3. What political issues do you feel strongly about? Look up the location of the local party headquarters that supports your position on an issue and go there to see what type of volunteer work you can do.
4. Find a bill online at your state government bill-tracking site that deals with an issue important to nursing or health care (e.g., tobacco-related, Medicare or Medicaid issues, or changes in the nurse practice act). Track the bill as it goes through the bill-making process. What legislators are key in its passage? Contact them by phone or letter to let them know that you either support or disagree with the bill. Did the bill pass?

References

1. Merriam Webster Online Dictionary. Retrieved November, 2013 from http://www.merriam-webster.com/

2. Dotson MJ, Dave DS, Cazier JA. Addressing the nursing shortage: A critical health care issue. *Health Marketing Quarterly,* 29(4):311–328, 2012.

3. Shaffer FA, To Dutka JY-H, Perspectives on credential evaluation: Future trends and regulatory implications. *Journal of Nursing Regulation,* 3(1):26–31, 2012.

4. Shaffer FA, To Dutka JY-H. Perspectives on credential evaluation: Future trends and regulatory implications. *Journal of Nursing Regulation,* 3(1):26–31, 2012.

5. Valentine NM. Communicating nursing's excellence and value: On the way to magnet. *Nursing Economic$,* 31(1):35–43, 2013.

6. The Magnetic pull: A staff report. *Nursing Management,* 41(2):38, 40–44, 2010.

7. Somers MJ, Finch L, Birnbaum D. Marketing nursing as a profession: Integrated marketing strategies to address the nursing shortage. *Health Marketing Quarterly,* 27(3):291–306, 2010.

8. American Nurses Association. Funding for Nursing Workforce Development Programs. Retrieved December 2014 from http://nursingworld.org/TitleVII–112thCongress

9. American Nurses Association of Colleges of Nursing. Nursing Faculty Shortage. Retrieved December 2014 from http://www.aacn.nche.edu/media-relations/fact-sheets/nursing-faculty-shortage

10. Ebner AL. What nurses need to know about health care reform. *Nursing Economic$,* 28(3):191–194, 2010.

11. Lung CJ. Support your political action committee: Contribute to the PAC and make sure your voice is heard in Washington. *American Society of Radiologic Technologist Scanner,* 42(3):56, 2010.

12. McKay ML, Hewlett PO. Grassroots coalition building: Lessons from the field. *Journal of Professional Nursing,* 25(6):352–357, 2010.

13. Aiken LH, Clarke SP, Cheung RB, Sloane DM, Silber JH. Educational levels of hospital nurses and surgical patient mortality. *Journal of the American Medical Association,* 290:1617–1623, 2003.

4

Issues in Delivering Care

The Health-Care Debate: Best Allocation of Resources for the Best Outcomes

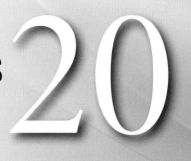

Linda Newcomer

Rob E. Newcomer

Learning Objectives

After completing this chapter, the reader will be able to:

- Briefly discuss the history of past attempts at health-care reform
- Identify the pros and cons of the Affordable Care Act
- Identify the position of the American Nurses Association (ANA) on health-care reform
- Explain the Affordable Care Act and its origins
- List the impending challenges to health-care reform
- Explain why nurses and prospective nurses need to know about health-care reform

100 YEARS OF CONTROVERSY

The conversation concerning health-care reform started over 100 years ago and is likely to continue as long as the quality of health care is less than ideal, the cost is more than expected, and the access remains less than 100 percent. Most recently, health-care reform and its legislative outcome, the Affordable Care Act (ACA), have been the subject of much public debate. Unfortunately, much of the conversation has continued to revolve around the political talking points, misinformation, and the trepidation of the people it affects.[1] The debate is likely to continue as long as there are disparate and strongly held ideologies on the role of government in the lives of U.S. citizens.

WHAT NURSES NEED TO KNOW

With the rapidly increasing volume of information addressing improvements in client care, new medical technology, and ever-evolving regulatory changes, a legitimate question that many nurses would ask before starting to read a chapter on health-care reform is, "Why?" Although a case could be made that every concerned citizen should be spending more time learning about the scope and implications of needed health-care reform, there are many important reasons this applies particularly to nurses.

The Institute of Medicine's (IOM) report, "The Future of Nursing: Leading Change, Advancing Health" (Chapter 15) recommended that "Nurses should be full partners, with physicians and other health care professionals, in redesigning health care in the U.S."[2] It is impossible to be a full partner in this process without knowledge of the history, scope, cause, and potential solutions to the issues.

More Than a Job

Some nurses say they just want to do their job and take care of their clients and go home at the end of the day without being involved in the political process. They need to understand that health-care policy affects clients, families, communities, and nurses every day. Health-care policy is about people, and nurses often care for the most vulnerable people every day—the very young, the old, and the ill. The decisions made in health-care policy decide which providers people can see, which clients can afford medications, which clients can receive preventive care or early diagnosis treatment, and ultimately, who lives and who dies. (See Chapter 19 for more details about the political process.) The decisions in the health-care policy arena will determine where nurses practice, what they are allowed to do, and their ability to be reimbursed for the services nurses provide at an individual and collective level.

Eliminating Waste

Many hospitals and providers have already begun the process of value-based purchasing (VBP), ensuring that health-care providers are held accountable for both cost and quality of care. VBP is a method of obtaining products and services at a lower price and has been used by private industry and the federal government for many years. By using mass purchasing power, they can negotiate lower prices and better quality of services, including health care. According to a report, value-based purchasing attempts to reduce inappropriate or ineffective care by identifying and rewarding the providers who perform best, possibly by using the National Database of Nursing Quality Indicators (NDNQI), along with other well-developed indicators as measurement tools.[3] It has been suggested that nursing-sensitive measures, those that promote optimal staffing and practice environment, could demonstrate what all floor nurses already know: adverse events and mortality are highly dependent on the quality and number of nursing staff.[4] (For more information, go to http://www.qualitynet.org/dcs/ContentServer?c=Page&

> *The decisions in the health-care policy arena will determine where nurses practice, what they are allowed to do, and their ability to be reimbursed for the services nurses provide at an individual and collective level.*

pagename=QnetPublic%2FPage%2FQnetTier3&cid=1228772237147.)

Nursing-sensitive value-based purchasing is tied directly to the fourth message identified in the Future of Nursing report: "Effective workforce planning and policy making require better data collection and an improved information infrastructure."[2] The information infrastructure will be developed and implemented whether or not nurses participate in the process. It is important for staff nurses to be a part of the conversation that decides on the data-collection tools that will determine adequate and appropriate nurse staffing levels.[4]

More Clients, Increased Demands

Full implementation of the ACA means an estimated 32 million new clients are going to have insurance and need primary care. Repeated studies have shown that nurse practitioners can safely provide 80 percent of the care provided by family practice physicians without any decrease in quality or health outcomes and with an increase in client satisfaction.[5] Even with the current numbers of nurse practitioners (NP) and family practice physicians, there will still be a shortage of primary care providers. As of mid-2013, there are still regulatory barriers preventing advanced practice nurses from functioning to the full extent of their education and being fairly compensated for their work.[6] Legislative decisions will be made at both the state and federal level that will either reduce or increase these barriers and compensation for NPs.

Registered nurses (RNs) are the largest single group of health-care providers in the United States. Nursing as a profession has not historically participated collectively in full partnership with other players in the health-care industry in determining health-care policy.[7] Voices of nurses need to be heard as advocates for health-care decisions that have the most positive impact on the clients for whom they care. To participate fully in the conversation and process of finding solutions to the current health-care problems, nurses—current and future—need to educate themselves on the economic, political, ethical/moral, and health outcome issues that drive health-care policy.

A BRIEF HISTORY OF HEALTH REFORM IN THE UNITED STATES

It is easy to think of health-care reform as just the latest in a series of political topics that provide a framework for political parties to air their differences. Health-care reform as a political issue actually surfaced in 1912 and has resurfaced periodically since that time. Although everyone wants good health care that is easily available and affordable, there is little consensus on how to accomplish it. The debates about health-care policy revolve around some of the most fundamental issues in a democratic government: roles of government and individuals, regulation versus the free market, right versus privilege, and federal versus state responsibility and control. Added to this mixture are powerful special interests, such as large pharmaceutical companies, insurance providers, and physician associations, which are all concerned with financial outcomes.

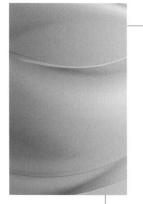

Issues in Practice

Resolving the Health-Care Reform Debate Using Critical Thinking

Although critical thinking is used in all aspects of decision-making, it is particularly important in resolving issues like the health-care reform debate.

As a way of looking at the world, critical thinking allows the nurse to consider new ideas and then evaluate those ideas in light of accepted information and her or his own value systems. Nurses are constantly making important decisions in both their professional and personal lives. By viewing critical thinking as a purposeful mental activity in which ideas are evaluated and decisions reached, nurses will be able to make ethical, creative, rational, and independent decisions related to client care.

Critical thinking, when applied to the health-care reform debate, is a powerful problem-solving tool. When used purposefully, it becomes a gestalt that allows the nurse to sort through the multiple variables that exist in the reform debate. Effective use of critical thinking is evident when nurses successfully apply their knowledge about the issue and come to a creative solution to a complex and multifaceted debate.

Questions for Thought

1. How much do you know about the ACA of 2010? Putting aside your ideological perspective and thinking about it critically, is the law helping the uninsured or hurting them?

2. What additional information about the ACA would be helpful in understanding its effects on health care? Where can you find additional information about it?

3. Have there been other recent issues in health care that you can apply critical thinking to?

Presidents Get Involved

As a presidential candidate of the Bull Moose Party in 1912, Theodore Roosevelt became the first national political figure to call for some type of reform for national health coverage. This call started the century-long quest for universal health care. It is reported that Franklin Delano Roosevelt (FDR), after starting a conversation about the establishment of national health insurance, retreated from including it in what became the Social Security Act of 1935, in large part due to the opposition from the American Medical Association (AMA). FDR instructed aides to begin working on national health insurance legislation, but he died before any bill was introduced.[8] One of the primary reasons health insurance became a benefit offered by employers at this time was because FDR implemented wage controls that capped how much employees could earn. Employers used health benefits as a way to attract employees since benefits were exempt from wage controls. Offering health care as a benefit was the first time the person who uses health care was separated from the one who pays for health care, a practice that is considered the norm today.

Harry Truman pressed Congress on multiple occasions to enact into law a plan known as the Truman-FDR plan. This plan proposed a single-payer public health insurance plan similar to the Canadian health-care plan. Again, powerful interests applied enough pressure so that Truman scaled back his original plan until it was reduced to providing health coverage only to the elderly.

In 1961, John F. Kennedy began his vigorous advocacy of a plan to provide health benefits to the elderly. This became the framework for the Medicare program. He was assassinated before he could see these new laws enacted. Lyndon Baines Johnson presided over passage of the Medicare and Medicaid Act in 1965, which was considered the most ambitious health insurance advance in U.S. history until the enactment of the ACA.

Richard Nixon is credited by many as the first president to attempt to hold down the rising cost of health care and health insurance through health-care reform. In 1973, he signed a law to encourage development of health maintenance organizations that were the first manifestations of managed care. A Republican, Nixon demonstrated that universal health insurance was not just a goal of the Democratic Party when he proposed private coverage for citizens through a federal mandate on employers and individuals.[8] Nixon believed a nationwide mandate that would require all citizens to have and pay for health insurance was necessary to reduce the cost of health insurance, but it was not popular with the majority of Americans. Nixon's proposed underlying structure for comprehensive health-care reform became the basis for the plan Mitt Romney would implement in Massachusetts and the framework that President Obama would pursue three decades later in developing the ACA.[9] The Watergate scandal and subsequent resignation of Nixon stopped any further progress in health-care reform from his administration. The increasing costs of health care and health insurance were to become a continuing concern in politics from this point forward, regardless of any plans or attempts to provide universal coverage.[8]

President Jimmy Carter introduced a health reform plan similar to Nixon's, including coverage for catastrophic illnesses or injuries. It had an employer's mandate and a replacement for Medicare and Medicaid to cover the elderly, disabled, and poor. This plan was united with a cost containment package directed at hospital and physician costs. The cost containment legislation passed the Senate in 1979 but was defeated in the House of Representatives.[8]

A call for universal health coverage did not reemerge in presidential politics until the presidency of Bill Clinton. In 1993 his wife, Hillary Rodham Clinton, took charge of a task force to reform health care and developed the Health Security Act of 1993. Again, powerful business interests intervened to scare the public and influence politicians, resulting in the failure of any significant health reform. The backlash and the divisiveness from this very public failure, in addition to other factors, helped the Republicans to reclaim control of the House and Senate in the midterm elections. This ended any presidential conversation on universal health coverage until the

> *A Republican, Nixon demonstrated that universal health insurance was not just a goal of the Democratic Party when he proposed private coverage for citizens through a federal mandate on employers and individuals.*

election of Barack Obama as president in November 2008.[9] (For more information about long-term political effects of the failed Health Security Act of 1993, go to http://www.princeton.edu/~starr/20starr.html.)

Historical Factors Related to Health Insurance

The first form of national insurance coverage was started in Germany under Chancellor Otto von Bismarck in 1883. Other countries in Europe soon followed. Anti-German sentiment in the United States was present at the time Theodore Roosevelt introduced the idea of national insurance coverage in the United States in 1912. This resentment has been cited as one of the reasons the idea did not make progress at that time. The original purpose of health insurance was to share the risk across a large group so that health care could be provided when needed. Providers could get paid without depending on the current financial ability of the person needing health care. With no government initiatives being considered, hospitals and physicians began to offer nonprofit private insurance plans in the 1920s and 1930s. This type of insurance required that the individual only be treated by the physician in the hospital with whom he or she was insured.[8]

In response to declining hospital occupancy during the Great Depression, the American Hospital Association established statewide Blue Cross insurance plans that provided hospital coverage at a choice of any hospital in the state. Soon, state medical societies began to provide Blue Shield insurance to cover physician services.[5] Because of wage and price controls during World War II, employers discovered they could legally use employer paid health insurance to compete for scarce employees. After WWII, unions began to negotiate for health benefits in their contracts. These factors encouraged the growth of private for-profit commercial insurance plans.[8]

Community Rating Versus Experience Rating

The original Blue Cross/Blue Shield insurance set premiums by what was called **community rating,** where rates were set by medical costs across a geographic area or region, or even across the whole nation. The commercial profit-based insurance companies introduced the concept of experience rating. An **experience rating** system is used to estimate how much a specific individual or group will have to spend on medical care within a very limited setting, such as an industry. This rating is based on how much the

person has already spent, what conditions are already present, and what risk factors a person has as compared to what would be considered a "normal" expenditure. Experience rating tailors health insurance policies to the specific group or individual rather than a geographic area, and these policies tend to have lower rates.

Experience rating was used as a competitive tool by setting low premiums for special organizations that had primarily young healthy employees. However, this scheme left other insurance companies and the government paying increasingly higher insurance rates for the elderly and those with chronic diseases. The elderly, who tend to have more age-related illnesses, were one of the groups hardest hit by use of experience rating. Community rating was unable to survive in an insurance market that was using experience rating. In 1945, the Blue Cross/Blue Shield providers outnumbered commercial insurance providers two to one. By 1955, commercial insurance providers outnumbered the "Blues." Legislation, including the exemption from taxes of employer-paid health insurance, was signed into law by Dwight Eisenhower in 1954, making the private for-profit insurance business once and forever part of the American health-care landscape.[8]

Because of the high cost of experience-rated insurance, by the late 1950s, fewer than 15 percent of people over the age of 65 had any type of insurance.[5] The federal and state governments' first attempts to fill in large gaps in the availability of health-care insurance for select groups in the population started with the Medicare and Medicaid legislation of 1965. First was the coverage of those persons over 65, the disabled, and children in poverty. In 1997, the Children's Health Insurance Program was created to extend the Medicaid coverage to many uninsured children and their parents.[8]

Government Gets Involved

Although the entry of the government into the health-care insurance industry assisted those people left behind by the private insurance companies, it also created a guaranteed source of income to the health-care industry. Health-care cost started rapidly rising when the availability of large sums of government dollars were being funneled into a system that rewarded health-care providers for increasing the number of services rather than positive health outcomes. Combined with the unrestrained use of new and increasingly complicated technology, health-care costs exploded, exceeding the inflation rate tenfold.[8]

The biggest expansion of Medicare since its initial enactment occurred under Republican president George W. Bush, who signed into law an unfunded prescription drug benefit bill. The bill increased seniors' access to prescription medications through the Medicare Part D program. The bill also provided subsidies to private companies to compete with Medicare such as the Medicare Advantage program. Proponents hailed the bill as the answer to seniors' financial problems with purchasing needed medications; however, opponents called the bill a giveaway to drug companies because it prevented, by law, Medicare from negotiating for discounts with drug companies or purchasing medications from other nations. Although providing additional services for seniors, the Medicare Part D bill was an unfunded mandate that increased the cost of providing these Medicare services and included no cost savings measures.[10]

Rising Costs Spur Reform

After the failed attempt at health-care reform in 1993, serious political discussion did not reemerge until the presidential campaigns for the 2008 elections. During this interval, many organizations interested in health-care costs and outcomes, such as the IOM, the Kaiser Family Foundation (KFF), and the World Health Organization (WHO), began to release reports about the rising cost of health care and the declining state of U.S. health care compared with other countries.[11–13]

In 2008, a large group of bipartisan veterans of the 1993–94 national health reform campaign met to discuss the future of health-care reform. All three leading Democratic presidential candidates had presented similar plans for comprehensive health reform. The Republican nominee, John McCain, produced a markedly different plan for health reform. Most of the attendees at the meeting believed that a Democratic president in 2008 would make a concerted effort to achieve comprehensive health reform. The group was less confident about *actually* achieving comprehensive health reform unless there was a Democratic congress.

> *Although the entry of the government into the health-care insurance industry assisted those people left behind by the private insurance companies, it also created a guaranteed source of income to the health-care industry.*

After a long discussion with expert advice from many quarters, a "ten commandments" for presidential leadership on health-care reform was produced. Its goal was to assist the president-elect to avoid the pitfalls of previous attempts to bring about health-care reform. The "ten commandments" included:

1. Clearly communicating the vision and goals to the public.
2. Keeping all the stakeholders at the table.
3. Tasking Congress to work out the details of the plan.
4. Involving the states.
5. Reducing partisanship.
6. Moving the legislation to a speedy completion.
7. Being politically forceful while moving the legislation forward.
8. Selecting advisors and spokespersons who the public trusts.
9. Limiting the scope of the reform legislation to a manageable size.
10. Getting the congressional leadership onboard early in the process.

President Obama was successful at achieving most of the commandments, except for managing the partisanship of a recalcitrant Congress.[8] (For more information, go to http://www.stthomas.edu/business/pdf/System_2009_Report.pdf.)

THE NEED FOR HEALTH-CARE REFORM

Four broad categories—economic issues, societal issues, ethical/moral issues, and health outcome issues—delineate the need for health-care reform. Another noteworthy issue concerns the inconsistent state policies for consumer protection. Investigations were conducted that revealed insurance companies carrying out such practices as canceling or denying claims after an insurance policy had been issued because of a client's costly disease, denying all claims for a period of time and then paying only those that were formally challenged by clients, and failing to pay claims for falsely discovered "preexisting conditions." The data collected across the nation demonstrated a

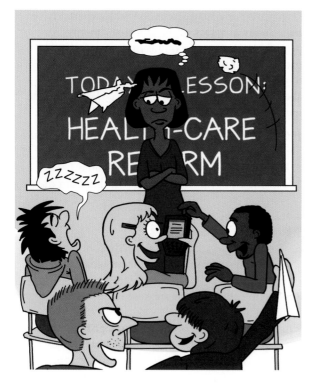

lack of self-regulation by the insurance companies and a lack of federal oversight and enforcement because the individual states are responsible for regulating insurance companies within their boundaries. Although some insurance companies' negative practices are blatantly unethical, other insurance companies claim that these negative practices are more appropriately due to regulations imposed by state and federal governments.

Economic Issues

The Organisation for Economic Co-operation and Development (OECD) is an international organization, representing 34 industrialized countries, that compiles and analyzes international health-care data.[14]

According to their recent reports, the United States spends two-and-a-half times more than the OECD average health expenditure per person. These figures can be misleading, however, since costs included in health-care expenditures include things such as paying for treatments not always available in other countries, cost of research that is funded in the United States in greater amounts than other countries, and the cost of self-medication and treatment.[15] U.S. health-care costs per person are twice as much as

France, for example—a country that is generally accepted as having a high-quality health-care system.[15]

Health-care costs have grown more rapidly than most other sectors of the economy, and its share of the national economy has increased disproportionally. Some critics suggest that the costs began to escalate once the Medicare act was passed and more government funds were available to provide health-care without restrictions. To get a balanced picture of health-care cost comparisons across nations, it is important to look at both expenditure as a percentage of gross national product (GNP) and expenditure per capita. The United States leads other countries in both measures. In 1970, total health-care costs in the United States were approximately $75 billion, or $356 per person. With the increase in spending to $8,233 per person for health care in 2010 and $2.6 trillion for total health-care costs, the share of the overall U.S. economy has risen from 7.2 percent in 1970 to 17 percent. Projections suggest that by 2020, this share will increase to 19.8 percent of GNP.[16] Predictions have been to expect health-care costs to rise as the baby boom generation begins to age and deal with many chronic conditions.

The large percentage of U.S. GNP that is spent on health-care costs limits the amount of money that is available for spending on education, improving the transportation infrastructure, and many other programs. The excessive health-care costs create a competitive disadvantage for American companies in the international market.

Impact of Ever-Increasing Costs

Health-care costs not only impact the national economy but also personal finances. The average American's salary increased 38 percent from 1999 to 2009. During this same period of time, the cost of health insurance premiums rose 131 percent.[17] A study found that in the United States, there were almost 700,000 bankruptcies per year due to excessive medical bills;[18] many of these people with high medical bills were well educated, owned homes, and fell into the middle-class income category. Over 75 percent of people filing for medical bankruptcy had health insurance at the beginning of their illness.[19] The truth is that just about anyone could be one bad diagnosis or one serious accident away from financial ruin.[20]

Societal Issues

Issues other than economics and politics can interfere with access to care and the quality of care. Health status can also be affected in part by social and economic conditions and the resources and support systems that exist in our neighborhoods, schools, and homes.

Socioeconomic Disparity

In 1999 at the request of Congress, the IOM studied the extent of the health-care disparities and their sources and suggested strategies for intervention.[21] They looked into racial and minority health outcomes, the percentages of racial/ethnic minorities who are uninsured, and the perceptions by minority populations of their access to health care and its quality. Although rising health-care costs cause many people to have difficulty paying their medical bill and to put off needed health care because of cost, the percentages are noticeably higher for those who have lower income and even higher for those without any insurance (public or private).

In 2010, a study by the KFF showed that only 10 to 11 percent of the non-elderly adult population with insurance or Medicaid had no regular source of health care. The rate among the uninsured was 55 percent. This same study showed that compared to non-elderly adults with insurance or Medicaid, the non-elderly adult without insurance was almost three times as likely to forgo needed health care and over six times more likely to not have care than those with insurance.

The data concerning insured and uninsured children is even more revealing. Children with no insurance are over 7 times more likely to have no regular care provider as compared to those with Medicaid and almost 10 times more likely than those with private insurance. In 2010, uninsured children in the United States did not receive needed health care 8 to 13 percent more often than those children with Medicaid or private insurance.[22]

Health-care costs have grown more rapidly than other sectors of the economy, and its share of the national economy has increased disproportionally.

What Do You Think?

Do you know someone who does not have health insurance? Do they avoid seeking health care for illnesses or injuries for which you would seek care?

Pervasive Disparity

Compounding these problems is the widening gap on health outcomes between the insured and the uninsured. The person with income below double the poverty level is three times more likely to be without health insurance within a year than those at four times the poverty level.[23] The socioeconomic conditions that have created the traditional health disparities are further causing the same groups to experience an ever-increasing loss of health insurance. Health-care disparities among minority groups undermine health-care outcomes for all aspects of care including access to care, quality of care, and efficiency of delivery of care, which lead to missed opportunities to help ensure long, healthy, and productive lives.[23]

Cost-Shifting

Health-care costs increase for everybody when the uninsured receive no preventive care. Without preventive care and early treatment interventions, individuals with chronic health problems and late-stage serious diseases end up being treated in a more expensive hospital setting rather than in a less expensive physician's office or clinic. Those costs accrue regardless of the person's ability to pay, and uncompensated costs are shifted to hospitals and health-care providers and eventually to those with insurance.

A study analyzed federal data and data from private sources for the year 2008. It was determined that the uninsured received $116 billion worth of care from hospitals, doctors, and other providers. The uninsured actually paid for only about one-third (37 percent) of the total costs of the care they received. Another one-third came from third-party sources, such as government programs and charities. Approximately $42.7 billion went unpaid and constituted uncompensated care. It is estimated that cost shifting this way costs those with insurance about $1,100 more per year in increase insurance premiums.[23]

The costs for the uninsured end up falling on taxpayers for government-supported programs or private insurers in the form of increased taxes and premiums. It is often referred to as the *hidden health-care tax*. In essence, those with health insurance end up paying twice—once for themselves and once for the uninsured.[24]

Health Outcome Issues

Despite spending significantly more for private pay and out-of-pocket costs for health care, the United States does not always have the best health outcomes in the world for some health concerns.[23] The single major differentiating factor between other developed countries and the United States is access to health care. These failures are not always due to the way in which health care is delivered. Societal issues such as drug use, obesity, poor lifestyle choices, and violence play a domineering role and do affect the measures. Some of the key measures in which the United States lags behind are:

- Mortality rates: the United States ranks 19th out of 19 wealthy countries.
- Americans with diabetes die younger than any of the other 19 countries.
- Americans have the worst survival rate after kidney transplants.
- Healthy life expectancy at age 60: the United States was tied for last among 23 countries.
- Infant mortality: America was 23rd out of 23 wealthy countries.[25]

Higher Mortality Rates

Despite the high levels of health-care spending in the United States, there are fewer physicians per capita than in most other developed countries. In 2010, the United States had only 2.4 physicians per 1,000 people, well below the average of 3.1 in developed countries. Most OECD countries have enjoyed large gains in life expectancy over the past decades. In the United States, life expectancy at birth increased by almost 9 years between 1960 and 2010. However, Japan had an increase of over 15 years, and the other OECD countries had an average increase of 11 years. In 1960, the life expectancy in the United States used to be 1.5 years *above* the OECD average; in 2012, it was more than 1 year *below* the average.[23]

An Obese Population

Obesity rates have increased in recent decades in all OECD countries, although there are notable differences. In the United States, the obesity rate among adults—based on actual measures of height and weight—was 35.9 percent in 2010, up from 15 percent in 1978. This is the highest rate among

> " *A study found that in the United States, there were almost 700,000 bankruptcies per year due to excessive medical bills.* "

OECD countries, and it is a lifestyle choice that significantly influences most of the key measures. The average for the 15 OECD countries with measured data was 22.2 percent in 2010. Obesity's growing prevalence foreshadows increases in the occurrence of weight-related health problems such as diabetes and cardiovascular diseases. There will be higher health-care costs in the future because of this trend.[23]

Moral/Ethical Issues

The idea that access to health care is a basic human right is supported by WHO,[24] the AMA Code of Ethics,[26] the ANA Code of Ethics,[27] and many religions.[28] Over 20,000 people die every year from medical problems that could be treated if they had had insurance.

Although almost everyone agrees that health care should be available to everyone without risking bankruptcy, the ethical issues focus on the most equitable way to ensure that it happens. Should those that have more economic advantages bear the bulk of the costs? Should those who choose a less risky healthy lifestyle pay less than those who don't? Should people pay for services they don't need because others need them? Do those who pay for the insurance or administer insurance programs get to create regulations to force those who make poor lifestyle choices to modify their behaviors? If a single-payer option is instituted, does the government get to force healthy lifestyles on individuals? Can they force people who are covered to get health care? Who gets to determine appropriate treatments, and how much will be paid to have them?

These questions and many others each come with consequences, regardless of the model selected. Nurses need to understand these issues if they are to be prepared to deal with them in the future.

The Morality of Shady Practices

Several of the OECD countries use private insurance companies to provide part or all of their health care. However, the United States, in addition to being the only wealthy industrialized nation not to provide basic health care to all citizens, is the only OECD country to allow private companies to profit from providing *basic* health care. The insurance companies in the other OECD countries make profits only on non-basic or sophisticated services that go beyond the basic care required by the government.[18]

Since all companies are run by humans, regulations need to be in place to prevent unscrupulous ones from trying to increase profits by selling **junk policies,** selectively withholding services, and delaying or denying services that are included in the policies. These insurance companies receive tax subsidies from the government, so regulating their practices should fall under government control.

Separate from the issue of whether or not our tax dollars subsidize the insurance companies are the ethics of increasing profit by limiting financial losses for covered services. These limits are usually spelled out in the policy, but most persons purchasing the policies have little understanding of the cost of a chronic or traumatic event and don't think it will apply to them. As most people understand it, the purpose of insurance is to spread the risk across the largest pool of people. It is accepted that some people will receive more care than others due largely to unforeseen medical needs. (For more information on "junk health-care policies," go to http://www.mcclatchydc.com/2013/12/19/212069/junk-insurance-comes-back-to-haunt.html or http://www.consumerreports.org/cro/magazine/2012/03/junk-health-insurance/index.htm or http://www.forbes.com/sites/danmunro/2013/11/12/estimate-of-junk-health-insurance-market-over-1200-plans-covering-almost-4-million-people/.)

In some cases, insurance companies have suddenly added policy limit caps to policies held by employees who have worked for the same company for many years and have had the same insurance plan. These employees have paid into the company-sponsored insurance for themselves and their families all during their employment. After years of paying their health insurance premiums regularly, they or their family could be left without sufficient insurance coverage if they exceed the cap. Subsequently, they may be unable to get new insurance that they can afford due to a preexisting illness. For people with high-cost chronic disorders such as hemophilia, lifetime caps pose a serious threat that affects health care, career choices, and financial stability.[23]

> *The costs for the uninsured end up falling on taxpayers for government supported programs or private insurers in the form of increased taxes and premiums.*

A study conducted investigating the effects of lifetime caps on employer-sponsored health insurance plans focused on the prevalence of lifetime limits, the number of people affected by them, and the costs of increasing or removing these limits from health insurance plans. The study pointed out that unless they were very wealthy, people with high medical expenses who lose their insurance usually had to resort to seeking Medicaid coverage.[29] Opponents of the ACA believe that those are exactly the types of scenarios in which government should step in rather than controlling all aspects of health care.

Another unethical practice of insurance companies is that of **rescission**—the cancellation of health insurance policies that are already in place. It is legal for insurance companies to cancel policies if the policyholder lied on the initial application to deliberately hide some preexisting condition or other important information. However, some companies have mechanisms or even whole departments in place whose sole job it is to try to find a technicality or error that would justify the retroactive cancellation of medical insurance policies for holders who developed illnesses that required expensive treatment and care.[30]

Lawsuit Opens the Door

In 2007, a court case brought to light the industry-wide but long-hidden practice of withdrawing coverage after expensive medical treatments were already approved.[31] The *Los Angeles Times* filed a suit to make the documents from an arbitration case public. Generally, arbitration cases are sealed and no information about the case can be made public under penalty of the law.

A decision by a judge opened up the documents from the arbitration case so that the insurance company had to make public its actions. The documents showed a direct link between cancellations of employee policies and financial gain for the insurance company. The information revealed that just one company had avoided paying about $35.5 million in medical expenses between 2000 and 2006 by revoking approximately 1,600 policies. The insurance company accomplished this by setting annual savings targets for its employees. The incentive was for revoking policies—employees were rewarded with bonuses for meeting and exceeding the targets.[30] The holders of these revoked policies were left with tens of thousands of dollars of unanticipated medical expenses after policy cancellations, and many of them were unable to receive lifesaving care. A Robert Wood Johnson Foundation research study found that there were documented deaths as a result of interrupting or ending treatment due to recision.[29] It was not an isolated case.

A 2008 congressional investigation into the problem of rescission found insurance was being canceled retroactively "over minor and/or unintentional discrepancies and omissions in a person's application materials or medical records when high cost health care claims were submitted."[32] Chief executives of three of the largest health insurance companies in the nation were called before this congressional committee. Even with only the incomplete documentation provided to Congress from the three companies, between 2003 and 2007, the companies saved more than $300 million from the practice of canceling policies.[32] Lawmakers were appalled and outraged as they listened to case after case of actual rescissions by these three companies.

> *Despite the high levels of health-care spending in the United States, there are fewer physicians per capita than in most developed countries. In 2010, the United States had only 2.4 physicians per 1,000 people, well below the average of 3.1 in developed countries.*

Horror Stories

After being diagnosed with an aggressive form of breast cancer, a nurse from Texas recounted losing her health insurance coverage. The reason she was given for the policy cancellation was because she had not disclosed a visit to a dermatologist for acne many years before, which the insurance company considered a preexisting condition for cancer. A sister of an Illinois man told Congress that he died of lymphoma after the insurer canceled his coverage. At the time, he had already been approved for a lifesaving bone marrow transplant. The rationale for the policy cancellation was failing to report gallstones and the possibility of an aneurysm that were on his chart after an x-ray many years before. This x-ray was never discussed with the client, and even the insurance company was never able to find any evidence that indicated intentional deception on the part of the client.[33]

When the executives of these three major insurance providers were each asked separately by the chairman of the committee if they were willing to limit the cancellation of policies to only cases where they could prove "intentional fraudulent misrepresentation," all three said they would not stop the practice. They noted that there were no state laws that prevented the practice of canceling the policies of clients with high-cost diagnoses and illnesses.[34]

Insurance Regulatory Issues

In the individual health insurance market, regulation is provided through a mix of state and federal endeavors. Although insurance regulation is primarily delegated to the states, the federal government often writes federal policies or protections that are supposed to be incorporated into the state regulations and enforced. One of the most recent of these federal attempts at consumer protections was the Health Insurance Portability and Accountability Act (HIPAA) of 1996. One of its key purposes was to allow employees to bring with them their health insurance policy when they changed jobs and prevent cancellations of polices due to preexisting conditions.

A research project also looked into the cancellation of polices when clients were diagnosed with severe expensive illnesses and how state and federal regulations were being enforced related to these practices. They looked specifically at the success or failure to implement and enforce the provisions of HIPAA.[29] Gaps were found in consumer protections in the state laws and regulations themselves. Enforcement was lacking in all the states they studied.[29]

Other investigations were conducted that revealed a common practice of insurance companies was to cancel or deny claims after an insurance policy had been issued because the client's disease and treatment became too costly. There were no rules or regulations to prevent this practice until passage of the ACA. Overall, the data collected across the nation demonstrated a severe lack of federal oversight and enforcement. Although some insurance companies' negative practices are truly ethical violations, others more appropriately are a result of lack of regulation or regulatory disputes.

A Lack of Information

Another important finding of the study was that none of the states collected enough information to really know what was happening in the insurance market. There was virtually no information about the already identified problem areas of cancellations of policies and denial of claims. They concluded that federal laws alone are not enough to protect people buying insurance.[29] A proactive approach to supervision and regulation enforcement is necessary for regulation enforcement at both the state and federal levels.

Four recommendations were offered based on the lessons learned from studying the case studies from across the nation. The researchers felt that the problems were sufficient enough that federal policymakers should address the regulation of health insurance markets, regardless of whether other national health reform is successful or not. The four recommendations are:

- To the extent states continue to regulate insurance under health reform, state laws must clearly and consistently reflect the federal standards.
- Direct outreach and support on consumer rights must be expanded.
- Regulators must collect more detailed data about the health insurance markets they regulate and use specific criteria on when to carry out a market conduct review.
- The federal government must take on a larger role to protect consumers.[30]

The Congressional Committee on Energy and Commerce reached similar conclusions after they conducted a study in 2008. They issued a memorandum in 2009 that included the following conclusions:

- The market for individual health insurance in the United States is fundamentally flawed.
- The current regulatory framework governing this market is a haphazard collection of inconsistent state and federal laws.
- Protections for consumers and enforcement actions by regulators vary widely, depending on where individuals live.

- Insurance companies take advantage of these inconsistent laws to engage in a series of controversial practices[31] (Table 20.1).

Considering this preceding information, there is overwhelming evidence showing there is a need for health-care insurance reform and an increase in regulation by outside entities. The question, of course, then becomes *how* to go about fixing this system. Some of these issues were addressed in the ACA, but many still remain unresolved. It may take a decade to determine the successes and failures of individual parts of the ACA law.[35]

What Do You Think?

How much did you know about health-care reform before reading this chapter? How much do your parents or elderly relatives know?

" After years of paying their health insurance premiums regularly, they or their family could be left without sufficient insurance coverage if they exceed the cap. "

THE DEBATE

The health-care reform debate rages at all levels, from family members sitting around the dinner table to the halls of Congress and the Oval Room of the White House. It is unlikely that the debate will end any time soon since the ideology of the progressives, mainly Democrats, and conservatives, mainly Republicans, is so different. Progressives believe that for-profit industries that are concerned about their bottom lines are not willing to sacrifice capital to take care of social needs and that the federal government should establish and run substantial social programs, such as for social security, health care, education, and welfare, in order to meet the needs of all citizens, especially those impoverished. They believe that the private sector does not have the will or the money to effectively meet these needs of the poor. An underlying belief is that persons controlling the private sector possibly are greedy and have more self-serving interests than those controlling government.

Yet, conservatives fear that too much government control will lead those in power to potentially abuse citizens' rights for their own gain. The idea is that those in government positions are equally at risk as those in the private sector of being

Table 20.1 **Selected Findings of the 2008 Congressional Investigation of Health Insurance Rescissions**

- Rescinding coverage on the basis of typos in the application form
- Rescinding coverage on the basis that individuals failed to disclose conditions they were unaware they had
- Rescinding coverage for family members incurring high-cost claims, even if they were not involved in the omission or discrepancy
- Investigating the medical histories of all enrollees diagnosed with certain high-cost illnesses or conditions
- Evaluating employees based on how much money they save the company by retroactively canceling policies
- Using a computer algorithm to identify women recently diagnosed with breast cancer to trigger an investigation into their records to find a pretext to rescind coverage

Sources: Prohibiting Rescissions Fact Sheet. Retrieved May 2013 from http://www.dmhc.ca.gov/Portals/0/HealthCareInCalifornia/FactSheets/fscirc.pdf; Prohibiting Rescissions in Women's Health. Retrieved May 2013 from http://www.nationalpartnership.org/site/DocServer/HCR_Prohibiting_Rescissions.pdf?docID=11241

self-serving, greedy, and ultimately immoral. Conservatives believe in individual liberty and personal responsibility and that the government is only responsible to ensure equal opportunity. They think that it is easier to influence a wider base of private enterprise by withholding support of problematic companies than it is to try and retrieve power given to a selected few in government. They believe it is a principle that motivated the Founding Fathers to design the government structure as they did. They are also currently very concerned about the large national debt and annual budget deficits that mean the cost of these programs will need to be paid for by future generations, thus reducing their ability to achieve the American dream. They say that the debt accrued by these programs will eventually cause the greatest harm to those they intend to protect. However, whatever side a person takes, it must be dependent on thoughtful reflection and a full consideration of all the facts rather than a reflexive reaction

to the other side's opinion. There are several issues both sides agree on:

- There needs to be a way to reform a health-care system without taking ever bigger slices out of the GNP.
- Successful reform of health care begins with the realization that there is no perfect health care system.
- Reform needs to be accomplished within a reasonable amount of time at an affordable price.
- Different approaches meet different needs and set different priorities.

All solutions proposed by either side will have both positive and negative aspects. The goal needs to be to find those actions, solutions, and measures that can improve the system and that have the fewest drawbacks. Each health-care system solution attempts to address the highest priorities in health care such as cost, quality, and the most inclusive coverage.

Proponents of the ACA

Proponents of the ACA focus on increasing access to health care for every citizen by removing all the barriers that are now in place and improving the quality of health care by establishing standards and outcomes for treatments. They believe that the cost of treating preventable chronic illness by early detection and prevention will cost much less than treating diseases and their complications in their late stages. It is their position that the limitations currently placed on individuals wishing to purchase health insurance from a poorly regulated industry that has engaged in unethical practices interferes with individual rights and the free marketplace and is discriminatory against minority groups, the working poor, and the middle class. They support the principle that the large health insurance companies who are currently running the health-care system produce increased costs and encourage waste. They believe that health should be paid for based on the quality of care and health-care outcomes rather than the fee-for-service method currently used. They see the ACA and its provisions as a way to eliminate these inadequacies and a means to accomplish their goals. (For more information, go to http://www.rasmussenreports.com/public_content/politics/current_events/healthcare/health_care_law.)

Commodity or Public Good?

The polls on American health care have consistently shown that Americans believe that health care is too expensive and that too many Americans go without needed care due to the lack of insurance. Those in favor of the ACA believe the national debate over reform centers around a philosophical disagreement about what roles the private and public sectors should play in the health-care system. They believe that health care should *not* be treated like just another commodity or service that can be bought and sold in a competitive free market. Rather, it should be considered a public good with the status of a right similar to education and Social Security. Both are administered as government programs and are funded and regulated by the government with the primary goal of providing a public good rather than earning profits for stockholders.

Benefits of the ACA

The proponents of the ACA project that as much as $850 billion will be saved on health care by reducing fraud and abuse, improving communication, and instituting stricter price controls. Reducing and/or eliminating unnecessary tests and treatments and improving efficiency could further reduce costs.[10] It will also eliminate the practice of cost shifting in which those with insurance and the government pay for the uninsured through higher premiums and taxes. Other proposed benefits of the ACA include the following

> *The (court case) information revealed that just one company had avoided paying about $35.5 million in medical expenses between 2000 and 2006 by revoking approximately 1,600 policies.*

Expanded Coverage for American Citizens

- Extends coverage for young adults who can stay on their parents' insurance until age 26
- Expands family planning eligibility for which states can apply
- Sets up insurance exchanges to offer citizens insurance at a competitive cost
- Increases the number of insured by as many as 32 million by 2019

Consumer Protection From Unfair Insurance Practices

- Requires insurance companies to issue or renew a policy regardless of any preexisting condition
- Prevents insurance companies from canceling insurance when the client develops a serious expensive illness

- Prohibits setting annual or lifetime limits (caps)
- Requires coverage of newly issued plans without a client co-pay
- Eliminates co-pays for preventive services such as mammograms and colonoscopies
- Eliminates co-pays for women's preventative services
- Requires coverage for those participating in clinical trials
- Closes the Medicare Part D gap on medications ("doughnut hole") for seniors
- Requires chain restaurants to display caloric content of the meals they serve

Administrative Regulations for Insurance Companies

- Requires simpler, more standardized paperwork, reducing insurance company costs
- Increases competition among insurance companies through insurance exchanges
- Prohibits discriminating against or charging higher rates based on gender or preexisting medical conditions. Age is a factor that can be considered.
- Requires insurance companies to reveal details about administrative and executive expenditures (e.g., salaries, perks, benefits, stock options, etc.)
- Requires insurance companies to spend 80 to 85 percent of policyholders' premium dollars on health costs and claims, leaving 20 to 15 percent, respectively, for administrative costs and profit
- Prohibits enforcing client eligibility waiting periods in excess of 90 days for group health plans
- Establishes a Consumer Assistance Program in each state to help citizens navigate the ACA regulations
- Mandates individual purchase of insurance to lower the cost of premiums
- Requires a broad-enough risk pool to keep costs low

Improving Health-Care Quality

- Establishes the Client-Centered Outcomes Research Institute
- Establishes a New Prevention and Public Health Fund to invest in proven prevention and public health programs; goal is to keep Americans healthy

- Establishes the Center for Medicare & Medicaid Innovation
- Establishes a new trauma center program
- Increases funding for community health centers
- Establishes new programs to support school-based health centers and nurse-managed clinics
- Creates incentives for Accountable Care Organizations (ACO) to meet quality thresholds with shared cost savings
- Establishes Community Care Transitions Program to decrease rehospitalization

Lowering Health-Care Costs

- Sets up a new federal agency, the Independent Payment Advisory Board (IPAB), to recommend how much to pay doctors and hospitals for procedures
  - The Board is intended to be independent but board members are appointed by the president and approved by the Senate.
  - The Board is tasked with containing and reducing increasing health-care costs.
- Links hospital payment to quality outcomes
- Links physician payment to quality outcomes
- Encourages integrated health systems to manage client care at all levels
- Establishes pilot programs to bundle payments
- Cuts government subsidies to insurance companies that operate Medicare Advantage plans without reducing any Medicare benefit
- Stops overpayment to some insurers
- Eliminates waste and fraud in the insurance system by aggressively pursuing cheaters
- Imposes health-care reform fees on pharmaceutical companies that will benefit from the increased number of covered people

Improving Workforce Health Care

- Establishes a National Health Care Workforce Commission
- Expands Public Health Service Commissioned Corps
- Expands primary care and nurse training programs
- Increases funding to National Health Service Corps
- Increases Medicaid payment rates to primary care physicians

- Assists with medical school debt of primary care physicians

Taxes and Funding Changes

- Raises Medicare tax for individuals earning more than $200,000/year and couples earning over $250,000/year from 2.9 to 3.8 percent
- Imposes excise tax on taxable medical devices
- Requires a 3.8 percent tax be applied to all sources of income, not just wages, with some exceptions
- Imposes a penalty on those who are able to and decide not to purchase health insurance
- Imposes a penalty on large employers that do not assist workers with health insurance
- Offers 2 years of tax credits to qualified small businesses to provide health insurance
  - New tax on extremely generous health plans. The hope is individuals who have to pay at least a percentage of their health costs will not abuse the medical system for unneeded care.[8]

> *There was virtually no information about the already identified problem areas of cancellations of policies and denial of claims.*

The ACA has been cited by some organizations and health policy experts as the most comprehensive health-care reform in the history of the United States. They believe it is one of the most far-reaching pieces of social policy since the Civil Rights legislation. Although it is acknowledged that a better national health reform law could probably have been written, it is the bill that passed.[8]

Opponents of the ACA

Opponents to the ACA agree that health-care reform is needed and also agree that everyone should have access to health care and health promotion interventions. They don't agree that this bill as it was passed is the most fiscally efficient way to achieve those goals. They point out that before passage of the bill, 85 percent of the population were covered by private health insurance, Medicare, and Medicaid, and most were satisfied with their insurance. They understood where the deficiencies in access to care occurred and believed it would be more cost-effective to address the needs of the 15 percent who needed help rather than change the system for the 85 percent who were insured.

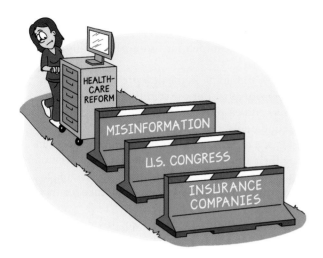

Commodity or Public Good?

Those who oppose the ACA also agree that health care is too expensive, but they disagree that government mandate for the same coverage for everyone regardless of need is the best way to achieve that goal. They believe strongly in a commonsense regulated but still free market system. The health-care insurance industry is one of the most regulated industries in the country, and those regulations are increasing the costs of insurance. Health care *should* be a service that can be bought and sold in a competitive free market based on the needs of the purchaser. Automobile insurance is treated that way. Why not health-care insurance?[10]

Drawbacks of the ACA

Skeptics believe that the ACA forces America's health-care system in the wrong direction by transferring vast powers to governmental bureaucrats. They believe that placing this control under government auspices will reduce competition, one of the main drivers of innovation and improvement. The free marketplace's law of supply and demand has been the key driving force for the tremendous success of the American capitalistic system in most areas of life, and the insurance industry should be left alone to either succeed or fail like any other business. They believe that a profit-driven business produces the best products at the lowest prices because businesses that are not efficient will fail in the marketplace.

The way the ACA bill was passed, government bureaucrats and decision-makers will control the money and decisions that should remain in the hands of individual clients and their families. Subsequently, it presupposes that the government decision-makers have a more compelling interest in the individual's needs and outcomes than insurance companies do. It takes away some of the states' rights to establish regulations and policies. They also believe that the law is fundamentally flawed because of the hasty way it was enacted with undefined provisions that leaves writing the rules and regulations under control of an unelected bureaucrat rather than those who actually represent the constituents. Other weaknesses of the ACA include the following

Effects on the Economy

- Slows economic growth by taking money needed for growth out of the economy
- Reduces employment because the cost of hiring employees will increase
- Suppresses wages because there is an option to reduce work hours to under 30 hours per week to avoid the employer mandate to provide insurance
- Raises taxes, which leaves less money for growing business
- Impedes an already staggering recovery
- Transfers money from productive private hands to the less efficient public sector
- Discourages work and savings by taking money from consumers for more taxes
- Does not really reduce spending because of "double counted savings" and historically government-run programs just cost more to operate
- Increases the federal deficit

Effects on Workplace Health

- Changes the nature of the employer–employee relationship due to the employer mandate
  - Employers will need to have detailed household information, such as family size and income for each family member, from each of their employees.
- Encourages employers to drop coverage due to increased cost of premiums or reduce work hours and avoid paying for insurance
- Increases the invasion of workers' privacy

Effect on Medicare and Medicaid

- Reduces payments to many Medicare providers relative to what they were receiving under the previous law while mandating increases in the coverage they provide

- Delays progress to repair existing unsustainable entitlement programs such as Social Security and Medicare
- Increases costs to low-income and minority senior citizens
- Threatens seniors' access to care by reducing the supply of providers

Effects on State's Rights

- Directly assaults the states' traditional rights to regulate health insurance. They believe that the powers the federal government have taken to implement this program are not supported by the Constitution and these rights belong to the states.
- Imposes unknown insurance costs on consumers, states, and the federal government. Unlike the federal government, states are required to balance their budgets. The unknown costs put states in a position of having to fund the programs imposed by the federal mandate without the funding to keep the programs running.
- Grants more discretionary authority to unelected federal bureaucrats to micromanage health insurance coverage than state legislatures have ever granted to state insurance regulators
- Fails to take into consideration the different health needs of different states or individuals

Effects on Health-Care Providers

- Increases costs of managing their practice because of the need to comply with an increased number of regulations and need for documentation
- Cuts payments to physicians across the board by 25 percent. Decreased reimbursements and increased costs risk a reduction in supply of health-care providers.
- Limits and loosens conscience protection for clients from unscrupulous providers
- Requires providers to make available services that are opposed to their religious beliefs

Effects on Insurance Providers

- Dooms insurance companies to failure because the rules for setting up exchange plans are too complicated—most insurance companies cannot meet the qualifications.
- Undermines competition among health insurance companies
- Creates ambiguity in the new preventive care requirements that impose significant penalties if insurers and employers do not comply with DHS requirements
- Puts at a disadvantage private business by restricting their ability to be profitable. This will eventually cause them to go bankrupt, ultimately leading to government-controlled health insurance for their workers.
- Increases the odds of eliminating private insurance companies, making the single-payer system controlled by government the only option
- Decreases incentive or innovation and improvement because the bureaucratic system will be unable to effectively manage such a large system
- Prevents insurance companies from meeting the needs of individuals and requires them to provide coverage the individual doesn't need. As a result, individual's premiums will be higher.

> " *Health care should be a service that can be bought and sold in a competitive free market based on the needs of the purchaser. Automobile insurance is treated that way. Why not health-care insurance?* "

Effects on the Public

- Forces younger, healthier individuals to pay higher premiums to cover the care of older, sicker adults. That is an additional financial burden on a generation that is already burdened with a poor job market and high education costs, which will significantly affect their ability to improve their lives.
- Requires care decisions to be made by unelected bureaucrats rather than individuals and families. That assumes that persons not involved in the care of the individual will make more caring and moral decisions than families will.
- Makes it more difficult to cover the uninsured because there will be fewer providers
- Massively increases the dependence on government programs at the cost of reduced private coverage.[14] They believe that setting up systems that make citizens dependent rather than independent is morally wrong.
- Requires individuals to pay for procedures and treatments that violate their religious beliefs

Although there have been several drafts of health-reform plans drawn up by the opponents of the ACA, they have never been introduced by the legislative bodies. However, opponents believe that an effective health-care reform plan would include:

- Providing individual tax deductions for all persons purchasing private health insurance similar to those provided for businesses
- Promoting new group purchasing arrangements based on individual membership organizations and various associations, including union, fraternal, ethnic, and religion-based groups
- Allowing insurance companies to sell policies across state lines without regulation to increase competition
- Allowing employers to convert their health-care compensation from a defined benefit package to a defined contribution system
- Improving consumer-directed health options (such as health savings accounts, health reimbursement arrangements, and flexible spending accounts) that encourage greater transparency and consumer control over health-care decisions
- Extending national preexisting condition protections in the non–group health insurance markets for those with continuous creditable coverage, thus rewarding responsible persons who buy and maintain coverage
- Setting up a fair competitive bidding process to determine government payment in traditional Medicare fee-for-service and Medicare Advantage programs
- Reviewing Medicare rules and regulations and eliminating those that unduly burden doctors and clients, such as the restriction preventing doctors and patients to contract privately for medical services outside of the traditional Medicare program
- Encouraging the states to set up mechanisms such as high-risk pools and risk transfer models that help lessen the problems of individuals who are difficult to insure
- Expanding states' ability to develop consumer-based reforms that enable states to customize solutions for their citizens
- Strengthening premium assistance in Medicaid to enable young families to obtain private health insurance coverage
- Improving client-centered health-care models for those on Medicaid

- Increasing federal and state efforts to combat fraud and abuse in Medicaid, including tightening eligibility loopholes in Medicaid for long-term care services
- Encouraging personal savings and the development of a robust private insurance market for long-term-care needs
- Making the ban on taxpayer-funded abortion permanent
- Making a permanent government-wide policy to ensure protection of the right of conscience among medical providers and personnel
- Halting all new tax increases and promoting tax cuts that would expand private insurance coverage and grow the economy
- Reforming medical malpractice laws to ensure strong patient protection while limiting trial lawyer fees and non-economic damages

(For more information, go to the Case Against Obamacare at http://www.heritage.org/research/projects/the-case-against-obamacare; Ferarra, P. Look out below, Obamacare chaos is coming. 2013. Retrieved September 2014 from http://www.forbes.com/fdc/welcome_mjx.shtml; The 4 best legal arguments against Obamacare. Retrieved May 2014 from http://reason.com/archives/2012/03/24/4-best-legal-arguments-against-obamacare.)

Many of those who oppose the ACA point out that it imposes numerous tax hikes that transfer more than $500 billion over 10 years out of the pockets of hardworking American families and businesses and into the pockets of a Congress that is not known for being careful about how tax dollars are spent. They believe that the spending on new entitlements and subsidies will discourage economic growth both now and in the future and removes peoples' incentive to work to reach their maximum potential while becoming participating members of society.

They want to see the current ACA replaced by a system that values limited intrusion of government on individual's daily lives and the free market. They want health-care decisions to remain with individuals and their families rather than relinquishing those decisions to unaccountable people they do not know. Additionally, they want to ensure that competition in both health care and health insurance industries continues to spur innovation and treatment effectiveness. Only in this way will there be true health-care reform that would reduce the number of the uninsured, improve the quality of and accessibility to care, make health care more affordable, and reduce the budget deficit.

What Do You Think?

Where do you stand on the health-care debate? Is there a middle ground where you see the positive aspects of some of the reforms in the ACA while understanding that there is room for improvement?

ANA POSITION ON HEALTH-CARE REFORM

The first Nursing's Agenda for Health Care Reform in 1991 was endorsed by over 60 nursing and other health organizations. This document underwent two significant updates. They recognized that the ongoing shortage of nurses and other health professions and a rapidly growing body of scientific research reinforced the critical need for change.[34] The ANA continues its strong commitment to its belief that health care is a human right. All persons should have access to affordable, high-quality health-care services when they need them. The health of individuals, the strength of society, national well-being, and the overall productivity of the United States will be positively impacted when there is accessible, affordable, and high-quality health care for all citizens. The updates made to the initial ANA document include:

> *The ANA continues its strong commitment to its belief that health care is a human right. All persons should have easy access to affordable, high-quality health-care services when they need them.*

- The ANA reaffirms its support for a restructured health-care system that ensures universal access to a standard package of essential health-care services for all citizens and residents.
- The ANA believes that the development and implementation of health policies that reflect the six IOM aims (i.e., safe, effective, client-centered, timely, efficient, and equitable) are based on outcomes research and will ultimately save money.
- The system must be reshaped and redirected away from the overuse of expensive, technology-driven, acute, hospital-based services in the model we now have to one in which a balance is struck between high-tech treatment and community-based and preventive services, with emphasis on the latter. The solution is to invert the pyramid of priorities and focus more on primary care, thus ultimately requiring less costly secondary and tertiary care.
- Ultimately, the ANA supports a single-payer mechanism as the most desirable option for financing a reformed health-care system.[34]

The recommendations from this 17-page Health System Reform Agenda addresses many of the issues that have been raised. The recommendations made in 1991 have been upheld as reasonable and necessary steps to correct a flawed health-care system, and the updates reflected the most current research and statistics. All major bipartisan health-care policy organizations, constituency groups, and many consumer advocacy groups have made policy recommendations that support the direction proposed by the ANA.[36]

The ANA believes that the new reforms are designed to move the country from a system that provides illness care to one that provides client-centered and preventive health care. This is the type of care that is provided best by nurses.[37] The ACA addressed the majority of the ANA Reform Agenda. However, the ACA does not explicitly declare health care a human right and does not provide for a single-payer system.[38] The AARP also agrees with the ANA concerning nurses, the amount and type of funding provided, and the administrative division responsible for the provisions.[39,40]

SUMMARY OF THE AFFORDABLE CARE ACT OF 2010

The original Patient Protection and Affordable Care Act (PPACA) contained 10 titles and was signed into law on March 23, 2010. The Health Care Education and Reconciliation Act (HCERA) of 2010 made amendments to the original 10 titles. The HCERA was signed into law on March 30 after being approved by the House and Senate on March 25, 2010. The term Affordable Care Act (ACA) refers to the PPACA as modified by the HCERA.

There are a total of 487 sections and 906 pages included in the ACA.

The verifiable final page count in the bill itself is 906, with an additional 109 pages of regulations written by DHS.[41] The length and complexity of the ACA is a testament to how comprehensive the changes are, addressing almost all aspects of the current health-care system. There are 10 titles or sections to the ACA:

Title I: Quality, Affordable Health Care for All Americans

Title II: The Role of Public Programs

Title III: Improving the Quality and Efficiency of Health Care

Title IV: Prevention of Chronic Disease and Improving Public Health

Title V: Health Care Workforce

Title VI: Transparency and Program Integrity

Title VII: Improving Access to Innovative Medical Therapies

Title VIII: Community Living Assistance Services and Supports Act (CLASS Act) (Repealed in January 2013)

Title IX: Revenue Provisions

Title X: Reauthorization of the Indian Health Care Improvement Act[42–46]

(See Table 20.2.)

Evaluating Health-Care Reform

With all the state-of-the-art diagnostic tests and treatments available in the United States, the highly respected and innovative doctors, and many of the world's best hospitals, the United States produces many of the significant advances in technology and

Table 20.2 What the ACA Does

Major Revisions	Date
Expanded Coverage	
• Extending coverage for young adults by allowing them to stay on parents' insurance until age 26	2010
• States can apply to expand family planning eligibility to same eligibility as pregnancy.	2010
• Insurance exchanges will be set up.	2013
• Congressional Budget Office (CBO) estimates as many as 32 million more people could have some form of health insurance by 2019.	
• Half through increased Medicaid coverage—eligibility increased up to 133 percent of poverty level	2014
• Half through private insurance exchanges	2014
Insurance Regulation/Consumer Protection	
• **Guaranteed Issue**	2010 new
• Insurers will be required to issue or renew a policy regardless of any preexisting condition.	2014 existing
• Should provide coverage for an additional 20 million	
• **Outlaws rescissions**	
• Insurer can no longer accept insurance payments as long as you are healthy and then find a reason to cancel your coverage when you become ill.	2010
• **Prohibits setting annual or lifetime limits**	2010 new
• Insurer can't terminate coverage because your illness became too expensive.	2014 existing
• Insurers are required to reveal details about administrative and executive expenditures.	2010
• Insurers must spend 80 to 85 percent of premium dollars on health costs and claims, leaving only 15 to 20 percent for administrative costs and profit.	2011
• New plans must cover without deductible:	
• Preventive services (i.e., mammograms and colonoscopies).	2012
• Women's preventative services.	
• Limits administrative costs	2012
• Top is 15–20 percent	

(continued)

Table 20.2 **What the ACA Does—cont'd**

Major Revisions	Date
• Requirement to use simpler, more standardized paperwork	
• Set up insurance exchanges for self-insured in each state	2013
• Prohibited from discriminating against or charging higher rates based on gender	2013
or preexisting medical conditions but not based on age	2014
• Prohibited client eligibility waiting periods in excess of 90 days for group health	2014
plans	
• Ensures coverage to those participating in clinical trials	2014
• Establish Consumer Assistance Programs in states	2014
• Individual Mandate	2014
• Required to have a broad enough risk pool to keep costs low	
Improving Quality and Lowering Costs	
• **Establish Client-Centered Outcomes Research Institute**	2010
• **Providing Preventive Care in coverage**	2010
• **New Prevention & Public Health Fund**	2010
• Invest in proven prevention & public health programs	2011-2020
• Closing the Medicare Part D gap on medications ("doughnut hole")	2011
• Establish Center for Medicare & Medicaid Innovation	2011
Improving Quality and Lowering Costs	
• Sets up a new federal agency, the Independent Payment Advisory Board	2011
• To recommend how much to pay doctors and hospitals for procedures	
• Independent board but appointed by the president	
• Tasked with containing and reducing increasing health-care costs	
• Establish new trauma center program	2011
• Increased funding for community health centers	2011
• Establish new programs to support school-based health centers and	2011
nurse-managed clinics	
• Create incentives for accountable care organizations to meet quality thresholds	2012
with shared cost savings	
• Community Care Transitions Program to decrease rehospitalization	2012
• Linking hospital payment to quality outcomes	
• Linking physician payment to quality outcomes	2014
• Encouraging integrated health systems	
• Pilot program to bundle payments	
Workforce Issues	
• Establish a National Health Care Workforce Commission	2010
• Expanded Public Health Service Commissioned Corp	2010
• Primary care and nurse training programs expanded	2011
• Increased funding to National Health Service Corp	2011
• Increase Medicaid payment rates to primary care physicians	2013
• Help pay medical school debt of primary care physicians	2013
Taxes and Other funding	
• Cuts taxpayer subsidies to insurers who operated Medicare Advantage plans	2011
• This does not reduce any Medicare benefit.	
• It stops overpayment to some insurers.	
• Has provisions for the elimination of waste and fraud	2011
• Fees imposed on drug manufacturers	2011
• Raises Medicare tax for individuals earning >$200,000 & couples earning	2011
>$250,000 from 2.9 percent to 3.8 percent	
• Imposes excise tax on taxable medical devices	2013

Table 20.2 **What the ACA Does—cont'd**

Major Revisions	Date
• Requires for the first time that 3.8 percent be applied to non-wage income with exceptions	2013
• Penalty on those who don't buy insurance, waived in 2014 because of problems with program rollout	2014
• Penalty on large employers that don't assist workers with health insurance	2014
• New tax on "Cadillac" insurance plans (extremely generous health plans)	2014
• The hope is individuals who have to pay at least a percentage of their health costs will not abuse the medical system for unneeded care.	
Other	
• Chain restaurants required to display caloric content	2010
• Two years of tax credits will be offered to qualified small businesses to provide health insurance	2013

Sources: ANA health reform timeline. Retrieved May 2013 from http://www.rnaction.org/site/PageServer?pagename= nstat_take_action_healthcare_reform&ct=1; Key features of ACA by year. Retrieved May 2013 from http://www. healthcare.gov

biomedical research. However, with a health-care delivery system that is fragmented, wasteful, inefficient, irrational, and unsustainably expensive, the United States continues to lag behind in many categories that define a healthy country.[47]

Health performance indicators that showed significant deterioration or no improvement since 2006 and 2008 include insurance costs and access to care, affordable care, primary and preventive care, hospitalizations from nursing homes, and rehospitalizations. Additional indicators that raise concerns are infant mortality; childhood obesity; safe care; client-centered, timely, coordinated care; and disparities. There is as much as a fourfold difference between the top and bottom performing hospitals, health plans, and geographic regions in the United States.[23] If the top performers in providing health care, quality of facilities, insurance coverage, and geographical areas are four times better than the bottom performers, the high performers should be able to provide the lessons and experience needed to lead the way to improvements. Unfortunately, the current fee-for-service system rewards the numbers of services and not high-quality outcomes.[48]

Along with identifying the health-care delivery issues that need to be improved, how it can be paid for in the most cost-effective way also needs to be addressed. There is no question that health-care costs are rising. One of the main reasons for this

problem has been anticipated since the late 1940s when the birth rate escalated after World War II. These baby boomers have significantly influenced costs as they aged, beginning with the increased costs of building schools and eventually, as the early baby boomers enter their older years, creating a huge demand for health-care services.

What was not anticipated was the recent recession, job losses, and the fact that many of them were unwilling or unable to save sufficient amounts to retire in good fiscal shape. Many lost their insurance when they lost their jobs and didn't have sufficient income to purchase insurance, which now costs more because of age and preexisting conditions. Therefore, some need to choose between health care, needed prescription drugs, and food. Additionally, the recession and job losses affect many more Americans who don't have the money to purchase individual insurance plans, especially without a job. For taxpayers and government budgets, programs such as Medicare and Medicaid must bear a greater share of financial coverage of health care than ever before. This means a larger share of government budgets is being absorbed by increased health-care costs.

Passage of the ACA did immediately provide some relief to those underinsured or uninsured, including closure of the "doughnut hole" or the drug coverage gap in Part D, where 6.3 million Medicare recipients have saved over $6.1 billion on prescription drugs since the enactment of the ACA.[49] Other popular benefits include the following:

- Medicare beneficiaries and Americans with private insurance took advantage of newly covered preventive services and screenings at no cost to them.
- Young adults up to age 26 can now be covered by their parents' private insurance due to extension of coverage provided under the ACA.
- Americans with preexisting conditions now cannot be refused health insurance because of their condition.
- Americans will no longer have limits on coverage or increased premiums due to age ratings.[50]

A private insurance carrier launched a patient-centered medical home (PCMH) program in 2011 with 3,600 primary care practices. In the first year of operation, the PCMH program saved $40 to $50 million in expenses when compared to the projected cost of care. Primary care physicians are no longer being paid by the number of services provided. Rather, they are being paid to deliver a healing relationship while collecting the data needed to manage their clients.[51]

The ACA has provisions that target many of the identified gaps in care, including reduced access, affordability, and support for innovations to make care more client-centered and coordinated.

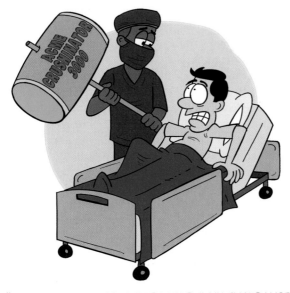

"THIS IS THE ONLY PROCEDURE YOUR JUNK INSURANCE POLICY ALLOWS FOR BREAKING UP KIDNEY STONES!"

There are also federal incentives to facilitate the adoption of meaningful use of health information technology.[23] Health information technology advances can decrease health-care costs through administrative cost savings related to record keeping and provision of data to compare effectiveness data, help identify root causes of problems, and identify ideal staffing problems. This same information technology (IT) could increase safety by having a portable electronic health record that prevents duplicative or inappropriate treatment because of a lack of complete information, potentially reducing medical errors. IT can increase the use of latest research and evidence by clinicians and allow clients the ability to compare treatments, facilities, and providers.[52] Clients and caregivers have input individually and collectively through organizations into setting the research agenda.[53]

FULL IMPLEMENTATION OF THE ACA

The passage of the ACA was a significant achievement but is not the end of the political battle.[54] Many states have attempted to overturn or not comply with the law because of the impact of it on their budgets. The landmark Supreme Court decision upholding the vast majority of the ACA on June 28, 2012, and the reelection of Barack Obama in November 2012 signaled that the ACA has a good chance of not being repealed.[55] However, the real and perceived success of its many provisions and demands for changes to it will depend upon many future factors.

What Still Needs to Be Implemented

States that choose to set up state exchanges were required to have them in place by October 1, 2013. The national eligibility for Medicaid increases to 133 percent of the poverty level at the beginning of 2014.[56] States that were planning to operate state-based exchanges had to submit an exchange blueprint to the federal Department of Health and Human Services (HHS) by December 2012, and states planning for a state-federal partnership had to submit by February 15, 2013. Seventeen states and the District of Columbia have declared their intent to establish state-only-based exchanges. Only 7 states have submitted plans to pursue a state-federal partnership exchange. As of March 2014, 26 states have indicated they will not create a state exchange, which will cause an initial default to a federally facilitated exchange.[57] (For more information, go to http://obamacarefacts.com/state-health-insurance-exchange.php.)

The rollout of the exchanges didn't happen as smoothly as hoped. The software programs created both access to information and sign-up issues, more people lost their insurance than actually signed up, there was a problem with the exchanges supplying incorrect information to insurance companies, and many people found that they still could not afford the cost. Problems occur in the rollout of many large government programs, so perceptions of the benefits of the program may change over time. Numbers recently released showed that some of those who did sign up for insurance were eligible for Medicaid. By March 31, 2014, the second deadline date, over 8 million individuals and families had enrolled in the ACA, which was the goal for this enrollment period.[58] To attract more people to sign up, new commercials were being aired targeting young adults.

Electronic Enrollment

All exchanges must allow consumers to apply for and enroll in coverage online, in person, by phone, by fax, or by mail. They must provide assistance that is language and culturally appropriate. There must be access to call centers and a website with information about insurance options and application assistance.[59] There should be a Navigator program to improve public awareness and facilitate enrollment (see Chapter 27). The computerized system must determine eligibility for public programs, premium tax credits, and cost-sharing subsidies for those purchasing insurance through the exchange.[60]

Some governors have refused to participate in the exchanges because, while early costs were to be paid from the federal budget, once the programs are established, the costs will need to be covered by state budgets, which could significantly influence their ability to balance their budgets without large tax increases. However, in many of the states that have established exchanges, large numbers of people have signed up for insurance. As this process moves forward, HHS will have to assume primary responsibility for operating exchanges in the states that opted out of the process. HHS will seek to coordinate with state agencies on multiple fronts, and although cooperation is not mandatory, it will be important to ensure effective and smooth operation.[61]

One of the least popular parts of the ACA—the individual mandate—was to go into effect in 2014, but its implementation has been delayed until at least 2016. The mandate has also been called *individual responsibility*, in that it acknowledges that everyone is in some state of health at any given time in their lives and everyone plans on growing older, which usually increases the need for health care. Paying for health-care insurance throughout a person's life span makes the costs more affordable for all in the long run. The insurance industry maintains that the only way to cover everyone who needs insurance, without being able to deny those with preexisting conditions, is to require persons who will pay to purchase insurance but not use it.[8] Without the individual mandate, the concern is that young people without chronic health problems would opt out of paying for insurance premiums until they became sick or were injured in an accident. Without the mandate, the cost of universal health care becomes prohibitively high for insurance companies and the government.[62]

Before the passage of the ACA, Republicans strongly supported the idea of the individual mandate for purchasing health insurance as a measure of the individual citizens being responsible for self-care.[63] The idea of the mandate is that all citizens would be required to purchase some type of health insurance to spread the cost out and lower premiums, which fits well with the Republican free market ideology. It is not a new idea. If a person owns an automobile, states have required an individual mandate for auto insurance for over 40 years. Like automobile insurance, the ACA allows individuals to select from a menu of policies that range from very expensive to relatively cheap; however, a driver has the option to give up his automobile, drivers license, and abstain from driving and thereby does not need to purchase insurance, whereas the ACA requires all individuals to have health insurance since all individuals have some state of health all the time.

The origins for the idea for an individual mandate for health insurance is most often credited from the severely conservative Heritage Foundation; however, they did not endorse the part of the mandate that allowed the government to set standards for insurance policies and regulations for the insurance industry.[64] They believe that the free market and individual insurance companies will regulate themselves. The mandate was also initially adopted and supported by most of the Republican Party; however, after it became part of the ACA, almost all these supporters changed their minds and now oppose it.[65]

Lack of Funding of the Provisions

There has been a continuing difficulty in getting funding for many of the provisions of the ACA. Even provisions that were originally funded in the law have had funding cuts in subsequent budgets. For instance, the National Healthcare Workforce Commission was established with a four-part mission to (1) serve as a resource for governments, (2) evaluate education and training activities to determine if demand for health-care workers is being met, (3) identify and make recommendations to address barriers to better coordination between federal and state agencies, and (4) encourage innovations to address population needs.[66] Although members have been appointed, no funds have been appropriated for this Commission and the members have been barred from meeting even at their own expense.

Changes in Financing

Although the ACA is referred to as health-care reform, it changes the way health care is financed and how outcomes can be improved.[67] As it is implemented, there will be a significant impact on federal revenues, direct or mandatory spending, and discretionary spending. Some of these changes in spending will be directly related to quality of care and health-care outcomes. Although the ACA is projected to bring in or save money to pay for itself and lower the deficit, many of the built-in costs of the ACA must be approved annually by Congress.[68] Congress can always refuse to fund a program that has already been voted into law.

Projected funding of many other ACA programs have been removed as a result of mandatory budget cuts. Two programs that are very important to nursing have suffered the same fate. First, a program was established in Section 5208 to support nurse-managed health centers that provided comprehensive primary care and wellness services to vulnerable or underserved populations. This section authorized

$50 million and money as necessary for the program. Congress allocated $15 million from another fund in 2011, but no appropriations were made after that date.[69] Research into many of the issues raised in the IOM report "For the Public's Health: Investing in a Healthier Future" was authorized by the ACA. However, funding and infrastructure development for the program were still not available at the time the report was published in 2012.[70]

What Happens if the ACA is Repealed?

An analysis of the projected data through 2019 determined the impact of repealing all or part of the ACA. For the ACA to work, it needed all three legs of the three-legged stool concept that the ACA was based on: guaranteed issue of insurance regardless of preexisting issues, the individual mandate, and the subsidies to make the insurance affordable.[69]

Based on the analysis, the following conclusions were reached:

- Repealing the requirement to buy insurance would mean more people would wait until they got sick to buy insurance in the new non-group exchanges, which would increase the average premium by 27 percent in 2019.
- Retaining the law's insurance reforms but repealing the subsidies and the requirement to purchase insurance would further discourage people from buying insurance when they're healthy. Premiums in 2019 would cost twice as much as projected under the law as a result.[71]
- Retaining the law but repealing the mandate would cover fewer than 7 million new people in 2019, rather than the 32 million projected to be newly covered by the law. Federal spending, however, would decline by only about a quarter under this scenario since the sickest and most costly uninsured are the ones most likely to gain coverage.
- Retaining only the insurance reforms in the law—repealing both the mandate and the subsidies—would not increase the number of people with insurance, leaving 55 million people uninsured in 2019.[72]

The Effect of Waivers on the Costs of the ACA

Some who are concerned about the costs of the ACA focus on how the waivers that are included in the law will affect how much the government will have to pay to cover new customers. There are six waivers granted under the ACA for various reasons to certain segments of the population (Box 20.1).

B o x   2 0 . 1

Waivers to the ACA

- **Medical loss ratio waiver** for mini-med (junk) health insurance plans used by the fast-food industry that experiences a high turnover rate in employees. This will likely be revoked by the time of full implementation of the ACA.
- **Annual limit waiver** also associated with "junk" policies used by the fast-food industry and was eliminated in 2014.
- **Medical loss ratio waiver** (adjustment) for entire United States is designed to counteract the possible effect of the ACA on limiting the number of insurance companies in any particular state. Maine is the only state that has officially applied for this waiver.
- **State innovation waiver** for states that develop health-care insurance plans that cover as much or more than the ACA at a lower cost.
- **Accountable care organizations (ACO) antitrust waiver** has not yet been developed. ACOs are similar to health maintenance organizations (HMO) who serve at least 5,000 Medicare clients with higher quality care at a lower cost than required by the ACA.
- **Individual mandate waivers** include the following groups or individuals:
  1. Contentious objectors based on religious grounds
  2. Members of a religious organization that provides health care as its main mission
  3. Some illegal immigrants, although they are not covered by the ACA and are unable to get care
  4. Incarcerated persons
  5. Individuals below the poverty line
  6. Members of a recognized Indian tribe
  7. Individuals suffering a "hardship" that affects their income
  8. All members of Congress and the congressional staff

Although it is difficult to estimate how many people may fall under the mandate waiver, it is estimated that between 9 and 12 percent of the population will qualify for them. However, many of these groups, such as prisoners, Indian tribe members, and Congress already have health insurance from other state or federal government programs.[73] Illegal immigrants are specifically barred from obtaining any health coverage, treatments, or care under the ACA plan, and it only makes sense that they should not have to pay for something they are unable to use. Also, registering for care under ACA would expose them to deportation. Interestingly, private insurance companies are willing to sell plans to illegal immigrants outside of the ACA restrictions. (For more information about waivers, go to http://heartland.org/policy-documents/six-types-obamacare-waivers or http://www.healthcare.gov/exemptions/ or http://www.forbes.com/sites/theapothecary/2012/07/09/obamacares-dark-secret-the-individual-mandate-is-too-weak/.)

Lack of Knowledge About the Provisions of the ACA

When evaluating the results of their Health Tracking Poll 3 years after passage of the ACA, the Kaiser Family Foundation (KFF) reports there has not been an increase in the public knowledge of the provisions of the ACA since 2010. More disturbing are the results that show that, while over half of Americans say they do not have enough information about the ACA to understand how it will affect them, that percentage rises to two-thirds in some of the key groups the law was designed to help.[1] The reason for this lack of knowledge seems to stem from the fact that most of what the public has heard for several years has been partisan debate.[39] Although the government and many organizations such as American Association of Retired Persons (AARP), the KFF, and others have created Web pages and materials to help educate people, these efforts have obviously not been effective enough in reaching or educating those in need of education.

In January 2013, a national survey of adults aged 18 to 64 who are under 400 percent poverty level was conducted and found that 78 percent of uninsured adults and 83 percent of the Medicaid expansion population were unaware of new options for insurance starting in 2014. This study also looked at communication needs, how best to help, outreach tools, and a cluster analysis of the diverse population. Three recommendations were made from this study: (1) use key facts to raise awareness, (2) emphasize core motivations, and (3) address skepticism.[74]

CHALLENGES FOR THE FUTURE

Many of the most popular provisions of the ACA are among the least widely recognized, including giving tax credits to small businesses to buy insurance, closing the Medicare "doughnut hole," and extending dependent coverage. One of the harsh realities of a two-party political system is that, sometimes, what is in the best interest of the public as a whole is not in the best interest of one or the other political party. As of May 2014, the Republican House of Representatives passed over 50 bills to repeal the ACA, none of which were successful.

Controlling the Costs of Medical Care

There are many concerns, some that started even before the provisions began to take place, that the ACA will not do enough to control costs. If insurance premiums continue to rise as much as they have in the past, it could endanger the very heart of the bill—to provide affordable health care to almost all. The political realities of trying to seek concessions from powerful financial interests in the health-care industry, without alienating them in the process, required politicians to accept less than was wanted. Many economists believe that the market control exerted by medical providers and drug companies is the primary dynamic driving up costs. Many reports point to the reality that procedures and medical products cost far more in this country than they do elsewhere.

The biggest loss for cost containment, without consideration of a single payer, may have been the loss of the "public option." Although the supporters of the public option promoted it primarily as competition with the private insurance companies to keep premiums down, some economists believed that its purchasing power in seeking lower rates from medical providers would have been its biggest potential financial impact,[75] while others believed that lack of competition would reduce

"Nurses need to remain vigilant and involved, particularly at the state level."

innovation needed to find most cost-effective tests and treatments.

Empowering Public Health

Clinical hospital-based medicine has for many years now separated itself from the public health community, which is primarily concerned with prevention measures and the health of the population at large.[5] The IOM addresses resource needs and ways to approach them in a predictable and sustainable manner that ensures a robust and sustainable health-care system for the entire population.[67] The summary of this report states that it is not sufficient to expect that changes in payment, access, and quality alone will improve the public's health. As a large proportion of the diseases overburdening our health-care system are preventable, the failure to develop and deliver preventive strategies through the public health system will continue to create a burden on the U.S. economy. The ACA recognizes this problem and addresses it in Titles II and VIII.

Health Literacy

The National Patient Safety Foundation (NPSF) produced a fact sheet in 2011 called "Health Literacy: Statistics at a Glance." They reported that 90 million adults in the United States are at risk due to limited health literacy.[72]

The full implementation of the ACA will mean that approximately 16 million more people will be added to the Medicaid roles. Lack of health literacy is present in all demographic groups but is more common in the same demographic groups that determine eligibility for Medicaid (i.e., lower socioeconomic status, limited education, and people with mental or physical disabilities). People with health literacy deficits will have difficulty in several ways. It will be difficult for them to understand the multiple types of coverage offered by the ACA and which one is best for them. They will find it difficult to make an informed choice and difficult to complete the complicated forms for eligibility. This group will have problems in initiating their own care and interacting with health-care providers to make their health-care needs known.[73]

Public Opinion

There is always an inverse relationship between public opinion and politics: Public opinion helps drive political decisions, and politics helps form public opinion.[74] Change is always a little frightening for people. In the midst of formulating comprehensive legislation affecting everyone's lives, it was easy to get people to start thinking about what they might lose, rather than understanding what benefits their families or the nation would gain,[10] mainly because they have experience with what they are currently doing but no guarantees that the promised gains will happen.

Social Determinants of Health

When looking at the determinants of health, it is important to consider the social determinants. Researchers have found that better health outcomes in life expectancy, infant mortality, and potential years of life lost were associated with the ratio of social spending to health services spending. The United States is one of only two OECD countries that spend less on social services than health services.[74]

Lessons From Other Countries

When anyone suggests that the United States should look to other countries to find solutions to its health-care problems, the first thing most often heard is "we don't want socialized medicine." This term has come to be associated with everything Americans don't want in terms of health care—long lines, government control, rationing of health care, death panels, and communism. The reality is that wealthy, technologically advanced countries that are just as committed as the United States is to equal opportunity, individual liberty, and the free market have found ways to cover all their citizens with basic health care, spend less money, have better health outcomes, and be more satisfied with their care than Americans.[18] By analyzing both positive and negative outcomes of health-care payment systems in other nations, the United States can design a system that ensures personal freedom while supporting those most in need.

Reforming American health care does not mean that the United States could or should copy any country's institutions exactly. Americans cannot *adopt* another country's structure, but they can *adapt* those approaches to America's inherited conditions.

> *It is part of the professional responsibility of nurses to educate themselves about the facts in the health-care debate.*

OPPORTUNITIES FOR NURSING IN HEALTH REFORM

In December 2011, 21 nurses were among 73 health-care professionals selected through the CMS Innovation Center as "innovation advisors."[75] They are responsible for testing projects to see if they can achieve CMS's triple aim of better health, better care, and lowered costs through continuous improvement.[44] President Obama has demonstrated his respect for members of the nursing profession and the role they can play in the health care of the future.

With the full implementation of the ACA and its corresponding increase in clients who will be seeking health care, advanced practice nurses will be in even greater demand as primary care providers. Studies have shown that advanced practice nurses can meet the primary care needs of large segments of the population, ranging from well-child evaluations for pediatric clients to screening for chronic diseases found in the elderly population. There will also be additional demands for qualified nurses in any number of health-care fields such as nursing informatics, case managers, and nurse navigators. There are potential roles for nurses that will be created by the ACA that do not even yet have names.

Nurses need to remain vigilant and involved, particularly at the state level. It is important that advanced practice registered nurses (APRNs) are included in any discussions of state revisions of nursing practice acts as key providers in the health-care system. They must be allowed to practice to the full extent of their education and capabilities and receive appropriate reimbursement. As decisions are being made on how to contain costs, nurses working every day with clients must participate in the process to ensure that nursing activities are identified and measured.

Registered nurses are the largest group of providers of care who directly impact client outcomes. It is part of the professional responsibility of nurses to educate themselves about the facts and the input of both sides of the health-care debate. A significant increase in percentage of registered nurses joining their primary professional organization, the ANA, would give nursing one of the largest and most powerful voices in the country. Nurses should work with both political parties on issues important to health care and be able to identify misinformation or distortion of facts and make sound judgments and decisions based on the truth. The American public trusts nurses to advocate for their best interests. They have been rated number one for the past ten years on the Gallup polls for most trusted and honored professions.

Conclusion

The debate about the best way to pay for health care and improve client outcomes will go on well into the future as the various components of the ACA are fully implemented or changed. With a law as extensive as this, it would be expected that provisions will be modified or eliminated as they are rolled out and unforeseen problems and unintended consequences become evident.

It is important that nurses have input into all phases of the implementation and outcome analysis of health-care changes. They were at the table when it was initially designed, and they need to be there when problems arise. Nurses have a wide range of knowledge and firsthand experiences in the health-care system at all levels, knowledge and experiences that are very useful and highly sought after by policymakers. The most effective way for individual nurses to make their voices heard is by joining a professional organization. Politicians respect groups with large numbers of votes. Nurses will feel the impact of health-care reform in multiple ways, such as increased numbers of clients, changes in facility organizational structures, and increased demand for more nurses. The old adage "If you're not part of the solution, you're part of the problem" was never so true as it relates to the nursing profession and health-care reform.

Critical-Thinking Exercises

1. Find one of your classmates whose opinion of the ACA differs from yours. Have a thoughtful discussion with him or her about health-care reform. Try to formulate a "middle ground" approach to reforming the health-care system.
2. Research "Myths about health-care reform." Make a list of at least 10 myths. Without stating that they are myths, read the list to several friends or relatives and ask them which ones they agree with. Are you surprised by their answers?
3. A May 2013 story in *U.S. News & World Report—Health* reported that men without insurance have a four times higher rate of advanced prostate cancer than men with insurance. The uninsured also have a much lower chance of surviving the disease (http://health.usnews.com/health-news/news/articles/ 2013/05/07/prostate-cancer-may-be-deadlier-for-the-uninsured). Do a Web search for other uninsured groups (e.g., women, children, elderly, etc.). Does the lack of insurance affect their health and well-being?

References

1. Kaiser Family Foundation. Public Opinion on Health Care Issues, Kaiser Health Tracking Poll Publication #8425-F: 2013 Retrieved April 2013 from http://www.kff.org

2. Future of Nursing, Campaign for Action: 10M Recommendations, 2011.

3. Agency for Healthcare Research and Quality. Theory and reality of value-based purchasing: Lessons from the pioneer, 1997. Retrieved April 2013 http://www.innovations.ahrq.gov/content.aspx?id=405

4. Kavanagh K, Cimiotti J, Abusalem S, Coty M. Moving healthcare quality forward with nursing-sensitive value-based purchasing. *Journal of Nursing Scholarship*, 44(4):385–395, 2012.

5. Bodenheimer T, Grubach K. *Understanding Health Policy—a Clinical Approach* (6th ed.). New York: McGraw Hill Lange, 2012.

6. Shalala DE. The Future of Nursing: Leading Change, Advancing Health, National Research Council. Washington, DC: National Academy Press, 2011.

7. Buerhasu P, DesRoches C, Applebaum S, Hess R, Norman L, Donelan K. Are nurses ready for health care reform? A decade of survey research. *Nursing Economic$*, 30(6):318–329, 2012.

8. McDonough J. *Inside Health Reform.* University of California Press, Los Angeles. 2012.

9. Balz D. Landmark: The Inside Story of America's Health-Care Law—the Affordable Care Act—and What it Means for Us All. *Journal of Public Affairs,* 2010.

10. Jacobs LR, Skocpol T. *Health Care Reform and American Politics: What Everyone Needs to Know.* Journal of Public Affairs. Oxford, England: Oxford University Press, 2013.

11. Hussey P, et al. How Does the quality of care compare in five countries? *Health Affairs,* 32(4), 2013. Retrieved April 2013 from http://content.healthaffairs.org/content/23/3/89.long

12. World Health Organization. The Right to Health: Fact Sheet No 323, 2012. Retrieved from http://www.who.int/whr/2002/en/

13. Institute of Medicine. *Insuring America's Health: Principles and Recommendations.* Washington, DC: National Academies Press, 2004.

14. Squires D. Multinational Comparisons of Health Systems Data, 2012. Commonwealth Fund. Retrieved April 2013 from http://www.commonwealthfund.org/~/media/files/publications/in-the-literature/2013/nov/pdf_oecd_multinational_comparisons_hlt_sys_data_2013.pdf

15. OECD Indicators. Health at a Glance, 2009. Retrieved April 2013 from http://www.oecd.org/std/leading-indicators/

16. Global issues: Health care around the world, 2012. Retrieved from www.globalissues.org

17. Nissen S. Escape Fire, Aisle C Productions & Our Time Projects, 2012.

18. Reid TR. *The Healing of America: A Global Quest for Better, Cheaper, and Fairer Health Care.* New York: Penguin Books, 2012.

19. Himmelstein D, Thorne D, Warren E, Woolhandler S. Medical bankruptcy in the United States, 2007: Results of a national study. *American Journal of Medicine,* 122:8, 741-746, 2009.

20. Tumulty K. The health-care crisis hits home. *Time,* 173:10, 26-31. 2009.

21. Institute of Medicine. *Unequal Treatment: What Health Care Administrators Need to Know About Racial and Ethnic Disparities in Healthcare.* Washington DC: National Academies Press, 2002.

22. Carrier E, et al. The uninsured and their health care needs: How have they changed since the recession? Kaiser Commission on Medicaid and the Uninsured, 2011.

23. The Commonwealth Fund. Why Not the Best? 2011. Retrieved June 2014 from http://www.commonwealthfund.org/publications/fund-reports/2011/oct/why-not-the-best-2011

24. Families USA. Hidden health tax: Americans pay a premium, 2009. Retrieved April 2013 from http://familiesusa.org/product/hidden-health-tax-americans-pay-premium

25. American Medical Association. Opinion 9.0651—Financial Barriers to Health Care Access, 2013. Retrieved April 2014 from http://www.ama-assn.org/ama/pub/physician-resources/medical-ethics/code-medical-ethics/opinion90651.page

26. American Nurses Association. Code of Ethics, 2001. Retrieved April 2013 from http://www.nursingworld.org/codeofethics

27. Pies R. Health care is a basic human right—almost everywhere but here. Physicians for a National Health Program, 2013. Retrieved April 2014 from http://www.pnhp.org/news/2011/march/health-care-is-a-basic-human-right-almost-everywhere-but-here

28. Life time and annual limits. US Department of Health and Human Services. Retrieved August 2014 from http://www.hhs.gov/healthcare/rights/limits/

29. Harbage P, Haycock H, Ledford M. Post claims underwriting and rescission practices. Robert Wood Johnson Foundation, 2012. Retrieved August 2014 from http://www.rwjf.org/content/dam/web-assets/2009/01/post-claims-underwriting-and-rescission-practices

30. Girion L. Health insurers tied bonuses to dropping sick policyholders, 2007. Retrieved from http://www.latimes.com/business/la-fi-insure9nov09,0,4409342.story

31. U.S. House of Representatives Committee on Energy and Commerce Hearing Memorandum, Supplemental Information for "Health Policies," June 16, 2009.

32. Girion L. Blue Cross praised employees who dropped sick policyholders, lawmaker said. *Los Angeles Times,* 2009. Retrieved April 2013 from http://articles.latimes.com/2009/jun/17/business/fi-rescind17

33. This American Life, Act Three. Restrictions May Apply, Transcript of program aired July 24, 2009. Chicago Public Media and Ira Glass.

34. American Nurses Association. ANA's Health System Reform Agenda, 2008.

35. MacGillis A. *Landmark: The Inside Story of America's Health Care Law and What It Means for Us All.* Perseus Books, New York, NY, 2010, pp. 1–8, 64–71.

36. The Commonwealth Fund. The path to a high performance U.S. health system: A 2020 vision and the policies to pave the way. Washington, DC, 2009. Retrieved August 2014 from http://www.commonwealthfund.org/

37. Robert Wood Johnson Foundation. Commission to build a healthier America—beyond health care new directions to a healthier America, 2009. Retrieved April 2013 from http://www.rwjf.org/en/research-publications/find-rwjf-research/2009/04/beyond-health-care.html

38. Trossman S. U.S. Supreme Court takes up ACA. The American Nurse. Retrieved August 2014 from http://www.theamericannurse.org/index.php/2012/06/06/u-s-supreme-court-takes-up-aca/

39. American Nurses Association. ANA policy & provisions of health reform law, 2010.
40. AARP Public Policy Institute. Nursing Provisions P.L. 111-148, the Patient Protection and Affordability Care Act, 2010.
41. Altman D. Pulling it together. Kaiser Family Foundation, 2013. Retrieved April 2013 from http://www.kff.org
42. Shakir F,. I want to be senate majority leader in order to make Obama a one-term president. Think Progress, 2012. Retrieved June 2014 from http://thinkprogress.org/politics/2010/10/25/126242/mcconnell-obama-one-term/
43. Klein E. 14 Reasons why this is the worst Congress ever. *Washington Post,* 2012. Retrieved June 2013 from http://ivn.us/2012/07/13/ezra-kleins-14-reasons-why-this-is-the-worst-congress-ever/
44. McCarter J. Obamacare unpopular unless it's not called Obamacare. Daily KOS, 2012. Retrieved August 2014 from http://www.dailykos.com/story/2012/06/25/1103100/-Obamacare-unpopular-unless-it-s-not-called-Obamacare
45. Giffey T. Is "Obamacare really that long?" Leader-Telegram, 2012. Retrieved April 2013 from http://www.leadertelegram.com/blogs/tom_giffey/article_c9f1fa54-d041-11e1-9d01-0019bb2963f4.html
46. Center for Medicare Advocacy. Medicare Facts & Fiction, 2013. Retrieved April 2013 from http://www.medicareadvocacy.org/medicare-facts-fiction-quick-lessons-to-combat-medicare-spin/
47. Howard B. 11 myths about health care reform. AARP, 2012. Retrieved June 2013 from http://www.aarp.org/health/health-insurance/info-09-2012/medicare-and-health-care-reform-myths.html
48. Krugman P. Understanding Medicare cuts. *New York Times,* 2012. Retrieved April 2013 from http://krugman.blogs.nytimes.com/2012/08/22/understanding-medicare-cuts/?pagewanted=p
49. Krugman P. Health reform myths. *New York Times,* 2010. Retrieved April 2013 from http://regator.com/p/234642699/paul_krugman_health_reform_myths/
50. Krugman P. Paying for health reform. *New York Times,* 2011. Retrieved April 2013 from http://krugman.blogs.nytimes.com/2011/12/12/paying-for-health-reform/
51. Rutenberg J, Calmes J. False "death panel" rumor has familiar roots. *New York Times,* 2009. Retrieved April 2013 from http://www.nytimes.com/2009/08/14/health/policy/14panel.html
52. Holan A. Politifact's Lie of the Year: "Death Panels," 2009. Retrieved April 2013 from http://www.politifact.com
53. Wilensky G. What can we really expect from healthcare reform? Eye on Washington, Healthcare Financial Management Association, 2009.
54. Daily Howler. Two (Republican) Women! Gail Wilensky and Betsy McCaughey present a punishing contrast, 2009. Retrieved April 2013 from http://www.dailyhowler.com/dh090809.shtml
55. Democratic Policy & Communication Center. Myth vs. Fact: IPAB and Medicare, 2012. Retrieved April 2013 from http://dpc.senate.gov/docs/fs-112-2-193.pdf
56. Watson B. The 5 biggest Obamacare myths explored, explained, and debunked. Daily Finance, 2012. Retrieved April 2014 from http://www.dailyfinance.com/2012/07/11/the-5-biggest-obamacare-myths-explored-explained-and-debunked/
57. Noble M. Paul Krugman and the single-payer system. 2009. Retrieved April 2013 from http://pnhp.org/blog/2008/10/13/nobel-laureate-paul-krugman-on-single-payer/
58. U.S. Department of Health & Human Services. Seniors saved over $6 billion as a result of the health care law. Retrieved April 2013 from http://www.hhs.gov/news/press/2013pres/03/20130321a.html
59. AARP. AARP at Third Anniversary Affordable Care Act Offers Many Benefits, Many More to Come, 2013. Retrieved April 2013 from http://www.aarp.org/about-aarp/press-center/info-03-2013/AARP-At-Third-Anniversary-Affordable-Care-Act-Offers-Many-Benefits-Many-More-to-Come.html
60. Arvantes J. New health care models take lessons from past reform efforts, . Retrieved April 2013 from http://www.aafp.org/news/payment-special-report/20120921specrpt-managed-care.html
61. Kocher R. Health care reform: Trends driven by the evolution of U.S. health care policy. Castlight, 2012. Retrieved April 2013 from http://www.castlighthealth.com/health-care-reform-trends-driven-by-the-evolution-of-u-s-health-care-policy/
62. Patient-Centered Outcomes Research Institute. National priorities for research and research agenda, 2012. Retrieved April 2013 from http://www.pcori.org/assets/PCORI-National-Priorities-and-Research-Agenda-2012-05-21-FINAL.pdf
63. Peck A. With millions still waiting for Sandy relief, Republicans reintroduce Obamacare repeal. Think Progress, 2013. Retrieved April 2013 from http://thinkprogress.org/health/2013/01/03/1394071/bachmann-repeal-obamacare/
64. Focus on Health Reform. Establishing health insurance exchanges: An overview of state efforts. Kaiser Family Foundation Report, 2013.
65. Cohen R. Kafkaesque Committee: The National Healthcare Workforce Commission, NPQ-Nonprofit Quarterly, 2013. Retrieved April 2013 from https://nonprofitquarterly.org/policysocial-context/21862-kafkaesque-committee-the-national-healthcare-workforce-commission.html
66. Redhead CS, et al. Discretionary spending in the Patient Protection and Affordable Care Act (ACA). Congressional Research Service Report for Congress, 2012.
67. Institute of Medicine. *IOM Summary for the Public's Health: Investing in a Healthier Future.* Washington, DC: National Academies Press, 2012.
68. Gruber J. Health Care Reform Is a "Three-Legged Stool." Center for American Progress, 2010. Retrieved April 2013 from http://www.americanprogress.org/issues/healthcare/report/2010/08/05/8226/health-care-reform-is-a-three-legged-stool/
69. Undem T, Perry M. Informing Enroll America's Campaign Findings from a National Study, 2013. Retrieved April 2013 from https://s3.amazonaws.com/assets.enrollamerica.org/wp-content/uploads/2013/11/Informing-Enroll-America-Campaign.pdf
70. MacGillis A. Landmark: The Inside Story of America's Health Care Law -The Affordable Care Act - and What It Means for Us All. Perseus Books, Washington DC, 2010, pp. 191–194.

71. National Patient Safety Foundation, Health Literacy: Statistics at-a-Glance, 2011.

72. Wizeman T. Health Literacy Implications for Health Care Reform: Workshop Summary. Washington, DC: National Academies Press, 2011.

73. Blumenthal D, Morone J. *The Heart of Power, Health and Politics in the Oval Office.* University of California Press, Los Angeles, 2010.

74. Bisognano M. Thinking along the continuum. IHI Leadership Blog, 2013. Retrieved April 2013 from http://www.ihi.org/communities/blogs/_layouts/ihi/community/blog/itemview.aspx?List=81ca4a47-4ccd-4e9e-89d9-14d88ec59e8d&ID=18

75. Gallup Poll. Honesty/Ethics in Professions, 2013. Retrieved April 2013 from http://www.gallup.com/poll/1654/honesty-ethics-professions.aspx

21

Spirituality and Health Care

Roberta Mowdy

Learning Objectives

After completing this chapter, the reader will be able to:

- Develop a working definition of *spirituality*
- Distinguish spirituality from religion
- Describe what is meant by the nursing diagnosis "spiritual distress"
- Describe research that supports the health benefit of spiritual practices
- Describe the relationship between spirituality and one alternative healing modality used within nursing

ROUGH SPOTS ALONG THE TRAIL

The road of life often is filled with twists and turns, ups and downs, and precipitous waysides. People who are facing potentially long-term or debilitating illnesses, confronting acute health crises, or suffering from loss and grief may find themselves reexamining the foundational beliefs they have held since childhood. Usually, at no other time in a person's life is he or she so focused on evaluating the spiritual self than during such crises. Yet the times when clients are most vulnerable also can be opportunities for personal and spiritual growth.

Nurses have the unique task of working with clients at various points throughout their life journeys. Often nurses encounter clients during the "rough parts of the trail." The holistic nursing perspective requires nurses to view each person as a bio-psychosocial being with a spiritual core. Each component of the self (i.e., physical, mental, social, and spiritual) is integral to and influences the others (Fig. 21.1). Nurses spend more time with their clients than do other health-care workers. Therefore, the spiritual needs of clients must be recognized as a domain of nursing care. Holism cannot exist without consideration of the spiritual aspects that create individuality and give meaning to people's lives.[1] Thus, nurses must be sure to address the spirit along with the other dimensions to provide holistic care.

NURSING AT LIFE'S JUNCTURES

It is universally true that the human life cycle is marked by a rhythm of transitions: birth, the entry of a child into society, puberty, sexual

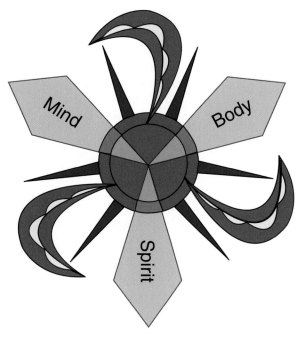

Figure 21.1 Components of the self.

awakening, entry into adulthood, marriage, parenthood, illness, loss, old age, and death. In all cultures there are other rhythms that people honor, such as the solar and lunar cycles, the agricultural cycle, and the reproductive cycles. These cycles constitute the rhythm of human life.

Developmental Crisis

All people recognize the importance of transitions and in some way have ritualized them through their religions or through custom. People learn from their own cultural groups how to behave during each transition, and each cultural group has conceptualized an understanding of these human experiences. Their importance is universally recognized.

Nurses primarily have contact with clients in the health-care setting within the context of these transitions. Developmental crisis theory holds that transitions are times of anxiety and vulnerability for families. Therefore, nurses are required to treat people who are going through transitions with great tenderness and care. It is a sacred trust for nurses to be allowed into a family system in transition. Clients and families may seek spiritual support or may feel spiritual abandonment. Ideally, nurses can help people identify and find the spiritual support they require.

Science as Magic

Over a long period of time, from the Enlightenment of the 17th century to the dawn of the 21st century, political leaders and educated people in Western cultures came to believe that all the answers to human suffering could be found in science and technology. For example, early in the 20th century, antibiotics were thought of as "magic bullets" that cured diseases and reduced suffering. People were eager to take part in research studies to solve their health-care problems.

It was in this context that the nursing profession embraced the Western scientific method as the measure for defining itself. Nurses believed, and some still do believe, that rigorous research involving testing of hypotheses would provide the theoretical base for the practice of professional nursing.

SOCIAL AND SCIENTIFIC EFFECTS ON SPIRITUALITY

More recently, the horrors of terrorism, global warming, major natural disasters, space exploration, and the mapping of the human genome are among changes that have given urgency to reconsideration of the question, "What does it mean to be fully human in the universe as it is now understood?" It is evident that science and technology cannot offer the solutions to all human problems; in fact, they have contributed to many of them.

What Do You Think?

Make two lists: a list of the problems that science and technology have caused during the last 20 years and a list of the problems that have been solved by technology and science. Which list is longer? Why?

To Be Fully Human

Science, electronic communications, and the great social experiments of the past two centuries are among the influences directing humans to a consciousness that individuals are connected to all peoples and to the whole of creation. There is a growing belief that all people share a common basic sense of existence that encompasses everyone and everything. This sense of oneness with the universe that is often associated with severe illness or injury and near-death experiences has the potential to produce profound changes in the way that people view themselves and the world around them. Some people who have had these experiences take life events less personally and tend to see the similarities in all people as if they were members of their family regardless of how different their external appearances may be. They may also experience a heightened compassion for the suffering of others, become involved in altruistic acts, or forgive others more easily. These actions often correspond to finding more meaning, richness, and joy in their lives. Many spiritual leaders believe this type of change is the essence of becoming more human.

In the realm of health care, the increasing awareness that true healing only occurs when there is a reintegration of the physical with the spiritual and the mental gives testimony to the need for increased emphasis on the spiritual aspect of care. Both health-care providers and clients need to recognize that spiritual traditions other than their own contain valuable insights into the nature of human beings and the oneness of creation.

Phenomenology

A feature of postmodernism is the realization that the concept of truth is relative, allowing for an appreciation of diverse perspectives on what is true. Since the mid-1980s, science, including nursing science, has expanded its ways of discerning truth, leaving behind traditional hypothetico-deductive, quantitative research. The emergence of **phenomenology** within the discipline of philosophy is one major influence that has led nursing to appreciate qualitative methods of discovery. As a philosophical approach to understanding truth, phenomenology parallels and is closely related to existentialism, advocating the view that consciousness determines reality and truth in space and time.

In the health-care setting, a phenomenological approach recognizes the belief that the client's observations may be more objective than those of the nurse: They are attached to the client's past experiences and knowledge, which include rich descriptions of the person's life transitions. In nursing, intuition has emerged as a phenomenon worthy of further investigation. This change in viewpoint coincides with increased interest in complementary and alternative therapies and with the importance of spirituality in healing and wellness.

> *Spirituality may be regarded as the driving force that pervades all aspects of and gives meaning to an individual's life.*

THE NATURE OF SPIRITUALITY

Spirituality is a broad and somewhat nebulous concept that has to do with the search for answers to certain questions and issues (Box 21.1). Similar concerns have been identified among children of various cultural backgrounds in research on the development of spirituality.

A Diverse Heritage

A rich heritage of spiritual practices, including systematic reflection for growth toward wholeness, is found in all the major religions of the world. The roots of the great traditions, including each religion's prayer practices, can be traced to the shift in human consciousness that occurred around 500 BC. During this period, many great teachers and spiritual leaders emerged, including Confucius; Lao-tzu; Siddhartha Gautama, who became the Buddha; Zoroaster; the Greek philosophers Socrates, Plato, and Aristotle; and the Hebrew prophets Amos, Hosea, and Isaiah.

St. Augustine, a Roman Catholic bishop who lived in North Africa during the 5th century, is credited with first identifying the relationships among contemplation, action, and wisdom within the Christian tradition. For Augustine, the contemplative life was properly focused on the discernment of truth and was open to all people. Augustine equated truth with God.

Hope Through Compassion

Spirituality is often defined as integrative energy, capable of producing internal human harmony, or holism. Other definitions refer to spirituality as a sense of coherence. Spirituality also entails a sense of transcendent reality, which draws strength from inner resources, living fully for the present, and having a sense of inner knowing. Solitude, compassion, and empathy are important components of spirituality for many individuals.

The concept of hope is central to spirituality. Spirituality may be regarded as the driving force that pervades all aspects of and gives meaning to an individual's life. It creates a set of beliefs and values that influence the way people conduct their lives. Spiritual activity involves introspection, reflection, and a sense of connectedness to others or to the universe. For many people, this connectedness focuses

Box 21.1

Spiritual Questions

Why Are We Here?
How do we fit into the cosmos?
What power or intelligence created and orders
   the universe?
What is the nature and meaning of divine or
   mystical experiences?
How are we to make meaning of suffering?
How are we to behave toward other people?
How are we to deal with our own shortcomings
   and failures?
What happens to us when we die, and where
   were we before we were born?

ultimately on a supreme being who is sometimes called God.

When providing spiritual care to their clients, nurses must base their actions on compassion, or sensitivity to the suffering of others. Compassion is a way of living born out of an awareness of one's relationship to all living creatures, a sensitivity to the pain and brokenness of others. The Greek word for *compassion* literally means "to feel in one's innards." Given this definition, one can easily see how compassion is part of spirituality and the life journey.

A Sense of Meaning

Traditionally, the term *spirituality* has been defined as a sense of meaning in life associated with a sense of an inner spirit. However, it is difficult to identify what such a spirit is like and how it can be observed. Spirituality can be defined from both religious and secular perspectives. A person with spiritual needs does not necessarily have to participate in religious rituals and practices.

Despite the lack of consensus regarding the definition of spirituality, several themes emerge from an interdisciplinary review of the literature:

- All human beings have the potential for spirituality and spiritual growth.
- Spirituality is relational.
- There is a necessary link among religion, moral norms, and spirituality.
- Spirituality involves lived experience; it is a way of life.

In some ways spirituality is a mystery. Although human beings can experience spirituality,

appreciate it, and grow in it, there is much about spirituality that cannot be explained or reduced to human language.

On the basis of these themes, spirituality is defined as a way of life, usually informed by the moral norms of one or more religious traditions through which a person relates to other persons, the universe, and the transcendent in ways that promote human fulfillment (of self and others) and universal harmony.

The Religious Perspective

From the religious perspective, spirituality can be defined as encompassing the ideology of the *imago dei* (image of God), or soul, that exists in everyone. The soul makes the person a thinking, feeling, moral, creative being, able to relate meaningfully to a supreme being and to others. This being or force may be called God, Allah, the divine creator and sustainer of the universe, the divine mystery, or other names that convey a profound sense of transcendence and awe. A religious perspective often entails a set of beliefs, or a creed, that helps explain the meaning of life, suffering, health, and illness. Most religions also incorporate and promote a set of positive values, such as charity to others, faith in a supreme being, and a requirement for a lifestyle that involves honesty, truth, and virtuous living. Persons who accept and follow the beliefs and tenants of their religion should be able to develop a deep spirituality that will ultimately lead to their self-actualization. Additionally, these beliefs can be crucial to a believer's physical well-being. (For more information on the relationship of spirituality and physical health, go to http://www.ncbi.nlm.nih.gov/ pubmed/15979795 or http://globalhealth.washington .edu/docs/Bezruchka%201.pdf.)

Religious Practice Gone Astray

Spirituality is often mistakenly understood to mean just religious practice; however, it should be considered in the broader sense of the term. Religion can be an approach to or expression of spirituality, and spirituality is a component of religion, but the two concepts are different.

It is quite possible for the members of a specific religion to be limited in their spirituality. Most people have known individuals who dutifully follow the rules of their religious tradition. They strongly believe that if they have adhered to the rules correctly, God will reward them with blessings such as health, success, affluence, social status, and power. For these individuals, adverse events like disease, death of a loved one, or loss of investments can be devastating because they are perceived as a failure in religious practice or punishments from God. On the other hand, there are many deeply spiritual persons who do not belong to any organized religion but who may be profoundly reflective about the meaning of their life and experiences.

Specific Values and Beliefs

Current religious leaders attempt to help a diverse population appreciate religious traditions other than their own. They point out that all the world's major religions seek to answer the same questions: "Why are we here?" "What does it all mean?" and "What, if anything, are we supposed to be doing with our lives?" All religions taken together can be perceived like a stained-glass window that refracts the light in different colors and offers reflections of different shapes. Each of the world's religions is different because it has evolved to respond to unique histories and different cultural developments.

Definitions of religion usually identify a specific system of values and beliefs and a framework for ethical behavior that the members must follow. Religion can be thought of as a social construct that reflects its cultural context and specific philosophical influences. A religion evolves within a specific cultural group, situated in history, and attempts to discern what the group beliefs are and how the group has come to understand God's commandments.

Religion, as an institutionally based, organized system of beliefs, represents only one specific means of spiritual expression. Participation in a religion generally entails formal education for membership, an initiation ceremony, participation in worship gatherings, adherence to set rules of behavior, participation in prescribed rituals, a particular mode of prayer, and the study of that group's sacred texts. Religious groups vary widely in their tolerance of intragroup diversity of beliefs and behaviors as well as their respect for the belief systems of others. In addition, a specific religious group may encompass a wide range of understanding of what its practices represent.

> *Occasionally, health-care professionals may encounter individuals whose spiritual practices are highly questionable or discomforting to witness (e.g., worshippers of Satan or those who seek to invoke harm to others through their prayers and rituals).*

Occasionally, health-care professionals may encounter individuals whose spiritual practices are highly questionable or discomforting to witness (e.g., worshippers of Satan or those who seek to invoke harm to others through their prayers and rituals).

The Secular Perspective

Although some people believe that secularism is synonymous with nonspirituality or even antispirituality, it is actually a philosophical approach that separates organized formal religion from government. The principle of secularism endorses the right of people to be free from governance by organized religious creeds and teachings and asserts the right to freedom from governmental imposition of one particular religion upon the citizens of a country. Secularism in the United States also acts to protect all organized religions and the people who belong to them from interference by the government.

Although the secular perspective separates religion from government, it is not necessarily nonspirituality. Secular spirituality is seen as a set of positive values, such as love, honesty, or truth, chosen by the individual to ultimately become that person's supreme focus of life and organizing framework. It is a type of spiritual ideology without an external religious structure or organization that emphasizes the search for an inner peace rather than a relationship with a divine being. People who seek a secular spirituality are often motivated by the wish to live a happy existence, which may or may not involve the need to help others. They believe in a human life that goes beyond the materialistic yet often they do not believe in a supreme being. For the individual who subscribes to secular spirituality, living a good life involves nurturing positive thoughts, emotions, words, and actions and believing that everything in the universe is mutually dependent.

Manifestation of Spirituality

The religious and secular perspectives can exist together in the totality of a person's life. A person's spirituality may be nourished by the ability to give and receive touch, caring, love, and trust. Spirituality may also entail an appreciation of physical experiences such as listening to music, enjoying art or literature, eating delicious food, laughing, venting emotional tension, or participating in sexual expression. In the context of a person's spiritual growth and development, a series of four developmental stages have been proposed for human spirituality:

- Stage 1: The chaotic (antisocial) stage, with its superficial belief system
- Stage 2: The formal (institutional) stage, with its adherence to the law
- Stage 3: The skeptic (individual) stage, with its emphasis on rationality, materialism, and humaneness
- Stage 4: The mystical (communal) stage, with its "unseen order of things"[2]

A SPIRITUAL TRADITION IN NURSING

Modern nursing has a rich legacy of the appreciation of spirituality in health and illness. Florence Nightingale's views of nursing practice were based on a spiritual philosophy that she set forth in *Suggestions for Thought*. She was the daughter of Unitarian and Anglican parents, and among her ancestors were famous dissenters against the Church of England. The skepticism fostered by her Unitarian upbringing may have influenced her to question and critique established religious doctrine. Her search for religious truth caused her to become familiar with the writings of Christian mystics (e.g., St. Francis of Assisi, St. John of the Cross) and also with various Eastern mystical writings, including the *Bhagavad Gita*.

> " *Nightingale saw no conflict between science and mysticism. To her, the laws of nature and science were merely 'the thoughts of God.'* "

The Lady of the Lamp

Most modern nurses consider Florence Nightingale (1820–1910) to be the mother of the nursing profession (see Chapter 2). Most know her as "the lady of the lamp," who almost single-handedly brought about sweeping changes in British medicine, care delivered on battlefields, and public health. Nightingale realized a call to care early in her life. She was a sickly child, and as the recipient of care from family members, she began to reciprocate in kind by nursing other sick relatives.

A Modern Prophet?

Nightingale sought places where she could learn to care for the sick and dying in a way that distinguished what she did from the work of common chambermaids. She attended the Institution of Deaconesses at Kaiserwerth in Dusseldorf, Germany. This was a Protestant training hospital that taught something akin to nursing as a call from God and a diaconal function. Through her time at Kaiserwerth and her contacts there, she came to believe that all persons on a mission or quest to become Christlike are given certain gifts and talents. Some say Nightingale was a modern prophet of God and saw herself as a liberated human being.

For Nightingale, spirituality involved a sense of a divine intelligence that creates and sustains the cosmos, and she had an awareness of her own inner connection with this higher reality. The universe, for Nightingale, was the embodiment of a transcendent God. She came to believe that all aspects of creation are interconnected and share the same inner divinity. She believed that all humans have the capacity to realize and perceive this divinity. Nightingale's God can be described as perfection or as the "essence of benevolence."[3]

The Thoughts of God

Nightingale saw no conflict between science and mysticism. To her, the laws of nature and science were merely "the thoughts of God." Spirituality for Nightingale entailed the development of courage, compassion, inner peace, creative insight, and other "Godlike" qualities. Based on this belief, Nightingale's convictions commanded her to lifelong service in the care of the sick and helpless.

Nightingale endorsed the tradition of contemplative prayer, or attunement to the inner presence of God. All phenomena, Nightingale believed, are manifestations of God. A spiritual life entails wise stewardship of all the earth's resources, including human beings. She saw physical healing as a natural process regulated by natural laws, and as she stated in her *Notes on Nursing*, "What nursing has to do . . . is to put the client in the best condition for nature to act upon him."[3]

Spirituality and Religion in Nursing Theory

As nursing sought to establish itself as a profession with a legitimate knowledge base, the concern with human spirituality was downplayed and even consciously ignored until the early 1980s. Typically, the spiritual domain is assigned to the art rather than to the science of nursing because its seemingly subjective nature is mistakenly equated with esthetics and intuition. Paying attention to the spiritual domain in providing holistic care depends on the beliefs and values of both the nurse and the client.

There are over 26 major nursing theories and conceptual frameworks that have been developed since the 1960s. Although 14 of them recognized the spiritual domain of health somewhere in their assumptions, only 2 theories mention it by name.

Energy Fields

Martha Rogers's Science of Unitary Human Beings is an example of a profoundly spiritual view of humanity that does not directly name the concept of spirituality. Rogers's framework suggests that there are unbounded human energy fields in interaction with the environmental energy field. Her spiritual definitions can also apply to the concept of the soul (discussed later). Rogers, who grew up in Tennessee amid fundamentalist Christians, was loath to be interpreted in that light; moreover, she had to establish her credibility at New York University during the 1950s, before nursing was accepted as a scientific discipline.

An Aspect of Holistic Health

Betty Neuman, in the later development of her theory, and Jean Watson are the only theorists who clearly acknowledged the impact of spirituality in the development of their theories (see Chapter 4). Watson alone defined and explained the spiritual terminology she used to discuss the spiritual aspect of holistic health.

Watson specifically identifies the awareness of the clients' and families' spiritual and religious beliefs as a responsibility of a nurse.[4] She advocates that nurses should appreciate and respect the spiritual meaning in a person's life, no matter how unusual that person's belief system may be. Watson states that

nurses have an obligation to identify religious and spiritual influences in their clients' lives at home and to help clients meet their religious requirements in inpatient settings. For example, nurses can facilitate clients' use of religious measures, such as the lighting of candles (real or electric), putting flowers and personal objects in the room, ensuring privacy, and playing music to promote increased comfort and relieve anguish.

Spiritual Distress

Since 1978, the North American Nursing Diagnosis Association (NANDA) has recognized the nursing diagnosis of spiritual distress.[5] It has most recently been defined as "disruption in the life principle that pervades a person's entire being and integrates and transcends one's biological and psychosocial nature."

Defining characteristics of spiritual distress include concerns with and questions about the meaning of life and death, anger toward God, concerns about the meaning of suffering, concerns about the person's relationship to God, the inability to participate in preferred religious practices, seeking spiritual help, concerns about the ethics of prescribed medical regimens, preoccupation with illness and death, expressing displaced anger toward clergy, sleep disturbances, and altered mood or behavior. Spiritual distress may occur in relation to separation from religious or cultural supports, challenges to beliefs and values, or intense suffering.

Illness as Punishment

Nurses should be aware that some individuals have been seriously harmed by their religious communities.

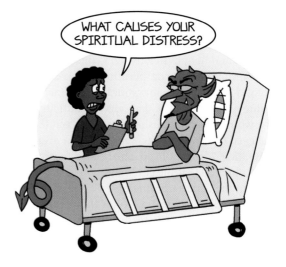

WHAT CAUSES YOUR SPIRITUAL DISTRESS?

Examples of harm might include being shunned or excommunicated, being told that they are evil, being forced into a rigidly controlled lifestyle by a cult, or being physically or sexually assaulted by members of the religious community. For these people, illness may be seen as punishment for some sinful action, and they may perceive any offer of spiritual support from the religious community as profoundly threatening. They may believe that God has abandoned them or that the idea of God is foolish or even destructive.

Given the rapid turnover of clients in most health systems, there may be little that the nurse can do other than to acknowledge their spiritual pain and accept them, with the assurance that "I am here for you now." If there is more time for contact, the nurse may be able to refer a client or family to appropriate support groups or clergy.

Going Against Tradition

At times clients make health-care decisions that conflict with the beliefs of their religious communities. These often produce high levels of spiritual distress that may affect both the mental and physical well-being of the client. Consider the following case study:

> When I was a nursing student in the early 1970s, I cared for a woman who was undergoing a therapeutic abortion because of several medical complications of her pregnancy. She had her first child before RhoGAM was available, and she, an Rh-negative mother, had borne an Rh-positive baby. She had only one kidney, and her physicians were concerned that the immunological complication of carrying a second Rh-positive baby would jeopardize that kidney's function. The decision was difficult for the woman and her husband to make, but they believed the first priority was to care for and raise their 7-year-old son. She needed to protect her kidney so that she could live and participate fully in the child's upbringing.
>
> The night before I cared for this woman, her clergyman came to the hospital and told her that she would go to hell for her decision. Being a devout church member, the woman

was extremely distressed the next day. The primary nurse assigned to this woman recognized the spiritual distress caused by the clergyman and requested that a hospital chaplain spend time with her. The chaplain talked and prayed with the woman for several hours. These actions brought great comfort to the woman, who proceeded with the abortion.

Clients often make choices that are difficult for nurses to accept. For instance, because of religious beliefs, clients may refuse commonplace treatments, such as blood transfusions, medications, and even minor surgeries. End-of-life decisions are often based on family members' spiritual beliefs and can be controversial among the health-care personnel who are involved in the decision. In some acute care settings, chaplains and psychiatrists conduct regular group sessions with staff nurses to assist them in understanding and accepting controversial client decisions. The Terri Schiavo case in Florida demonstrates how well-meaning people with strong religious beliefs can be diametrically opposed when it comes to end-of-life decisions.

> " *At times clients make health-care decisions that conflict with the beliefs of their religious communities. These often produce high levels of spiritual distress that may affect the client's mental and physical well-being.* "

The Human Energy System and the Soul

Most religious traditions include a concept called "the soul." Religious traditions usually offer explanations of what the soul is, how and when human beings acquire a soul, and what happens to the soul after death, but "soul" need not be a religious concept.

Images of the Soul

Thomas Moore, a psychotherapist who has written extensively about spiritual development, describes the soul "not as a thing, but a quality or a dimension of experiencing life and ourselves. It has to do with depth, value, relatedness, heart, and personal substance . . . [not necessarily] an object of religious belief or . . . something to do with immortality."[6] Yet Moore observes that the soul must be nurtured, and religious practices can provide that nurturance. For Moore, spirituality is the effort a person makes to identify the soul's worldview, values, and sense of relatedness to the whole of the person and of creation. The work of the soul is the quest for understanding or insight about major life questions.

Some people may depict the soul as an image of the person that extends several feet beyond the physical self, or characterize it by color and energetic movement. Many people believe that the soul enters the body at some point during gestation and leaves the body at approximately the moment of death. Reincarnation, or the return of a soul for many earthly lifetimes, is a concept encountered in many religious frameworks, including certain mystical traditions within Judaism and Christianity, although not all denominations subscribe to it. The reason for the soul's return to earthly life is to learn, to develop, and to be purified. Some traditions express this process in terms of earning an improved position in the spiritual world to become closer to God after the final judgment.

The soul would seem to be an exquisitely precise and vast center for communication. Souls have the capacity to communicate with one another, with all living things, and with the divine source of all energy. Their capacity is not limited by the laws of physical matter. Some alternative modalities of healing rely on energy movement through the soul.

Examples of therapies that capitalize on knowledge of the soul and the movement of a divinely generated energy, life force, or grace (*chi* in Chinese, *ki* in Japanese, *prana* in Indian traditions) include therapeutic touch, Reiki, and shiatsu. Energy can move in many directions. When a person needs it, energy can be drawn from its divine source into the person. Excess energy can be moved from one person to another, and the flow of energy throughout the person's energy field can be balanced to achieve a state of health.

Human Energy Centers

Some alternative healing practices that use colors, herbs, aromas, and crystals can be regarded as consistent with a paradigm of repatterning the human energy field or altering the flow of energy throughout the person's body. The circulation of divine energy may be thought of as coming from God and circulating through all living things, the earth, and all the celestial bodies, thus interconnecting all creation.

Religious traditions of India and other Eastern cultures teach that the human energy system contains seven energy centers, or chakras. These can be considered the primary openings in the human energy system through which energy flows. Each center has or controls a unique type of energy and spirituality that it allows to enter or leave the body. The root chakra is located at the base of the torso or the perineum, and its energy has to do with the material world. The crown chakra, the highest level of energy at the top of the head, relates to spirituality.

Examining the religious art of many cultures, over many centuries, artists depict these areas of their subjects' bodies in similar ways. For instance, holy people are depicted with vivid, large, or colorful hearts, and their heads are surrounded by halos. At the very least, the chakras represent a paradigm for ordering the archetypal issues of human life.

What Do You Think?

What sources of religious energy do you have? When and how do you use them?

Communication Between Worlds

Some individuals seem to be more aware of the nonphysical or spiritual realms than others. Many people have had a precognition or déjà vu experience during their lives. However, nurses may have more opportunities to glimpse a different reality than laypeople. Nurses have been involved in research on the near-death experience for more than 20 years.

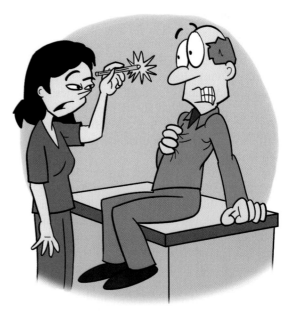

"SIR, THE BRIGHT LIGHT YOU SEE
IS MY PENLIGHT, NOT THE AFTERLIFE."

The Near-Death Experience

Across religious and cultural traditions and throughout history, a common near-death experience has been documented, but only since the early 1980s has it gained credence among Western health professionals.

Many clients describe the experience of near death as a sensation of floating in the air while visualizing their body lying below on a hospital bed, at the scene of an accident, or where the near death occurred. They often watch health-care personnel who are working to resuscitate the body. The person then experiences being drawn into a tunnel, perhaps accompanied by other forms or spiritual beings, and moving toward a bright light that exudes great energy or love. They also describe a communication with the light being, generally identified as God, about whether they are to remain there or return to the earthly body.

Obviously, in cases of near death, the decision is made to return. Individuals who have experienced near death often report that they have developed a great inner peace, that they no longer fear death, and that their lives have been transformed by what they experienced.

Nurses who spend much of their time working with clients who are near death, such as hospice nurses, are most likely to have witnessed the experience of deathbed visions and gained a glimpse of a different realm of reality. Dying clients who are having a deathbed vision are often aware of multiple realities: the tangible here and now that family members and caretakers can observe and "the other side," where they see loved ones who have died and are waiting for their arrival.

Some medical researchers attribute near-death and deathbed experiences to progressive hypoxia in specific brain centers. However, others give the experiences a spiritual interpretation. Could a husband, for example, really come to meet his wife of many years past? A vast amount of literature on angels and spiritual guides emphasizes that people need not feel alone or frightened by future situations or crises. Angels and other spiritual guides are available to comfort them just for the asking.

Some authorities believe that children are more open to communication from the spiritual world than adults because they have not yet been contaminated by the laws of natural science that are generally accepted by Western society.

Spirituality in Children

Some authorities believe that children are more open to communication from the spiritual world than adults because they have not yet been contaminated by the laws of natural science that are generally accepted by Western society. Nurses can watch for and nurture spirituality in children. When a nurse is open to such an occasion and acts on it, an opportunity for transcendent and reciprocal spiritual growth is available to both the child and the nurse.[7] Children may be conscious or unconscious participants in a spiritual life. By their mere presence, their demonstrations of love, their ability to draw love from their family and friends, and their expression of awe of the natural world, children provide strong aspects of spirituality to the world. Children express their spirituality primarily through behaviors. They imitate ritual and use symbols in imaginative play. They question with innocence and intent. Children express values and make value judgments. They use art, dance, song, and movement to express joy, despair, awe, and wonder; to deal with suffering; and to question meaning in their experiences. Children who have developed and are supported in spiritual and religious expression or practices develop a framework for the understanding of social relations and the natural world.[7]

Mysticism

Mystics are people believed to have a different relationship to time, space, matter, and energy than most of the population. It seems that they are able to understand the real nature and full capability of their souls and can apply that knowledge and ability to the physical world, producing changes that science has difficulty explaining and that some call miracles. For example, a current-day Hindu holy man in India named Sai Baba generates ash that has brought miraculous healing to some people who have touched it. Also, many healing miracles were documented by physicians and scientists during the lifetime of the Italian Franciscan priest Padre Pio before his death in 1968.

The common message of mystics from around the world is that people are to live lives of love and compassion for all. The extraordinary love and compassion that most mark the early life of the Dalai Lama, a Buddhist holy man, is depicted in the historical films *Seven Years in Tibet* and *Kundun*.

SPIRITUAL PRACTICES IN HEALTH AND ILLNESS

The way that nurses care for and nurture themselves influences their ability to function effectively in a healing role with another person or client. Spirituality is an important component of a life's journey. Tending to matters of the soul aides a person in living a healthy lifestyle and is fundamental to integrating spirituality into clinical practice.

Nurturing the Spirit

Caring for their spirits or souls requires nurses to pause, reflect, and take in what is happening within and around them, to take time for themselves, for relationships, and for other things that animate them. Maintaining and nourishing one's spiritual disposition can be achieved in a variety of ways, and nurses give the same suggestions that they themselves use to heal internally.

"Care of the spirit is a professional nursing responsibility and an intrinsic part of holistic nursing."

Spiritual Assessment Questions

Nurses may have some difficulty assessing the spiritual status of a client. Some questions that facilitate gathering this information include:

- What is strength for you?
- Where can you get your strength?
- Who gives you strength?
- How can you increase your inner strength?
- What does peace mean to you?
- Where do you feel at peace?
- Who makes you feel more peaceful?
- What situations will increase your sense of peace?
- When do you feel most secure?
- Where do you get your security from?
- Who makes you feel secure?
- How can you increase your security?[1]
- To support the "whole" person, health-care providers should be willing and able to address their client's spiritual needs. How do you feel about discussing such matters with your clients?

- If you feel uncomfortable about addressing the issue of spirituality, is there someone with whom you can discuss these matters and perhaps alleviate your discomfort so you can better serve your clients?

A Professional Responsibility

Care of the spirit is a professional nursing responsibility and an intrinsic part of holistic nursing. Nurses must become confident and competent with spiritual caregiving, expanding their skills in assessing the spiritual domain and in developing and implementing appropriate interventions. A caring relationship with a client is necessary to show the person that he or she is significant. Effective spiritual care requires self-awareness, communication, trust building, and the ability to give hope.[8]

The nursing profession must understand and support holistic care. Therefore, spirituality and the delivery of spiritual care become fundamental content areas for nursing students.[9] What the nurse needs is a set of social, psychological, and personal skills combined with sensitivity, open-mindedness, and tolerance. The skills will include such things as listening, responding appropriately, correctly identifying emotional states, showing accurate empathy, and so forth. The sensitivity will enable her to detect the sometimes subtle cues given by the patient, the open-mindedness will prevent the nurse from automatically interpreting what she sees and hears in terms of her own worldview and beliefs, and the tolerance will enable the nurse to accept beliefs expressed and requests made, which may not accord with her own sentiments. Guidelines and policies must be developed to fully support nurse educators in their endeavors.

A persistent barrier to the incorporation of spirituality into clinical practice is the fear of imposing particular religious beliefs and values on others. Nurses who integrate spirituality into their care of others need to recognize that, although each person acts out of and is informed by her or his own spiritual perspective, acting from this foundation is not the same as imposing these beliefs and values on others. In fact, many practitioners believe that the more grounded they are in their own spiritual understandings, the less likely they are to impose their values and beliefs on others.

A number of organizations and agencies encourage the incorporation of spiritual practices into health care (Boxes 21.2 to 21.4).

Prayer and Meditation

Prayer and meditation are spiritual disciplines practiced in many traditions, both cultural and religious. Appreciating the personal nature of these disciplines, the nurse, with respect and sensitivity, can help clients remember or explore ways in which they reach out to and listen for God or the absolute. Recalling the place and meaning of prayer and the ways in which they experience the presence of and communion with God or the absolute, provides clients with a rich resource.

In the clinical setting, both the nurse's and the client's understanding of prayer will determine its role. Clarifying the client's understanding of and need for prayer is part of holistic nursing. Some clients want others to pray with or for them, whereas others do not believe in prayer. Nurses should support each client's request and needs for prayer, which may mean inviting others to take part in various forms of prayer with and for the client, or simply praying with the client themselves. Facilitating the appreciation and practice of prayer in a client's life is an important aspect of caring for the spirit.

Relief Through Imagery

When a person is physically confined to a hospital room, the practice of imagery may enable him or her to experience another space. Imagery can take a person to a temple, an ocean, a place of religious worship, a breakfast nook, or any "sacred space"—that is, a life-giving and healing place for the client. In this other space, the client may feel more comfortable in spirit and more able to engage in prayer or meditation. Family and friends, as well as other clients and other staff, may be resources in this practice of imagery.

Exploring as many aspects of the prayer experience as possible enriches both the nurse's and the client's understanding of the nature and place of invocation. Sacred or inspirational readings, music, drumming, movement, light or darkness, aromas, and time of day are among the many factors that may be important considerations in meditation.

The client's method of reflection, in all of its fullness and meaning, nurtures the spirit, and the nurse may be able to support the client's prayer or meditation needs by facilitating changes in the environment or schedule. It is wise to remember that merely the process of listening to and appreciating self-reflection of another nurtures the spirit and acknowledges the spiritual dimension of that person.

Relaxation Response

The relaxation response and prayer have been demonstrated to affect illnesses. The ability of people to participate in their own healing through prayer or meditation may use a source of healing power called *remembered wellness*, sometimes also called *the placebo effect*. It is based on the belief that all people have the capacity to "remember" the calm and confidence associated with emotional and physical health and happiness. As a source of energy that can be tapped into, remembered wellness should not be regarded suspiciously but instead should be used for healing. However, its effectiveness depends on the individual's belief system.

Remembered Wellness

Remembered wellness depends on three components: belief and expectation of the client, belief and expectation of the caregiver, and belief and expectation generated by a caring relationship between the client and the caregiver. A warm and trusting relationship seems to enhance the effectiveness of the care provided.

Everyone involved in providing health care is in a position to use remembered wellness as an energy source to enhance the healing process. One thing health-care providers can do to promote healing is to speak positively of treatments and medications being

---

Box 21.2

American Holistic Nurses' Association

The American Holistic Nurses Association (AHNA) was founded in 1980 by a group of nurses dedicated to bringing the concept of holism to every arena of nursing practice. They define holism as wellness—that state of harmony between body, mind, emotions, and spirit—in an ever-changing environment.

The AHNA offers certification in holistic nursing and has endorsed programs in aromatherapy, interactive imagery, and healing touch.

Source: Visit the AHNA website at http://www.ahna.org.

Box 21.3

Parish (Congregational) Nursing

Parish (congregational) nursing is a movement of the past two decades in which churches, synagogues, mosques, and other faith communities designate nurses to serve their membership. Parish nursing is viewed as a healing ministry, and parish nurses are attuned to spiritual issues raised by health transitions and the healing nature of spiritual practice. They may assist people to remain in their own homes, connect them with other health services for which they are eligible, or provide needed health teaching and support. At times their role is simply to be present with them.

The International Parish Nurse Resource Center is located in St. Louis, Missouri. They can be contacted at 314-918-2559, 314-918-2527, or on the Internet at http://www.parishnurses.org.

given to clients is adapted to their specific levels of knowledge and anxiety. Basically, the client is not told about *all* the potential side effects in great detail, particularly those that commonly have a psychological component like headaches, back pain, and shortness of breath. Other experts believe that the contextual informed consent approach may invalidate consent forms and destroy the nurse–client relationship, which is built on trust. (For more information on the nocebo effect, go to http://www.the-scientist.com/?articles.view/articleNo/36126/title/Worried-Sick/.)

What Do You Think?

Is the practice of contextual informed consent ethical? Under which system of ethical thinking is it more likely to be considered ethical? Utilitarianism or deontology? How would you approach a client who was anxious about the side effects of a medication or a surgical procedure?

used. For example, positive reinforcement occurs when the nurse refers to the client's medication as the "drug your doctor prescribed to help your heart" or the food tray as "nutrition to help your body fight your infection."

The Nocebo Effect

In contrast to the placebo effect, the "nocebo" (negative placebo) effect is the fulfillment of an expectation of harm. If a client is told something bad is going to happen to them and believes it, the likelihood of it happening increases. It is also an effect that health professionals can cause. Examples of the nocebo effect include advising clients that a medicine will probably make them sick, telling them that chemotherapy will drain their energy and cause more of their hair to fall out, or informing them that a certain percentage of people die from a given procedure. Such warnings can actually bring about the complications. Any teaching about the side effects of medications has the potential to produce a nocebo effect, and there really is no way to prevent it. It creates a difficult ethical dilemma for the nurse, who is caught between the obligation of beneficence (do no harm) and the obligation of informed consent (see Chapter 6 for more detail).

Some have proposed a middle ground called *contextual informed consent,* where the information

A Quiet Focus

Sometimes called *transcendental meditation* (TM) or *mantra meditation,* the relaxation response entails 20 minutes, twice each day, of quiet meditation with the eyes closed, focusing on a word or image that is spiritually meaningful to the person. When an intrusive thought enters the person's consciousness, the person should lightly dismiss it, as if gently blowing a feather away, and return to the meditation word or image. Over time, individuals who use this method have lowered blood pressure, decreased incidents of dysmenorrhea, and reduced chronic pain; this practice has brought about improvement in a number of illnesses.

Peace Through Awareness

Relaxation, meditation, visualization, and hypnosis can help seriously ill clients, including many with cancer. Meditation is a technique of listening. However, listening is not a passive process. Rather, it is a way of focusing the mind in a state of relaxed awareness to pay attention to deeper thoughts and feelings, to the products of the unconscious mind, to the peace of pure consciousness, and to deeper spiritual awareness.

Some teachers of meditation suggest that the person select a spiritually symbolic word (e.g., God, love, beauty, peace, Mary, Jesus) on which to focus, whereas others suggest watching a candle flame. Still

Box 21.4

International Center for the Integration of Health and Spirituality

The International Center for the Integration of Health and Spirituality (ICIHS) in Rockville, Maryland, disseminates research on the benefits of spiritual practices to health professionals through their publication, conferences, and speakers. For further information about this resource, contact ICIHS at http://www.encognitive.com.

others teach practitioners to focus on their breathing. All these methods are intended to bring the person to a deeply restful state that frees the mind from its usual chatter. This is the experience of being centered. People may experience spiritual insights, but more often they experience a gradual enhancement of well-being.

Visualizing an Outcome

Visualization is the practice of meditating with an image of a desired outcome or the process of attaining it. It is preferable that the image be selected by the person using it rather than someone else. For example, a person with a tumor might visualize miniature miners mining the unhealthy tissue and carting it away. Hypnosis is the process of suggesting an image of a desired reality to someone. Both these techniques have been demonstrated to stimulate the immune system.

Researchers have also observed that some seriously ill people believe that they deserve their illness as a punishment for something they did in the past. Helping them forgive themselves often brings about dramatic improvements in their conditions. Releasing fear and hate has a similar effect. This process reflects back to Nightingale's belief that nurses need to help clients get out of the way of their own healing.

It might seem logical to conclude that clients who do not recover from illness, or who die, have failed to help themselves or did not adequately use their spiritual powers. That is not the case. Spiritual modes of healing do not always lead to cure. Spiritual healing takes a much broader view and includes enhanced comfort and an inner peace with disability or death.

Therapeutic Touch

The human touch can make the difference between life and death."[9] Therapeutic touch (TT) is an active alternative healing modality that involves redirecting the human energy system. In recent years, TT has been retrieved from ancient traditions, studied, and refined.

Altered Wave Patterns

As a healing practice, TT is consistent with the Science of Unitary Human Beings developed by Martha Rogers. The Science of Unitary Human Beings defines people as energy fields interacting with the larger environmental energy field. The energy fields are characterized by patterns of waves. One way of altering the wave patterns of the human energy field is to use TT to move energy into and through it in deliberate ways.

The practitioner of TT acts with the intent of relaxing the recipient, reducing pain and discomfort, and accelerating healing when appropriate. Early controlled studies showed that the hemoglobin levels of a group of clients who received TT increased significantly more than the levels in a control group who did not receive TT.

The TT practitioner should approach the client with compassion and the intent to heal, and the recipient of care ideally approaches the healing encounter with receptivity and openness to change. The practitioner of TT first centers and then assesses the state of the recipient's energy field, noting energy levels and movement around the chakras. Cues may be determined through physical sensations in the practitioner's hands, direct visualization, inner awareness, or other intuitive modes of insight.

After assessing the recipient, the TT practitioner, working from the center of the client's energy field to the periphery, directs energy from the environment into the client's field as needed, then stimulates energy flow through the client's field, clears congested areas in the energy field, dampens excess energetic activity, and synchronizes the rhythmic waves of the energy flow, depending on the client's needs. The practitioner is not diverting his or her own energy into the client because it would be detrimental to the practitioner. Rather, the TT practitioner redirects the client's energy field or directs energy from the environment outside the client.

An Expression of Care

Families and friends may need encouragement to share physical expressions of care and concern in the sometimes intimidating hospital environment. Nurses may encourage them with statements such as, "It's okay to hold her hand; you won't interfere with the tubes." "He mentioned that you give a wonderful back rub; would you like to give him one today?" "She seems to know when you are in here holding her hand." "I can show you how to massage her feet." "Would you like to brush her hair?"

Persons vary in their degree of comfort with touch and the conditions in which they may want to share touch. The

> *Therapeutic touch (TT) is an active alternative healing modality that involves redirecting the human energy system.*

nurse's own feelings about and comfort with touch help in assessing the place and potential use of touch in the client's situation. At times when words cannot be found, or in circumstances in which people are more comfortable with physical expression than with words, touch is a powerful expression of spirit and an instrument of healing.

Issues in Practice

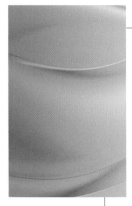

Religious Issues Versus Care Issues

Angie and Edward are a young couple with two teenage children. They are a close and loving family who have a large network of family and friends. The entire family is active in their church, school, and other community groups.

Alan, 15 years old, has just been severely injured in a high school soccer game. Angie and Edward are summoned to the hospital where they are told that Alan has multiple fractured bones and possible internal injuries. While they are waiting for the surgical team to arrive, the couple keeps vigil at their son's bedside in the pediatric intensive care unit (PICU). The surgeon informs the distressed parents that there is evidence that Alan's injuries are more serious than previously diagnosed. Alan has active internal bleeding and will need a blood transfusion to survive. Although genuinely devastated, the parents adamantly refuse to sign for the lifesaving blood transfusion, stating that they are Jehovah's Witnesses and that receipt of blood is against their religion. The surgeon asks you, Alan's nurse, to get the parents to change their minds. You talk with the couple, but they continue to refuse to sign the surgical consent form.

Questions for Thought

1. What are the primary underlying spiritual principles involved in this dilemma?
2. Do Alan's parents have the right to refuse their consent for a blood transfusion on the basis of religious beliefs?
3. Do you think that Alan being a minor (under 18 years old) makes a difference in this situation?
4. What actions do you think the charge nurse should take?
5. How would you resolve this dilemma?

NURSING AS A PROFESSION OR VOCATION

Although the nursing profession is deeply rooted in religious traditions, modern nursing has spent considerable energy attempting to distance itself from this aspect of its history. Nursing as vocation has given way to nursing as profession (see Chapter 1). The current health-care system has required nurses to shift their identity from vocation to profession in order to achieve appropriate value in a system that is increasingly economically oriented.

Nursing as Spiritual Calling

Nursing is much more than the mere secular enterprise the modern world perceives it to be. Perhaps it is time that nurses reevaluate the work they do and consider it a vocation—that is, a life calling in the spiritual sense of that word. The world's religions consistently allude to the symbolic and deep meaning of the work that nurses do. Nursing practice has the capacity to be richly imaginative and to speak to the soul on many levels. It can be carried out mindfully and artistically, or it can be done routinely and unconsciously, like any other job. When nursing is practiced with deep consciousness and purpose, it nurtures the nurse as well as the client.[9]

Some experts perceive that nursing is directly connected to the nurse's fantasy life, family myths, ideals, and traditions. The profession of nursing may be one way nurses sort out their major life issues. Although the choice of nursing as a career may often seem to have been serendipitous, in the spiritual context it is reasonable to question whether anything really happens by accident. As nurses practice nursing, they craft themselves, undertaking the soul's lifetime work of self-definition and self-identification.

When the Well Runs Dry

As with most professions, at times it may become difficult, even impossible perhaps, to feel good about the work that one is doing. Negative attitudes about work are detrimental to a person's self-development and often cause people to become overly invested in the surface trappings of work, such as money, power, and success. The phenomenon of burnout among nurses has been identified and studied for many years (see Chapter 10). Burnout can be viewed from a spiritual perspective, in which the well runs dry, energy fields become unbalanced, or the person experiences a

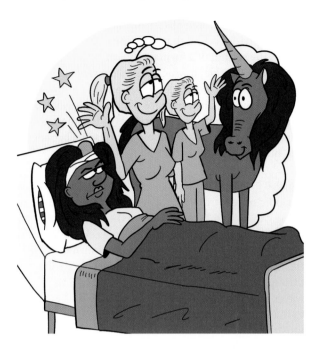

prolonged "dark night of the soul," or even feels that the nurse's life work is devoid of meaning.[8,10]

People working in the helping professions, whose work is rooted in compassion and concern for others, are prone to depression and burnout. A concerted effort at spiritual development, or the nourishment of the soul, is essential to nurses' overall mental and physical well-being.

Maintaining Balance

As discussed above, the integration of the mind, body, and soul is required for a balanced, productive, and fulfilled life. Because of the close interconnection of the three elements any time one becomes imbalanced, the other two are affected. For example, high levels of anxiety or emotional stress of the mind increases the pulse and blood pressure and have been linked to peptic ulcers and chest pain in a person with an otherwise healthy body. Similarly, a physical illness or injury can cause anxiety and depression in a person with a usually healthy mind.

Self-Restoration

To maintain an internal state of balance, the first thing nurses need to do is take time to feed their spirit. Daily prayer or meditation is an important source of insight and energy. Belonging to a group or community that actively pursues spiritual growth is also a powerful source of spiritual nourishment. Many individuals find that their spirits are nourished within the setting of a formal religion, although not necessarily the one in which they were reared. It is not uncommon for people to seek a faith community in midlife or later life, perhaps after being away from one for many years. The experience of trying various religions and modes of worship is by itself a broadening, nurturing experience.

A Sense of Sacredness

Periodic retreat from the hustle and bustle of modern living can be highly restorative to the spirit. A retreat may be for a few hours, a half-day, a weekend, a week, or longer. For some people, keeping a journal is a retreatlike experience. For others, it may be a stroll through a beautiful park, a few hours watching waves on a beach, or a trip to the woods. Retreat is most effective when time is consistently set aside for introspection and reflection rather than for tasks.

> *People working in the helping professions, whose work is rooted in compassion and concern for others, are prone to depression and burnout.*

A sense of sacredness can infuse everyday life with meaning and zest if nurses open themselves to it. It is a part of normal human activity to celebrate seasonal and family holidays with specific rituals, music, decorations, group gatherings, and foods. These types of activities honor life cycles that are greater than the individual and nurture important relationships that serve as a **support system.**

Enjoy Special Moments

Many people have routines for their weekends or days off that allow time for self-restoration. These special activities may include making a large country breakfast while listening to favorite music; baking cookies, bread, or a pie; sitting for an extended period of time in a favorite easy chair; or even playing a physically demanding sport like basketball. Many people have favorite coffee mugs or dishes or special objects in their homes that are not only beautiful but may also remind them of loved ones, wonderful trips, religious experiences, or other events that nourish them each time they view the object.

One of the most spiritual aspects of a person's life is the enjoyment of beauty. It costs little or nothing to plant or cut flowers or to listen to music. It is in these moments that a person's creativity and insight are most evident.

Regaining the Center

The hectic modern world continually urges people to enhance their capacity for dealing with multiple concerns at the same time.[11] Some people even define success by looking at how many tasks they can juggle simultaneously. *Multitasking* is the buzzword for the health-care environment of the 21st century. Nurses must be able to talk on the telephone, send faxes and e-mails, surf the net, and use a word processor for entering client data at the same time that they are developing care plans, evaluating clients, answering call lights, supervising unlicensed assistive personnel, and providing physicians with information.

Although this is highly productive, the more nurses multitask, the more disconnected they become from themselves. Multitasking can be thought of as the antithesis of spiritual nurturance. Spirituality is about personal wholeness, whereas multitasking is about fragmentation.[10] When nurses slow down and center their energy fields, they have the capacity to be fully present and the ability to attend with complete consciousness to their loved ones, colleagues, and clients.[12]

Conclusion

Spirituality within the nursing context needs to be seen as a broad concept encompassing religion but not equated with it. Fundamental to this concept is a search for meaning within life and its particular events, such as ill health. Nursing students need to be made aware of the many forms that spiritual distress may take.[13]

Nurses are in an ideal position to provide spiritual care that positively affects the mental and physical health of their clients. To be able to focus clearly on clients' spiritual needs, nurses must first consider their own spirituality as a starting point for self-knowledge. The means of supporting clients with spiritual problems must be explored. Teaching methods should be participatory and student centered. The means of assessing and meeting spiritual needs hinges on effective communication skills and determines whether the nurse is "being with" the client as opposed to merely "being there." The meaning of the holistic moment emerges through the synergistic interaction among its elements (Fig. 21.2). Just as a person is greater than the sum of her or his parts, so is the holistic moment greater than the sum of its parts, namely spirituality, presence, and relationship to others.[11]

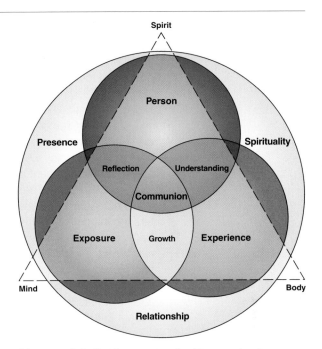

Figure 21.2 Elements involved in experiencing spirituality and presence in the nurse–client relationship. (Adapted from Rankin EA. Finding spirituality and nursing presence. *Journal of Holistic Nursing,* 24[4]:286, 2006.)

Critical-Thinking Exercises

Mrs. Jan Steiner, 73 years old, has outlived two husbands. Ted, her second husband, died 20 years ago. Reared in the Roman Catholic faith, Mrs. Steiner converted to Judaism when she married Ted. Her two daughters by her first husband were also reared in the Roman Catholic tradition. One of them, Kathy, continues to practice her religion. The other daughter, Judith, is Unitarian.

Mrs. Steiner experienced a stroke 2 years ago that left her moderately disabled. At that time she moved into a long-term care facility. She was still able to read and to enjoy visits with friends and family, but a second stroke 3 months ago left her incontinent and aphasic.

Mrs. Steiner has just had a major heart attack. Although bypass surgery could extend her life, she has never articulated any end-of-life desires. Her daughters are in conflict over how Mrs. Steiner's medical management should proceed. Kathy strongly believes that as long as Mrs. Steiner is alive, life should be actively supported. It would be morally wrong to do less than that. Judith, on the other hand, believes that what has been the "life" of Mrs. Steiner is essentially over and it is a waste of resources to merely delay the inevitable. The nursing staff, as they attempt to facilitate communication between the family and the medical staff, feel caught in the middle.

- What are your own spiritual beliefs about the proper approach to Mrs. Steiner's medical management?
- Analyze the positions of Kathy and Judith from both their ethical and spiritual contexts.
- What resources are likely to be available in the hospital or the community to help the daughters come to a decision?

Bypass surgery is not performed, and Mrs. Steiner returns to her long-term care facility. Her overall condition continues to deteriorate, and within 3 months she is very near death. She seems to have little awareness of her surroundings and does not consistently recognize or respond to her daughters.

- Knowing the religious divergence within Mrs. Steiner's family, how might the nursing staff facilitate their preparation for the death of their mother and her funeral?
- What would happen within Mrs. Steiner's circle of family and friends if any "side"—Catholic, Jewish, or Unitarian—"won" in planning her end-of-life care?
- Have you seen blending of religious traditions in rituals of marriage or burial? What are the advantages and disadvantages of such an approach?
- What might be the outcomes of handling their mother's death in a strictly secular or nonsectarian way and allowing all relatives and friends to mourn privately in accordance with their own spiritual traditions?

References

1. Clarke J. A critical view of how nursing has defined spirituality. *Journal of Clinical Nursing,* 18(12):1666–1673, 2009.
2. Hussey T. Nursing and spirituality. *Nursing Philosophy,* 10: 71–80, 2009.
3. Swinton J, Pattison S. Moving beyond clarity: Towards a thin, vague, and useful understanding of spirituality in nursing care. *Nursing Philosophy,* 11(4):226–237, 2010.
4. Nightingale F. *Notes on Nursing.* New York: Dover, 1969. (Originally published in 1860.)
5. Watson J. *Nursing: Human Science and Human Theory of Care: Theory of Nursing.* New York: National League for Nursing, 1988.
6. North American Nursing Diagnosis Association I. Nursing Diagnosis: Definitions and Classification, 2012–2014. Philadelphia: NANDA I Publications, 2012.
7. Moore T. *Care of the Soul: An Inspirational Programme to Add Depth and Meaning to Your Everyday Life.* New York: Harper Perennial, 2012.
8. Mueller C. Spirituality in children: Understanding and developing interventions. *Pediatric Nursing,* 36(4):197–208, 2010.
9. Campbell D. Spirituality, stress, and retention of nurses in critical care. *Dimensions of Critical Care Nursing,* 32(2):78–83, 2013.
10. O'Brien ME. *Spirituality in Nursing.* Sudbury, MA: Jones & Bartlett Learning, 2011.
11. Dolamo BL. Spiritual nursing. *Nursing Update,* 34(4):22–24, 2010.
12. Shores CI. Spiritual perspectives of nursing students. *Nursing Education Perspectives,* 31(1):8–11, 2010.
13. Paley J. Religion and the secularization of health care. *Journal of Clinical Nursing,* 18(14):1963–1974, 2009.
14. Young Y, Koopsen C. *Spirituality, Health, and Healing: An Integrative Approach.* Sudbury, MA: Jones and Bartlett Learning, 2011.

22 Cultural Diversity

Joseph T. Catalano

Learning Objectives

After completing this chapter, the reader will be able to:

- Define *culture* and identify its expression
- Compare and contrast the "melting pot" and "salad bowl" theories of acculturation
- Identify the components of an accurate cultural assessment
- Distinguish between primary and secondary cultural characteristics
- List and define the key aspects of effective intercultural communication
- Name two sources of information about transcultural nursing

TRANSCULTURAL NURSING

Culture is a powerful influence on how nurses and clients interpret and respond to health care and to each other. Both nurses and clients expect to be treated with respect and understanding for their individuality no matter what their cultural origins. Nurses who understand essential characteristics of transcultural nursing will be able to provide competent and culturally sensitive care for clients from all cultural backgrounds.

WHAT IS CULTURE?

Culture is defined and understood in several ways. Culture may be seen as a group's acceptance of a set of attitudes, ideologies, values, beliefs, and behaviors that influence the way the members of the group express themselves.[1] It is a collective way of thinking that distinguishes one relatively large group from another over generations. For example, members of a political party, although diverse in other ways, may be viewed as belonging to a particular culture because of their beliefs and ideologies. These are often handed down from parents to children over generations. Cultural expression assumes many forms, including language; spirituality; works of art; group customs and traditions; food preferences; response to illness, stress, pain, **bereavement**, anger, and sorrow; decision-making; and even world philosophy.

A Powerful Influence

An individual's cultural orientation is the result of a learning process that literally starts at birth and continues throughout the life span. Behaviors, beliefs, and attitudes are transmitted from one generation to the next. Although expressions of culture are primarily unconscious, they have a profound effect on an individual's interactions and response to the health-care system.

When Cultural Traditions are a Barrier to Care

Mrs. Su Sung, who is 74 years old, is brought into the emergency department (ED) by her family because of "very bad indigestion that won't go away." Three family members (a middle-aged man and woman and a younger woman) accompany the elderly lady. They are discussing her condition in a mixture of English and another language the nurse does not recognize. Because the client does not seem to understand any English, the nurse attempts to address the family. The younger woman speaks only broken English but manages to explain that the client is her grandmother and that she is accompanied by her mother and father, who speak even less English than she does. By default, the granddaughter serves as the translator. After much prompting, she explains that her grandmother arrived in the United States for a visit only 2 days ago from a small mountain village in Korea where she has lived all her life. She had been having periodic episodes of "indigestion" for several weeks before the visit and used traditional herbal teas prescribed by the local healer to treat her condition. On the basis of further assessment and a diagnostic test, it is determined that Mrs. Sung had an extensive myocardial infarction at least 1 week before her trip and is currently in a mild state of congestive heart failure (CHF).

She is given medications for the chest pain and CHF and is started on anticoagulant medications in the ED. She is then transferred to the coronary care unit (CCU), where she is scheduled to have a coronary angiography the next day. The angiogram shows multiple blockages in her coronary arteries and extensive myocardial damage. Because of her age and the extensive damage to her heart, the physician thinks it would be too risky to attempt bypass surgery and decides to monitor her closely and treat her medically until she is stable enough to have a balloon angioplasty.

When the CCU nurse assigned to Mrs. Sung enters the room at the beginning of her shift the day after the angiogram, she finds the client covered with four heavy blankets and a bedspread and sweating profusely. When the nurse attempts to remove the excessive bedcovers, the client's daughter protests vehemently in Korean and puts the blankets back on as soon as the nurse leaves the room. The daughter seems to think that her mother is sick because she is too cold and gives the elderly woman hot herbal drinks from a thermos bottle she has brought from home.

When the granddaughter arrives, the nurse explains to her why excessive heat is harmful to the client's cardiac status and why she needs to follow the diet restrictions prescribed by the physician. The ingredients of the herbal drinks are unknown, and there may be some serious interactions with the numerous medications the client is receiving. The granddaughter translates this information to her mother, who seems to become even angrier with the nurse. Although she outwardly seems to comply with the restrictions, she continues the traditional folk treatments in secret, believing the Western hospital food is bad for her mother's health.

Mrs. Sung is very quiet and hardly ever asks for help. When she does talk to her family, the conversation is usually about the airplane flight to the United States and the belief that high altitude probably caused all Mrs. Sung's problems.

Her condition gradually deteriorates during her hospitalization, despite all the medical treatment. The nurse and physician tell the family about the client's worsening condition and the likelihood that she will not survive the hospitalization, but they refuse to relay the information to the client.

Although this situation is fictitious, it demonstrates some of the potential problems that nurses may encounter when interacting with clients who come from a strong traditional cultural background. Culture is, among other things, a belief system that has been developed over a person's lifetime and, like all strongly held belief systems, is difficult to

> " *Culture is not a monolithic concept. Any individual probably belongs to several subcultures within his or her major culture.* "

change. In the case of Mrs. Sung, it is easy to see the futility of attempting to change her belief system in a short period of time with a limited number of inter-actions. It is also important to consider the effect of the family. Rather than encouraging the client to make an exception to her way of thinking in order to follow care recommendations, the family reinforced the client's beliefs.

Concepts of Culture

Culture is not a monolithic concept. Any individual probably belongs to several subcultures within his or her major culture. Subcultures develop when mem-bers of the group accept outside values in addition to those of their dominant culture. Even within a given culture, many variations may exist.[1] For example, it is logical to conclude that people who live in the United States all belong to the American culture; this com-monality is a part of every citizen's identity. However, teenagers living in the rural areas of Oklahoma may find it difficult to re-late to teenagers raised in the inner city of Philadel-phia. Even though they speak the same language and share a cultural per-spective, their past experi-ences, in terms of where in the country they grew up, are so diverse that it may be difficult for them to relate to each other.

Many individuals who migrate to the United States from other countries now cling tenaciously to their traditional cultural practices and languages, resulting in a phenomenon called multiculturalism.

Culture can be envisioned as a flawed photocopy machine that makes duplicates of the original document with minor modifications. As a society attempts to preserve itself by passing down its values, beliefs, and customs to the next genera-tion, slight variations in the practices inevitably occur. For the most part, the key elements of the culture remain intact. However, other elements change greatly due to influences from both within and outside the group.

Diversity

Diversity is a term used to explain the differences between cultures. The characteristics that define diversity can be divided into two groups: primary and secondary.

1. Primary characteristics tend to be more obvious, such as nationality, race, color, gender, age, and religious beliefs.

2. Secondary characteristics include socioeconomic status, education, occupation, length of time away from the country of origin, gender issues, residen-tial status, and sexual orientation. These may be more difficult to identify, yet they may have an even more profound effect on the person's cultural identity than the primary characteristics.[2]

When individuals make generalizations about others based on the obvious primary characteristics or the less evident secondary characteristics, they are stereo-typing the other person. Stereotyping is an oversimplified belief, conception, or opinion about another person (or group) based on a limited amount of information.

MELTING POT VERSUS SALAD BOWL

The United States has traditionally been considered a melting pot of world cultures. Early in the history of the United States, most people who came from distant lands were eager to be assimilated into American culture. Many people Americanized their names, shed their tradi-tional dress, learned American manners and customs as quickly as possible, and made valiant efforts to learn English without the benefit of formal school-ing—all so they could "fit in" with their new homeland. Until recently, most people who immigrated to this country were very willing to acculturate (i.e., to alter their own cultural practices in an attempt to become more like members of the new culture). The end result was a blending, or melting pot, of cultures.[3]

Multiculturalism

Since the early 1970s, the practice of intentional ac-culturation by immigrating cultures seems to have fallen by the wayside. Many individuals who migrate to the United States from other countries now cling tenaciously to their traditional cultural practices and languages, resulting in a phenomenon called *multi-culturalism*.[3] Rather than blending smoothly into the bigger pot as former immigrants have done, the modern immigrants maintain their own unique flavors and textures, much like the ingredients in a large tossed salad. As an ever-growing phenomenon, multiculturalism is something that health-care providers need to be aware of; they must learn ways of adapting their health practices to allow for these diversities.

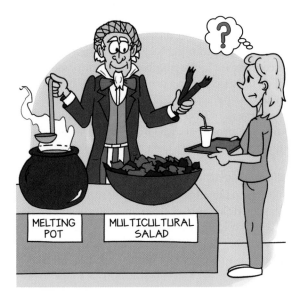

Drawbacks and Benefits

There are drawbacks and benefits to both approaches. In the era of the melting pot, individuals who attempted to retain their native beliefs, customs, and languages were often ridiculed, scorned, and generally made to feel they were outsiders to the mainstream culture. When they did become homogenized into the American culture, learned the language of the dominant society, and made an effort to be seen as belonging, they were more likely to be accepted as equals and quickly advanced up the socioeconomic ladder.

Cultural Relativism

The current salad bowl trend has the advantage of allowing individuals in the dominant culture to gain an appreciation of other cultures for their unique contributions to society. The drawback of the salad bowl is that it tends to create pockets of culturally different individuals who live in but have only minimal interaction with mainstream American society. If they do not speak the language or decide not to participate in the customs of the dominant culture, unfortunately, it can be challenging for them to advance their socioeconomic status.

The salad bowl process has also given rise to cultural relativism among some groups. Cultural relativism occurs when members of a strong cultural group understand their culture and group members

only from their own viewpoint rather than from that of the larger culture.[4] It is based on the belief that one's own culture, native customs, religion, and even language are the best in the world and all others are in some way inferior. People who hold to cultural relativism do not try to understand the larger culture's unique characteristics, values, and beliefs. For example, in many Western societies, dogs and cats are considered to be pets, but in some non-Western cultures, they are viewed as a food source. If a small cultural group persists in the practice of eating cats and dogs even though the majority culture where they now live does not view this practice as acceptable, then they would be practicing cultural relativism. (For more information on cultural relativism, go to http://faculty.uca.edu/rnovy/Rachels—Cultural%20Relativism.htm.)

Heritage Consistency

Some cultural groups manage to blend the melting pot and the salad bowl together through a rather complex process called *heritage consistency*. Ostensibly, they "Americanize" by wearing business suits, speaking English, eating American food, and engaging in traditional American hobbies. However, when they are at home, or with groups from their nation's culture, they speak their native language, wear traditional clothes, eat native meals, and generally follow their native customs.

What Do You Think?

Identify and rank by priority at least five of your own health-care values (e.g., exercise, immunizations). Identify five health-care values of a culture with which you are familiar. How do these values compare with your own?

This approach to acculturation has the advantages of allowing them to fit in and advance within the larger culture, while retaining many of the cultural elements that feel like home, which provides a sense of stability in their lives. It does, however, create in some individuals a type of cultural confusion that may lead to increased tension and anxiety.

U.S. ETHNIC POPULATION TRENDS

In contrast to most other major nations, the population of working and young people in the United States is increasing even as the baby boomer generation ages.

This trend is due to the United States' relatively high birth rate, with nearly 4.3 million births in 2007. This was the highest birth rate in over 45 years, due in part to the influx of new immigrants, who tend to have more children than those who have been living in the United States for more than one generation. A report by the Pew Research Center shows a decline in birth rate from 2008 to 2010, attributed primarily to the recession; however, this trend is beginning to reverse as the economy continues to recover. (For more information, go to http://www.smithsonianmag.com/specialsections/40th-anniversary/The-Changing-Demographics-of-America.html#ixzz2htPeYqjE or http://www.pewsocialtrends.org/2012/11/29/u-s-birth-rate-falls-to-a-record-low-decline-is-greatest-among-immigrants/.)

A Population Shift

According to U.S. Census Bureau statistics, in the year 2010 (the last year data were available), approximately 120 million, or 38 percent, of the entire U.S. population was composed of minority groups, up from 33 percent in the year 2006.[5] If current trends continue, it is projected that by the year 2043, the Caucasian population will be a minority group, constituting 48.9 percent of the total U.S. population. In states such as California, the white population may be a minority as early as 2030. These shifts will require a redefinition or rethinking of the term *minority,* as it is currently defined as racial or ethnic groups that compose less than 50 percent of the population.[6]

Contributing to the rapid growth in minority populations is the number of immigrants coming to the United States; however, from 2002 to 2012, the numbers have actually decreased from 1,059,364 to 1,031,631. Currently, the largest numbers of immigrants are from Asia, Mexico, and Central and South America. Fewer immigrants have come from Africa and Europe than in previous years.[7]

The Need for Transcultural Nursing

The percentage of minority nurses does not reflect the national population trends. Despite efforts on the part of the National League for Nursing (NLN), American Association of Colleges of Nursing (AACN), and other organizations concerned with nursing education, the number of minority nurses has risen only slightly in 10 years to approximately 13 percent from 10.7 percent of the registered nurses (RNs) practicing in the United States. The percentage of men who are RNs has fallen slightly from 5.8 percent to 5.4 percent over the past decade. The latest reported statistics from the NLN in 2012 demonstrate a marked increase in the number of minority students enrolled in basic nursing programs, from 29 percent in 2009 to 33 percent in 2012. In a perfect world, the percentage of RNs from various minority groups should be approximately 33 percent and would mirror the percentage from each minority group.[8]

Culturally Competent Care

Despite the relatively low number of minority nurses, it is expected that nurses from one culture should be able to give culturally competent care to individuals from any other culture. Health care is considered culturally competent when health-care providers and institutions are able to provide care for clients that meet the clients' cultural needs. Ultimately, cultural competency leads to high-quality care to every client regardless of language, race, or ethnic background.

> *Despite the relatively low number of minority nurses, it is expected that nurses from one culture should be able to give culturally competent care to individuals from any other culture.*

Being on the front lines of health care, nursing is the one profession that is continually confronted with cultural changes that result from ethnic shifts in the population. Nurses now recognize they can no longer use traditional ethnocentric models to guide their practice and protocols. Nurses are leading the way in promoting an understanding of individuals from other cultures and improve the overall quality of health care for everyone.

Coverage for Minorities

The Medicare and Medicaid laws that evolved out of the social programs of the 1960s have increased the number of culturally diverse clients with whom nurses come in contact. Historically, many minority groups tend to be among the poorest segments of the population and have the lowest percentage of insurance coverage. Before the Medicare and Medicaid legislation that expanded government-funded health care to cover all welfare recipients, some ethnic minorities were unable to afford health care and were seen in the health-care setting only when severely ill. Ethnic minorities are now covered by these laws and, by their increasing numbers in all levels and areas of health care, have prompted nurses to become more sensitive to the transcultural aspects of their work. The ACA of 2010 has also increased insurance coverage for the number of minorities who fall into the working-poor class so that they are now being seen more regularly in the health-care system.

Since the 1970s, transcultural nursing has become an important subject in most nursing programs. However, nursing education lagged behind in taking steps on the path to seeking a true integration of cultural competence into daily practice. Nursing education with incentives from accrediting entities are now moving to incorporate cultural competency into their curricula. As technological and transportation advances bring more and more people from different cultures closer together, there will be an increased demand for nurses who can practice effectively in a culturally diverse society.[9] Many challenges still lie ahead.

DEVELOPING CULTURAL AWARENESS

Developing cultural awareness is the first step in becoming a culturally competent nurse. One of the main challenges for nurses who practice in a culturally diverse environment is to understand the client's perspective of what is happening in the health-care setting. From a cultural viewpoint, it may be very different from what the nurse believes is occurring.

Awareness Begins at Home
A nurse develops cultural awareness only when he or she is able to recognize and value all aspects of a client's culture, including beliefs, customs, responses, methods of expression, language, and social structure. However, merely learning about another person's culture does not guarantee that the nurse will have cultural awareness. Nurses must first understand their own cultural backgrounds and explore the origins of their own potentially prejudiced and biased views of others. Several tools have been developed to measure a person's cultural awareness.

Cultural awareness begins with an understanding of one's own cultural values and health-care beliefs. To those unfamiliar with a particular culture's health-care beliefs, many of the health-care practices may appear meaningless, strange, or even dangerous.

Beliefs about health care are based in part on knowledge and are often related to religious beliefs. For example, if a particular society has no knowledge of bacteria as a cause of infection, antibiotics may seem useless in achieving a cure for the disease. With that in mind, if a society believes the illness is caused by evil spirits entering the body as the result of curses by witches or medicine men, practices such as incantations; use of ritualistic objects like bones, feathers, or incense; and even bloodletting and purgatives to release the spirit from the body are acceptable approaches to achieving a cure.

Cultural Belief Systems
Cultural belief systems are highly complex. For example, some Native American groups attributed twin births to witchcraft and believed that one of the twin infants had to die so that the other might live. These beliefs and practices are usually kept as closely guarded secrets among the group's members, and there may even be some type of sanction or punishment for members who reveal the belief.

The Purpose of Tradition
Many cultural beliefs develop over time from a trial-and-error process that has both benefits and drawbacks. For instance, several Native American tribes that live in the Western desert have developed the practice of keeping infants in cradle boards until they begin walking. This practice, from a safety viewpoint, protects the crawling infant from injury and bites from creatures that are commonly found in the desert, such as scorpions, rattlesnakes, and poisonous insects or lizards. However, the practice tends to delay the leg muscle development of the child and increases the incidence of hip dysplasia because of the child's position in the cradle board.

Some cultural beliefs have a primary purpose of explaining unusual or unpredictable events. For example, many traditional Vietnamese Americans believe that mental illness results from some action that offended one or more of the gods. They also believe that a family member who is mentally ill brings disgrace on the family, and thus knowledge of the illness must be kept secret, especially from strangers. As a result, traditional shamans, or priest-doctors, are sought to attempt to appease the offended deity through rituals and prayers. Only with great reluctance will a traditional Vietnamese American family seek therapy or medication for a mental illness.

Cultural Values

Several sources of the development of cultural values include religious beliefs, worldviews and philosophies, and group customs. The values that underlie any particular culture are powerful forces that affect all aspects of a person's life, ranging from individual actions and decision-making to health-care behaviors and life-goal setting. Values, which are discussed in Chapter 6, are the ideals or concepts that give meaning to an individual's life. They are deeply ingrained, and most individuals will strongly resist any attempt to change their value structure.

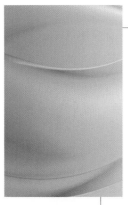

Issues Now

Minority Nurses Needed for the Future of Nursing

Recruiting, retaining, and reshaping the role of minority nurses has been a primary concern of the health-care industry for almost a decade. Initiatives have been implemented by both the private sector and governmental agencies to increase the numbers of minority nurses and meet the needs of the ever-shifting client demographics.

The last comprehensive study of minority nurses conducted in 2008 shows that there has been only a slight increase in the number of minority nurses since 2000. Based on the estimated number of 3.1 million licensed RNs in the United States, the following percentages are found in each minority group:

- African American: 5.4 percent (167,400)
- Asian, Native Hawaiian: 5.8 percent (179,800)
- Hispanic: 3.6 percent (111,600)
- American Indian or Alaska Native: 0.3 percent (9,300)
- Multiracial: 1.7 percent (52,700)
- Men: 9.6 percent (322,200)

Hospitals have been the primary employer of minority nurses and recognize that their employment is a matter of survival. In the competition to attract clients, hospitals cannot afford to have clients feel uncomfortable because of cultural diversity issues. A recent survey showed that 88 percent of minority nurses are employed in nursing, whereas only 82 percent of nonminority nurses are. Also, 85 percent of minority nurses are working full-time, but that number drops to 65 percent for nonminority nurses.

Although hospitals and health care in general acknowledge the need for more minority nurses, some nurses are experiencing barriers to their career mobility. Although the core issues are not unlike those that all nurses experience—understaffing, frustration with paperwork and regulations, and unappreciative administration and physicians—they also feel that their ethnic background may be hindering their chance for promotion. Sometimes their capabilities are questioned because of their differences, and that is a big deterrent.

The role of minority nurses continues to develop as an issue for the future of health care. Not only are they desired employees because of the changing demographics of the population, but also many in the health-care system believe that diversity in their nursing staff will increase the quality of care for the increasing numbers of minority clients. To help recruit nurses and retain those who are already practicing, several organizations have been established that nurses can contact. The National Coalition of Ethnic Minority Nurse Associations and the Tennessee Hospital Association's Council on Diversity are available for assistance. (For more data on minority nurses, go to http://www.aacn.nche.edu/media-relations/fact-sheets/enhancing-diversity.)

Sources: Nursing Statistics 2009. Retrieved December 2010 from http://www.minoritynurse.com; Percentage of Students Enrolled in Basic Nursing Programs 2008–2009. Retrieved December 2010 from http://www.nln.org/research/slides.

Cultural values are neither right nor wrong; they exist in a culture as the result of a long-term process of development that can often be traced back to a need for group survival. However, when judged from the perspective of other cultures, they may seem strange or perhaps harmful. Nurses sometimes feel uncomfortable when dealing with clients who have unfamiliar cultural beliefs and different expectations of the outcomes of the health care being provided. As a result, nurses may unconsciously transfer their own expectations of care from their own cultural background and disregard those of the client. This approach often leads nurses to fail when trying to change health-care behaviors in minority groups.

Recognizing Health-Care Practices

Although all nurses strive to provide the highest quality health care possible, a report by the Institute of Medicine (IOM) indicates that multicultural health care often falls short of the mark. Most nurses are conditioned to address the problems that are obvious and within their line of sight, but sometimes it is necessary to take a step back and look at the bigger picture. Interprofessional collaboration provides a wider view and higher quality culturally competent care.

Changing the Client's Values

It is important to recognize that one of the primary functions of nurses is to change clients' values about health care. It is not an easy task. The first step, always, is to recognize that the nurse comes from a particular culture that has its own set of health-care values. Like all values, these have developed over time and are dependent on the nurse's education, upbringing, religious beliefs, and cultural background.

The next step is to identify the culture of the client and recognize specific health-care practices that are both similar to and different from those of the nurse. The nurse must then make a decision about whether it would be constructive or even possible to change the client's belief on a specific matter and if the end result would be beneficial enough to put forth the necessary effort.[10]

When Is Persuasion Appropriate?

For example, many cultures have strong values concerning pregnancy and the birth of children. In traditional Middle Eastern families, the birth process is valued as an event strictly involving women, and the father is usually not present to either witness or assist

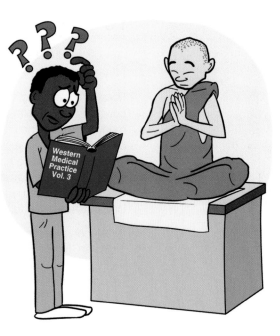

in the delivery. However, midwives and obstetric nurses from the current American culture place a high value on the father's participation in the birth event as a way of promoting stronger family ties and starting the bonding process as soon as possible. The nurse who takes care of a Middle Eastern family must determine whether to try to convince the father to stay in the delivery room during the delivery. In any event, the ultimate outcome remains relatively unchanged. Even without the father in the delivery room, the child is delivered safely, and only the bonding process with the father is delayed.

In the southwest and southern plains of the United States, some American Indian tribes believe strongly in the effectiveness of "medicine bags" and special leather or beaded necklaces in protecting infants from harm and promoting their growth. It is not unusual to observe infants wearing these types of necklaces when they come to the traditional Western medical clinics for care. The main concern of providers in these clinics is the possibility of the infant choking if the necklace should become entangled, but this practice is so ingrained in certain members of the culture that they will refuse to remove the necklaces or they may remove them for the clinic visit and then put them back on after the visit. Because of the ethical principal of autonomy or self-determination, the most health-care providers can do is teach the parents about the potential dangers of the necklaces and hope they will reconsider the risk. Forcibly removing the necklace will break down the trusting relationship with the provider and probably anger the parent of the child.

Assessing Culture

Obtaining accurate cultural assessments can be time-consuming and difficult. However, the only way nurses can avoid imposing their cultural values and practices on others and develop plans of care based on their knowledge about others' beliefs and customs is to make a concerted effort to obtain this information. Several cultural assessment tools for clients have been developed—some short and directed, others lengthy and complicated. One of the most thorough cultural assessments developed to date is based on Purnell's Model for Cultural Competence (Box 22.1). Although this tool is lengthy, it can provide a reliable overview of the client's culture. Nurses should not neglect completing an assessment of their own culture as well.

Beginning the Assessment

Most busy nurses do not have the time to complete this assessment on every client from a different culture. However, the following key questions can serve as a starting point for a cultural assessment:

- Why do you think you are ill? What was the cause of the illness?
- What was going on at the time the illness started?
- How does the illness affect your body and health?
- Do you consider this to be a serious illness?
- If you were at home, what type of treatments or medications would you use? How would these treatments help?

Box 22.1

The 12 Domains of Cultural Assessment: Purnell's Model for Cultural Competence

I. Overview, inhabited localities, and topography overview
   A. Heritage and residence
   B. Reasons for migration and associated economic factors
   C. Educational status and occupation
II. Communications
   A. Dominant language and dialects
   B. Cultural communication patterns
   C. Temporal relationships
   D. Format for names
III. Family roles and organization
   A. Head of household and gender roles
   B. Prescriptive, restrictive, and taboo behaviors
   C. Family roles and priorities
   D. Alternative lifestyles
IV. Workforce issues
   A. Culture in the workplace
   B. Issues related to autonomy
V. Biocultural ecology
   A. Skin color and biological variations
   B. Diseases and health conditions
   C. Variations in drug metabolism
VI. High-risk behaviors
   A. High-risk behaviors
   B. Health-care practices

VII. Nutrition
   A. Meaning of food
   B. Dietary practices for health promotion
VIII. Pregnancy and childbearing practices
   A. Fertility practices and views toward pregnancy
IX. Death rituals
   A. Death rituals and expectations
   B. Responses to death and grief
X. Spirituality
   A. Religious practices and use of prayer
   B. Meaning of life and individual sources of strength
   C. Spiritual beliefs and health-care practices
XI. Health-care practices
   A. Health-seeking beliefs and behaviors
   B. Responsibility for health care
   C. Folklore practices
   D. Barriers to health care
   E. Cultural responses to health and illness
   F. Blood transfusions and organ donation
XII. Health-care practitioners
   A. Traditional versus biomedical care
   B. Status of health-care providers

Source: Purnell LD, Paulanka BJ. *Transcultural Health Care*. Philadelphia: F. A. Davis, 1998, with permission.

- What type of treatment do you expect from the health-care system?
- How has your illness affected your ability to live normally?
- If you do not get better, what do you think will happen?

Because clients from different cultures may feel uncomfortable revealing information about cultural beliefs, values, and practices to strangers, it is a good idea to begin your assessment by asking some general questions. A client is more likely to trust a nurse who demonstrates interest in that person as an individual. Only after a warm and trusting environment has been established will a client be willing to reveal the more personal aspects of his or her culture to the nurse.

Understanding Physical Variations

Physical assessments made on individuals from other cultures require a certain level of cultural awareness and competence. Although the assessment techniques used for different individuals may be identical, the nurse needs to know the basic biological and physical variations among ethnic groups.[11] The interpretation of assessment findings may be affected by ethnic variations in anatomical structure or characteristics (e.g., children from some Asian cultures may fall below the normal growth level on a standardized American growth chart because of their genetically smaller stature).

Issues in Practice

Cultural Aspects of Organ Donation

"Sarah, are you going to ask them?" The tall, haggard third-year trauma resident stood across the desk from me and eyed me with apprehension.

"Well," I sighed, "He's medically suitable and has been declared brain dead. So, yes, I'm going to ask them." I had been coordinator of the New Mexico Organ Procurement Organization for more than 2 years and had asked families for permission to obtain organs for transplantation literally hundreds of times.

"But they're Navajo," he said.

"Organ donation is an option for them," I replied. "They deserve to be offered the option at the very least."

"Can I come in with you?" he asked. "There are a lot of them in there."

"Sure," I said. When a traditional Navajo came to the hospital for treatment with "white man's" medicine, often the whole family came too.

So, after reviewing the client's case file to identify the legal next of kin and doing a few laps around the intensive care unit (ICU) to work out my adrenaline, the resident and I went into the ICU conference room to approach a traditional Navajo family for consent for organ donation.

As I entered the room, 13 pairs of dark eyes looked up at me. I ran through in my head all the things I had learned regarding the American Indian culture in my training. Keep it low-key. Don't make prolonged eye contact. American Indians are stoic in their grief. I took a deep breath, let the resident introduce me, and we began our conversation.

The family was young, and the patient had never married, so the oldest daughter was making the decisions. She had a lot of good questions for me, as did the rest of the family, and I sat on the floor in front of them with my knees drawn up to my chest and talked with them for a long time.

"You know we're Navajo?" one of her brothers asked me. "Organ donation is against our beliefs."

"I realize that," I said. "But you have the option to save a life, possibly as many as three lives, and I wanted to let you know."

"Our uncle got a kidney transplant last year," the oldest daughter said while looking at her brother. "I think we owe something back. Can we have some time to talk about this?"

I thanked them for their time, expressed my condolences again, and left the room with the resident.

Once we were back on the unit, the resident got excited.

"Oh, man. I think they're going to say yes," he said, shifting from one foot to another. "That would be so awesome to have the first Navajo donor here."

I could see the story starting to form in his head and smiled at him when I saw the anticipation and hopefulness in his eyes. *I helped with that American Indian donor. It was so cool.*

Just then, the doors to the ICU swung open and a pair of elderly, withered-looking American Indian women walked into the unit and right up to the desk where I was sitting. They inquired as to which room my client was in and went into the room after I told them. They hovered at the client's bedside for several minutes, regarding the beeping medication pumps, the monitors, and the ventilator with disdain.

(continued)

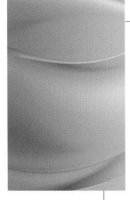

Issues in Practice continued

"Don't get your hopes up," I said to him under my breath.

Silently, the pair left the unit through the doors they had just entered, making eye contact with no one and showing no emotion.

"Who are they?" the resident asked.

"I believe those were the tribal elders," I said.

He looked at me with disbelief. "What do we do now?"

"Now we wait," I said.

I kept myself busy shuffling papers and returned a couple of phone calls. I was playing Free Cell on the computer when the oldest daughter appeared around the corner. I could tell she had been crying.

"Can we see the doctor in our room?" she asked.

"Sure, wait here and I'll go get him," I said.

I went around the corner where he was lounging with his feet propped up on the desk. He was chatting with the unit clerk. "I really think they're going to do it," he said.

"The family wants to see you," I interrupted.

When he looked at me, I saw a question mark on his face. I returned the look with one of my own. Having been in this situation a couple of times before, I had a feeling I knew what the outcome would be.

We walked around the corner, and he went into the conference room with the family, and I returned to my desk to wait.

Two minutes later he was back. He slumped into the chair beside me. "They declined," he sighed disappointedly. "What do I do now?"

"You," I said, "are done. Thank you very much for all your time and hard work. I've got to do some paperwork and call in the decline, and then I'm going home."

He sighed again and then patted my leg. "Well, good effort."

Questions for Thought

1. Was it ethical to ask the family about organ donation when American Indian beliefs generally prohibit it? Do you know of any American Indian organ donors?

2. Was there another possible approach to seeking permission from the family?

3. Why are American Indians opposed to organ donation when they routinely accept organs for transplantation?

Source: Sarah T. Catalano, coordinator, New Mexico Organ Procurement Organization.

Changes in skin color may also affect the interpretation of assessment findings (e.g., cyanosis in people with a light versus a dark complexion). To determine whether the client's skin color is normal or abnormal, the nurse must know what constitutes the normal color for a particular ethnic group. In assessing for cyanosis, the nurse may need to examine the client's oral mucosa and may also need to measure capillary refill times to determine whether the client has cyanosis.

As with all assessments, the ultimate goal of cultural assessment is to provide the best care possible for the client.[11] A fundamental belief that nurses hold to strongly is that all clients have a right to self-determination, including the customs, practices, and values that emanate from their culture. By considering both the cultural and ethnic variables of each client, nurses will avoid practice that is ethnocentric and conducted strictly from the nurse's cultural viewpoint.

PROVIDING CULTURALLY COMPETENT CARE

Transcultural Understanding

Cultural competence has become a buzzword in the health-care system. The term has several divergent definitions, with little consensus among cultural experts. However, cultural competence as it relates to nursing can be regarded as the provision of effective care for clients who belong to diverse cultures, based on the nurse's knowledge and understanding of the values, customs, beliefs, and practices of the culture.

What Do You Think?

Using Purnell's cultural assessment tool, assess your own cultural background. In what areas of your own culture are you lacking knowledge?

Providing culturally competent care requires the development of certain interpersonal skills that allow nurses to work with individuals and groups in the community. The primary skills required for cultural competence include communication, understanding, and sensitivity. Although the basic types of cultural skills are similar, their application within and between cultural groups may differ greatly. The development of cultural competence is not a one-time skill to check off on a skills checklist; rather, it is an ongoing process that continues throughout the nurse's career.[12]

Transcultural Communication

The ability to communicate is the foundation on which culturally competent care is built. The most obvious barrier to culturally competent care for the non-English-speaking client is the lack of a common language (Box 22.2). Communication is a highly complex process that requires both verbal and nonverbal exchanges. Nonverbal communication includes (but is not limited to) body language, facial expressions, eye contact, personal space, touch and body contact, formality of names, and time awareness. Other factors that affect communication are volume of voice, tone, and acceptable greetings. Often clients communicate differently with family and friends than they do with health-care personnel. Nurses should be aware that in some cultures (e.g., those with a strong caste system, which involves a class structure), communication between those in the upper and lower classes may be affected by tradition. For example, some cultures hold the role of women in health care in high esteem, whereas other cultures may consider women in health care as the bottom rung on the ladder. The U.S. Department of Health and Human Services has developed standards for Culturally and Linguistically Appropriate Services (CLAS) (Box 22.3).

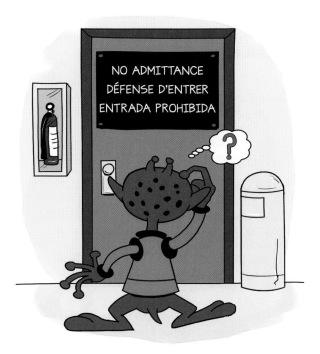

Box 22.2

Guidelines for Communicating With Non-English-Speaking Clients

1. Use interpreters rather than translators. Translators just restate the words from one language to another. An interpreter decodes the words and provides the meaning behind the message.
2. Use dialect-specific interpreters whenever possible.
3. Use interpreters trained in the health-care field.
4. Give the interpreter time alone with the client.
5. Provide time for translation and interpretation.
6. Be aware that interpreters may affect the reporting of symptoms, insert their own ideas, or omit information.
7. Avoid the use of relatives who may distort information or not be objective.
8. Avoid using children as interpreters, especially with sensitive topics.
9. Use same-age and same-gender interpreters whenever possible. However, clients from cultures who have a high regard for elders may prefer an older interpreter.
10. Maintain eye contact with both the client and the interpreter to elicit feedback and read nonverbal clues.
11. Remember that clients can usually understand more than they express; thus, they need time to think in their own language. They are alert to the health-care provider's body language and may forget some or all of their English in times of stress.
12. Speak slowly without exaggerated mouthing, allow time for translation, use active rather than passive tense, wait for feedback, and restate the message. Do not rush; do not speak loudly. Use a reference book with common phrases, such as *Roget's International Thesaurus* or *Taber's Cyclopedic Medical Dictionary.*
13. Use as many words as possible in the client's language and use nonverbal communication when unable to understand the language.
14. If an interpreter is unavailable, the use of a translator may be acceptable. The difficulty with translation is omission of parts of the message; distortion of the message, including transmission of information not given by the speaker; and messages not being fully understood.
15. Note that social class differences between the interpreter and the client may result in the interpreter's not reporting information that he or she perceives as superstitious or unimportant.

Source: Purnell LD, Paulanka BJ. *Transcultural Health Care: A Culturally Competent Approach* (3rd ed.). Philadelphia: F. A. Davis, 2008, with permission.

Box 22.3

U.S. Department of Health and Human Services' Culturally and Linguistically Appropriate Services (CLAS) Standards

Standard 1: Health-care organizations should ensure that patients/consumers receive from all staff members effective, understandable, and respectful care that is provided in a manner compatible with their cultural health beliefs and practices and preferred language.

Standard 2: Health-care organizations should implement strategies to recruit, retain, and promote at all levels of the organization a diverse staff and leadership that are representative of the demographic characteristics of the service area.

Standard 3: Health-care organizations should ensure that staff at all levels and across all disciplines receive ongoing education and training in culturally and linguistically appropriate service delivery.

Standard 4: Health-care organizations must offer and provide language assistance services, including bilingual staff and interpreter services, at no cost to each patient/consumer with limited English proficiency at all points of contact and in a timely manner during all hours of operations.

Standard 5: Health-care organizations must provide to consumers/patients in their preferred language both verbal offers and written notices informing them of their right to receive language assistance services.

Standard 6: Health-care organizations must assure the competence of language assistance provided to limited English proficient patients/consumers by interpreters and bilingual staff. Family and friends should not be used to provide interpretation services (except on request of the patient/consumer).

Box 22.3

U.S. Department of Health and Human Services' Culturally and Linguistically Appropriate Services (CLAS) Standards—cont'd

Standard 7: Health-care organizations must make available easily understood patient-related materials and post signage in the languages of the commonly encountered groups and/or groups represented in the service area.

Standard 8: Health-care organizations should develop, implement, and promote a written strategic plan that outlines clear goals, policies, operational plans, and management accountability/oversight mechanisms to provide culturally and linguistically appropriate services.

Standard 9: Health-care organizations should conduct initial and ongoing organizational self-assessments of CLAS-related activities and are encouraged to integrate cultural and linguistic competency-related measures into their internal audits, performance-improvement programs, patient satisfaction assessments, and outcome-based evaluations.

Standard 10: Health-care organizations should ensure that data on the individual patient/consumer's race, ethnicity, and spoken and written language are collected in health records, integrated into the organization's management information systems, and periodically updated.

Standard 11: Health-care organizations should maintain a current demographic, cultural, and epidemiological profile of the community as well as a needs assessment to accurately plan for and implement services that respond to the cultural and linguistic characteristics of the service area.

Standard 12: Health-care organizations should develop participatory, collaborative partnerships with communities and utilize a variety of formal and informal mechanisms to facilitate community and patient/consumer involvement in designing and implementing CLAS-related activities.

Standard 13: Health-care organizations should ensure that conflict and grievance resolution processes are culturally and linguistically sensitive and capable of identifying, preventing, and resolving cross-cultural conflicts or complaints by patients/consumers.

Standard 14: Health-care organizations are encouraged to regularly make available to the public information about their progress and successful innovations in implementing the CLAS standards and to provide public notice in their communities about the availability of this information.

Source: National standards on culturally and linguistically appropriate services (CLAS). Office of Minority Health website. Retrieved April 2013 from http://minorityhealth.hhs.gov/templates/browse.aspx?lvl=2&lvlID=15

Nonverbal Responses

Nurses who work with non-English-speaking clients need to develop alternative ways to measure a client's understanding rather than depending only on a verbal response. Nurses must be cautious when interpreting the nonverbal responses from some cultural groups, which may respond to all questions with a yes, a nod, or a smile. In the American culture, this response usually indicates understanding and **compliance**. However, particularly in Asian cultures, nodding and smiling can be signs of respect for the nurse's position or an attempt to avoid confrontation. For example, see the quoted scenario on page 557.

Speech Patterns

The use of silence by some cultural groups has led to misunderstandings in the health-care setting. For example, Asian Americans consider silence to be a sign of respect, particularly for elders, whereas Arab Americans and the English use silence to gain privacy. Among many people in Europe (e.g., the French, Russians, and Spanish), silence often indicates agreement.

Variations in communication style also account for misunderstandings and miscommunications. Factors such as loudness, intonation, rhythm, and speed of speech all are important in communication. Among certain cultural groups, American nurses have a reputation for speaking at a rapid rate and for using medical jargon. Some nurses also have a reputation for their tendency to increase the volume of their voices when communicating with clients who do not speak English, as if talking more loudly will increase understanding.[12]

On the other hand, groups such as American Indians and Asian Americans speak more softly and

Issues Now

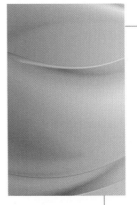

Informed Consent Requires Understanding

Sinwan Ho is an elderly woman from an Asian culture who speaks very little English. She was admitted to the Gastromed Health Care Center for a routine colonoscopy and polypectomy, which was performed on May 20, 2003, by Lawrence Kluger, MD. During the procedure, the bowel was perforated. The next day Ms. Ho underwent a laparotomy with removal of the damaged part of the colon and the formation of a colostomy.

Ms. Ho was readmitted on September 2, 2003, to have the colostomy closed and the colon reconnected. She recovered well, but several years later she began experiencing abdominal pain and gastrointestinal symptoms. It was determined that lesions had formed in the reconnected bowel and were closing the bowel. On April 20, 2006, Ms. Ho was readmitted and another colostomy was performed. Later that year on September 6, 2006, the colostomy was again closed with reconnection of the bowel. The client had a total of five surgeries related to the first routine procedure.

Dr. Kluger was initially sued for malpractice, but the court could not find conclusive evidence that he had committed any medical errors, and the case was dismissed as a "bad outcome."

Later a suit was filed on behalf of Ms. Ho. According to her testimony and that of a friend, Kenneth Lee, she had not been properly informed of the possible complications of the procedure in language that she could understand. She did sign the informed consent form when it was handed to her. The court determined that lack of clear communication of the possible complications was a deviation in the standard of care.

In further testimony, Dr. Kluger admitted that he knew the client did not speak much English and that he had made no attempt to find an interpreter to help explain the procedure and the possible complications such as bowel perforation and colostomy. However, his lawyer argued that because the possibility of an intestinal perforation with a resulting colostomy is so low, revealing that information did not meet the state's requirement as a "reasonable degree of medical probability."

The court ruled that Dr. Kluger's failure to adequately communicate the complications of the procedure did not meet the requirement for malpractice. However, it did rule that there was a case for medical negligence based on the premise that failure to disclose what a reasonable and prudent client would want to know is a deviation from a standard of care.

In 2010, the hospital's insurance company settled the case for an undisclosed sum, imposing a gag order on all parties and without acknowledging wrongdoing by the hospital or the physician.

Source: Ho v. Kluger, A.2d, 2009 WL2431591 (N.J. App., August 11, 2009). Retrieved November 2013 from http://www.leagle.com/decision/In%20NJCO%2020090811191

may be difficult to hear even when the nurse is standing at the bedside. These groups may misinterpret the louder, more forceful tone of the American nurse as an indication of anger. Arab American groups are often noted for their dramatic communication styles. Nurses may misinterpret this behavior as hostility, when in reality the client is merely trying to demonstrate a point using an emotional communication style. To prevent misunderstandings, nurses need to analyze their own speech patterns and consciously modify their tone and pace when working with different cultural groups.

Personal Matters

Nurses also need to recognize that certain groups are much less willing to disclose private matters or personal feelings than others. In general, clients from American or European origins tend to be less secretive about almost all issues because the practice of sharing has been encouraged from an early age. However, many Asian cultures, particularly the Japanese, are highly reluctant to discuss personal topics with either family or health-care providers. Other groups, such as Mexican Americans, discuss personal issues openly with friends and family members but are reluctant to do so with health-care providers, whom they do not know well.

Even within these groups there are wide variations. American women probably constitute one of the most open groups when it comes to expressing personal feelings, whereas American men tend to have much more difficulty with this type of communication.

Open-Ended Language

It is common for nurses to presume that clients trust them instantaneously simply because they are nurses and should answer even the most personal questions without hesitation. As discussed earlier, it may be

"An English-speaking nurse gave a non-English-speaking Asian client preoperative instructions about how to prepare an abdominal surgical site. She thought that she had shown the client how the bottle of povidone-iodine, a powerful skin disinfectant, was to be used in scrubbing the area. The client smiled and nodded throughout the instruction. When asked whether he had any questions, he did not respond. The nurse took the silence to mean that he had no questions. When the nurse left the room, the client promptly drank the whole bottle of povidone-iodine. Fortunately, the error was discovered immediately, and no long-term complications occurred from the accident."

much more productive to start the communication process with small talk and general, nonthreatening questions to establish a trustworthy rapport. Often the use of open-ended questions and statements allows the client to express beliefs and opinions that would be difficult to discover through closed-ended questions that the client can answer with a simple yes or no.

As the level of trust increases, the client will be more likely to reveal important information in the more sensitive areas of the assessment. In addition, sensitivity to the nonverbal aspects of the communication process allows nurses to use behaviors that increase trust and to avoid gestures, facial expressions, or eye contact that may relay a message of superiority, hostility, anger, or disapproval.

Touch Misinterpreted

A leading cause of miscommunication is touching clients from different cultures in ways that they consider inappropriate.[12] American nurses are taught early in their first nursing classes, usually on physical assessment or basic skill courses, that it is necessary to "lay on hands" in order to provide quality care. Students who are reluctant to palpate the femoral pulses of their laboratory partner or remove a client's shirt to auscultate anterior heart and breath sounds may receive a failing grade for the course.

However, touching in other cultures conveys a number of alternative meanings, ranging from power, anger, and sexual arousal to affirmation, empathy, and cordiality. For example, it is generally not acceptable for men and women to touch in many Arab cultures, except in the privacy of the home and in the context of marriage. American women nurses who palpate pulses, listen to breath sounds, or palpate for tactile fremitus when assessing men from an Arab culture may be communicating a message that they never intended.

Some groups, such as Mexican Americans and Italian Americans, who frequently touch and hug family members and friends, are much less receptive to touching by strangers during health-care examinations, particularly if the health-care provider is of the opposite gender. In these situations it is extremely important for the nurse to explain, before the particular physical contact occurs, what he or she is going to do and why it should be done. The nurse should also avoid any unnecessary contact, such as palpation of femoral pulses when the client has pneumonia.

Personal Space

Closely related to the issue of touch is the concept of personal space. Personal space is a zone that individuals maintain around themselves in most casual social situations. When a person's personal space is violated, it often creates a generalized feeling of discomfort or threat, which causes the person to move away from the offending individual. Nurses routinely violate clients' personal space when performing physical assessments or providing basic care.

The distance required to maintain a comfortable personal space varies widely from one culture to another. People who belong to the European, Canadian, or American cultures usually require between 18 and 22 inches of distance for a comfortable personal space when communicating with strangers or casual acquaintances. In contrast, individuals from the Jewish, Arab, Turkish, and Middle Eastern cultures may require as little as 3 to 5 inches of personal space when talking with another person and often interpret physical closeness as a sign of acceptance. In addition, they prefer to stand face-to-face and maintain eye contact when they are talking.

It is easy to understand why misinterpretations in communication might arise. A client from a Middle Eastern culture might judge an American nurse to be cold and aloof, although she is merely maintaining a comfortable personal space from the client. Likewise, an American nurse may feel physically threatened by the close communication style of a Turkish American client and continually back away from the client in an attempt to reestablish his or her personal space.

> *Nurses who work with non-English-speaking clients need to develop alternative ways to measure a client's understanding rather than depending only on a verbal response.*

Eye Contact

Similarly, eye contact communicates different messages to different cultures. Among American and many European cultures, making periodic eye contact during conversations indicates attentiveness to the communication and is a means of measuring the person's sincerity. Common sayings such as, "Look me in the eye and say that," and admonitions for public speakers to make eye contact with the audience emphasize the underlying positive value these cultures place on eye contact. Lack of eye contact may be interpreted as inattention, insincerity, or disregard.

In contrast, some American Indian cultures believe that the eyes are the windows of the soul and that direct eye contact by another may be interpreted as an attempt to "steal the soul" from the body. Between American Indian men, direct eye contact is a sign of challenge and aggression and may precipitate a violent physical confrontation. Among some South American cultures, sustained eye contact is a sign of disrespect, whereas in other cultural groups, particularly Mexican Americans, eye contact with a child is believed to convey the *mal de ojo*, or "evil eye." Many childhood and adult illnesses among these cultures are attributed to the effects of the evil eye, and practices such as tying red cloths or strings around children's wrists are used to ward off illnesses. Eye contact, a routine part of American culture, has diverse and powerful meanings to clients from other cultures.

The complexity and importance of communication should never be underestimated when working with clients from diverse cultures. Merely speaking a language does not encompass the entirety of communication. Awareness of the meanings of gestures, body positions, facial expressions, and eye movements is essential in culturally competent communication.

LOOKING DEEPER

Several other elements must be considered for effective transcultural nursing, including passive obedience, cultural synergy, building on similarities, and conflict resolution. The term *passive obedience* refers to a type of behavior that develops when clients from a different culture believe that the nurse is an authority figure or expert in health-care matters. Although many cultures may display this type of behavior to some extent, it is most commonly seen among Asian American groups. These cultures try to cope with the uncertainty of their health status and the threat of an authority figure by becoming passively obedient. Rather than asking questions they think will reveal their lack of knowledge or confusion about some health-care issue or that they believe may challenge the authority of the nurse, they become passively obedient and compliant.

Cultural Conflicts

It is inevitable that conflicts will arise from time to time when a nurse cares for clients of different cultures. It is important to recognize that the origins of many conflicts reside within the individual. Nurses may label clients from other cultures as noncompliant, when in reality the nurse has an incomplete understanding of the client's culture or unrealistic expectations for behavior.

> " *. . . touching in other cultures conveys a number of alternative meanings, ranging from power, anger, and sexual arousal to affirmation, empathy, and cordiality.* "

What Do You Think?

Think of the last client for whom you provided care. What were the cultural differences that affected the care you gave? What measures did you use to overcome these? What might you have done differently to improve care?

Other common reasons for noncompliance among culturally diverse clients include the lack of external symptoms of disease, inconvenient or painful treatments, and lack of external support from family members or close friends.

Respect for Healing Traditions

The nurse first needs to ask the client what traditional treatments are used in dealing with this disease. In some cases, in which the traditional treatments are similar to the ones used by the health-care facility, the nurse may be able to demonstrate this similarity to the client.

In other cases, the treatments may be very different. However, if culturally based alternative treatments do not interfere with the prescribed treatment plan or threaten the client's health, they can be used simultaneously with the standard medical treatments. For example, nurses who work in the American Indian health-care system and hospitals have become accustomed to finding bone fragments, feathers, and leather medicine pouches in the beds of their clients.

Cultural Synergy

Cultural synergy is a term that implies that health-care providers make a commitment to learn about other cultures and to immerse themselves in those cultures. Nurses who work actively to develop cultural synergy tend to be more successful in the delivery of competent transcultural care. Nurses achieve cultural synergy when they begin to selectively include values, customs, and beliefs of other cultures in their own worldviews. The first step in cultural synergy is the desire to know everything about another culture and to purposely establish relationships with individuals from other cultures.[13]

More Alike Than Different

Closely related to cultural synergy is the recognition that cultures are much alike in many aspects. It seems that most books and publications written about cultural diversity present only the diversity of cultures and not the similarities. Although recognition of cultural differences is important, it should be just one step toward the ultimate realization that there are more similarities than differences among diverse cultures.

Many colleges offer courses in comparative religions identifying the many similarities of the fundamental beliefs that underlie the major religions. However, many college courses on cultural diversity have not evolved past the point of identifying cultural differences. Perhaps this is due in part to the salad bowl approach to cultural communication that exists in current society. Perhaps a new approach to acculturation, based on the similarities between cultures rather than on the differences, should be developed.

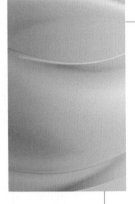

Issues in Practice

Case Study: Cultural Conflict Within a Family

In 1990, Jose Bisigan, aged 87 years, and his wife Carmen, aged 85, sold their small restaurant and immigrated to Los Angeles from a small town in the Visayan region of the Philippines. They came to join their firstborn daughter, a nurse named Felicia, aged 54; her husband; and their three children, ages 10, 13, and 18. Mr. Bisigan speaks limited English and is in a poststroke rehabilitation unit. Since the stroke, he has had mild aphasia, mild confusion, and bladder and bowel continence problems. His hypertension and long-standing diabetes are controlled with medication and diet. His wife, daughter, and grandchildren have been supportive of him during this first hospitalization experience. Mr. Bisigan's family has cooperated with the health team, often agreeing with minimal resistance to the prescribed treatment management. The rehabilitation team recommended subacute rehabilitation treatment as part of the discharge plan.

As a businessman and the elder in the family household, Mr. Bisigan is looked to for counsel by the immediate and extended family. Mr. Bisigan's status, however, has caused friction between Felicia and her husband, Nestor, an American-born Filipino who works as a machinist. Nestor has accused Felicia of giving excessive attention to her mother and father. Felicia's worries about her parents' health have made Nestor very resentful. He has increased his already daily "outings with the boys." Felicia maintains a full-time position in acute care and a part-time night shift position in a nursing home.

Mr. Bisigan's discharge is pending, and a decision must be made before Medicare coverage runs out. Felicia has to consider the possible choices available to her father and the family's circumstances and expectations. Mrs. Bisigan, who is being treated for hypertension, has always deferred decisions to her husband and is looking to Felicia to make the decisions. Because of her work schedule, the absence of a responsible person at home, her mother's health problems, and intergenerational friction, Felicia considers nursing home placement. She is, however, reluctant to broach the subject with her father, who expects to be cared for at home. Mrs. Bisigan disagrees with putting her husband in a nursing home and is adamant that she will care for her husband at home.

Felicia delayed talking to her father until the rehabilitation team requested a meeting. At the meeting, Felicia indicated that she could not bring herself to present her plan to put her father in a nursing home because of her mother's objection and her own fear that her father will feel rejected. Feeling very much alone in resolving the issue about nursing home placement, she requested the team to act as intermediary for her and her family.

Questions for Thought

1. Identify cultural family values that contribute to the conflicts experienced by each family member.

2. Identify a culturally competent approach the team can use when discussing nursing home placement with the Bisigans.

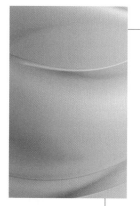

Issues in Practice continued

3. How might the rehabilitation program be presented to Mrs. Bisigan and still allow her to maintain her spousal role?

4. Discuss at least three communication issues in the family that are culture-bound and suggest possible interventions.

5. Identify psychocultural assessments that should be done by the rehabilitation team to have a greater understanding of the dynamics specific to this family.

6. Identify health promotion counseling that might be discussed with the Bisigans' grandchildren.

7. Identify and explain major sources of stress for each member of this household.

Source: Purnell LD, Paulanka BJ. *Transcultural Health Care: A Culturally Competent Approach* (3rd ed.). Philadelphia: F. A. Davis, 2008, with permission.

INFORMATION SOURCES FOR TRANSCULTURAL NURSING

Like all practice areas in the profession, transcultural nursing is also striving to increase the quality of care by using best practices based on evidence-based practice (EBP). Through the rapid growth of research and information sources on transcultural nursing, new models and theories have been developed. However, these new theories and models may lead some individuals to assume that clients can be categorized by race, culture, and ethnicity. The reality is that individual clients cannot be put into culturally specific boxes or labeled by virtue of their culture or skin color. People are individuals and the criteria identified for a particular cultural group do not accurately describe every client who belongs to that racial, ethnic, or cultural group.

From a Conference . . .

With the rapid growth of a minority population in the United States, there is an increasing interest in cultural diversity and transcultural nursing. The origins of the current transcultural movement can be traced back to 1974, when a transcultural conference on communication and culture was held at the University of Hawaii School of Nursing. Following the success of this conference, a series of transcultural conferences was planned over the next year to bring together nurses, sociologists, anthropologists, and other social scientists to discuss issues that would eventually form the basis for transcultural nursing.

Not long after the Hawaii conference, the Transcultural Nursing Society was organized. It was incorporated in 1981 and began publishing its semi-annual official journal, *Journal of Transcultural Nursing*, in 1989. It is now a peer-reviewed quarterly journal that provides information on all aspects of culture and nursing. It is now providing articles online. In 1976, the American Nurses Association (ANA) recommended that multicultural content be included in nursing curricula. Since then, the ANA, in conjunction with the Expert Panel on Global Nursing and Health, has developed Standards of Practice for Culturally Competent Nursing Care (2010) (see http://www.tcns.org/files/Standards_of_Practice_for_Culturally_Compt_Nsg_Care-Revised_.pdf).

. . . to a Specialty

Since the 1980s, more and more universities and colleges have started offering graduate degrees in transcultural, cross-cultural, and international nursing. Graduates are now able to become certified transcultural nurses (CTNs) by completing oral and written examinations offered by the Transcultural Nursing Society. Nurses do not need to be from minority groups to obtain the CTN qualification.

Society has not remained stagnant during this period of development and organization. Growing numbers of immigrants, changing governmental regulations, and grassroots movements all have contributed to the pressure placed on nursing to recognize and effectively care for clients from different cultures.

Conclusion

The major changes in U.S. demographics that began in the 1980s—and have been accelerating ever since—require nurses to provide culturally sensitive care. A fundamental belief of professional nursing holds that all individuals are to be cared for with respect and dignity regardless of culture, beliefs, or disease process. Therefore, nurses must actively seek multicultural education.

However, nurses need to keep in mind that cultural assessments and decisions about care are relative to the nurse's own personal experiences, beliefs, and culture. There is a natural tendency to unconsciously stereotype individuals from other cultures on the basis of one's internal value system. There is also a tendency to batch all individuals from one culture into a single group, when in reality there may be wide variations within the group.

It is a well-accepted belief that nurses who value cultural diversity will deliver higher-quality care. Nurses who have a high level of cultural knowledge and sensitivity maximize their nursing interventions when they become coparticipants and client advocates for individuals who might otherwise be lost in an impersonal health-care system. Only when nurses can understand the client's perspective, develop an open style of communication, become receptive to learning from clients of other cultures, and accept and work with the ambiguities inherent in the care of multicultural clients will they become truly culturally competent health-care providers.

Critical-Thinking Exercises

- Try this experiment. Without letting them know what you are doing, walk up to your classmates and note at what distance they start backing away from you (personal space). If you have classmates that are from a different culture or ethnic group than you, is the personal space distance different from those of your own culture?
- Look up the census data for your city or town for the years 2000 and 2010. Has the percentage of culturally different individuals changed? Is that change obvious in what you hear and see in your city or town? How?
- What cultural group do you belong to? Identify and list five traditions or cultural practices that you and your family follow.
- Is it possible for people from a different culture to use both the salad bowl and melting pot approach to cultural integration at the same time? Provide an example of how this might occur.
- List the elements of culturally competent care that you have developed so far in your career. What other skills do you need to work on to become fully culturally competent?

References

1. Wilkes L, Jackson D. Enabling research cultures in nursing: Insights from a multidisciplinary group of experienced researchers. *Nurse Researcher,* 20(4):28–34, 2013.

2. Nairn S, Hardy C, Harling M, Parumal L, Narayanasamy M. Diversity and ethnicity in nurse education: The perspective of nurse lecturers. *Nurse Education Today,* 32(3):203–207, 2012.

3. Fassler M. Melting pot management: Treat diversity at the workplace as boon, not bane. *Modern Healthcare,* 15;40(7):25, 2010.

4. MacNab YC, Malloy DC, Hadjistavropoulos T, et al. Idealism and relativism across cultures: A cross-cultural examination of physicians' responses on the Ethics Position Questionnaire (EPQ). *Journal of Cross-Cultural Psychology,* 42(7):1272–1278, 2012.

5. United States Census Bureau, Quick Facts. Retrieved April 2014 from http://quickfacts.census.gov/qfd/states/00000.html

6. Cooper M. Census officials citing increasing diversity say U.S. will be a plurality nation. *New York Times,* 2012. Retrieved April 2013 from http://www.nytimes.com/2012/12/13/us/us-will-have-no-ethnic-majority-census-finds.html

7. Yearbook of Immigration Statistics: 2012. Retrieved April 2013 from http://www.dhs.gov/yearbook-immigration-statistics-2012-legal-permanent-residents

8. Minority Nursing Statistics. Retrieved April 2013 from http://www.public.iastate.edu/~monica66/wbtu/teachingunit/statistics.html

9. Strunk JA, Townsend-Rocchiccioli J, Sanford JT. The aging Hispanic in America: Challenges for nurses in a stressed health care environment. *Medical/Surgical Nursing,* 22(1):45–50, 2013.

10. Cordon C. Structural inequality and diversity in nursing. *Minority Nurse,*12(1): 30–35, 2012.

11. Vasiliou M, Kouta C, Raftopoulos V. The use of the Cultural Competence Assessment Tool (Ccatool) in community nurses: The pilot study and test-retest reliability. *International Journal of Caring Sciences,* 6(1):44–52, 2013.

12. Helena BJ. How cultural competency can help reduce health disparities. *Radiologic Technology,* 84(2):129–147, 2012.

13. American Association of Critical-Care Nurses. The AACN Synergy Model for Patient Care. Retrieved April 2013 from http://www.aacn.org/wd/certifications/content/synmodel.pcms?menu=

Impact of the Aging Population on Health-Care Delivery

23

Joseph Molinatti

Learning Objectives

After completing this chapter, the reader will be able to:

- Analyze and discuss the effect of health care over a person's life span
- Relate current economic conditions to the increasing cost of health care
- Evaluate the effects of educating the older population about the need to maintain a healthy lifestyle
- Demonstrate an understanding of the long-term results of the passage of the Affordable Care Act on the health status of future aging populations
- Interrelate the elderly population's view of spirituality and how it impacts their health-care status

THE SILVER TSUNAMI

The health-care system currently used in the United States was designed primarily to treat acute illness and injury. Today, the health-care system is evolving to provide high-quality care for chronic illnesses and adapt to behaviors and personal issues of an aging population. This rapid growth in the older population has been coined the "silver tsunami," as it increases the demand for health services focused on chronic disease, comorbid status, and the unique health promotion needs of older adults. However, the truth of the matter is that the vast majority of the elderly are relatively healthy and manage their chronic conditions at home.[1] Although their concept of what it means to be healthy is different from the expectations of younger people, as long as they can continue to live their lives independently, they consider themselves to be in good health.

Nurses in today's health-care system are dealing with a rapidly aging population as the first "baby boomers" (adults born between 1946 and 1964) become 65 and older. Over 37 million people in this group (60 percent) will have one or more chronic conditions by 2030.[1] Older adults are at a much higher risk for chronic illness, which includes diseases and conditions such as obesity, diabetes, coronary artery disease (CAD), chronic obstructive pulmonary disease (COPD), arthritis, dementia, coronary vascular disease (CVD), cancer, osteoarthritis, and depression.[2] Even though the majority are able to remain in their homes, generally speaking, the older population has more hospitalizations, more admissions to nursing homes, and is the most likely to lose the freedom of living in their own homes; therefore, the possibility of experiencing low-quality care increases simply be-cause they are participating in the health-care system more frequently.[3]

A Major Killer
Since the older population is living longer, chronic disease has become a major problem and a leading cause of death. The health-care system is continually increasing its focus on the chronic disease process. Nearly half of Americans aged 20 to 74 have some type of chronic condition.[4] Each year, 7 out of 10 Americans die from chronic diseases, with strokes accounting for more than 50 percent of all the deaths. Chronic disease accounts for more than 36 million deaths globally per year.[5]

All the major health organizations have identified obesity and dia-betes as a major health concern. Over 25 percent of people with chronic conditions are limited in one or more activities. Arthritis is the most common cause of restricting activity, while diabetes continues to be the leading cause of kidney failure and blindness among adults. The reality is that chronic diseases have no measureable cures. The best that can be hoped for is to treat the symptoms and slow down the diseases' progress.

Chronic disease management has changed over the years, which allows for a better approach for those with chronic illness. In line with the approach advocated by the Affordable Care Act (ACA), the newer management programs emphasize prevention and wellness throughout the health-care system, particularly in community care.[5]

Self-Care
In Dorothea Orem's model of nursing, individuals are responsible for their own care.[6] Callista Roy's model talks about how the choices people make help them adapt to illness and maintain wellness[7] (see Chapter 3).

> *The reality is that chronic diseases have no measureable cures and the best that can be hoped for is to treat and control the symptoms and to reduce the speed of the disease's progressions.*

As people age, the ability to perform activities of daily living often decrease if any type of illness occurs that impinges on their physical and/or mental function. It is evident that the majority of adults would prefer to reside in their own community and home as long as possible. Being in a familiar environment makes the older adult more apt to remain independent and have a sense of comfort and belonging. Often, when inde-pendence is removed from older adults, they do not have a family support system to help them. States that invest in home support services for the elderly have re-duced the number of clients receiving long-term insti-tutional care and overall spending in their Medicare programs.[8]

Health-Care Coverage
Health expenditures in the United States has neared $2.6 trillion in 2010, over 10 times the $256 billion spent in 1989.[9] In past few years, the growth rate in expenditures has been declining slightly as com-pared to the late 1990s and early 2000s. However, the expenses are expected to multiply faster than the national inflation rate for the foreseeable future.[10] The total health-care spending has accounted for 17 percent of the nation's gross domestic product.

Medicare and Medicaid account for a large portion of this expenditure. Medicare is a federal gov-ernment–sponsored health-care program developed primarily for senior citizens over the age of 65, those with end-stage renal disease, and disabled persons who are eligible to receive Social Security benefits because of their contribution to the Social Security system dur-ing their working years. To maintain consistent and uniform coverage across the county, the program is run and maintained by the federal government and is divided into Part A, which covers hospital care; Part B, which covers medical insurance; and Part D, which covers prescription drugs. Participants in the program may be required to pay a deductible and a small co-pay for medical services.

Medicaid differs in that it is primarily for low-income families and low-income individuals. There is much variability in who qualifies for Medi-caid and the benefits that are available because it is administered and managed by the individual states,

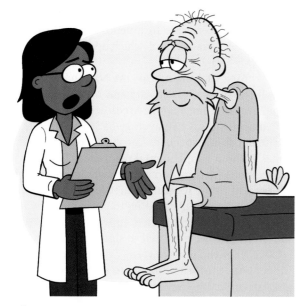

"YOUR CHART INDICATES YOU'RE 34 YEARS OLD. WE NEED TO TALK ABOUT WELLNESS AND PREVENTION!"

which receive matching funds from the federal government. Some states are very restrictive in who can receive benefits and may require that clients have virtually no income and meet other criteria such as passing drug screening tests and demonstrating the inability to find a job. In states with more progressive Medicaid programs, clients can receive services such as hospitalization, x-rays, laboratory services, midwife services, clinic treatment, pediatrics care, family planning, nursing services, in-home nursing facilities for clients over age 21, and medical and surgical dental care. A large percentage of Medicaid expenditures go for nursing home care and children. (For more information, go to http://www.diffen.com/difference/Medicaid_vs_Medicare or http://answers.hhs.gov/questions/3094 or http://www.medicare.gov/Pubs/pdf/11306.pdf.)

Employers are faced with a growing need to increase their expenditures in premiums for family coverage for their employees, and as a result, they are hiring more part-time employees who are not required to be covered. Although the trend in rising unemployment has started to reverse slightly in recent years, many individuals are overqualified for the work and or these jobs are still at the lower end of the pay scale, which leads to an overall lower income for middle-class Americans. As a result, there is greater government health-care spending through the Medicaid program, which covers low-income families.[9]

Medicare not only covers the elderly but also those with disabilities. Both state and federal budgets are being affected by these increased costs.[10] Medicare also covers some costs for those who need a skilled nursing facility or require rehabilitation and those individuals who receive the service from Centers for Medicare and Medicaid Services (CMS) nursing home after a qualifying hospital stay.[11] To qualify for such coverage, there needs to be a certain amount of time spent in a hospital prior to the admission to a skilled facility. Conversely, only Medicaid clients who are in a facility that is certified by the government are eligible for Medicaid coverage.

Individuals who have multi-morbid problems require longer hospital stays. The trend in recent years is to reduce reimbursement to hospitals and health-care providers such as physicians and nurse practitioners for the Medicare clients they are seeing. Since the midterm 2010 elections, some state legislatures have attempted to further decrease reimbursement to health-care providers.[12,13] Reducing Medicare reimbursement to providers who are caring for the elderly has caused some providers to stop accepting new Medicare clients and increases the numbers of elderly clients that providers—who are still willing to accept Medicare clients—must see.[2]

Health-Care Ruling

When the Supreme Court issued its ruling upholding the ACA in 2013, it had a favorable effect for seniors on Medicare. A large segment of the older population expressed a sense of relief regarding their health-care options.[14] When the ACA was passed by Congress in 2010, the changes in coverage were spread out over a number of years. If the bill had not been reaffirmed by the Supreme Court as being constitutional, none of the provisions would have been implemented, leading to a marked decrease in coverage for seniors and a pullback on coverage for the currently uninsured.

Now that health-care reform is in effect, new goals have been set by the government that may change the attitude of American citizens about the role of the government in their lives. After a disastrous rollout of the ACA website in October of 2013, large numbers of the public sector developed doubts regarding the health-care reform law. Over the next few months, the ACA website was fixed and increasing numbers of citizens began enrolling in large numbers, meeting the goal of 8 million enrolled by the

March 31, 2014, deadline. Although President Obama had promised that people could keep their old health-care plans if they wanted, the ACA actually set minimal standards for what needed to be covered in health-care plans, which meant that health-care plans that did not meet the standards of the law were canceled.

The reality is that the ACA is a work in progress that will take several years to reach its full potential. Although there is a blueprint for it, no one really knows what it will look like when it is totally implemented. There will be problems that come up along the way to its full implementation and changes that need to be made in the law. All citizens, including the elderly, need to keep abreast of the changes and developments that occur as the ACA progresses. One of the best ways to keep current is to monitor websites such as http://www.dailykos.com/story/2013/11/08/1254122/-Official-ACA-Numbers-Expect-between-40K-400K-Actual-Enrollments# or http://www.abta.org/care-treatment/support-resources/the-affordable-care-act.html, which update information on a weekly basis.

Max Richtman leads the National Committee to Preserve Social Security and Medicare, and he believes that the average Medicare beneficiary will continue to save an average of $650 a year, a significant sum, especially for seniors on fixed incomes without supplemental insurance. The ACA also expands Medicaid to anyone who earns up to 133 percent of the federal poverty level, or $14,856 for a single person. According to projections by the Congressional Budget Office, approximately 17 million people are expected to sign on to Medicaid by 2022. (For the most current Congressional Budget Office information, go to http://www.cbo.gov/latest/Health-Care/Affordable-Care-Act.)

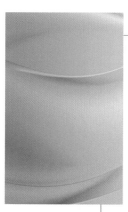

Issues Now

Interdisciplinary Approach Improves Care Outcomes for Elderly Clients

Researchers at the Mount Sinai School of Medicine in New York City investigated the use of a Mobile Acute Care for the Elderly (MACE) service provided by the hospital. They compared it with the general medical services offered through their in-patient services to see if there were any significant differences in outcomes for elderly clients. The research design was a prospective, matched cohort study, and the tool used was a three-item care transition measure.

The MACE team was made up of a geriatrics attending physician, a geriatrics fellow, a geriatric nurse coordinator, and a social worker. The goal of the program was to help clients avoid the complications of long-term hospitalization that often result from being bed-bound and physically inactive. The MACE team attempted to discharge elderly clients to their previous living arrangements as quickly as possible and to provide safe, seamless continuity of care from hospital to home.

The research population consisted of clients who were 75 years or older. Selection was based on the criteria of being admitted because of an acute illness. They were divided into two groups: one went to the MACE service and the other to the regular in-patient care setting. Clients were matched for age, diagnosis, and ability to ambulate independently. A total of 173 matched pairs of clients participated in the study from November 2008 through August 2011.

The results of the study indicated that the elderly clients who were treated in the MACE program were less likely to experience adverse events such as falls, pressure ulcers, restraint use, and catheter-associated urinary tract infections, and they had shorter hospital stays than clients receiving the traditional hospital care. They also had a higher level of satisfaction with the experience. However, treatment with the MACE interdisciplinary, team-based, client-centered model of acute care did *not* reduce the rate of rehospitalization within 30 days. The functional status for both groups was the same. The researchers concluded that the use of a coordinated, interdisciplinary model of care, such as the MACE service, can improve the care outcomes among hospitalized older adults.

Source: Hung WW, Ross JS, Farber J, Siu AL. Evaluation of the Mobile Acute Care of the Elderly (MACE) Service. *JAMA Internal Medicine,* 173(11) 1–7, 2013. Retrieved April 2013 from doi:10.1001/jamainternmed.2013.478

ACA Phased In

Although some of the provisions of the Affordable Care Act had already been implemented by 2015, 2014 was the year when the most noticeable changes became effective. One key provision will assist couples to save more of their assets in qualifying for Medicaid. In the past, a spouse often had to decrease his or her assets in order to qualify for Medicaid.

The ACA has also sparked the interest of the Gerontological Society of America (GSA) regarding the multiple provisions that will affect the aging population across the country.[15] The GSA believes that the elderly should have a high quality of life that is focused on client-centered care. It also believes that in order for the vision to be successful, federal and state policies must expand the health-care options of the older adult to include in-home and other care that enables them to live independently as long as possible. Members of the GSA will continue to inform policymakers about the growing health-care needs of the older population of adults.[15] Older adults and their caregivers need support and resources to better understand their needs and to make the most of Medicare and other benefit programs.[16]

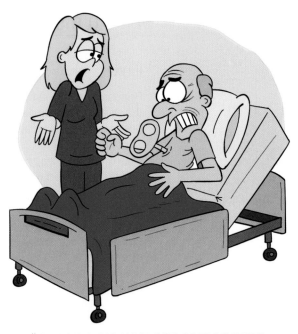

"THIS WAS THE ONLY TYPE OF PACEMAKER COVERED UNDER OBAMACARE!"

What Do You Think?

Has the Affordable Care Act improved or hurt health care in the United States? Since the implementation of the ACA, have you experienced any advantages or disadvantages in the health-care system?

Recent data indicates that older adults now account for 26 percent of all physician office visits, 35 percent of all hospital stays, 34 percent of all prescriptions, 38 percent of emergency medical services responses, and 90 percent of all nursing home use.[16] As the implementation of the ACA unfolds, experts on aging have an important opportunity to make certain that the law impacts the well-being of not only seniors but also those of all ages. Its emphasis on prevention and lifelong wellness fits well with the goals and philosophy of nursing.

Longevity Increases Health-Care Cost

The older population is living longer. Their newfound longevity is the result of a combination of factors, including new technology, availability of life-sustaining medications, better educated and higher-quality health-care professionals, newly built health-care facilities, and higher-quality long-term care. The national expenditure for prescription medications is now at 10 percent of the total health-care cost.[17] The national expenditure for all the advanced care modalities is now 75 percent of the nation's health costs.[4] Administrative cost accounts for an additional 7 percent of health-care expenses.

With the increase ease of use of and access to technology, there are many older adults who are using the Internet and mobile health technologies. These technologies offer opportunities to provide screening and treatment that the elderly might not otherwise seek or be able to access because of lack of transportation or limited mobility. For example, there is now a smartphone application that can support detection, monitoring, and self-management of illnesses.[18] The emerging Medicare accountable organizations are beginning to integrate geriatric mental health as components of health coaching and chronic disease management for clients with complex, high-cost health conditions.[18]

Research shows that the amount of health-care spending associated with acute care is very different from the costs of long-term care. Most older adults are relatively successful at remaining independent and functional within the community setting.[19]

Healthy People 2020

The Healthy People 2020 program, under the auspices of the U.S. Department of Health and Human Services (HHS), focuses on the improvement of health for the totality of the American population. The goals of Healthy People 2020 are to promote quality of life, healthy development, and healthy behaviors across the life span. It provides comprehensive material on disease prevention and health promotion with appropriate goals and objectives within a measureable time frame.[5]

There are many tools that the Healthy People program uses for strategic management by the federal and state governments, local communities, and many other public- and private-sector organizations to aid in maintaining healthy people. A set of objectives and target dates are used to measure progress for health issues in specific populations and serve as a foundation for prevention and wellness activities across various sectors and within the federal government. It serves as a model for measurement at the state and local levels.[5]

Chronic disease affects the older population by decreasing their quality of life, which ultimately leads to higher cost of health care. Chronic conditions cause debilitation and pain. Effective public health strategies currently exist to help older adults remain independent longer, improve their quality of life, and potentially delay the need for long-term care.[20]

Population Growth

America's population has increased markedly due in part to the increase in life span. The country's concerted effort to control infectious diseases through immunizations and antibiotics, improved sanitation, contamination-free drinking water, and safe food supply have contributed to population growth. Public recognition of health hazards such as tobacco use, secondhand smoke, the non-use of seat belts, and unsafe motor vehicles has also contributed to longevity.[14]

There were only 3 million people ages 65 years or older (3 percent of the population) in 1900.

In the year 2000, the 65-year-and-older group numbered 35 million (12.4 percent of the total population), or 1 in 8 people. The fastest growing segment of the population is the age bracket above the 65 and older group—the age 85 and older, which is projected to increase from 50,000 in 2000 to 1 million in 2050.[21]

As the older population increases, health-care providers must understand the needs and outcomes of care for this population. Current research focuses on the most effective ways of using interventions or programs affecting chronic diseases such as diabetes and arthritis. Many older adults have multiple concurrent chronic or acute diseases. These are further complicated by a poor client psychological response because of their declining mental conditions, limited financial resources, lack of transportation, and the grieving process. Living arrangements become challenging, particularly if they live far away from relatives or lack a strong support system.[2]

Today's elderly population has relatively easy access to high-quality health care. As the ACA is phased in over the next few years, health care will become more accessible to those in need. The health-care costs for the elderly population accounts for 36 percent of U.S. health care expenditures: $72 billion from Medicare, $20 billion from Medicaid, and $10 billion from other sources. Health care consumes as much as 20 percent of the income of elders, who average $1,500 in out-of-pocket expenses per year. Most health-care expenditures are made in the last 6 months of life.[21]

> *The older population is living longer. Their newfound longevity is a result of a combination of factors, including new technology, availability of life-sustaining medications, better educated and higher-quality health-care professionals, newly built health-care facilities, and higher-quality long-term care.*

THE IMPACT OF AN AGING POPULATION

As discussed above, the growing elderly population in the United States is having major economic consequences for the country, especially for the federal and state programs that help support the health care of the elderly. The median annual income of elderly men is $15,000 and for women, $8,500. The elderly living below the poverty level is 11 percent, with 27 percent categorized as near poor. Women statistically account for 74 percent of poor elders whose only source of income is Social Security. About half have pensions and 12 percent subsist on Medicaid.[22] The demographic shift of people over age 65 who make up an increasingly large percentage of the population is not a temporary phenomenon associated only with aging of the baby boomer generation. It is a permanent fixture of the American population and will have a long-term impact on the economy.[23]

Long-Term Effects on Nursing

As more of the elderly seek health care, the nursing shortage will only become more pronounced. Currently, the median age of nurses is 46, which indicates that over 50 percent of the nursing workforce is reaching retirement age. It is projected that there will be a shortage of between 200,000 and 800,000 registered nurses (RNs) by 2025. In addition, reforms in health care will flood the health-care system with millions of newly insured clients, further increasing the need for highly educated nurses.

Burden on the Health-Care System

An aging population will place an increased burden on an already stressed health-care system. As the shortage becomes worse, nurses will need to work back-to-back shifts under highly stressful conditions. These types of working environments have been shown to cause long-term fatigue, accidents and injury, and increased job dissatisfaction. Research has demonstrated that nurses who work multiple shifts make more mistakes and have a higher incident of medication errors. The overall quality of client care decreases, and nurses who are overstressed begin to leave the profession, which only makes the shortage worse.

The nursing education system has made valiant efforts to increase the number of graduates from their programs. Although they have increased the number of graduates significantly over the past 10 years, they still are not meeting the demand created by older nurses who are retiring and the increasing number of elderly clients.

What Do You Think?

Have you had any direct experiences of the nursing shortage, such as low staffing on a unit? How was the situation handled?

> " *Research has demonstrated that nurses who work multiple shifts make more mistakes and have a higher incident of medication errors.* "

Lack of Geriatric Specialists

As more and more of the aging population enters the health-care system, there is an increasing need for practitioners who specialize in elderly care. The medical community has been slow to respond to this trend, providing nursing with a golden opportunity. Almost all nursing programs today have a course on the care of the elderly. Advanced degree programs are offering degrees and certification in gerontology for nurse practitioners. The reality of the future health-care system is that almost all nurses, except for those working in pediatrics and obstetrics, will be providing care for older clients. With the projected shortage of primary care physicians, nurse practitioners are in a perfect position to fill this need.

The ACA places an increased emphasis on the integration of client care. It requires that chronic diseases are linked with preventive measures such as screening, counseling, education, and the social determinants of healthy behaviors. True integrated preventive care also involves community services such as immunization and outreach programs. This type of holistic approach to care of the elderly is the foundation of nurse practitioner education.

Additionally, there are increasing numbers of the elderly who come from other cultures and who do not speak English. To meet the needs of this population, nurses will be required to provide high-quality care in multicultural and multilingual settings (see Chapter 21). In addition, effective treatment of the variety of mental disorders associated with chronic illness must be part of any care provided. This will also require additional screening and monitoring because these mental disorders are progressive. Mental disorders are the leading cause of compromised self-care and self-management of the elderly at home.

Special Education Needs

To provide better holistic care, nurses today must educate the older population. This education is important in improving the health of the community and the everyday lives of the elderly. Because many of the elderly have limitations such as reduced hearing and visual acuity, poor memory, and disorientation, nurses need to use specialized education techniques to be effective. The goal of all education is to change behavior. Many elderly find changing very difficult because their current behavioral patterns have developed over their lifetimes.

One technique that has proven effective is the positive continuous reinforcement procedure that can be easily employed in professional practice. Repetition combined with positive reinforcements such as praise, a pleased look, or another type of reward are all positive reinforcements. When the positive reinforcement is linked to a change in behavior, it becomes a motivator. Use of this technique can help build a positive learning environment, add interest and even excitement to the learning sessions, and increase a supportive pattern of trust and communication (see Chapter 12).

In developing an effective teaching plan, it is important to remember that all individuals, but particularly the elderly, bring their life experiences to a learning situation. These experiences are based on their religion, gender, ethnicity, economic class, age, sexuality, and mental and physical abilities. Any health teaching must acknowledge and build upon these experiences. Learners also have a set of values that must be identified and incorporated into teaching. In any educational process, a power disparity exists between teachers and students that must be carefully formed by the instructor. In order for teachers to adhere to this delicate balance, they must have authority over their students. This disparity may be amplified by a student's cultural background (see Chapter 22). Recognizing this disparity and creating an atmosphere where the learner does not feel threatened and feels free to ask questions is key to his or her understanding and remembering the content being taught.

> *The goal of all education is change in behavior. Many elderly find changing very difficult because their current behavioral patterns have developed over many years.*

Disaster Preparation

Recent disasters, such as Hurricane Sandy, pointed out the special needs of the elderly population in a disaster situation. The damage produced by Sandy was horrific, destroying many homes and key infrastructure. It required a massive evacuation of people from certain areas. (For details on disaster planning, see Chapter 26.) Disaster planning often does not include any special preparation for the elder population, who may be more profoundly affected because of mobility limitations and chronic diseases that decrease their abilities to cope with major disasters. During evacuations, many elderly leave behind life-sustaining medications and assistive devices that they need for their normal daily activities. Although the ability to move them quickly to a rescue center may save their lives, it has a profound effect on their levels of orientation and quality of life. Often these shelters consist of large rooms with rows of cots with little ability to meet the health needs of the elderly.[21] In addition to the disaster planning measures found in Chapter 25, planning for the elderly and disabled should include:

- Assembling a team of relatives or neighbors who can aid in moving larger immobile individuals safely. It should include at least one individual who can move or carry heavy objects such as mobility devices or life-support equipment.
- Providing one or more of the team members with a key to the elderly person's house.
- Naming one or more of the team members as a legal health-care decision-maker in case the primary decision-maker is injured in the disaster.
- Assembling a "to go" emergency kit in a sturdy tool box or small suitcase that, in addition to the supplies listed in Chapter 25, also contains at least 7 days' worth of items the disabled person routinely uses, such as medications, adult diapers, ostomy supplies, sanitizing supplies, syringes for diabetics, dressings for those with wounds, and sterile water. Keep the kit near the door that is commonly used for exiting the residence.
- Keeping commonly used mobility assist devices such as wheelchairs, crutches, and canes near the door of exit.
- Knowing how to get to the nearest special needs shelters.
- Having a list of the elderly or disabled person's everyday routine, including times of medicines, treatments, and dressing changes, along with the supplies in case caregivers become separated.

For more information about preparation for care of the elderly in emergencies, go to http://www.fema.gov/news-release/2013/03/26/elderly-need-special-plans-be-ready-disaster or http://www.fema.gov/news-release/2013/03/26/elderly-need-special-plans-be-ready-disaster.

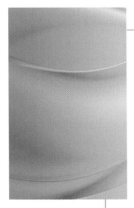

Issues in Practice

A Research Investigation in the Spirituality of the Elderly

This study investigated the concept of spirituality in the well elderly who live within a community setting and live independently in either Southern California or the New York metropolitan area.

The purpose of this study was to investigate the concept of spirituality in the well elderly and their perceived ideas, needs, and concerns. Twenty-six volunteers participated in an unstructured interview. The participants responded to a list of questions pertaining to the role of spirituality in their everyday lives. The data was grouped into respective themes and categories.

Qualitative research methodology explored the meaning of spirituality for the well elderly living within a community setting. The sample size was 26 individuals, ages 65 to 85, who were asked nine open-ended questions used during a face-to-face interview (Box 23.1).

Box 23.1

Spirituality Questions and Answers

1. "When I say the word *spirituality*, what does the word mean to you?"
   Answered themes: God, faith, religion, one with nature, church
2. "How is spirituality important in your life?"
   Answered themes: Prayer, keeping in touch with self, fascination with other religions, oneness with nature
3. "Are there people, activities, resources that help you meet your spiritual needs?"
   Answered themes: Church, synagogue, family, cultural experiences, friendship
4. "In what way might your definition of spirituality be applied to your life?"
   Answered themes: Respect for life, creation of life
5. "How has spirituality influenced your life?"
   Answered themes: Closer to God, attending mass, a child of a Holocaust survivor
6. "Are you aware of the concept of spirituality?"
   Answered themes: Visiting Israel, church, saints, Ten Commandments
7. "Have you ever had any experience(s) that was particularly spiritually significant to you?"
   Answered themes: Only one responded and spoke of his comrades in a foxhole and God being present. Someone spoke of an out-of-body experience and seeing Jesus Christ and told to return to her body.
8. "Over time, has the concept of spirituality taken on a different meaning in your life?"
   Answered themes: Sense of spirituality grew over time and relationships, more prayer; simply growing older meant an increased spiritual need and the need to be part of a spiritual community.
9. "What factors influenced your decision to pursue your spiritual needs?"
   Answered themes: Friendship, prayer, religious affiliation, hospice volunteer[25]

Issues in Practice continued

The results indicated that regardless of a person's history, age, gender, work background, or religious upbringing, spirituality played an important role in their daily lives. Also, they feel a powerful influential spiritual force guides them during periods when they may be lonely or suffering from a feeling of being isolated. Each participant was aware of the significance of spirituality, the important role it played in his or her life. The elderly felt that they had knowledge of the various modalities and how spirituality plays a significant role in real-life practices. These real-life experiences included prayer and helping others.

Research Design

Qualitative research methodology was the method used to explore the meaning of spirituality for the well elderly who are living within a community setting, the significance spirituality has in their lives, and how nurses understand the well elderly's spiritual needs.

Transcription analysis and descriptive interview questions were used to analyze the beliefs, meaning, and purpose in life based on grounded theory. Grounded theory was used so that there would be accurate data collection and proper coding through the entire process of this research.

Findings

There are two groups of thirteen—26 participants in total. One group was in New York and one was in California. Of the participants in the New York group, there was one African American and of the participants in the group in California, one was Hispanic. The rest in both groups were Native Americans. Most participants identified themselves as Catholic (5), Jewish (5), Lutheran (1), Unitarian (1), or Baptist (1). California participants included 5 females, 8 males. Most participants identified themselves as Catholic (8), Episcopalian (1), Protestant (1), Christian (1), and no religious affiliation (2).

Summary

The results of the spirituality research study indicated that regardless of family history, gender, age, and religious affiliation, spirituality played a role in their daily lives. The well elderly had knowledge of various modalities of spirituality. This knowledge of spirituality has been integral within their life.

Study conducted in 2012 by Joseph Molinatti, PhD, RN.[21a]

Questions for Thought

- In your care of the elderly, have you found that they have a better developed sense of spirituality than younger clients? What do you attribute the difference or lack of difference to?
- Do you believe that a strong sense of spirituality helps elderly clients recover more quickly? Give examples of when you have experienced spirituality in elderly clients.
- Was the sample size of this study adequate to produce reliable results? Does the demographic division of subjects have an effect on the study results?

Appreciating the Older Population's Spirituality

Older people prefer to remain independent and within their own homes. To an older adult who is either well or ill, this freedom may have a spiritual connection. With aging and changes in health status, many of the elderly find new meanings for their existence. They make preparations for their vertical transcendence from life to death.[22]

Some nurses have difficulty in their role when managing the needs of the elderly or dying client due to a conflict they may have in coping with their own fears of death. By understanding their own belief systems, nurses may feel more comfortable in addressing the client's spiritual needs. The needs the nurse can respond to and assist with include psychological, physical, spiritual, or emotional support.[24] Nurses must be committed to understanding and be able to assess the importance spirituality plays in elderly clients' daily lives, whether living at home, in a community setting, hospital, or long-term care facility (see Box 23.1).

When nurses provide spiritual support to any client during a time of illness, the client develops a sense of balance with the life he or she has lived. The same holds true for the elderly adult. Nurses know how important it is for the elderly to be comfortable physically, but they also need to take into consideration their spiritual needs. Using spiritual strategies improves the individual's self-esteem and relationships with others and with God. These strategies include using empathy and open-ended questions such as, "What you've been saying indicates that you are distressed about your condition. Have you given any thought to why it has happened to you?" or allowing the client to vent religious or spiritually oriented concerns, and supporting the client's spirituality by promoting the use of prayer and scripture, encouraging family to participate in rituals and prayers, or helping the client understand the etiologies of spiritual distress as they work through the grieving process. Using these strategies will help elderly clients find meaning and hope in their lives.[25] (For more information on spiritual strategies, see Chapter 20.)

What Do You Think?

Have you ever had a client ask you to pray with him? How did you handle the request? If you haven't fielded that request, how would you handle it?

Our society today seeks more information on spirituality for themselves and for other members of their families. Only a limited number of books and nursing programs provide information on spirituality in health care (see Chapter 21).

In the past, there has been controversy as to whether or not spirituality should be included in a nursing curriculum. There were some educators who were not convinced that a nurse should attempt to deal with a client's spiritual needs. Rather they feel that area of care belongs to the clergy or those who are trained in pastoral services. Nursing has a relatively short history of incorporating spirituality into health care. However, historically, the concept of spirituality has always been essential to nursing care, often referred to as *psychosocial care*.[26] If nurses are not trained formally in spirituality, clients will not believe that the nurse possesses expertise in this area.

Spirituality in Nursing Education

By being formally educated in spirituality, the nurse will have the necessary skills to establish trusting relationships with clients. Today, more and more nurse educators are integrating spiritual concepts into education to help students understand the importance of spirituality in nursing practice.[27]

Students should be prepared in nursing school to provide spiritual care, understand how it affects the growing older population, and the risks for chronic illness. When viewing spirituality from the nursing perspective, it is important to determine how spiritual care should be taught and implemented in a nursing education program. Just as food and rest are universal needs, so are spiritual needs.[28] Spirituality courses could be taught in the first or second year for a baccalaureate program. This would expose students to these important spiritual issues early in their education and practice.[29]

The spirituality content does not always need to be taught as a separate course; instead, it can be included as part of another course such as an introduction to nursing or integrated moral theology course.[30] The more nurses understand about the lived experience of the healthy elderly, the better equipped they will be to provide for the total needs of the individual. Adding to this body of knowledge would enable faculty to better prepare nurses for the assessment and intervention of the spiritual needs of both the healthy and ill elderly. Research on spirituality has been on an increase as it relates to the terminally ill, those with chronic illness, and those with incurable diseases. However, there remains limited information on how spirituality relates to the older population living independently.

The history of nursing has shown that nurses care for clients by providing physical and comfort care. Nurses identify themselves as the ones who nurture clients through caregiving, providing high-quality care, and determining how the outcome will affect the client.

Nurses are beginning to include spirituality in their care and are gaining more knowledge in this arena. The Joint Commission on Accreditation of Healthcare Organizations (JCAHO) has established a standard of client care that includes spiritual and emotional care for clients. JCAHO states that the client's spiritual assessment is to include identification of spiritual practices important to them.[31]

Spirituality has many connotations to each individual. One can view spirituality through the sunrise and the sunset, and it can include compassion and selflessness, altruism, and the experience of peace within ourselves.[31] All these factors can contribute some meaning to one's existence and create new challenges for individuals on a daily basis.

A person does not have to be religious to be spiritual. Spirituality exists across the life span and does increase as a person gets older. Within nursing and nursing research, spiritual integrity is as important as any human need.[32] Spirituality can be viewed as a basic human need and is important because it has the potential to promote quality of life, especially to the elderly. As one ages, there is a need to hold on to something that has a meaningful purpose in life, whether this basic need is family, friends, or items that have spiritual meaning.[33]

Aging is a true journey that includes existential and spiritual companions that may or may not be sought but are always available to everyone (young or old).[34]

> *" Spirituality has many connotations to each individual. One can view spirituality through the sunrise and the sunset, and it can include compassion and selflessness, altruism, and the experience of peace within ourselves. "*

A study was conducted that found that as people age, they become more spiritual. This study showed that there was a correlation between age and high spirituality scores. Individuals with high spirituality scores had identified spiritual practices and experiences that they connected to physical trauma that affected emotions and bodily awareness.[35]

What nurses need to understand is that spirituality may entail an appreciation of physical experiences such as listening to music, walking along the beach, enjoying art or literature, eating good food, enjoying life, laughing, venting emotional tension, or participating in sexual expression.[36] Often as a person ages, material things become less significant; however, there is an increased interest in satisfaction of life. Some older adults may even have mystical experiences that may be a response to events in their past lives and the many recent changes they have experienced.[37]

Effects of Spirituality on Health

Spiritual practices may improve coping skills, increase social support systems, provide hope, promote healthier behaviors, and produce a sense of relaxation. Alleviating stress, promoting healing, and practicing spirituality all have a positive influence on our immune, cardiovascular, and nervous systems.[38] There are researchers who believe that certain beliefs, attitudes, and practices associated with being a spiritual person help maintain a healthy lifestyle by including faith, hope, forgiveness, and a strong social support system in their daily activities. Some studies show that prayer may have a noticeable impact on health and healing.[39]

For the most part, both the ill and the well elderly populations see the importance of spirituality and prayer as a way of keeping in touch with their inner selves. Other life elements that meet spiritual needs include family, church, synagogue, holiday gatherings, hobbies, and friendship. As people grow older, they are more apt to hold on to family memories (e.g., pictures, ornaments, treasures).

Conclusion

The older population is growing and living longer but has chronic diseases such as dementia, heart disease, and diabetes. The economic impact of this growing population has increased the cost of health-care coverage to $2.6 trillion in the United States within the past 2.5 years. Employers are faced with the need to increase medical insurance coverage for employees and their families. The increase in cost of health care for the older population is on the rise because of new technology, more drug availability, and increase in health providers' salaries.

The aging population has an impact on almost all segments of the health-care system. It is straining resources and requiring a shift in paradigm from an illness-oriented system to a prevention-and-maintenance-oriented system. For nurses, it is a realization that they will be taking care of increasing numbers of elderly clients and they must learn new modalities of communication and treatment. In the short term, it will worsen the nursing shortage, but it is also providing new opportunities for nurse practitioners interested in the care of the elderly.

Critical-Thinking Exercises

- Develop a care plan for a client who has a nursing diagnosis of "spiritual distress." What type of assessments would indicate this diagnosis?
- Write a teaching plan for a group of elderly clients outlining the benefits of the Affordable Care Act for them as it is phased in over the next several years.
- How do you think the rapidly increasing aging population will affect your nursing practice?
- Does your nursing program have a class that deals specifically with issues of the elderly? Go to the Internet and look up programs that offer a degree in gerontology.
- Use the spirituality questions in Box 23.1 to evaluate one of your elderly relatives or friends. How did the answers compare to the answered themes?

References

1. AHA American Hospital Association. When I'm 64: How boomers will change health care, 2007. Retrieved April 2013 from http://www.worldcat.org/title/when-im-64-how-boomers-will-change-health-care/oclc/131744039

2. Leuven-Van KA. Population of aging: Implication for nurse practitioners. *Journal for Nurse Practitioners,* 8(7), 2012.

3. Martin G, Schoeni RF, Andreski PM. Trends in the health of older adults in the United States, 2012 Retrieved January 2013 from http://www.ncbi.nlm.nih.gov/pmc/articles/PMC3342521/

4. Centers for Disease Control and Prevention. Rising healthcare costs are unsustainable, 2011. Retrieved January 2013 from http://www.cdc.gov/workplacehealthpromotion/businesscase/reasons/rising.html

5. Finkelman A, Kenner C. *Professional Nursing Concepts: Competencies for Quality Leadership.* Burlington, MA: Jones and Bartlett Learning, 2013, pp. 201–229.

6. Catalano, JT. *Nursing Now! Today's Issues, Tomorrow's Trends.* Philadelphia, PA: F.A. Davis, 2012.

7. Wilkinson JM, Treas LS. *Fundamentals of Nursing Theory, Concept, and Application.* Philadelphia, PA: F.A. Davis, 2011.

8. Older Adults-Healthy People. Retrieved January 2013 from http://www.healthypeople.gov/2020/topicsobjectives2020/overview.aspx?topicid=31

9. Center for Medicare and Medicaid Service, Office of the Actuary, National Health Statistics Group. National Health Care Expenditure Data, January 2012. Retrieved January 2013 from http://www.cms.gov/Research-Statistics-Data-and-Systems/Statistics-Trends-and-Reports/NationalHealthExpendData/index.html?redirect=/nationalhealthexpenddata/

10. Robert Woods Johnson Foundation. High and rising health care costs: Demystifying U.S. healthcare spending, 2008. Retrieved January 2013 from http://www.Kaiseredu.org/Issue-Modules/US-Health-Care-Costs/Background-Brief.aspx

11. Paying for nursing home care. Retrieved January 2013 from http://www.medicare.gov/what-medicare-covers/part-a/paying-for-nursing-home-care.html

12. Yoffe E. Please t*ake the gold watch. Please! Journal for Nurse Practitioner,* 554–559, 2011. Retrieved 2013 from http://www.slate.com/articles/life/silver_lining/2011/04/please_take_the_gold_watch_please.html

13. Walker EP. Washington week: Medicare cut averted in nick of time. *Journal of Nurse Practitioner,* 554–559. Retrieved January 2013 from http://www.medpagetoday.com/washington-watch/washington-watch/30392

14. Span P. What the health care ruling means for Medicare, 2012. Retrieved January 2013 from http://newoldage.blogs.nytimes.com/2012/06/28/what-the-health-care-ruling-means-for-medicare/?_php=true&_type=blogs&_r=0

15. Geriatric friendly provisions in the Affordable Care Act. Retrieved September 2014 from http://www.americangeriatrics.org/files/documents/Adv_Resources/Geri.Friendly.Provisions.ACA.pdf

16. The American Geriatrics Society. Geriatrics health professionals leading change, improving care of older adults (2012 Policy Priorities). Retrieved January 2013 from http://www.americangeriatrics.org

17. Martin AB. Growth in US health spending remained slow in 2010; Health share of gross domestic product was unchanged from 2009. *Health Affairs,* 31(1):208–219, 2012. Retrieved January 2013 from http://content.healthaffairs.org/content/31/1/208.abstract

18. Bartels SJ, Naslund JA. The underside of the silver tsunami—older adults and mental health, 2013. Retrieved January 2013 from doi:10.1056/NEJMp1211456.

19. Horgan S, LeClair K, Donnelly M, Hinton G. Developing a national consensus on the accessibility needs of older adults with concurrent and chronic, mental and physical health issues: a preliminary framework informing collaborative mental health care planning. *Canadian Journal on Aging* 28(2):97–105, 2009.

20. Altman D, Levitt L. The sad history of health care cost containment as told in one chart. Health Affairs Web Exclusive, 2003. Retrieved January 2013 from http://www.ncbi.nlm.nih.gov/pubmed/12703559

21. Lundy KS, Janes S. *Community Health Nursing: Caring for the Public's Health.* Burlington, MA: Jones and Bartlett, 2009.

21a. Perinotti-Molinatti, J. The Significance of Spirituality in the Elderly. An unpublished dissertation. Argosy University/Sarasota, Sarasota Florida, November, 2012.

22. Cora VL. In Lundy KS, Jones S: *Community Health Nursing: Caring for Public's Health.* Sudbury, MA: Jones and Bartlett, 2009, *856–891.*

23. Public Health and chronic disease. Retrieved September 2014 from http://www.apha.org/NR/rdonlyres/9A621245-FFB6-465F-8695-BD783EF2E040/0/ChronicDiseaseFact_FINAL.pdf

24. Young J. Obamacare 2013: Obama's legacy tied to healthcare reform that bears his name. Huff Post Business, 2013. Retrieved January 2013 from http://www.huffingtonpost.com/2013/01/19/obamacare-2013_n_2474417.html

25. Heammermeister J, Peterson M. Psychosocial and health-related characteristics of religious well being. *Journal of Christian Nursing,* l(33):33–37, 2001.

26. De Young S. Spiritual care and unprepared nurse. *Journal of Christian Nursing,* 32:1986.

27. Clarke J. A critical view of how nursing defined spirituality. *Journal of Clinical Nursing,* 18:1666–1673, 2009. Retrieved January 2013 from doi:10.1111/i1365-2702.2008.02707.

28. Catanzaro AM, Mc Mullen K. Increasing nursing students' spiritual sensitivity. *Journal Christian Nursing,* 33:33–37, 2001.

29. Gallia KS. Teaching spiritual care: Beyond content. *Nursing Connection,* 9(3):29–35, 1996.

30. Koenig HG. *Spirituality in Patient Care: Why, How, When, and What.* Philadelphia: Templeton Foundation Press, 2007, p. 175–187.

31. Lewis D. The Joint Commission and spiritual care. Presence: An internal journal of spiritual growth, 2008. Retrieved January 2013 from http://Info.sdiworld.org/post/the-joint-commission-and-spiritual care

32. Pillow W. Spirituality beyond science and religion. Bloomington, IN: iUniverse, 2012. Retrieved September 2014 from http://www.huffingtonpost.com/deepak-chopra/a-new-creation-story-beyo_b_759933.html

33. Carson VB. *Spiritual Dimensions of Nursing Practice.* Philadelphia, PA: WB Saunders,1989.

34. Molinatti-Perinotti J. The significance of spirituality in the elderly. Dissertation.com., Boca Raton, FL, 2005.

35. Mowat H. Ageing, health care, and the spiritual imperative. . Retrieved January 2013 from www.sach.org.uk/agm04_hm.pdf

36. Wolman R. Spirituality: What does it mean to you? *New Age Journal,* (Sept/Oct):79–81, 1997.

37. Mowdy R. In JT Catalano (Ed.): *Nursing Now! Today's Issues, Tomorrow's Trends.* Philadelphia: F.A. Davis, 2012.

38. Oman D, Reed D. Religion and mortality among the community dwelling elderly. Retrieved September 2014 from http://ajph.aphapublications.org/doi/abs/10.2105/AJPH.88.10.1469

39. Benner DG. Spirituality and the awakening self. Grand Rapids, MI: Brazos Press, 2012. Molinatti J. The significance of spirituality in the well elderly. Published abstract. Indianapolis, IN: *Sigma Theta Tau International,* 2012.

Nursing Research and Evidence-Based Practice

24

Sharon Bator

Sheryl Taylor

Joseph T. Catalano

Learning Objectives

After completing this chapter, the reader will be able to:

- Discuss the necessity of nursing research as an essential component of comprehensive client care
- Describe ways in which nursing research can be used to enhance communication and understanding between cultures
- Describe the steps of the quantitative research process to generate further research
- Identify websites that facilitate accomplishing each of the steps of the quantitative research process to generate further research
- Demonstrate the ability to identify the basic similarities and differences related to qualitative and quantitative research designs
- Identify at least four strategies that may help promote implementation of valid research findings in clinical settings
- Describe the barriers to evidence-based practice
- Define and describe the concept and utility of evidence-based practice
- Discuss the research-practice gap as this relates to nursing research and identify some ideas for promoting change

A UNIQUE BODY OF KNOWLEDGE

One characteristic that defines a profession is the creation of a unique body of knowledge and related skills to guide its practitioners. There are many ways of obtaining knowledge. In the nursing profession, the development of a distinct body of nursing knowledge is an ongoing process. Nursing has a long and dignified history as a service and caring profession. It is well established that over 150 years ago, Florence Nightingale initiated practice-based health care when working with soldiers in the Crimean War. Nursing as a scientific discipline continues to evolve, and nurse scientists have been producing research since nursing's earliest days. Nursing research is essential to the development of the discipline of nursing and is essential for an evidence-based foundation for clinical practice. As with every profession, nursing continues to evolve to meet the needs of a changing society and the rapid development of new health-care technology.

Nursing education, in order to keep pace, had to enhance its teaching of research techniques through ongoing formal development. Nurses at all educational levels are responsible for understanding research and using it to improve client care.

From Research to Evidence-Based Practice

Using research is essential to improving quality of care for clients. In the 1970s, research became a formal part of educational institutions. In the 1990s, evidence-based medicine (EBM) or evidenced-based health care (EBHC) became the gold standard for physician care. It was the active application of the current best evidence to make the optimal decisions about the treatment of individual clients using statistical data to estimate the risk-benefit ratio that was supported by high-quality research on population samples. To broaden its application from medicine to nursing and to the other health-care professions, the name was changed to evidenced-based practice (EBP) and included an increased emphasis on improving the quality of care for both individuals and groups and improving health-care outcomes.

Nursing, which had always been involved in conducting research to some degree, shifted its focus from the mere production of research to its use in developing and using EBP in the practice setting. EBP expanded the range of research from strictly quantitative studies to also include qualitative studies that were better able to measure and understand certain elements of health care that revolved around a client's personal views of care, such as quality of life, spirituality, and religious and philosophical values. Through the integration of individual clinical expertise and client preferences, with the best available information developed from systematic research, EBP became the gold standard for nursing practice.

Whether originating from medicine, nursing, or other health-related disciplines, the U.S. Department of Health and Human Services' lead agency, the Agency for Healthcare Research and Quality (AHRQ), was given the task of improving the quality of health care and client safety and improving the efficiency of the system. Currently only 10 to 15 percent of U.S. health-care providers consistently use standardized evidence-based care. Because of the poorer outcomes experienced by those facilities not using EBP, they had a resulting 30 percent increase in cost of operation over facilities that do use EBP.

Studies show that it takes approximately 20 years to fully embed research findings into facility-wide client care. One solution to speed up the process of incorporating EBP into client care was developed by the AHRQ. It created a framework that uses the following three steps: (1) knowledge creation, (2) diffusion of the evidence, and (3) dissemination and adoption (institutionalizing) of the change. This framework creates a multidisciplinary map for education and practice to establish parallel paths whose ultimate goal is improved client outcomes. However, there are barriers that have to be overcome before EBP can be fully used to improve outcomes. One barrier has been the use of the traditional trial-and-error method of developing new nursing knowledge.

TRIAL AND ERROR

In the past, much of what constituted the practice of nurses was based on the edicts of those in authority. Nursing practice focused on doing exactly what was prescribed by the person in charge, usually the physician. Before the profession started building its own body of knowledge, it made sense to rely on the judgment of those who had more education and were considered by society to be authorities on the issues of health and illness and with whom nurses worked closely.

Experiential learning, also called the *trial-and-error process,* was used for many years in developing the knowledge, skills, and techniques nurses used in the promotion of health and healing. These practices were then passed on from one practitioner to the next. The trial-and-error method was used by scientists before the development of the scientific method and the research process. Those using the experiential method searched for knowledge within the universe of what was known about illness and healing. It served as the primary source of health-care knowledge for many years.

Today, the trial-and-error process has been replaced by the scientific inquiry and the formal research process that not only increases new knowledge but also demonstrates what is best in nursing practice. Research is the approach by which nursing knowledge may be judged much more reliable and transferable than that afforded by authority, tradition, or past experience. Nursing as a science depends on valid research evidence to support best practice. Research provides the crucial link between theory and practice.

This chapter presents an overview of pertinent issues regarding the critical nature of research as scientific support for the profession of nursing. It is directed primarily toward those who are consumers of research to increase their understanding of the research studies they read and to be able to identify good research from poor research. It also includes frameworks and models to perform nursing research, as well as common websites helpful for conducting, implementing, and disseminating research.

NURSING RESEARCH DEFINED

Nursing research can be defined as a systematic process for answering questions through the discovery of new information with the ultimate goal of improving client care.[1] Another commonly used definition for research is that it is a complex process in which knowledge, in this case in the form of discovery, is transformed from the findings of one or more studies into possible nursing interventions, with the ultimate goal of being used in clinical practice.

Research shows which approaches to nursing care are most effective and which do not work. Regardless of any barriers that might hinder discerning what works and does not work in nursing, all health-care disciplines are expected to use evidence-based practice. It is an expected fundamental competency in nursing. Also, nursing research is a key element in defining nursing as a profession and therefore must be embraced by nursing professionals. As one of a number of professions involved in providing health care, nursing accepts responsibility for discovering and defining its uniqueness among the health-care professions.

The Goals and Purposes of Inquiry

A major goal of nursing research is to expand and clarify the body of knowledge unique to the discipline of nursing. Scientific inquiry is the tool of choice for achieving the goals of professional clarification, justification, extension, and collaboration (Fig. 24.1). The purpose of nursing research is "to test, refine and advance the knowledge on which improved education, clinical judgment, and cost-effective, safe, ethical nursing care rests."[2] Nurses are held accountable for their actions and must be able to defend the interventions they use by relying upon strong empirical evidence. At the very minimum, nursing care must be safe and effective. With contemporary health-care cost-containment issues, nursing interventions are also expected to demonstrate practicality and cost-effectiveness. Nursing will not reach its full status as a profession until scientific inquiry becomes as much a part of daily practice as caring interventions.

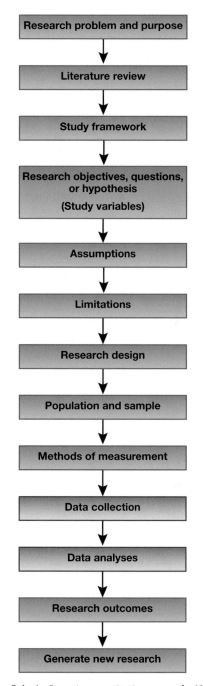

Figure 24.1 Steps in quantitative research. (Source: Burns N. *Building an Evidence Based Nursing Practice.* Philadelphia: FA Davis, 2013, p. 470.)

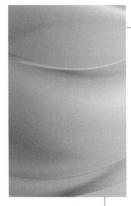

Issues Now

Big Bucks for Nursing Research in Health-Care Reform Act

If you had $1.1 billion, what type of research would you conduct? That's the amount that was made available for health-care research with the passage of the American Recovery and Reinvestment Act of 2009 and further clarified in the Affordable Care Act of 2010. If health-care reform is not repealed as promised by the opposition party in the legislature over the next few years, the sum may be increased to as much as $10 billion by the year 2019 and will be administered through the Patient-Centered Outcomes Research Trust Fund. Of course, not all of it is just for nursing research, but nursing will certainly get its share of the pie. Originally the money was to be spent in 18 months, but cooler heads recognized that was not realistic, so now it will be given out at the rate of several hundred million per year until it is gone.

How do you get the money? You must submit a research proposal similar to the ones that have been used for many years for all federal grants. Nursing will be up against stiff competition from the pharmaceutical and biomedical industries, which have well-developed research writing abilities. However, the distribution of the money will not rely totally on the federal government. The health-care reform bill contains provisions that change the oversight of funding from the Federal Coordinating Council of Comparative Effectiveness Research to a new organization called the Patient-Centered Outcomes Research Institute. This is a public-private partnership organization that will base funds distribution on the Institute of Medicine's (IOM's) list of 100 initial priorities.

Projects to be funded must come under the designation of comparative effectiveness research (CER). Best practices development is a key in receiving funding. In addition to the usual ethical compliance and regulatory documentation, researchers will also have to demonstrate that they are pursuing good clinical practice (GCP). GCP guidelines are much more specific about the elements of research protocol. In addition to documenting research methodologies, all researchers will be required to spell out in detail each aspect of the trial. The Research Institute will provide the tools required for the project. To start with, required information includes personal qualifications, curriculum vitae, institutional review board (IRB) submission, and approval documentation, tracking logs, and participant enrollment. These documents must all be in a regulatory binder that can be used by others at the research site when the principal investigator is unable to conduct the research.

The IOM's 100 priorities are not individually ranked in any particular order. They are divided into groups of 25, or "quartile" groups, according to the primary focus of the research. Many of the categories are community based because most health issues occur away from the hospital and outside the physician's office or clinic. Box 24.1 lists the top 10 areas that may interest nurses who wish to apply for some of the research money.

Issues Now continued

Box 24.1

Nursing's Top 10 IOM Priorities for Research

1. Preventing and treating overweight and obesity in children and adolescents through school-related interventions such as healthy meal programs, vending machines that sell healthy snacks, and physical activity.
2. Developing more effective treatment strategies for atrial fibrillation by comparing treatments such as surgery, catheter ablation, lifestyle changes, and medications.
3. Identifying risk factors and preventing falls in older adults through primary prevention methods such as exercise, balance training, and various clinical treatments.
4. Evaluating the effectiveness of comprehensive home-care programs for children and adults with severe chronic disease, particularly in minority and ethnic populations that have been identified as having ongoing health disparities.
5. Comparing the effectiveness of hearing loss treatments for children and adults in minority groups and ethnic populations; evaluating various methods, including, but not limited to, assistive listening devices, cochlear implants, electric-acoustic devices, rehabilitation methods, sign language, and total communication techniques.
6. Preventing obesity, hypertension, diabetes, and heart disease in at-risk groups such as the urban poor, Hispanic, and American Indian populations; comparing the effectiveness of strategies, including, but not limited to, pharmacological interventions, improved community environment, making healthy foods available, or a combination of interventions.
7. Reducing or eliminating health-care associated infection (HAI) in adults and children by testing various techniques, particularly where invasive devices such as central lines, ventilators, and surgical procedures are used.
8. Determining the best methods for early detection, prevention, treatment, and elimination of antibiotic-resistant organisms (e.g., methicillin-resistant *Staphylococcus aureus* [MRSA]) in both community and institutional settings.
9. Determining the best treatments for early detection and management of dementia to be used by caregivers in the community setting.
10. Publishing and distributing the findings of CER so that clients, physicians, nurses, and others can use the data to establish best practices. For examples of research studies that have been funded, go to http://www.shadac.org/news/share-funds-research-aca-implementation-through-8-new-grant-awards

Sources: Doherty RB. The certitudes and uncertainties of health care reform. Annals of Internal Medicine, 152(10):679-682, 2010; Eastman P. IOM workshop: US clinical research needs major transformation. Institute of Medicine. Oncology Times, 31(22):39-41, 2009; Elwood TW. Health reform and its aftermath. Journal of Allied Health, 39(2):65-71, 2010; Health care reform and clinical research: Gold rush or drug bust? Millions available, but long-term impact questioned. Clinical Trials Administrator, 8(5):49-53, 2010; Initial National Priorities for Comparative Effectiveness Research. Committee on Comparative Effectiveness Research Prioritization, Institute of Medicine. Washington, DC: National Academies Press, 2009. Retrieved May 2013 from http://www.nap.edu.

Beyond Clinical Practice

Some authors would limit the scope of nursing research to the clinical practice of nursing. In its fullest meaning, however, nursing research involves a systematic quest for knowledge designed to address any questions and solve any problems relevant to the profession, including issues related to nursing practice, nursing education, and nursing administration.[3]

Redefining the Client

Nurses know that clients are more than just individuals receiving nursing care within selected clinical settings. Nursing clients are family units, communities, organizations, institutions, corporations, local and state agencies, and citizens of a country and of the global community. To accurately measure how effectively it meets the needs of an expanding and diverse consumer base, the nursing profession must integrate an expanding and diverse body of scientific knowledge into its daily practice. Nurses must focus on promoting better understanding of the research process and encouraging their colleagues to seek the evidence needed to explain, modify, and improve nursing practice.

Setting Priorities and Directions

Clinical decisions and the resulting nursing interventions are justified by scientifically documented findings. Using nursing research, nurse investigators address issues related to cost, safety, quality, and accessibility of health care and look ahead to establish priorities and to define the future direction of the nursing profession. Recently, the IOM established a list of 100 research topics that are based on CER. Many of these are community oriented and fit well with both the directives of the Affordable Care Act and nursing's holistic approach to health care.

For many years, the American Nurses Association (ANA) has been a major contributor to setting goals and priorities for the profession. On its website (http://www.ana.org) is posted the organization's major expectations for the use of research in nursing. Nursing research can also be used to shape health policy in direct client care, within an organization, and at the local, state, and federal levels.

The ANA supports nursing research with a variety of resources such as the Research Toolkit. The ANA has developed a research agenda to guide the association in identifying priority areas. For more information, go to http://www.nursingworld.org/Research-Toolkit.

The Research Problem

Nurses in all areas, including clinical practice, education, law-making, and research, must be able to identify and state research problems. A clear statement of the research problem, whether it is a completely new area or one that has been the subject of previous research, is the first step in the scientific process and the foundation of the rest of the research study. The research problem can be identified through the problem-solving process, the nursing process, the research process, or the evidence-based practice process.

The four major concepts of all nursing theories—client (person), health, environment, and nursing (see Chapter 3)—should also be considered in identifying areas of interest that the nursing profession views as the core of its value system. The Population, Intervention, Comparison and Outcome (PICO) question flows naturally from nursing's values. An example of a PICO question that incorporates using client, environment, nursing, and health values can be seen in this scenario. A higher-than-average incident of infections has been found in infants (the population) in the neonatal intensive care unit. The infants are provided care by RNs who have artificial fingernails (intervention of interest). The incident of infections was lower before the RNs started wearing the artificial fingernails (intervention of comparison). After a new policy was implemented that artificial fingernails could no longer be worn by the staff, the number of infections decreased back to the average (positive vs. negative outcome).

Crossing Cultural Boundaries

One critical requirement for a dynamic profession is to understand and address cultural issues involved in nursing care and to understand the various cultures within the communities where nurses practice. There is also a need to look beyond perceptual and geographic boundaries in the promotion of dialogue, investigation, and collaboration with the many international nursing colleagues in the interest of culturally sensitive and global concerns. Culturally related issues provide numerous opportunities for nursing research (see Chapter 22).

DEVELOPMENT AND PROGRESSION OF RESEARCH IN NURSING

The Origin of Nursing Research

Florence Nightingale is viewed as the person who first elevated nursing to the status of a profession. In her first book, *Notes on Nursing* (1859),[4] she introduced the concept of research to the profession and expanded it in her subsequent publications. Nightingale believed in the importance of "naming nursing" through the collection and use of objective data. She also used this data to prove that there was a need for wide-ranging health-care reforms, including clinical practices, treatment of injured soldiers, and nursing education. Nightingale recognized the positive impact of combining strong logical thinking and empirical research in developing a sound scientific base on which to build the practices of the nursing profession.

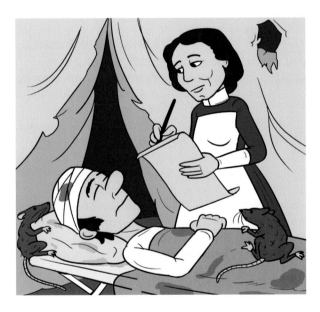

Methodical Observation

As the first recognized nurse epidemiologist, Florence Nightingale systematically collected objective data and in 1855 described environmental factors that affected health and illness. During the Crimean War, appalled by what she observed in the care of injured soldiers, Nightingale was forward-thinking enough to implement and then demand scientific inquiry in the practice setting. She methodically gathered facts, eventually supporting her claims that lack of cleanliness, fresh air, proper rest, and adequate nutrition

contributed to high levels of disease and death seen in the frontline "hospital" during the war.

As a result of her research, she petitioned forcefully for more supplies, better food, and cleaner conditions. She also successfully used the written media of the time, providing information and statistics to reporters for publication, which gave her observations and demands public support. Her strong advocacy for better care and improved environmental conditions lowered the mortality rate among wounded soldiers from 42 to 2 percent. Her work during the 1800s was not fully appreciated until more than a century later.[4]

The Development of Research

Even today, the full importance of this one woman's work to the profession of nursing is still being evaluated. Nightingale had few professional role models, relatively little education, a military organization that doubted her value, and meager financial support. In view of these challenges, her accomplishments were phenomenal. It is interesting to speculate about how much more progress would have been made in building the unique body of nursing knowledge if other nurses of her time had heeded Nightingale's earliest call for research.

A Look at Nursing Education

During the 1940s, many studies concerning nursing education came to the forefront because of the tremendous demand for educated nurses during World War II. Nursing education practices were evaluated in a study commissioned by the National Nursing Council for War Service. Findings from this study and others at the time uncovered weaknesses in nursing education. This relatively new wave of research spawned several other studies that looked at nurses' functions, roles, attitudes, acceptance, and interactions with clients.

A Center for Nursing Research

Several events that occurred during the 1950s prompted those conducting nursing research to carve out an ever-expanding path for the profession of nursing that continues to widen today. Nurses with advanced degrees were increasing in numbers, and a center for nursing research was formed at the Walter Reed Army Institute of Research.

Creation of the American Nurses Foundation and the journal *Nursing Research* allowed publication of nursing research findings that gave both a face and a voice to the studies. Many of these studies became the mirror and the microscope through which nurses studied themselves. This self-appraisal was an unprecedented research approach for any profession.

New Terminology for Nursing

In the 1960s, phrases such as *conceptual framework, conceptual model,* and *nursing process* made their first appearances in textbooks and other nursing literature (see Chapter 3). Nursing leaders, now becoming more focused on theoretical support for nursing, continued to lament the relative lack of research.

Many professional nursing organizations set priorities for research during this time. It was also during this time that another visionary nurse heeded the call to logical reasoning and empirical research. Virginia Henderson, one of the early nursing theorists, defined the role of nursing as being "to assist individuals (sick or well) with those activities contributing to health, or its recovery or to a peaceful death, that they perform unaided, when they have the necessary strength, will, or knowledge; to help individuals carry out prescribed therapy and to be independent of assistance as soon as possible."[4]

Nightingale recognized the positive impact of combining strong logical thinking and empirical research in developing a sound scientific base on which to build the practices of the nursing profession.

This definition was so conceptually clear that it was accepted by the International Council of Nurses (ICN) in 1960, and Henderson's work went on to identify many relevant research questions for the practice of professional nursing.

A Growth in Research Programs

In the 1970s, the number of graduate nursing programs experienced tremendous growth, and so did the number of nurses conducting research. Increases in the number of ongoing research studies pointed out the need for an improved way to publicize those studies. Three more research journals were developed: *Advances in Nursing Science, Research in Nursing and Health,* and the *Western Journal of Nursing Research.* During this time, the research focus began to shift from the study of nurses to the study of client-care needs. Clinical challenges were identified as having the highest priority for nursing research, a trend that continues today.

A Source of National Data

The 1980s witnessed another information explosion with the continued growth rate of research-trained, graduate school-educated nurses and the introduction of computers. Research and writing were both enhanced by electronic databases and the expanding World Wide Web. In 1983, the American Nurses Association created the Center for Research for Nursing.

The mission of this center is to serve as a source of national data for the profession. In 1986, the National Center for Nursing Research (NCNR) at the National Institutes of Health was established by congressional mandate. The mission of this organization is to support clinical (applied) and basic research to create a scientific foundation for the care of individuals across the life span. During the 1980s, a journal with the specific intention of providing research directed toward the practicing clinical nurse took form in *Applied Nursing Research.*

A New Focus on Practice

In 1993, the NCNR was awarded full institute status, and the National Institute of Nursing Research (NINR; http://www.ninr.nih.gov) came into being. In 1996, NINR had a reported $55 million budget, and it was poised to promote and support research priorities established during that decade. Since the late 1990s, studies have become more focused on the practice of nursing, the outcomes of nursing and other health-care services, and the building of a stronger knowledge base by replicating previous research using a variety of settings and situations.

THE NEXT STEP IN NURSING PRACTICE: CRITICAL DISCERNMENT

Because of the volume of literature being published by all health-care professions, including nursing, it is important to develop critical discernment skills. Critical discernment requires the nurse to understand the research process and to sift through and carefully assess all available and credible research findings. Once the research has been analyzed and judged, recommendations for using the best practice techniques can be made on the basis of best evidence.[5]

Evidence-Based Practice

Today, the movement to achieve cost-effective, high-quality care based on scientific inquiry generates the drive for evidence-based practice (EBP). Evidence-based practice is one of today's high-priority nursing issues.

Although nurses have been using evidence-based nursing practice in some form since the early days of nursing, it is only recently that the process has become formalized and widespread as a methodology. The current use of EBP in nursing requires a transition from nursing care that is based on opinions, past practices, and tradition to a practice that is based on scientific research and proven evidence. The goal of nurses using EBP is to obtain the best information available and to integrate it into their day-to-day nursing practice. Such practice includes the client's values and self-determination in providing care, as well as those of the client's family. The ultimate goal of EBP is to improve the quality of care.

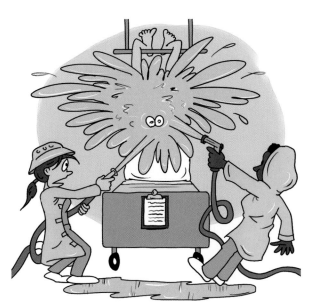

"ARE YOU SURE THIS NEW BATH TECHNIQUE WAS ON THE EVIDENCE-BASED PRACTICE LIST?"

Evidence Reports

Nurses can use numerous sources when incorporating EBP into their care provision. Research reported in the literature is a primary source of high-quality information, but not the only one. Other sources include expert opinion, collaborative consensus, published standards, historical data, local quality assurance studies, and institutional reports, including cost-effectiveness and client and family preferences and input. The key to using these various sources of information is the ability to grade or rank them so that nursing practice is based on the *best* information available. A list of sites that provide information about research findings in nursing is found in Box 24.2.

Evidence reports located at these sites provide a scientific basis for a disease or a nursing practice and then integrate that data into actions used in practice. Most sites will help synthesize previous and current knowledge related to the topic, review the information for quality and documentation, explain how EBP is currently being used, and discuss how useful the EBP is to the clinical practice. The reviews in evidence reports are more detailed than a typical literature review and include broad-based information translated into specific approaches to client care. Currently there is a substantial database, and new data are constantly being added to the site.[6]

What to Look For

Nurses should look for several key elements in evidence reports when attempting to integrate EBP into their care. The first part of the report should include a structured summary statement of the problem, practice, or disease that describes what is in the evidence report. The second part should comprise a lengthy and detailed analysis of the published and unpublished data, including reviews of articles and reports, the populations included in the studies, and the nature of the nursing actions investigated. One of the most important elements in the second part of the evidence report is the ranking or grading of the quality of the evidence.

The level of quality of the evidence is sometimes referred to as the "level of recommendation for use" and answers the nurse's question, "Is this information of high enough quality so that I can use it in my practice?" Integrative reviews in evidence reports should provide both the type of evidence included and the strengths and consistencies of the information.

Types of Evidence Used

Five types of evidence can be present in an evidence report, ranked from I (strongest) to V (weakest):

I. Meta-analysis of multiple well-designed, controlled studies that examines and synthesizes many studies to find similar results

Useful EBP Websites

U.S. Resources Related to the Steps of the Nursing Research Process	Website: Go to Information Under Research	Quoted Items of Interest Extracted From the Websites
American Nurses Association (U.S.)	http://www.nursingworld.org	Research Toolkit: Helps provide evidence-based care that promotes quality health outcomes 1. Asking the question 2. Acquiring information 3. Appraising the evidence 4. Essential nursing resources 5. Research glossaries 6. Critique a research article 7. Education about evidence-based practice and research 8. Comparative effectiveness research/ patient-centered outcomes research 9. Subjects protection 10. Research funding 11. Research organizations 12. ANA's research agenda 13. National Database of Nursing Quality Indicators (NDNQI) 14. International Council of Nurses (ICN) evidence-based practice resource 15. Research repository [members only-login required]
Joanna Briggs Institute (Australia)	http://www.joannabriggs .edu.au	The Joanna Briggs Institute (JBI) is the international not-for-profit research and development arm of the School of Translational Science based within the Faculty of Health Sciences at the University of Adelaide, South Australia. The institute collaborates internationally with over 70 entities across the world. The Institute and its collaborating entities promote and support the synthesis, transfer, and utilization of evidence through identifying feasible, appropriate, meaningful, and effective health-care practices to assist in the improvement of health-care outcomes globally.
Sigma Theta Tau International	http://www.nursingsociety.org	Research library Nursing library Research grants Call for abstracts Research initiatives

B o x 2 4 . 2

Useful EBP Websites—cont'd

U.S. Resources Related to the Steps of the Nursing Research Process	Website: Go to Information Under Research	Quoted Items of Interest Extracted From the Websites
		Research Resources Honor society archives Chapter archivist information PUBLICATIONS Books RNL Magazine Worldviews STTIconnect STTI Newsletter Journal of Nursing Scholarship GLOBAL ACTION Global initiatives STTI and the UN Nursing organizations Faculty summit Global Ambassador Program
AHRQ, Agency for Healthcare Research and Quality (U.S.)	http://www.ahrq.gov and http://www.innovations.ahrq.gov	
Institute for Healthcare Improvement (care bundle information)	http://www.ihi.org	The Institute for Healthcare Improvement is a small organization with a very big mission: improvement of patient care. It has many free resources. Learn from experts at IHI conferences and seminars. Virtual programs Get trained in improvement skills
National Guideline Clearinghouse (U.S.)	http://www.guidelines.gov	NGC is a public resource for evidence-based clinical practice guidelines. It shows a relationship to AHRQ. Has annotated bibliographies Learn AHRQ evidence reports: hospital-acquired conditions; mobile device resources Also has http://www.hhs.gov
University of Minnesota, Evidence-Based Health Care Project	https://www.lib.umn.edu/indexes/moreinfo?id=4219	Welcome to Evidence-Based Practice: An Interprofessional Tutorial Excellent tutorial
CINAHL	http://www.ebscohost.com/cinahl/	
EBSCOhost	http://www.ebscohost.com/	
National Library of Medicine	http://www.nlm.nih.gov/	

Continued

Box 24.2

Useful EBP Websites—cont'd

U.S. Resources Related to the Steps of the Nursing Research Process	Website: Go to Information Under Research	Quoted Items of Interest Extracted From the Websites
Certificate of Confidentiality, NIH	http://grants.nih.gov/grants/policy/coc/	
HIPAA-related issues, NIH	http://privacyruleandresearch.nih.gov/ and http://www.hhs.gov/ocr/hipaa/guidelines/research.pdf	
IRB material, NIH	http://www.pre.ethics.gc.ca/english/policystatement/policystatement.cfm	
U.S. Office of Human Research Protections (OHPR)	http://www.hhs.gov/ohrp/	
U.S. Office of Research Integrity	http://ori.dhhs.gov/	
Women and minorities in clinical research, NIH policy	http://grants2.nih.gov/grants/funding/women_min/guidelines_update.htm	
World Health Organization, informed consent templates	http://www.who.int/rpc/research_ethics/informed_consent/en/	
Internal validity information	http://www.socialresearchmethods.net/kb/intval.php	This is Trochim's website. Includes table of contents, navigating, foundations, sampling, measurement, design (internal validity); establish cause and effect; single group threats; multiple group threats; social interaction threats Introduction to design Types of design Experimental design Quasi-experimental design Relationships among pre-post designs
Research randomizer	http://www.randomizer.org	
Research randomizer	http://www.random.org	
Social research methods: Sampling	http://www.socialresearchmethods.net/kb/sampling.htm	
Software for sampling plans	http://www.samplingplans.com/software.htm?src=overture	

Sources: A guide to evidence-based practice on the Web. United States Department of Health and Human Services, 2013. Retrieved June 2013 from http://www.samhsa.gov/ebpwebguide/; Hopp L, Rittenmeyer L. *Introduction to Evidence-Based Practice: A Practical Guide for Nursing.* Philadelphia: FA Davis, 2012.

II. At least one well-designed experimental study with a random sample, control group, and intervention

III. Well-designed, quasi-experimental studies, such as nonrandomized controlled, single-group pretest or post-test, cohort studies, or time series studies

IV. Well-designed nonexperimental studies, such as comparative and correlational descriptive studies and controlled case studies

V. Case reports and clinical examples

The strength and consistency of evidence are also ranked on a five-point scale ranging from A (best) to E (poorest). In general, a "B" or higher should be present before a nurse integrates the data into EBP. The rankings are as follows:

A. There is type I evidence or consistent findings from multiple studies of types II, III, or IV.

B. There is type II, III, or IV evidence, and the findings are generally consistent.

C. There is type II, III, or IV evidence, but the findings are inconsistent.

D. There is little or no evidence, or there is type V evidence only.

E. Panel consensus: Practice recommendations are based on the opinions of experts in the field.

One potential problem in using these ranking systems is that they may not be the best method of analyzing the strength of the evidence. In nursing, much of the research is qualitative or descriptive, or even narrative, because of the difficulty in performing controlled studies with large groups of clients. The nurse needs to check the consistency of the results, even though there may not be any type I, II, or III studies in the evidence report.[5]

The next section of the evidence report focuses on clinical practice and should include practice-focused guidelines or recommendations for specific clinical interventions. Often this section begins with a statement such as, "There is very good evidence that . . ." or "There is no evidence that . . ." The practices outlined should be specific and relevant to the care being given.

The last section of the evidence report is the report source. Reports should be specific and current and should come from high-quality, refereed professional journals.

Evaluating an Evidence Report

The nurse can evaluate the evidence report by asking three questions. Only after answering these questions will the nurse be able to decide if the information should be incorporated into his or her practice.

1. *Is this the best available evidence?* Best sources include peer-reviewed journals and reports no more than 3 to 5 years old.

2. *Will the recommendations work for my practice given the client population and problems?* If the study population is of young adult white men and the nurse's primary work population is elderly women, the data generated may not apply.

3. *Do the recommendations fit well with the preferences and values of the clients I commonly work with?* If the values of the nurse's primary group vary greatly from those of the study group, it is likely the recommendations may not work well.

Nurses can locate evidence reports from numerous sources

> *The key to using these various sources of information is the ability to grade or rank them so that nursing practice is based on the best information available.*

Clinical Journals

Evidence-Based Nursing (http://ebn.bmj.com/)
Online Journal of Clinical Innovations (http://www.nursingworld.com)
Reformatted STTI *Online Journal for Knowledge Synthesis in Nursing* (http://www.nursingsociety.org/Publications/Newsletter/) (Must be a member to access)

Other Sources

National Guideline Clearinghouse (U.S. Agency for Healthcare Research and Quality): A repository for clinical practice guidelines (http://www.guideline.gov)
The Cochrane Collaboration (international): Develops and maintains systematic reviews
State University of New York (SUNY) website: Lists the best sites for information (http://www.cochrane.org/)

Best Practices

Although some use the terms *evidence-based practice* and *best practice in nursing* interchangeably, there is some difference between the two. Most of the time, *best practice* is defined as clinical nursing actions that are based on the "best evidence" available from nursing research. It has the goals of infusing nursing practice with research-based knowledge and applying the most recent, relevant, and helpful nursing interventions into the nurse's day-to-day practice. The purpose is to achieve client care outcomes that exceed the basic standards of care. To be considered a best practice, there must be empirical data from multiple institutions that are using the practice and it must be published in a professional journal. On the other hand, evidence-based practice is more geared to the goal of generating high-quality research that can be used to build best practices; however, conceptually there is a high degree of overlap between the two terms.

Moving Forward

When nurses begin to take the next step and integrate EBP and best practices into the care they provide, they will make a major leap toward raising the level of professionalism in nursing practice. Through the use of EBP and best practices in nursing, the quality of client care will improve when that care is based on validated evidence that focuses on what works best.

Currently, nurses have been given the responsibility not only to conduct research but also to evaluate, critique, and apply the research findings of other nurses and health-care professionals in their own practice. Understanding research is more than merely learning simple methods of inquiry. Research skills are expected from nurses at all levels, whether beginning or advanced. For the novice, this means being able to do literature searches and select articles to critique. The ability to read, understand, and critique research articles is the first step in upgrading clinical practice.

THE RESEARCH PROCESS

Long before graduation, nursing students often notice something in the clinical setting that grabs their attention. They may simply wonder if a different approach would work better in a particular situation or if the best technique is currently being used and what evidence exists to support a particular technique or intervention as "best."

As newcomers to the profession, students may question interventions or solutions that seasoned nurses often take for granted. Students may see the experienced nurse's familiar world differently,

and their minds may be open to possibilities that those in the field for many years cannot see. Questioning the status quo is a key first step in the research process. Applying critical thinking to a problem often leads to visualization of a research project, the development of a plan, the implementation of that plan, and finally, sharing of the findings with others. This process follows a logical progression from abstract ideas to concrete actions.

Research Designs

The word *design* implies both creativity and structure. The design for a research study can be seen as a road map or a recipe. It serves as a fairly flexible set of guidelines that will provide the researcher with answers to the questions of inquiry.

What Do You Think?

Have you seen any clinical procedures in your clinical rotations that could be improved? How would you design a research project to prove your belief?

> " *Understanding research is more than merely learning simple methods of inquiry.* "

To choose a research design, the nurse must first develop a vision of the overall plan for a study, including a general idea of the type of data needed to answer the research question. The design is a critical link that connects the researcher's framework with appropriate types of data. The level of preexisting knowledge in the area of inquiry also helps determine the research design. If little is known about a specific subject, an exploratory study may be the best method for uncovering new information. In exploratory research, there is usually more interest in the qualitative characteristics of data. Hypotheses are usually not required for these studies.

If the researcher is looking at variables that are independent or objective or that demonstrate cause and effect, a quantitative design is most suitable. If the research question invites discovery of meanings, perceptions, and the collection of subjective data, a qualitative design should be used.

Quantitative Versus Qualitative Research

Historically and in the tradition of scientific inquiry, quantitative experimental research designs were the most highly respected. These designs are guided by a somewhat rigid set of rules that give the most importance to the *process* of inquiry. However, the past 15 years have seen a growing interest in, and respect for, qualitative approaches in research, especially in the social sciences. Social researchers see human interactions as complex, highly contextual, and too intricate to be studied using a rigid framework or standard instrument. Also, attempting to conduct quantitative research on human subjects often produces serious ethical dilemmas. It is often very difficult to obtain approval for this type of research from the institutional review board or the institution's human rights committee, which determines the ethical status of human research.

Qualitative Designs

The purpose of qualitative inquiry is to gain an understanding of how individuals construct meaning in their world, visualize a situation, and make sense of that situation. For example, to nurses, the concept of "caring" is very important, yet the nurse will probably perceive caring differently than the client. The nurse researcher wishing to measure "caring interventions" might find this concept very difficult to quantify, but a qualitative method could yield much usable information.

Because of the nature of nursing and the usual subject matter (human beings), qualitative designs are best suited to answer questions that interest nurses. The most commonly used of these designs are shown in Box 24.3.

Semistructured interviews using open-ended questions and observations are the most commonly used data collection methods in qualitative studies. Knowledge generated by qualitative research answers questions related to the meaning and understanding of human experiences.

Questioning the status quo is a key first step in the research process.

Quantitative Designs

Quantitative designs use approaches that seek to verify data through prescriptive testing, correlation, and sometimes description. These designs imply varying degrees of control over the research material or subjects. Control of the research design can range from very tight to somewhat loose.

The design in quantitative research becomes the means used for hypothesis testing. The design also optimizes control over the variables to be tested and provides the structure and strategy for answering the research question. More highly controlled quantitative designs try to demonstrate causal relationships, and more flexible designs address relationships between and among variables. Whether qualitative or quantitative research is being conducted, it is important to remember the basic steps of the research process. For more detail on this process, go onto the ANA website toolkit (http://www.nursingworld.org). It has Web information for each of the research process steps listed in the figure.

In quantitative experimental design, a comparison of two or more groups is required. The groups under study must be as similar as possible so that results can be credited to the treatment of the variables and not to differences between the groups. The independent variable is the one managed or manipulated by the researcher. The dependent variable *depends on*, or is altered as a direct result of, the researcher's manipulation. Box 24.4 summarizes and classifies quantitative research designs.

In research, it is good to remember that neither the quantitative nor the qualitative research design is better than the other. Each research approach is useful in different ways, and both expand understanding of health care and the nursing profession. What *is* important is to choose the methodology that best addresses the questions the researcher is asking and collects whatever data are most useful.

NARROWING THE RESEARCH-PRACTICE GAP

More and more, nurses are becoming academically astute in the area of research. Unfortunately, education alone does not ensure transfer of what is learned in the classroom into the daily practice of nursing.

B o x   2 4 . 3

Qualitative Research Designs

Phenomenology
Ethnography
Grounded theory
Historical studies
Case studies

Box 24.4

Quantitative Research Designs

Experimental Designs
Pretest/post-test control group
Post-test only control group
Solomon four group

Quasi-experimental Designs
Nonequivalent control group
Time series

Pre-experimental Designs
One group pretest/post-test

Nonexperimental Designs
Comparative studies
Correlational studies
Developmental studies
Evaluation studies

Meta-analysis Studies
Methodological studies
Needs-assessment studies
Secondary analysis studies

Survey Studies
One-shot case study

Like the basic but critical skill of sterile asepsis, research will become a part of each nurse's practice only when it becomes a part of each nurse's ideology.

Two Different Cultures

Academic and practice arenas are often, in reality, two entirely different cultures. The critical and creative thinking so valued and promoted in the academic environment may fall victim to time and budget constraints within the clinical setting. To support what is best for clients, clinical practice areas such as hospitals must find ways to ensure that research finds safe harbor in the culture of practice. The implementation of research in practice will depend on inquisitiveness, development of cognitive skills, the ability to question one's own practice, and professional discipline. Nurses must also understand that sometimes research findings may conflict with practices rooted in tradition.[7]

Barriers to Research in Practice

Even though research is becoming more widely accepted than in the past, some experts are still asking, "Why generate more research when the research already generated has not been adapted to practice?" The research-practice gap remains a bewildering challenge to the nursing profession.

An Isolated Skill

A challenge to the use of research in practice is that research skills are often taught to nursing students in isolation from other nursing subjects. Learning in this way seems to broaden the division between research and practice by separating the two elements early in the nurse's professional development and education. Recommendations by the IOM's report on the future of nursing and documents from major professional nursing organizations point to the need to focus inquiry on and link research findings to clinical practice early in the education process. If these practices are adopted by and incorporated into nursing education, the research-practice gap should shrink and eventually be eliminated.

There has been an emphasis on nursing research for more than two decades, and nurses on the front lines of clinical practice are beginning to actively use research as a way to improve their practice. The interrelationship of clinical practice to EBP is outlined in Box 24.5.

Lack of Understanding

There are several barriers to the implementation of research in the health-care setting. Some researchers do not understand practice issues from the bedside nurse's viewpoint. As a result, nurses who attempt to use research studies to answer practice questions may feel that the research does not provide the practical solutions for which they are looking.

On the other hand, some nurses skilled in clinical practice may not be skilled in conducting research. Practicing clinical nurses may lack the knowledge to understand or interpret the language of research. Published research often appears so abstract and complicated that the message cannot be

B o x   2 4 . 5

Essential Features of Professional Nursing and Relationship to Evidence-Based Practice

Professional Nursing	EBP
Provision of a caring relationship that facilitates health and healing	Honoring client preferences and values in shared decision-making
Attention to the range of human experiences and responses to health and illness within the physical and social environments	Determining the applicability of evidence to an individual patient and his or her context
Integration of assessment data with knowledge gained from an appreciation of the patient or the group	Gathering individual or local data and situating them with evidence from the research of groups
Application of scientific knowledge to the processes of diagnosis and treatment through the use of judgment and critical thinking	Using clinical expertise and appraisal of the best available evidence of effectiveness to select the most appropriate nursing intervention
Advancement of professional nursing knowledge through scholarly inquiry	Using the evidence syntheses to identify gaps in knowledge and the need for further research
Influence on social and public policy to promote social justice	Advocating for policy that assures equal access to effective treatment and the incorporation of patient values and preferences in policy decisions
Assurance of safe, quality, and evidence-based practice	Questioning traditional practices and using the best available evidence to drive safe, high-quality care while discarding ineffective practices

Source: American Nurses Association. *Nursing's Social Policy Statement: The Essence of the Profession.* Silver Spring, MD: Nursingbooks.org. 2010.

found in the bottle. The information should be easily accessible to those who provide direct care to clients. Researchers must find ways of packaging the conclusions so that practicing nurses may easily understand and implement clinical solutions to the care issues they are facing.

What Do You Think?

Have you read a research report that you really did not understand or could not apply to clinical practice? Was it due to overly complicated language in the research report or a lack of knowledge on your part? What did you do about it?

Entrenched Practices

Entrenched nursing practices present another challenge. In the not-too-distant past, traditional nursing practices appear to have had a half-life longer than uranium. A few nursing traditions remain so widely accepted as fact that they are never questioned and therefore evade the scrutiny of testing. Best practice may never become evident without testing approaches to practices that have been accepted as necessary, preeminent, and sacrosanct.

Lack of Incentive

Historically, due to the real challenge of budget limitations, very few hospitals or other agencies have offered encouragement or rewards to nurses who are willing to seek out and use research findings in an effort to improve practice. One survey, conducted to identify barriers to implementation of research from clinicians' perspectives, revealed "insufficient authority and insufficient time" as the two obstacles most often cited.[1] However, these roadblocks are beginning to crumble because of accreditation requirements by the Joint Commission and recommendations from the IOM.

Resistance From Managers

Some researchers suggest that unit managers may view an environment of updates and change as unfavorable to maintaining a committed and cohesive staff. Some describe change as a threat to the constancy necessary for safe and expeditious client care.[8] Nurses willing to incorporate best practice evidence into clinical protocols must have confidence in their own professional judgment and the courage to stand up to nurses who find comfort in unchanging traditional practices.

Incorporating Best Practice

Several strategies can help nurses conduct and use research for the improvement of nursing care, such as attending conferences in which clinical research findings and ideas for practice are presented. Other strategies proposed include but are not limited to:

1. Incorporating research findings in textbooks, basic and continuing nursing education programs, and clinical policy and procedure manuals.
2. Explicitly connecting research use to institutional goals and objectives.
3. Developing joint committees between colleges of nursing and hospital nursing departments.
4. Inviting staff nurses to find and present summaries and abstracts during unit meetings and clinical case conferences, in an effort to increase the interest of colleagues working on their units.[9]

Almost all of the most widely read, clinically focused nursing journals have added research or EBP sections or routinely include research articles. These increase the ease of access to research, ensure a wider distribution of current clinical research findings, and promote the incorporation into clinical settings of best practices based on credible evidence. This mission serves the profession by simplifying some of the language of research and by giving voice to the importance and practical nature of clinical research.

COMPARATIVE EFFECTIVENESS RESEARCH

Improvement of client care is the primary reason for conducting nursing research. It is important to continually update research priorities based on client outcomes in both the hospital and the community setting. Past research often compared two treatments to determine which was more effective but never took the next step in translating the findings into the practice setting. CER emphasizes the need to use research to establish best practice standards and to sustain research that has proven effective.

Systematic Reviews

Systematic reviews present summaries of past research on a particular topic that are easy to read and understand. The role of such reviews has become more important as the volume of health-care literature has expanded. Other factors favoring reviews include the inconsistent quality of some research produced, the increased number of treatment approaches resulting from the availability of numerous pharmaceuticals, increasing numbers of health-care products on the market today, and the exponential growth of health-related technology.

> *Systematic reviews present summaries of past research on a particular topic that are easy to read and understand.*

Consideration of these factors has prompted the proposal that systematic reviews of existing literature replace primary research as a main source of evidence for clinical decision-making. One review of this type could replace many individual studies and free those making clinical decisions from finding, interpreting, and evaluating a collection of published primary research reports and articles.

Some believe that systematic reviews should represent the "gold standard" in research summaries. However, those eager to jump on the review-only bandwagon need to keep in mind that methods currently used for literature review may not most accurately reflect some of the nursing research being reviewed. The challenge exists in the "narrowly defined concept of what constitutes good evidence."[10]

Primary Research

What about only using nursing research studies as a source of information? One recurring criticism of primary nursing research is that much of it is accomplished as single studies. Some nursing researchers point to the fact that many excellent qualitative studies are not further validated by more rigorous quantitative studies. Other nursing leaders continue to urge nurse researchers to make replication studies a high research priority, particularly for research addressing clinical nursing issues. A single study is rarely adequate for making a decision to incorporate a new procedure or technique in a nurse's clinical practice.[11]

A Practical Angle

Evidence-based practice is believed to constitute the best of practice. Health-care administrators have become interested in it because of its potential to increase quality of care and decrease the cost of health-care delivery. Standards of nursing practice, clinical guidelines, and routine performance audits promote the use of research findings to some degree. The rapidly growing availability of electronic databases and increased emphasis on the teaching of research in nursing curricula, along with such support organizations as the Cochrane Collaboration (http://www.cochrane.org) and the Centre for Health Evidence (http://www.cche .net), all promote the expectation that nurses must be able and willing to use evidence to inform their practice.

How Useful Is It?

Successful implementation of EBP also depends on how practical and useful the information is to the practicing nurse. The usefulness of information requires the nurse to evaluate several factors, including potential benefits versus possible harm, cost-effectiveness, availability of ongoing support resources, and willingness of the health-care staff and clients to accept change.

With the emphasis on the urgency for implementing EBP, critical and creative thinking have become even more important for the following reasons:

- Nurses must access, understand, evaluate, and disseminate a rapidly expanding body of nursing and other health-related information.
- Nurses must be able to recognize commonalities and uncover inconsistencies regarding the values of the profession, the values of the organization that employs them, the needs of clients for whom they advocate, and even the popular culture that exerts pressure on the public's ability to make safe choices.
- Nurses recognize that it takes critical and creative thought to support research into complex health-care issues and to promote successful implementation of changes in professional practice.

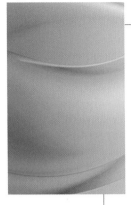

I s s u e s   i n   P r a c t i c e

Short Staffing in an Emergency

Halley had been working on the medical-surgical unit since her graduation from an associate degree in nursing (ADN) program 2 months ago. She had also had clinical rotations while in nursing school and felt comfortable and confident with the unit's procedures and her own skills. One Sunday evening, the house supervisor stopped her just before the beginning of her shift and explained that the registered nurse (RN) on the eight-bed maternity unit was going to be late because of a family emergency. Due to the overall short staffing on weekends at this hospital, Halley would need to be pulled to the maternity unit for no more than 2 hours to cover the RN position and pass medications until the regular nurse could arrive for her shift. That would leave the medical-surgical unit short staffed, but it was relatively quiet and only about three-quarters full.

Halley hurried to the maternity unit and received an abbreviated report from the staff who were waiting to go home. All the clients were stable, and the only potential problem was a client in the emergency department (ED) who was 36 weeks pregnant and might be in the early stages of labor. Although they hadn't received a report on the client in the ED, the departing staff joked that it would probably be the next morning before "anything happened."

After conducting an abbreviated initial assessment of the clients on the maternity unit, Halley called the ED to receive a report on their client. The client was a 36-year-old woman who had three children, ages 12, 9, and 2 years. The ED nurse also reported that the client's old charts revealed a history of "precipitous labor" (a very rapid labor with the sudden birth of the baby). Given the client's history and the relatively short time of her last delivery, Halley recognized that she did not have the skills or experience to provide safe care for this client.

Halley called the nursing supervisor and explained that she would need a nurse more experienced in obstetrics to help admit and care for this new client. The supervisor responded that the whole hospital was short of nurses and she had no one she could send. Halley would just have to do her best until the regular maternity unit nurse arrived.

A few minutes later, the ED nurses brought the client to the maternity unit. After she was transferred to a unit bed, Halley did an initial admission assessment with the following results: blood pressure 166/123; pulse 134; contractions 2 to 3 minutes apart, regular and strong; fetal heart rate 166, faint but regular; amniotic fluid leaking from the vagina. After making her assessment, Halley again called the supervisor and demanded that she come to the maternity unit immediately to help with this client, who Halley felt was going to deliver her baby very soon. The supervisor responded that she was in the middle of a code blue in the intensive care unit and that Halley would just have to hang on for the half hour or so until the maternity nurse was due to arrive.

Questions for Thought

1. What are the primary underlying ethical principles involved in this dilemma?
2. How do an individual nurse's ethical obligations differ from those of a hospital's administration?
3. What type of research data would help resolve this issue?
4. Do you think this case study reflects a realistic situation?

Essential Features

The goals of EBP include cost-effective practice based on the data produced by research, the dissemination of data, and the implementation of best practice interventions into the nurse's practice. The following have been identified as essential features of EBP:

- EBP is problem-based and within the scope of the practitioner's experience.
- EBP narrows the research-practice gap by combining research with existing knowledge.
- EBP facilitates application of research into practice by including both primary and secondary research findings.
- EBP is concerned with quality of service and is therefore a quality assurance activity.
- EBP projects are team projects and therefore require team support and collaborative action.
- EBP supports research projects and outcomes that are cost-effective.[12]

Evidence-based researchers conduct systematic reviews of existing literature. These reviews are necessary because of the large quantity of healthcare literature already in existence that has not been assimilated into practice. The mission of EBP researchers is to evaluate and present the available evidence on a specific topic in a clear and unbiased way. Clinical recommendations evolving from this process present nurses with sound decisions based on evidence of best practice. Consequently, researchers not only will know what questions have been satisfactorily answered, but also will be better able to identify where gaps in the knowledge still exist.

Networking: Where to Begin

As more evidence becomes available to guide practice, agencies and organizations are developing EBP guidelines. The Agency for Healthcare Research and Quality funds several EBP centers that are accessible through its website (http://www.ahrq.gov) and sponsors a National Guideline Clearinghouse where abstracts for EBP are available (http://www.guideline.gov). The American Pain Society (http://www.ampainsoc.org), the Oncology Nursing Society (http://www.ons.org), and the Gerontological Nursing Interventions Research Center (http://www.nursing.uiowa.edu/

excellence/evidence-based-practice-guidelines) also provide material. The Best Practices Network presents information from several organizations and is available at http://www.best4health.org.

RESEARCH ROLES BY EDUCATIONAL LEVEL

Leaders and educators within the profession of nursing agree that there is a role for every nurse in research, regardless of level of education. A minimal requirement for all 21st-century nurses is the ability to develop *and use* basic research skills. Nurses striving to improve their individual practice are increasingly committed to building a body of knowledge specific to nursing. Findings from scientific inquiry define the unique and valuable roles and the challenges of nursing.

Areas of Competency

One of the hallmarks of success in the field of research is the identification of research competencies for nurses at each educational level of preparation. In its classic document *Commission on Nursing Research: Education for Preparation in Nursing Research*, the American Nurses Association (ANA) identified research competencies for each classification of the nursing education program. It is presumed that professional nurses committed to lifelong learning will cultivate their research expertise throughout their careers. Following are the expected research roles by educational level.

> *Leaders and educators within the profession of nursing agree that there is a role for every nurse in research, regardless of level of education.*

Associate Degree Nursing Graduate

1. Demonstrates awareness of the value or relevance of research in nursing
2. Assists in identifying problem areas in nursing practice
3. Assists in collection of data within an established structured format

Associate degree nurses are expected to demonstrate an awareness of the value of research in nursing by becoming knowledgeable consumers of research information and by helping identify problems within their scope of nursing practice that may warrant exploration.

Baccalaureate Degree Nursing Graduate

1. Reads, interprets, and evaluates research for applicability to nursing practice
2. Identifies nursing problems that need to be investigated and participates in the implementation of scientific studies
3. Uses nursing practice as a means of gathering data for refining and extending practice
4. Applies established findings of nursing and other health-related research to practice
5. Shares research findings with colleagues

Nurses with a baccalaureate education are expected to be intelligent consumers of research by understanding each step of the research process to interpret, evaluate, and determine the credibility of research findings. The baccalaureate nurse is able to distinguish between findings that are merely interesting and findings supported by enough data to be included in the nurse's practice. Baccalaureate-prepared nurses also participate in one or more phases of research projects. These nurses must be alert to and uphold the ethical principles of any research involving human participants and oversee the protection of individual rights as specified in the ANA Code of Ethics.[13]

Master's Degree in Nursing

1. Analyzes and reformulates nursing practice problems so that scientific knowledge and scientific methods can be used to find solutions
2. Enhances quality and clinical relevance of nursing research by providing expertise in clinical problems and by providing knowledge about the way in which these clinical services are delivered
3. Facilitates investigation of problems in clinical settings by contributing to a climate supportive of investigative activities, collaborating with others in investigations, and enhancing nurses' access to clients and data
4. Investigates for the purpose of monitoring the quality of nursing practice in a clinical setting
5. Assists others in applying scientific knowledge in nursing practice

Doctorate Degree in Nursing or a Related Discipline

1. Provides leadership for the integration of scientific knowledge with other types of knowledge for the advancement of practice
2. Conducts investigations to evaluate the contributions of nursing activities to the well-being of clients

3. Develops methods to monitor the quality of nursing practice in a clinical setting and to evaluate contributions of nursing activities to the well-being of clients

Graduate of a Research-Oriented Doctoral Program

1. Develops theoretical explanation of phenomena relevant to nursing by empirical research and analytic processes
2. Uses analytical and empirical methods to discover ways to modify or extend existing scientific knowledge so that it is relevant to nursing
3. Develops methods for scientific inquiry of phenomena relevant to nursing[12]

ETHICAL ISSUES IN RESEARCH

Although guidelines that govern human behavior have always been a part of recorded history, the need for ethical standards in research came to the public's attention in a dramatic way following World War II, when evidence of the Nazis' medical experimentation and torture of selected groups of victims was revealed.

The Nuremberg Code

During the trials of Nazi war criminals, the U.S. secretary of state and the secretary of war discovered that the defense was trying to justify the atrocities committed by Nazi physicians as merely "medical research." As a result, the American Medical Association was asked to develop a code of ethics for research that would serve as a standard for judging the Nazi war crimes. This standard remains valid to this day and is known as the Nuremberg Code (Box 24.6).

National Research Act

Ethical issues are critical to all research, and researchers from all disciplines are bound by ethical principles that protect the rights of the public. One set of principles addressing the conduct of research came from the 1974 National Research Act. This act established the National Commission for Protection of Human Subjects in Biomedical and Behavioral Research.

Part of that act mandated the establishment of institutional review boards (IRBs), whose primary responsibility is to safeguard, in every way, the rights of any individual participating in a research study. IRBs are panels that review research proposals in detail to ensure that ethical standards are met in the

B o x   2 4 . 6

Articles Adapted From the Nuremberg Code

1. The voluntary consent of human subjects is absolutely necessary.
2. The experiment should yield fruitful results for the good of society.
3. The experiment should be so designed and based on results of animal experimentation and knowledge of . . . the disease or problem under study that the anticipated results will justify performance of the experiment.
4. The experiment should be conducted so as to avoid all unnecessary physical and mental suffering and harm.
5. No experiment should be conducted where there is an a priori reason to believe that death or . . . injury will occur.
6. The degree of risk . . . should never exceed that determined . . . by the importance of the problem to be solved by the experiment.
7. Proper preparations should be made . . . to protect the experimental subject against even remote possibilities of injury, disability, or death.
8. Only scientifically qualified people must conduct the experiment. The highest degree of skill and care should be required through all stages of the experiment.
9. During the course of the experiment, the subject should be at liberty to bring the experiment to an end.
10. During the course of the experiment, the scientist . . . must be prepared to terminate the experiment at any stage.

Source: Adapted from Trials of War Criminals before the Nuremberg Military Tribunals under Control Council Law No. 10, Vol. 2, pp 181-182. Washington, DC: U.S. Government Printing Office, 1949.

protection of human rights. The mission of the IRB is to ensure that researchers do not engage in unethical behavior or conduct poorly designed research studies.

Every university, hospital, and agency that receives federal monies must submit assurances that they have established an IRB composed of at least five members. These members should reflect a variety of professional backgrounds, occupations, ethnic groups, and cultures in an effort to uphold complete and unbiased project reviews.[14]

Code of Ethics for Nurses

The profession of nursing also has its own code of ethics to which all nurses are legally and ethically bound. The development of this code was initiated by the ANA board of directors and the Congress on Nursing Practice in 1995. In June 2001, the ANA House of Delegates voted to accept a revised Code of Ethics, and in July 2001 the Congress on Nursing Practice and Economics voted to accept the new language, resulting in a fully approved document called "Code of Ethics for Nurses With Interpretive Statements." A read-only version of this document is available at http://nursingworld.org/MainMenu Categories/EthicsStandards/CodeofEthicsforNurses/ Code-of-Ethics.aspx. Specific ANA position statements on selected ethics and human rights issues may be viewed at http://www.nursingworld.org/ mainmenucategories/ethicsstandards/ethics-position-statements (see Chapter 6).

Nurses must use the moral authority given to them by their license and position in the health-care structure to guard against anyone who tries to minimize the importance of that responsibility or who, for any reason, attempts to convince nurses to set aside their responsibilities. Nursing research most often addresses the needs and behaviors of human beings. Embedded in nurses' professional code of ethics is the charge to protect every person from harm. This responsibility extends beyond nursing *research* to include any client-related issue, any type of behavioral or biomedical research, and any questionable procedure.

In nurses' position of trust with clients, nurses possess a great deal of influence over a population that is especially vulnerable because of health issues and needs. This unique position of trust gives nurses a higher responsibility to protect and defend those in their care.

Informed Consent

Protection of human subjects underpins the conduct of research and implies that individuals have the information they need to make informed decisions. They have the right to be fully informed, not only about the care they receive, but also about any research in which they participate. Informed consent is both an ethical and a legal requirement in the research process. The ethical principle of self-determination is central to the process.

Besides those with special health considerations, certain groups of individuals are considered particularly vulnerable, owing, in part, to their lack of ability to give informed consent or their potential susceptibility to coercion. These groups include children, the mentally handicapped, elderly individuals, those with terminal diseases, the homeless, prisoners, those with terminal illnesses, and those who may have altered levels of consciousness as the result of a disease, medication, or sedation.

Nurses are well aware of the need for informed consent and the provision of information before procedures. This knowledge can serve nurses well in their obligation to obtain informed consent before conducting research.

The language of the consent form must be clear and understandable, written in the primary language of the client, and designed for those with no more than an eighth-grade reading level. Technical language should never be used. The Code of Federal Regulations states that subjects must never be asked to waive their rights or to release the investigation from liability or negligence. It is important to note that various institutions and researchers, in an extended effort to protect research participants, include more than the 12 key elements listed in Box 24.7.

> " *The Code of Federal Regulations states that subjects must never be asked to waive their rights or to release the investigation from liability or negligence.* "

Process Consent

In qualitative research, an important concept is process consent, which requires that the researcher renegotiate the consent if any unanticipated events occur.[15] An example of this might be a situation in which two parents with a small child in the hospital have given consent for the taping and study of "a day in the life of a hospitalized toddler."

During taping of the event, the parents are informed by the physician that a diagnosis is being questioned and their child must subsequently undergo an unexpected lumbar puncture. The parents may become visibly upset by this turn of events. In such a case the researcher should find a way of reconfirming the couple's ongoing interest in being part of the research study. When this family is given the opportunity to renegotiate the original agreement, the nurse researcher is confirming his or her role of advocate and proceeding in the best interest of all participants.

Detecting the Ethical Components of Written Research

It may be difficult to critique the ethical features of written research reports, but if there is evidence that permission to conduct the study was granted by an IRB, it is highly likely that the participants' rights were protected. Nurses have the responsibility of protecting the privacy and dignity of every individual, and the integrity of the nursing profession depends on doing what is right even when no one is watching. Box 24.8 provides the guidelines for critiquing ethics in research.

IMPLEMENTING RESEARCH IN THE PRACTICE SETTING

Knowledge that is generated by research and then translated into policy and procedure becomes the ultimate guide to the scientific practice of nursing. A primary responsibility of every nurse conducting research is the distribution of the findings (evidence) that have application in the client-care setting. Conversely, the professional responsibility of every nurse caring for clients requires that all nursing interventions be planned on the basis of reliable research findings.

Nursing research is of no value to the profession, or to the client, if the practice supported by the research is not used in the clinical setting. Unlimited opportunities for the generation and the dissemination of new knowledge exist in nursing, but the truly daunting task addresses the challenge of transforming that knowledge into practice.

The Call for Implementing Research

Research is critical to the professional practice of nursing. The Joint Commission's accreditation guidelines specify that client-care intervention must be based on information from scientifically valid and timely sources.

The mandate of the modern health-care system is that nurses make practice decisions based on the best scientific information available. Standard VII of the ANA Standards of Clinical Nursing Practice states that "the nurse uses research findings in practice." Nurses may participate in research activities in

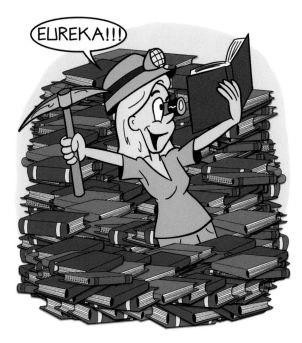

B o x 2 4 . 8

Guidelines for Critiquing the Ethical Features of Research

1. Was the study approved by an IRB?
2. Was informed consent obtained from every subject?
3. Is there information regarding anonymity or confidentiality?
4. Were vulnerable subjects used?
5. Does it appear that any coercion may have been used?
6. Is it evident that potential benefits of participation outweigh the possible risks?
7. Were participants invited to ask questions about the study and told how to contact the researcher, should the need arise?
8. Were participants informed how to obtain results of the study?

Source: Nieswiadomy RM. *Foundations of Nursing Research* (5th ed.). Upper Saddle River, NJ: Pearson/Prentice Hall, 2008. Adapted by permission of Pearson Education, Inc.

Approaches to Using Research

Nursing is not the only profession that is transforming research into practice. Almost every health-care discipline is trying to close the research-practice gap. They often identify significant difficulties involved in the changeover. Currently there are several models to help nurses apply research findings that support EBP. One model that appears both practical and relatively uncomplicated is found in Box 24.9.[17]

Promoting Change

Nurses must promote an environment conducive to change. In many hospitals, maintaining the status quo often appears to carry incentives that may intimidate even the most intuitive and confident change agent. The professional nurse committed to using "best evidence" to provide the best client care can be most effective by finding simple approaches that create an environment receptive to new research findings. Some helpful tactics include:

- Reading clinical journals regularly but also critically. Nursing professionals are well informed and believe in the concept of lifelong learning.
- Attending clinically focused nursing conferences where the latest client-care interventions are presented and discussed.

B o x 2 4 . 7

Key Elements of Informed Consent

1. Researcher is identified and credentials presented.
2. Subject selection process is explained.
3. Purpose of the research is described.
4. Study procedures are discussed.
5. Potential risks are identified.
6. Potential benefits are described.
7. Compensation, if any, is discussed.
8. Alternative procedures, if any, are disclosed.
9. Assurances regarding anonymity or confidentiality are explained.
10. The right to refuse participation or withdraw from the study at any time is assured.
11. An offer to answer all questions honestly is made.
12. The means of obtaining the study results is described.

Source: Nieswiadomy RM. *Foundations of Nursing Research* (5th ed.). Upper Saddle River, NJ: Pearson/Prentice Hall, 2008. Adapted by permission of Pearson Education, Inc.

a number of ways. They can conduct reviews of literature, critique research studies for the possibility of application to practice, or "[use] research findings in the development of policies, procedures and guidelines for client care."[16]

Box 24.9

Rosswurn and Larrabee Model for Application of Nursing Research

Assess the need for practice changes:
(a) Involve all nurses that have a stake in the intervention or change.
(b) Identify problems associated with the current practice.
(c) Compare available information.

Link the problem intervention and outcomes:
(a) Identify possible interventions.
(b) Develop outcome indicators.

Produce best evidence for consideration:
(a) Conduct a review of existing literature.
(b) Compare and contrast the evidence found.
(c) Determine feasibility (including cost in dollars and time).
(d) Consider benefits and risks.

Design a proposed practice change:
(a) Define the anticipated change.
(b) Identify necessary resources.
(c) Develop a plan based on desired outcomes.

Implement and evaluate the proposed change:
(a) Conduct a pilot study.
(b) Assess the process and the outcomes.
(c) Make a decision to alter, accept, or reject the proposed change.

Support the change with ongoing evaluations of the outcomes:
(a) Communicate the desired change to those involved.
(b) Conduct in-service education sessions.
(c) Revise standards of practice (policy/procedures) reflecting the change.
(d) Monitor the ongoing process and results.

Source: Rosswurm M, Larrabee J. A model for change to evidence-based practice. *Journal of Nursing Scholarship*, 31(4):317-322, 1999, with permission.

- Learning to look for evidence that clearly supports the effectiveness and the feasibility of updating nursing interventions.
- Seeking work environments that promote the use of research findings and evidence-based care.
- Collaborating with a nurse researcher. Apprenticeship to one who masters a skill is an old but venerated means of learning that skill.

- Learning to critically scrutinize the status quo. Many worthwhile ideas for change come from those students and nurses "in the trenches" and at the bedside.
- Pursuing the possibility of proposing and implementing a project. If the nurse finds a research-based idea for clinical care interesting, then taking the steps to research it can be productive.

Conclusion

Modern health care has become so complex and demanding that simple trial-and-error approaches do not provide the high-quality information required for the safe, effective, and economical care demanded by well-informed consumers. The nursing profession is quickly moving away from the "I do it because it's always been done this way" method of care to scientifically rooted care practices based on research. As a result, nurses are gaining increased recognition as key members of the health-care team.

Also, nurses are now required to be able to analyze and evaluate research findings to determine which studies are of high quality and therefore can be used as a guide for nursing practice. Similarly, nurses are required to contribute to the body of nursing knowledge by participating in nursing research studies conducted at their facilities. It is presumed that nurses with advanced degrees will initiate and conduct high-quality research.

The ability of nurses to make thoughtful use of research is an important first step in the development of EBP. Society's call for cost containment, high-quality care, and documented outcomes of health-care services will continue to fuel the engine of positive health-care developments. As nursing looks to its future, research and EBP will become increasingly more important factors that guide and inform the day-to-day practice of nurses.

GLOSSARY OF TERMS USED IN RESEARCH

Best practices Clinical nursing actions that are based on the "best evidence" available from nursing research.

Bias An influence that produces a distortion in the results of a research study.

Case study An in-depth qualitative study of a selected phenomenon involving a person, a group of people, or an institution.

Causal relationship A relationship between variables in which the presence or absence of one variable (known as the "cause") will determine the presence or absence of the other variable (known as the "effect").

Collaboration A cooperative venture among those with a common goal.

Comparative effectiveness research (CER) A method to determine the priority of research topics developed by the IOM, based on client outcomes both in and outside the institutional setting.

Conceptual framework A framework of concepts that demonstrate their relationships in a logical manner. Although less well developed than a theoretical framework, this framework may be used as a guide for a study.

Conceptual model A set of abstract constructs that explains phenomena of interest.

Correlation The degree of association between two variables.

Empirical evidence Objective data gathered through use of the human senses.

Epidemiologist One who studies the distribution and determinants of health and illness and the application of findings as a means of promoting health and preventing illness.

Ethical standards Standards determined by principles of moral values and moral conduct.

Ethnography A qualitative research approach involving the study of cultural groups.

Evidence-based practice (EBP) The selective and practical use of the best evidence, as demonstrated by research, to guide health-care implementation and decisions.

Experimental research design A quantitative research design that meets all of the following criteria: an experimental variable that is manipulated, at least one experimental and one comparison group, and random assignments of participants to either the experimental or the comparison group.

Exploratory study The descriptive examination of available data to become as familiar as possible with the information.

Grounded theory An inductive approach to research using a systematic set of procedures to develop a theory that is then supported by, or "grounded in," the data.

Historical study Qualitative research involving the systematic collection and synthesis of data regarding people and events of the past.

Hypothesis A formal statement of the expected relationship between variables in a selected population.

Informed consent Consent to participate in a study given by one who has full understanding of the study before the study begins. Informed consent is based on the principle of the right of each individual to self-determination.

Institutional review board (IRB) A panel established at an agency, such as a hospital or university, to review all proposed research studies and to set standards for research involving human subjects.

Metaparadigm The broadest perspective of a discipline giving an overview of the key theoretical models.

Nonprobability sampling A sampling process in which a sample is selected from elements of a population through methods that are not random. Convenience, quota, and purposive sampling are examples.

Nuremberg Code A code of conduct that serves as one of the recognized guides in the ethical conduct of research.

Nursing research A process that permits nurses to ask questions directed at gaining new knowledge to improve the profession, including elements of client care.

Phenomenology Qualitative research studies that examine lived experiences through descriptions of the meanings of such experiences by the individuals involved.

PICO question A question in which *P* represents "population" or "patient"; *I* stands for "phenomenon of interest"; and *CO* stands for "comparative" and "outcome."

Primary research source A report or account of a research study written by the researcher(s) conducting the study. In historical research, a primary source might be an original letter, diary, or other authenticated document.

Process consent A version of informed consent that supports renegotiation when a situation originally consented to undergoes change.

Qualitative research design A systematic but subjective research approach implemented to describe life experiences and give them meaning.

Quantitative research design A systematic and objective process used to describe and test relationships and evaluate causal interactions among variables.

Quasi-experimental design A type of experimental design in which there is either no comparison group or no random assignment of participants.

Random sample A selection process that ensures that each member of a population has an equal probability of being selected.

Reliability The dependability or degree of consistency with which an instrument measures what it is intended to measure.

Replication study A research study designed to repeat or duplicate earlier research. A different sample or setting may be used while the essential elements of the original study are kept intact.

Research design A blueprint for conducting a research study.

Research process A process that requires the comprehension of a unique language and involves the ability to apply a variety of research processes.

Review of literature An exploration of available information to determine what is known and what remains unknown about a subject.

Sample A subset of a population selected to participate in a study as representative of that population.

Scientific inquiry A logical, orderly means of collecting data for the generation and testing of ideas.

Theoretical framework A framework based on propositional statements derived from one theory or interrelated theories.

Validity The ability of an instrument to measure the variables that it is intended to measure.

Variable Any trait of an individual, object, or situation that is susceptible to change and that may be manipulated or measured in quantitative research.

Critical-Thinking Exercises

• Obtain and read both a qualitative and a quantitative research article. What are the main differences between the two articles? What are the similarities? Which produced the more reliable data?

• Identify the problem statement in each research article. Are they clearly stated? Do they contain more than one idea? How do they form the foundation for the research?

• Look up the topics of the two articles on one of the EBP websites. Was either article listed as a high-quality resource?

• Select a procedure or some problem you have encountered in your clinical rotations. Write a research problem statement for the issue. What type of research would be most appropriate for this issue?

• Reread the two articles you have selected. What, if any, are the ethical issues involved? How does the researcher deal with them?

• Read about the Nuremburg Trials (such as at http://www.u-s-history.com/pages/h1685.html). How do the results of these trials affect nursing research today? What were the primary violations the defendants were accused of?

References

1. Houser J. *Nursing Research: Reading, Using and Creating Evidence.* Sudbury, MA: Jones and Bartlett Publishers, 2011.

2. American Association of Colleges of Nursing. The research-focused doctoral program in nursing: Pathways to excellence, 2010. Retrieved May 2013 from http://www.aacn.nche.edu/

3. Polit DF, Beck CT. Nursing Research: *Generating and Assessing Evidence for Nursing Practice.* Philadelphia: Lippincott Williams & Wilkins, 2011.

4. Beyea S, Slattery M. Historical perspectives on evidence-based nursing. *Nursing Science Quarterly,* 26(2):152-155, 2013.

5. Brown R. *Nursing Evidenced Based Practice.* Richmond, VA: Virginia Commonwealth University Libraries, 2013.

6. Ogiehor-Enoma G, Taqueban L, Anosike A. Evidence-based nursing: 6 Steps for transforming organizational EBP culture. *Nursing Management,* 41(5):14-17, 2010.

7. Corchon S, Watson R, Arantzamendi M, Saracíbar M. Design and validation of an instrument to measure nursing research culture: The Nursing Research Questionnaire (NRQ). *Journal of Clinical Nursing,* 19(1-2):217-226, 2010.

8. Latimer R, Kimbell J. Nursing research fellowship: Building nursing research infrastructure in a hospital. *Journal of Nursing Administration,* 40(2):92-98, 2010.

9. Krugman M. Translating research into practice. *Journal for Nurses in Staff Development,* 2012. Retrieved June 2013 from DOI: 10.1097/NND.Ob013e31825f8f15.

10. Reinhardt JP. Research methods in evidence-based practice: Understanding the evidence. *Generations,* 34(1):36-42, 2010.

11. Schifferdecker KE, Reed VA. Using mixed methods research in medical education: Basic guidelines for researchers. *Medical Education,* 43(7):637-644, 2009.

12. Rahman A, Applebaum R. What's all this about evidenced-based practice? *Generations,* 34(1):6-12, 2010.

13. Oh EG, Kim S, Kim SS, et al. Integrating evidence-based practice into RN-to-BSN clinical nursing education. *Journal of Nursing Education,* 49(7):387-392, 2010.

14. Rid A, Schmidt H. The 2008 Declaration of Helsinki: First among equals in research ethics? *Journal of Law, Medicine and Ethics,* 38(1):143-148, 2010.

15. Hopp L, Rittenmeyer L. *Introduction to Evidence-Based Practice: A Practical Guide for Nursing.* Philadelphia: FA Davis. 2012.

16. Munten G, van den Bogaard J, Cox K, Garretsen H, Bongers I. Implementation of evidence-based practice in nursing using action research: A review. *Worldviews on Evidence-Based Nursing,* 7(3):135-157, 2010.

17. Newton JM, McKenna LG, Gilmour C, Fawcett J. Exploring a pedagogical approach to integrating research, practice and teaching. *International Journal of Nursing Education Scholarship,* 7(1):1-13, 2010.

Integrative Health Practices

Lydia DeSantis

Joseph T. Catalano

Learning Objectives

After completing this chapter, the reader will be able to:

- Describe the interrelationship between integrative health practices and alternative and complementary practices
- Compare the philosophy and objectives of alternative and complementary healing modalities with those of conventional Western medicine
- List major reasons why a growing number of people use alternative and complementary healing modalities
- Describe major types of alternative and complementary healing modalities
- Summarize methods by which nurses and clients can obtain information about alternative and complementary healing modalities
- Evaluate a client for use of alternative and complementary healing modalities
- Identify the strengths and weaknesses of alternative and complementary healing modalities

A DIFFERENT KIND OF HEALING

Complementary and alternative health-care practices, now called *integrative practices,* have been widely used by a large percentage of the population. Their popularity continues to increase dramatically with clients of all ages and backgrounds. Integrative practices include a range of traditional therapies and treatments that are not usually used or taught in conventional Western health care. Although some use the terms *alternative health care* and *integrative health care* synonymously, integrative care is more inclusive. It attempts to integrate the best of Western scientific medicine with a broader understanding of the nature of illness, healing, and wellness. It also includes complementary and alternative practices but goes beyond to include the care of the whole person, focusing upon health rather than illness.

Based upon evidence from research, integrative practice also involves the individual in his or her own care to achieve the highest level of health and well-being. Integrative health practice is highly inclusive, "integrating approaches to treatment from the allopathic, complementary, alternative, psychological, spiritual, environmental, nutritional, and self-help arenas."[1] With integrative health practices, clients are aided in using their illness crises as the starting point to making positive changes in their lives and reaching their full potential in wellness. It is important for nurses to have a solid understanding of this type of health care to ensure their clients' safety and well-being and to be supportive of their practices.

According to the World Health Organization (WHO), 80 percent of the world's population uses what Americans call "alternative" practices as their primary source of health care. Because of the widely accepted use of these practices, WHO has officially sanctioned the

611

incorporation of "safe and effective [alternative] remedies and practices for use in public and private health services." Currently, between 34 and 42 percent of Americans (60 to 83 million people) use alternative and complementary healing practices, as do 20 to 75 percent of people in western Europe, 33 percent in Finland, and 49 percent in Australia.[2]

The trend toward alternative practices has continued to grow in the United States since the 1990s. Studies show that 40 percent of people have developed an increasingly positive attitude toward alternative practices, whereas only 2 percent had more negative opinions. Both the general public (72 percent) and health maintenance organizations (HMOs; 73 percent) expect consumer demand for this area of health care to remain moderate to strong. Approximately 25 percent of the medicines used in modern therapy are derived from herbal plant sources used in traditional native healing practices. Although there has been rapid growth in biomedical knowledge and technology during this time period, the demand for alternative therapies continues to increase.[2]

Issues Now

The Federal Government Supports Integrative Medicine

The U.S. Health Resources and Services Administration (HRSA) announced in 2012 the availability of two grant programs aimed at developing integrative medicine. The two grants will provide funds in the sum of $3.3 million over the next 3 years. About $2.5 million will be provided to 16 programs ($150,000 each) to incorporate integrative medicine in medical residency programs. To qualify, programs must demonstrate how evidence-based integrative medicine content is being used in existing preventive medical residencies. The second grant will provide $800,000 to establish a national coordinating center for integrative medicine (NcclM). The goal of the center is to provide technical aid to and evaluate the progress of the developing IMR programs. It is also tasked with analyzing the efficiency of integrative medicine (IM), opening the door to a wider participation in its development.

The 2010 Affordable Care Act (ACA) has several provisions that will benefit integrative medicine and complementary and alternative medicine (CAM). With its emphasis on preventing insurance companies from denying coverage, ACA includes a provision that clients who are participating in clinical trials using alternative health-care methods cannot lose their coverage. Under the new law, insurance companies are required to cover all routine costs of medications and treatments used during the trial. The goal of the law is to make trials available to clients who otherwise might not be able to participate and to make it easier for researchers to conduct successful trials that will improve health care and treatments for others.

However, certain criteria must be met. First, the client must be categorized as "qualified." This means that the client must be authorized by his or her health-care provider for participation. The provider must also provide "medical and scientific information establishing that the individual's participation in such trial would be appropriate."

Second, the clinical trial must be "approved." An approved clinical trial, ranging from phase I to phase IV, is conducted to advance the prevention, detection, or treatment of cancer or other life-threatening disease or condition. The trial must meet at least one of three conditions: it must be federally funded or approved, approved by the Food and Drug Administration (FDA), or conducted by the federal government.

The bill also includes provisions to prevent insurance companies from discriminating against CAM practitioners. Practitioner coverage now includes acupuncturists, chiropractors, and naturopathic doctors who may prescribe dietary supplements. Some CAM practitioners believe the new provisions open the door for future growth of alternative health-care practices.

One overriding goal of Affordable Care Act (ACA) is to educate the public about methods to prevent illness and improve health-care status. To achieve this goal, the law supports the development of wellness plans to be implemented through community health centers, particularly in lower-income and underserved areas. These centers will provide wellness assessments, health education, and a

(continued)

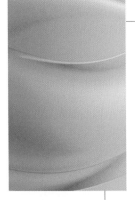

Issues Now _{continued}

selection of dietary supplements that have FDA-approved health claims. Some supplements that will be made available are folic acid, calcium, vitamin D, omega-3, and multivitamins. Supplements will be targeted for "at-risk" groups, such as calcium and vitamin D for older clients.

Another section of the new law promotes increased participation for CAM practitioners in the development of health-care policy. A new National Healthcare Workforce Commission will be created and will work with the U.S. Department of Health and Human Services. One of its projects is to create community health teams, which must include licensed CAM practitioners.

The law is new, and many questions still need to be answered. Some of the answers will come from research and through the pilot programs that are built into the health-care reform bill. However, it is certain that alternative health-care practices will be involved in future health-care developments.

Sources: CAM, supplements included in health care reform bill. Food and Drug Administration (FDA). Legislation, Government, Industry News. Retrieved November 2010 from http://www .naturalproductsinsider.com; Healthcare reform includes alternative medicine, dietary supplements. Nutritional Outlook, 2010. Retrieved April 2013 from http://www.nutritionaloutlook.com; Hoback J. Health care reform to impact CAM, supplements. Natural Foods, 2010. Retrieved April 2013 from http://naturalfoodsmerchandiser.com; Oberg B. What does health care reform mean for alternative medicine? 2010. Retrieved April 2013 from http://www.examiner.com; Perkins C. What does health care reform mean for alternative medicine? Holistic Health Talk, 2010. Retrieved November 2010 from http://www.holistichelp.net; Weeks J. Inclusion criteria fuels concern in proposed integrative medicine specialty . . . plus more. *Integrative Medicine: A Clinician's Journal,* 11(4):12–16, 2012.

DEFINING INTEGRATIVE HEALTH PRACTICE

Integrative health practice finds its origins in the definition of health presented by the WHO: Health is "a state of complete physical, mental and social well being and not merely the absence of disease or infirmity."[2] It is client focused. The integrative approach to health is based on the belief that clients, after an illness or injury, have the capability to regain their overall health and maintain wellness during their life spans. The work of the practitioner using integrative health practices is to become familiar with each client's particular health needs and then personalize their care using the full range of elements that affect health, including physical, mental, spiritual, social, and environmental factors. Taking into consideration the complex relationship between mind, body, and spirit, alternative health care addresses both the short-term care needs and long-term issues of the client.[3]

Integrative health care has the potential to affect the health status of clients across the spectrum of the health-care system. For nursing practice, it includes the ability to incorporate conventional health-care diagnoses and treatments with evidence-based practice (EBP), nonconventional alternative and complementary treatments, environmental factors, and nutritional therapies into their nursing skills set. Nurses must be able to bring to clients an awareness of how emotional, spiritual, cultural, and environmental factors in their lives affect their health and long-term well-being. On the clients' part, they need to develop a personal understanding of the causes and meanings of their illnesses and be willing to make a commitment to the healing process. Only then will they achieve the best outcomes from their treatments.[1]

Integrative health care practices differ from complementary and alternative practice in that integrative health care looks past the mere treatment of symptoms and attempts to identify and treat the underlying cause of the illness. However, alternative and complementary modalities are an essential element in achieving the goal of integrative health. Integrative health care is moving toward becoming a specialty of its own. There are a number of postgraduate programs on integrative health: the Arizona Center for Integrative Medicine (United States), the British College of Integrative Medicine (United Kingdom), the European University Viadrina (Germany), and the National Institute of Integrative

Medicine (Australia). This chapter will focus primarily on discussing alternative and complementary treatment modalities, keeping in mind that they are one element in an integrative approach to wellness.

DEFINING ALTERNATIVE AND COMPLEMENTARY HEALING

Several definitions are used for alternative and complementary health-care practices. They are sometimes defined as practices outside of conventional, science-based Western medicine and not sanctioned by the official health-care system. A considerable range of practices and concepts is included in alternative and complementary healing. These practices are generally used in place of conventional practices or used to enhance the effectiveness of standard medical treatments. The glossary at the end of this chapter outlines many of these practices.

An Outdated Definition

There is no universally accepted definition. Many alternative health-care practices originated a number of years ago within cultural belief systems and healing traditions. A commonly used definition in the United States for alternative and complementary modalities comes from the National Center for Complementary and Alternative Medicine (NCCAM), an agency of the National Institutes of Health. The NCCAM definition is "those treatments and health-care practices not taught widely in medical schools, not generally used in hospitals, and not usually reimbursed by medical insurance companies."

This definition is quickly becoming outdated. Several medical and nursing schools now include courses on alternative and complementary health-care practices. Also, the practice of alternative medicine is gradually becoming part of conventional health care. Physicians, nurses, and other health-care professionals are responding to the growing public use of these practices by incorporating selected modalities into their own client care. Physicians have begun referring clients to a variety of alternative healers and using alternative therapies for their own health.

A Holistic Basis

For the purposes of this discussion, alternative and complementary medicine is defined as the understanding and use of healing therapies not commonly

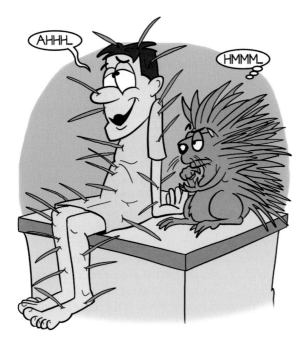

considered part of Western biomedicine. The focus here is mainly on methods of self-care, wellness, self-healing, health promotion, and illness prevention. Therapies and practices are called *alternative* when used alone or with other alternative therapies, and *complementary* when used with conventional therapies.

The use of the term *healing* is preferred to *medicine*. Integrative health care and alternative and complementary modalities typically are based in holistic philosophies, which go beyond treatment or cure of the physiological and psychological dimensions of care commonly associated with modern, scientific biomedicine. *Holism* refers to treatment of the whole person (body–mind–spirit) in that person's environmental context (i.e., physical, biological, social, cultural, and spiritual).

What Do You Think?

Do you use any alternative health-care practices? What are they? Why do you use them?

USE OF INTEGRATIVE THERAPIES

Although forms of integrative therapies have been used for many years in the United States, the passage of the ACA of 2010 has the potential to increase its use even more. Section 2706 of the ACA makes it illegal for insurance companies to discriminate against clients who use integrative therapies. Providers of integrative therapies must be reimbursed by the insurance companies at the same rates as providers of traditional procedures. There are other references to integrative therapies in the wellness and prevention sections of the ACA. The one sticking point is that the individual states can write their own language concerning which practitioners receive how much reimbursement for integrative practices.

Who Uses Them

In most national studies of alternative therapy users, ethnic and racial minorities are underrepresented, particularly among persons who do not speak English. Such exclusions raise questions about whether the use rate of alternative therapies in the United States may exceed 42 percent because the use of alternative therapies among immigrant populations and those with lower incomes tends to be high. Many such populations have grown up with these therapies as "folk" medicine, and their worldviews encompass different concepts of health, illness, and healing. Conversely, alternative health-care practices are most popular among women, people aged 35 to 49 years, people with higher educational levels (some graduate education), and those with annual incomes of more than $50,000.[2]

Why Their Use Has Increased

Three general theories have been advanced to explain the growing use of integrative healing: (1) dissatisfaction with conventional health care, (2) a desire for greater control over one's health, and (3) a desire for cultural and philosophical congruence with personal beliefs about health and illness. Many other client-specific reasons have also been postulated, such as belief in the effectiveness of integrative therapies and the individual's health status (Box 25.1). The rising cost of conventional health care may play a role as well.

Dissatisfaction

The increasing use of integrative therapies is due in part to the feeling that conventional health care is unable to deal with major health problems or improve a person's general health. People who have a high degree of distrust in conventional health care often rely primarily on integrative therapies. This lack

Box 25.1

Reasons for Use of Integrative, Alternative, and Complementary Modalities

People use integrative and alternative therapies alone or together with conventional health care for a variety of reasons. There is no single predictor of use, and the reasons for use may vary from situation to situation. Persons who seem to benefit the most from the alternative approach are those who:

- Prefer a personal relationship with healers.
- Refuse to give up hope and hopefulness, regardless of the illness or life state.
- Desire to focus on wellness, health promotion and maintenance, and illness prevention.
- Are concerned with gentle alleviation and management of suffering and illness rather than aggressive management of the end-stage of life through technology, medications, surgery, and other invasive procedures.
- Wish to participate actively in decision-making about their health care
- Believe in the holistic aspects of existence rather than in the primacy of biological and physiological aspects.
- Are "culture creatives"—persons at the leading edge of innovation and culture change who have been exposed to alternative lifestyles and worldviews compatible with those from which alternative and complementary modalities and theories have arisen.
- Share cultural and philosophical views similar to those from which alternative and complementary modalities have developed.

Source: Austin JA. Why patients use alternative medicine. *Journal of the American Medical Association,* 279:1548, 1998. From Aspen Reference Group. *Holistic Health Promotion & Complementary Therapies Manual* (1st ed.). ASPEN, 1998. Reprinted with permission from Delmar Learning.

of trust has increased recently for several reasons, including:

- Conflicting information from health-care-related studies and clinical trials about risk prevention and health promotion. For example, clients no longer know what to believe about salt intake, normal cholesterol levels, alcohol use, or hormone replacement therapy.
- Continuing emphasis of conventional health care on curative rather than preventive aspects of care. The lack of emphasis on illness prevention limits the ability of individuals to live long lives relatively free of disability from major chronic illnesses, such as arthritis, diabetes, cancer, and cardiovascular disease.
- Growing concern about costs, safety, and access to conventional health care. Many people are concerned about the increased incidence of hospital-acquired diseases, the many deadly medication errors committed over the past few years, the ever-increasing number of invasive procedures, antibiotic-resistant bacteria, and reliance on impersonal technology.

Desire for Control

Some people who use integrative therapies believe conventional care is too intolerant, authoritarian, and impersonal. They feel that some conventional health-care professionals lack sensitivity to the wishes of clients and their families when developing treatment plans. Clients believe they should be partners in decision-making about their care rather than just having decisions handed down to them.

In the United States, the majority of people report being reluctant to tell conventional health-care professionals that they use integrative therapies. Although almost all (89 percent) who use integrative therapies do so under the supervision of an integrative healer, about half of this same group do not consult a conventional health-care professional before they begin. Fourteen percent of persons see both conventional health-care professionals and integrative healers. Similar patterns of self-care and nondisclosure to conventional health-care professionals are found throughout the industrialized world.[4]

Holistic Philosophy

Conventional health care is often faulted for its limited focus on the physiological dimension of health and curing to the exclusion of the unity of mind–body–spirit healing. Another negative characteristic of conventional health care is its excessive dependence on medicine, surgery, and technology rather than on the more natural and noninvasive alternative approach that focuses on self-care and self-healing.

Belief in Effectiveness

Clients who use alternative therapies do so because they believe those therapies will work, either alone or when combined with conventional treatments. Persons who consider their health to be poor or who have chronic illnesses report greater benefits from alternative than conventional health care and are more likely to try both at the same time. Referral from conventional health-care professionals, friends, or other users of integrative therapies is also a prominent reason for the simultaneous use of both systems. For many clients, integrative therapies simply make them feel better than conventional health care does.

Cost of Alternative Care

Estimated costs of alternative medicines (herbs and nutritional supplements), diet products, equipment, and books and courses totaled $33.9 billion in 2007 (the last year a comprehensive national survey was conducted). Sixty-seven percent of HMOs cover one or more alternative and complementary healing (ACH) modalities, but coverage is uneven and varies regionally. Chiropractic is the most common covered service (65 percent), followed by acupuncture (31 percent), massage therapy (11 percent), and vitamin therapy (6 percent). HMOs expect to increase coverage for acupuncture to 36 percent, acupressure to 31 percent, massage therapy to 30 percent, and vitamin therapy to 27 percent. The most important reasons for adding coverage for these services are public demand, legislative mandate, and demonstrated clinical effectiveness.[5]

CLASSIFYING INTEGRATIVE METHODS

The underlying goals of any type of health care include preventing illness, promoting and maintaining health, and caring for people while alleviating the suffering caused by illness. However, despite these common elements, health-care practices vary profoundly in their modalities (technologies), practitioner education and monitoring, underlying concepts (models) of health and illness, modes of care delivery, and social and legal mandates to provide care. Because of the large number of variables, a confusing array of health-care systems, practitioners, and healing modalities has developed. Two systems that can be used to help define and classify alternative and complementary therapies are the Healing Matrix and the NCCAM classification.[4]

The Healing Matrix

The Healing Matrix (Table 25.1) contrasts conventional and alternative modalities and practitioners. The alternative modalities shown are (1) representative of those most commonly known by the general public, (2) sought in the United States and the industrialized world, and (3) practiced most often by conventional health-care professionals, including nurses.

> *The increasing use of integrative therapies is due in part to the feeling that conventional health care is unable to deal with major health problems or improve a person's general health.*

A Cross-Section of Care

Modalities in column 1 of the Healing Matrix are technologies that cut across various healing systems. The technologies are arranged vertically from the most concrete to the most abstract. The remaining columns include various healing modalities from conventional, marginal, and alternative healing systems.

Physical Manipulation Technologies. These are also known as "bodywork therapies." They are administered by a therapist or by the clients themselves as part of a self-care program. They include health rituals and breathing exercises to better bring about the union of body–mind–spirit.

Ingested or Applied Substances. A number of substances, including herbs, vitamins, and other nutritional supplements, and dietary regimens have the goal of helping the body heal itself, rid itself of toxins, and promote general health and wellness.

Energy Therapies. These modes of treatment maintain or restore health through the balancing of energy flow in the body. The goal is to restore the natural movement of vital forces or life essences that may have been disturbed by diseases or psychological factors.

Table 25.1 **The Healing Matrix**

Technologies	Orthodox	Marginal	Intuitive	Integrative
Physical manipulation	Surgery	Chiropractic	Rolfing	Craniosacral alignments
Ingested or applied substances	Physical therapy	Homeopathy	Feldenkrais	Massage therapy
Uses of energy	Pharmacology	Vitamin therapy	Naturopathic remedies	Yoga, aikido, tai chi
Mental	Laser surgery	Acupuncture	Herbs	Reflexology
Spiritual	Psychiatry	Acupressure	Flower remedies	Aromatherapy
		Secular or spiritual counseling	Reiki	Diet alternatives
		Established support groups (e.g., 12-step programs)	Magnetic or polarity healing	
			Therapeutic touch	Chakra balancing
			Self-help groups	Radionics
			Visualizations	Use of color, gems, and crystals
			Affirmations	Psychic, spiritual, or intuitive healing

Source: Adapted from Engebretson J, Wardell D. A contemporary view of alternative healing modalities. *Nurse Practitioner,* 18:51, 1993.

Mental (Psychic) and Spiritual Therapies

Included in these therapies are group or individual counseling techniques that help the client develop or attain spiritual and personal growth. Examples include intuiting, revelations, visualization, astrological and other readings, and invoking the spirit world.

Conventional Health Care

The modalities listed in column 2 (orthodox [conventional]) are part of the official health-care system in the United States. They are based on knowledge rooted in scientific and biomedical principles.

Licensed Integrative Care

The modalities in column 3 (marginal) are generally learned through the study of the standard curricula in institutions of higher education. Integrative healers practicing such modalities are usually licensed by the state, and most have credentialing and a professional body that sets standards for their practice. These modalities are not considered conventional therapies in the United States but may be part of conventional health-care systems in other nations.

For example, acupuncture is an essential mode of treatment in traditional Chinese medicine, which, along with biomedicine, forms the conventional health-care system in the People's Republic of China. In 1997, the National Institutes of Health Consensus Panel on Acupuncture reviewed research studies and other information on its safety, efficacy, and effectiveness. The studies showed sufficient evidence to approve acupuncture as an intervention for adult general and dental postoperative pain and to treat nausea and vomiting associated with chemotherapy.[6]

Intuitively Based Care

The modalities presented in columns 4 and 5 are less physiological. They are based on a more intuitive type of knowledge. Most alternative healers practicing such modalities are self-taught, have learned through working with more experienced practitioners, have attended courses or workshops on particular modalities, or have learned by a combination of methods. The integrative modalities in the bottom cell on the far right have the most intuitive knowledge base; that is, insights about the spiritual or physical self are gained through direct revelations or interpreted by another.[7] These include readers (e.g., astrologers or seers) and spiritual healers in touch with divine forces.

The NCCAM Classification

In 1992, Congress mandated the establishment of an Office of Alternative Medicine in the National Institutes of Health to enhance the study of ACH. In 1998, the Office became the NCCAM. Its mission is to conduct and support basic and applied research and training and to disseminate ACH information to conventional health-care professionals, alternative healers, and the public.

Complementary and alternative medicine (CAM) is defined by the NCCAM as those practices not commonly included in or used by conventional medicine. Five major categories of CAM are defined and subdivided into practices that (1) fall under CAM, (2) are found in conventional health care but reclassified as behavioral medicine, and (3) are overlapping—that is, they can fall in the domain of either CAM or behavioral medicine. Table 25.2 summarizes the NCCAM classification.

Category I

Category I includes alternative systems of theory and practice developed outside Western biomedicine. For example, acupuncture and Oriental medicine are grounded in traditional Chinese medicine. Also included in this category are traditional indigenous systems, which include all medical systems other than acupuncture and Oriental medicine that developed outside of Western biomedicine. It also includes unconventional Western systems not classified elsewhere that were developed in the West but are not considered part of biomedicine, such as homeopathy.

Finally, this category includes naturopathy, an unconventional medical system that has gained prominence in the United States. This eclectic approach consists of various natural systems, such as herbalism, lifestyle therapies, and diet as therapy.

Table 25.2 **Categories of Alternative Practice**

I. Integrative Medical Systems	
Traditional Oriental Medicine	
Acupuncture	Herbal formulas
Diet	Massage and manipulation (Tui Na)
External and internal Qi Gong	Tai chi
Traditional Indigenous Systems	
Ayurvedic medicine	Traditional African medicine
Curanderismo	Traditional Aboriginal medicine
Central and South American	Unani-tibbi
Kampo medicine	Siddhi
Native American medicine	

CAM	Overlapping
Alternative Western Systems	
Homeopathy	Anthroposophically extended medicine
Naturopathy	
Orthomolecular medicine	

Table 25.2 **Categories of Alternative Practice—cont'd**

II. Mind–Body Interventions

CAM	Behavioral Medicine	Overlapping
Mind–Body Methods		
Yoga	Hypnosis	Art, music, and dance therapies
Tai chi	Meditation	Humor
Internal Qi Gong	Biofeedback	Journaling

CAM		
Religion and Spirituality		
Confession	Nontemporality	"Special" healers
Nonlocality	Soul retrieval	Spiritual healing

CAM		Overlapping
Social and Contextual Areas		
Caring-based approaches (e.g., holistic nursing, pastoral care)		Community-based approaches (e.g., Native American "sweat" rituals)
Intuitive diagnosis		Explanatory models
		Placebo

III. Biologically Based Therapies

Phytotherapy or Herbalism

Aloe vera	Echinacea	Ginseng	Mistletoe
Bee pollen	Evening primrose	Green tea	Peppermint oil
Biloba	Garlic	Hawthorne	Saw palmetto
Cat's claw	Ginger	Kava	Witch hazel
Dong quai	Ginkgo	Licorice root	Valerian

Special Diet Therapies

Atkins	McDougall	Fasting	Paleolithic
Diamond	Ornish	High fiber	Vegetarian
Kelly-Gonzalez	Pritikin	Macrobiotic	
Gerson	Wigmore	Mediterranean	
Livingston-Wheeler	Asian	Natural hygiene	

Orthomolecular Therapies

Single Nutrients (Partial Listing)

Amino acids	Folic acid	Lysine	Niacinamide	Thiamine
Ascorbic acid	Glutamine	Manganese	Potassium	Tyrosine
Boron	Glucosamine sulfate	Magnesium	Selenium	Vanadium
Calcium	Iodine	Medium-chain triglycerides	Silicon	Vitamin A
Carotenes	Inositol	Melatonin	Glandular products	Vitamin D
Choline	Iron	Niacin	Riboflavin	Vitamin K
Fatty acids	Lipoic acid		Taurine	

(continued)

Table 25.2 **Categories of Alternative Practice—cont'd**

Pharmacological, Biological, and Instrumental Interventions		

Products

Antineoplastons	Cone therapy	Hyperbaric oxygen
Bee pollen	Enderlin products	Induced remission therapy
Cartilage	Enzyme therapies	Ozone
Cell therapy	Gallo immunotherapy	Revici system
Coley's toxins	H_2O_2	

Procedures/Devices

Apitherapy	Electrodiagnostics	Neural therapy
Bioresonance	Iridology	
Chirography	MORA device	

IV. Manipulative and Body-Based Methods		

Chiropractic Medicine

Massage and Bodywork		

Acupressure	Feldenkrais technique	Reflexology
Alexander technique	Osteopathic manipulative therapy (OMT)	Rolfing
Applied kinesiology	Pilates method	Swedish massage
Chinese Tui Na massage	Polarity	Trager bodywork
Craniosacral OMT		

Unconventional Physical Therapies		

Colonics	Heat and electrotherapies	Light and color therapies
Diathermy	Hydrotherapy	

V. Energy Therapies		

Biofield Therapies

External Qi Gong	Healing touch	Reiki
Healing science	Huna	Therapeutic touch

Bioelectromagnetically Based Therapies*		

Alternating and direct current fields	Magnetic fields	Pulsed fields

*Unconventional use of electromagnetic fields.

Source: Adapted from National Center for Complementary and Alternative Medicine. Classification of Alternative Medicine Practices, 2010. Available at: http://www.ncbi.nlm.nih.gov/pmc/articles/PMC2592334/

Category II

Category II includes mind–body practices, religion and spirituality, and social and contextual areas. Mind–body medicine involves a variety of approaches to health care and contains three subcategories. Mind–body systems are seldom practiced alone but are usually combined with lifestyle interventions.

Mind–body methods may be used as a supplement to a traditional medical system. They are sometimes used in conventional health-care practices; however, they are characterized as CAM when used for conditions for which they are not normally prescribed. Religion and spirituality include treatments directed toward biological functions or clinical conditions. Social and contextual areas include treatment methods that are not included in other categories, such as cultural and symbolic interventions.

Category III

Biologically based therapies include products, interventions, and practices that are natural in origin and biologically based. They may or may not overlap with conventional medicine and its use of dietary supplements.

Phytotherapy, or herbalism, is the use of plant-derived products for purposes of prevention and treatment. Diet therapies use special diets to reduce risk factors or treat chronic diseases. Orthomolecular medicine is the use of nutritional products and food supplements that are not included in other categories for prevention and treatment of disease. Pharmacological, biological, and instrumental interventions are those not covered in other categories and administered in an unconventional manner.

Category IV

Manipulative and body-based methods include body manipulation, body movement, or both. Chiropractic care specializes in adjustments and manipulation of the spine, returning the body to its optimal alignment. This type of care is most often used when people have pain in their lower back, shoulders, and neck. However, chiropractic is often considered to be holistic and these manipulations may also improve the overall state of wellness.

The ancient healing art of acupressure was first recognized in Asia approximately 5,000 years ago. The acupressure practitioner uses his or her fingers to gradually press key points throughout the body. It is believed that this pressure will stimulate the body's own healing mechanisms. It can also be self-performed to relieve stress and tension, boost the immune system, reduce some types of pain, and improve health. (For a diagram of the acupressure pressure points and more information, go to http://acupressure.com/articles/acupuncture_and_acupressure_points.htm.)

Category V

Energy therapies are based on manipulation of biofields with bioelectromagnetically based therapies. Biofields include energy systems and energy fields internal and external to the body that are used for medical purposes. Bioelectromagnetics is the use of electromagnetic fields in an unconventional manner for medical reasons.[4] Although it is called *therapeutic touch* (TT), there is no actual contact with the body or only very light touch. The use of TT is believed to redirect energy flow and treat pain and disease. Research shows that in some individuals TT is effective on wound healing, pain, and anxiety, but the reports of results have been mixed.

COMPARING CONVENTIONAL, ALTERNATIVE, AND INTEGRATIVE PRACTICES

Many similarities exist among integrative, alternative, and conventional health care. As they attempt to achieve similar goals, they overlap in methodology, even though the methods are derived from different concepts of healing and different theoretical models. Table 25.3 summarizes characteristics often cited as common to alternative healing and contrasts them with those usually associated with conventional health care.

A Reductionist Philosophy

In general, conventional medicine focuses on the physical or material part of the person, the body. It is concerned with the structure, function, and connections or communication between material elements that compose the body, such as bones, muscles, and nerves. Conventional medicine generally views all humans as being very similar biologically. Disease is seen as a deviation from what is generally considered to be a normal biological or somatic state.

Conventional medicine is sometimes considered reductionist because it tends to reduce very

Table 25.3 **Contrasts Between Conventional and Integrative Health Care**

Conventional	Integrative
Chemotherapy	Plants and other natural products
Curing/treating	Healing/ministering care
Disease category	Unique individual
End-stage	Hope/hopefulness
Focus is on disease and illness	Focus is on health and wellness
Illness treatment	Health promotion and illness prevention
Individual is viewed as disease category	Individual is viewed as unique being
Nutrition is adjunct and supportive to treatment	Nutrition is the basis of health, wellness, and treatment
Objectivism: person is separate from disease	Subjectivism: person is integral to the illness
Patient/client	Person
Practitioner as authority	Practitioner as facilitator
Practitioner paternalism/client dependency	Practitioner as partner/person empowerment
Positivism/materialism: data are physically measurable	Metaphysical: entity is energy system or vital force
Reductionist	Holistic
Specialist care	Self-care
Symptom relief	Alleviation of causative factors
Somatic (body biologic and physiologic) model	Behavioral-psycho-social-spiritual model
Science is only source of knowledge and truth	Multiple sources of knowledge and truth
Technological/invasive	Natural/noninvasive

complex entities (humans) to seemingly equal and more simple beings who are all anatomically and physiologically similar. From this perspective, it is believed that all individuals will respond in more or less the same ways to causative agents, such as bacteria and viruses, and respond similarly to common treatments, such as medicines and surgery. In other words, a person with measles, cirrhosis of the liver, or breast cancer will have the same course of illness as other persons with those illnesses and will respond to treatments in basically the same manner.

Diagnosis by Category

Conventional medicine has developed extensive disease categories, and great emphasis is placed on diagnosis and cure based on the assessment of physical signs and symptoms. Most newly developed medications, when they are in the human testing phase, are tested on men between the ages of 25 and 35 years, with the presumption that they will work similarly in women, elderly people, and children. That presumption is not always accurate, and there is a growing trend at pharmaceutical companies to test medications on groups of persons for whom they are more likely to be used.

Integration of Nonmaterial Factors

The physical body is the primary focus of conventional medicine. Because of this almost exclusive focus on the physical body, conventional medicine often does not consider or include the nonmaterialistic aspects of health and illness in diagnosis and treatment decisions. Thus, spiritual, psychological, sociocultural, behavioral, and energy system aspects play little or no role in conventional medical treatment.

Although there has been some movement to a more holistic approach to client care in traditional medical schools (doctors of medicine [MD]), overall conventional medical practice does not generally view the client as an integrated person-body that is affected simultaneously by both material and nonmaterial factors during everyday life. The integration of these elements is often not viewed as significant to the person's state of wellness or illness; therefore, therapies based on the concept of holism are not deemed to be essential in treatment. However, schools of osteopathic medicine (doctors of osteopathy [DO]) have been producing physicians with a holistic view of client care for many years. One major difference between the MD's and DO's medical educations is that the DO programs require 300 to 500 hours of study and practice of integrative practices, including hands-on manipulation of the human body.

The Holistic Approach

In contrast, the integrative and alternative approach views the person-body as consisting of multiple, integrated elements that incorporate both the materialistic and nonmaterialistic aspects of existence. These elements include the physical (material), spiritual, energetic, and social bodies. This view allows for various interpretations of how the different components of the person-body interact and function to affect health and illness and respond to different therapeutic interventions.

> *Most newly developed medications, when they are in the human testing phase, are tested on men between the ages of 25 and 35 years, with the presumption that they will work similarly in women, elderly people, and children. That presumption is not always accurate.*

The Multiple-Body View

The integration of multiple aspects into a unified but distinctly individual person-body results in the belief that the person-body responds as a whole to factors that affect its state of well-being. Although the signs and symptoms of illness for one person are similar to another person's, they may indicate different underlying causes based on variable risk factors. From this viewpoint, diagnostic measures and interventions cannot be based on only one aspect of the person's being but must be tailored to the person-body of each individual.

A Capacity for Self-Healing

A variety of integrative modalities are often needed to diagnose and treat each individual holistically. It often is not obvious when the health problems of the physical body correspond to the dynamics of the energetic body or when the energetic body merges with the spiritual body, and how they all are eventually integrated into the psychosocial body. The mediating role of the psychosocial body in the integrative approach emphasizes each person's capacity for self-healing. The importance of the mind–body interaction to elicit the placebo response and the need for clients to participate actively in the monitoring and maintenance of their health and well-being are positive factors in the diagnosis and treatment of their illness.

The multiple-body view found in some alternative health-care practices requires an eclectic approach to health promotion and maintenance. The diagnosis and treatment of illness from a multiple-body view require more than dependence on a single healing tradition centered on a one-body concept or on a fixed set of diagnostic criteria. The integrative approach requires active participation of both well and ill persons to better promote health or diagnose and treat disorders, rather than passive acceptance of a diagnosis and treatment plan from conventional health-care professionals. The goal is lifelong wellness.

Combining Modalities

The integrative philosophy includes both the material and nonmaterial aspects of the individual, stimulation of the self-healing forces, and the determination of a person's unique needs. It uses the concepts and treatment modalities of both alternative and conventional healing traditions simultaneously. These modalities are based on different worldviews or concepts of reality and address the individual healing needs of each person.

For example, acupuncturists may also use massage and other types of bodywork and energy-system methods; chiropractors may incorporate diet, herbs, and other kinds of naturopathic methodologies into chiropractic spinal manipulations; and massage therapists may include mind–body techniques such as meditation, imagery, and visualization. These alternative modalities are used to treat various client symptoms while integrative practices attempt to select the best of both conventional and alternative treatments and combine them to produce a long-term state of health[7] (Box 25.2).

What Do You Think?

Name someone you know or know of who has gotten better after an illness although not expected to. Why do you think this happened?

The concept of a multiple-body individual is central to integrative healing. Healers function as facilitators in the promotion of health and healing (Box 25.3). In contrast, conventional therapy relies primarily on the concept of the physical-body individual, and conventional health-care providers function as experts in determining the meaning of physical signs and symptoms of health or illness and prescribing interventions to promote health or cure illness. The concepts of wellness and holism, self-healing, energy systems, nutrition, and plant-based

Box 25.2

The Principles of Integrative Medicine

1. A partnership between client and practitioner in the healing process
2. Appropriate use of conventional and alternative methods to facilitate the body's innate healing response
3. Consideration of all factors that influence health, wellness, and disease, including mind, spirit, and community as well as body
4. A philosophy that neither rejects conventional medicine nor accepts alternative therapies uncritically
5. Recognition that good medicine should be based in good science, be inquiry driven, and be open to new paradigms
6. Use of natural, effective, less-invasive interventions whenever possible
7. Use of the broader concepts of promotion of health and the prevention of illness as well as the treatment of disease
8. Training of practitioners to be models of health and healing, committed to the process of self-exploration and self-development

Source: Lemley B. What is integrative medicine? 2013. Retrieved April 2013 from http://www.drweil.com/drw/u/ART02054/Andrew-Weil-Integrative-Medicine.html

Box 25.3

Defining Integrative Healers

Integrative healers are conventional health-care professionals who incorporate hands-on alternative and complementary modalities into their conventional client care and are sometimes called *integrative practitioners*. They should undergo the same educational, certification, and licensing processes as both conventional and alternative healers for the modalities they use.

Creating a universally applicable definition of integrative healers is extremely difficult because of the wide variety of healing traditions in use and the number of specialized healing techniques contained within them. The difficulty is compounded by the fact that many alternative healers incorporate various modalities from different healing traditions into their practices. For example, chiropractors commonly use therapeutic touch, acupuncture, acupressure, massage therapy, and naturopathic or homeopathic therapies. Massage therapists may combine multiple types of massage (e.g., Alexander, Swedish, Trager, and sports) with therapeutic touch, aromatherapy, reflexology, nutritional supplements, and electromagnetic therapies. The growing use of alternative practices by conventional health-care professionals is demonstrating the trend toward alternative healing practice.

medicine can be used to compare and contrast integrative and conventional methods of healing.

Wellness and Holism

The term *wellness* is often used interchangeably with *good health,* generally meaning an absence of disease or illness; however, in the context of this chapter, it includes much more. The term *holism,* first used in discussion of systems theory, is often defined as the totality or entirety of a system that is more than the sum of its parts. The system being looked at in health care is the human person.

Therapy From Outside

Wellness, from the perspective of traditional medicine, tends to focus on individuals who are seen as being at risk for illness. Prevention often begins when signs or symptoms arise and is directed at alleviating them rather than treating or removing their underlying cause. Because of the strong belief in the ethical principal of autonomy or self-determination, at-risk individuals are often permitted to engage in risky behaviors as long as conventional health care can find treatments or palliative measures for the symptoms of diseases it cannot prevent. For example, a client who smokes develops a chronic cough but does not yet have any of the smoking-related diseases (i.e., emphysema, bronchitis, lung cancer). This person would likely receive from a nonholistic physician a strong warning about smoking, but the major focus of care would be to provide the client with medication to eliminate the cough. From this perspective, the absence of an active specific disease is considered synonymous with wellness.

Because the focus of traditional medicine is on individual body systems or organs, it is considered to be reductionist (breaking apart) rather than holistic. It emphasizes the biological–physiological (body) dimension of the client and treats only the disease process for which signs and symptoms are already evident. The cause of illness is usually attributed to external forces or risk factors that "invade" the body from the surrounding physical, social, or biological environments.

> *The human spirit incorporates the values, perception of meaning, and purpose in life that can positively or negatively affect the ability to heal and achieve wellness.*

From the biomedical view, treatment usually centers on identifying potentially dangerous or invading agents and then destroying, immobilizing, or extracting them from the person's body. Interventions consist mainly of chemotherapeutic agents (medications), surgery, or other externally imposed treatments to prevent a person considered at risk from becoming ill or to prevent signs and symptoms from becoming full-blown diseases.

Therapy From Within

In contrast to traditional medical care, the integrative model views wellness as a state in which individuals are in harmony or balance with their internal and external worlds. A holistic understanding of wellness is much broader than the traditional concept of health. It implies that the client is aware of his or her present and future state of health in all of its aspects (physical, mental, emotional, spiritual, environmental, social, and occupational). To be able to achieve a true state of wellness requires the

clients to maintain, alter, balance, and evaluate their health in each one of the health aspects.

This approach to wellness forms a common thread in nursing models or theories of health (see Chapter 3). Integrative modalities hold that wellness can rarely be imposed on a person by an outside entity or agent. Rather, wellness is achieved mainly by individuals through the process of self-care. The individual assumes responsibility for maintaining his or her own state of health or wellness. The individual, when ill, works to return to a state of wellness by restoring both the internal and external (environmental) states of balance and harmony.

For example, in the case of the smoker who does not yet have an active disease process, the integrative health-care provider would also treat the cough but would spend much more time with the client to attempt to determine which stressors in his life trigger the urge to smoke. The integrative provider would likely offer the client methods either to reduce or eliminate these stressful situations. The provider would discuss with the client ways to stop smoking, including use of stop-smoking aids, hypnosis, and smoking cessation groups to help him gain control over his addiction and return to a healthy balanced state of life.

External disruptions—such as work stress, personal tragedy, a troublesome interpersonal relationship, or illness of a parent, spouse, or child—are seen as capable of affecting internal harmony and producing signs and symptoms of physical, emotional, or spiritual illness. This provides a holistic view of individuals in which they are one with their internal and external environments, thereby requiring holistic care. Treatment must address the whole individual (body–mind–spirit) in an environmental (physical, biological, social, cultural, and spiritual) context.

Spirituality is an essential part of holistic treatment (see Chapter 21). The human spirit incorporates the values, perception of meaning, and purpose in life that can positively or negatively affect the ability to heal and achieve wellness. From this perspective, health (balance or harmony), or the absence of illness, is but one aspect of wellness.

Self-Care

In the integrative model, first-level measures involve self-care aimed at wellness and can generally be performed independently. Some examples include exercising, eating a well-balanced diet, nurturing the spirit, getting enough sleep, cleaning the house, using defensive driving measures, doing breast or testicular self-examinations, applying sunscreen when outside, eliminating destructive habits, and practicing good hygiene.

The next level of self-care requires seeking the assistance of others to achieve balance in self and the environment. This level includes getting help to find satisfying employment, seeking prenatal care, taking parenting classes when pregnant, going to community meetings to address environmental safety and citizen quality-of-life issues, seeking conventional health screening examinations (e.g., mammography and dental checkups), obtaining glasses to correct myopia, and getting vaccinations and keeping them up to date. Alternative measures, such as acupuncture and energy therapies, can also be used in this level of care.

The third level of self-care requires a high degree of specialist assistance from integrative and alternative healers to deal with major disruptions in internal or external well-being. Measures from this level focus on the spiritual dimension and include searching for personal awakening, enlightenment, and self-actualization. Effective modalities to achieve this goal are often rooted in other systems of health care such as traditional Chinese medicine and spiritualism. In some cases, individuals may require the use of both alternative modalities and conventional health care when a single treatment modality is no longer effective.

Self-Healing

Integrative, alternative, and conventional health care all include the belief that the body has the capacity to heal itself. The integrative and alternative systems place self-healing as the central principle of their models and see it as the basis of all healing. Thus, integrative and alternative healers focus on helping people determine why the cells of their body are sick and search for imbalances from a holistic perspective.

> *Healers who believe in the therapeutic effectiveness of interventions and are able to convey that belief to their clients achieve more positive responses than healers who remain skeptical about the interventions they are prescribing.*

Conventional health care views the ability of the body to self-heal primarily through the normal process of replacing cells; examples include the physiological and biological processes involved in wound healing. Conventional care approaches the concept of body self-healing by questioning why the cells are not replacing themselves and attempts to facilitate healing through external means, which are potentially invasive, such as surgery or medications.

The Placebo Response

Conventional health practitioners tend to dismiss the effects of healing after integrative and alternative modalities have been used by attributing them to the placebo response. They feel that healing takes place only because the individual believes the treatment is effective. In conventional medicine, the term *placebo* has come to signify a type of sham treatment instituted to please difficult or anxious clients, or a sugar pill given when health-care professionals have nothing more to offer the client. In biomedical clinical research, a placebo is an inactive or nontreatment given to the control group under the assumption that it will not change any physiological responses and will therefore prove the effectiveness of the active treatments.

What Do You Think?

What are the ethical issues involved in using placebos? If you were being given a placebo and you found out, how would you feel? What if you improved with the placebo? Would you still feel the same way?

The placebo response plays an important part in the testing of new drugs. The commonly used double-blind study requires that neither researchers nor study participants know which group is receiving the study drug and which group is receiving an inert substance (placebo). At the conclusion of the study, researchers compare results and decide whether a higher percentage of the experimental group experienced the hoped-for results from the active medication than the control group received from the placebo. However, clinical studies have shown that some participants respond positively to placebo medications between 30 and 70 percent of the time. The clients with the highest positive results from placebos include those with:

- Pain from chronic disease, such as cancer, arthritis, back pain, angina pectoris, and gastrointestinal tract discomfort.
- Autonomic nervous system disorders, such as phobias, psychoneuroses, depression, and nausea.
- Neurohormonal disorders, such as asthma, other bronchial airflow conditions, and hypertension.

How Does It Work?

Researchers do not have a good understanding of the mechanism by which the placebo response produces positive results. Some believe that the placebo effect is at work in all therapeutic intervention regardless of whether the intervention is an alternative or a conventional treatment. Four possible factors have been examined:

- An endorphin-mediated response
- Belief of the client
- Belief of the healer
- The client–healer relationship
- Remembered wellness

Endorphin-Mediated Response. Endorphins are the body's natural painkillers; they are released primarily when a person experiences fear, stress, or pain. Endorphins work by binding with opioid receptor sites in order to reduce pain as well as cause a change in mental status, such as a degree of euphoria. There are over 20 types of endorphins; however, the beta-endorphins are the most powerful with an effect stronger than morphine. Relaxation therapies and other types of stress-reducing and stress-controlling techniques are believed to promote the release of endorphins that relieve pain. When experimental groups were given medications that block the release of beta-endorphins, clients with postoperative dental pain reported an increase in pain.

Belief of the Client. A person's belief in the effectiveness of the therapy is an important factor in its success and may be just as important as the therapy itself. Studies of client compliance in taking prescribed beta-blocker heart medications, conducted in the first year after myocardial infarction, showed that mortality rates were almost equal for those failing to take either the beta-blocker or the placebo. Mortality rates for both these groups were higher than the rates for those who faithfully took their prescribed medications or placebos.

Belief of the Healer. Healers who believe in the therapeutic effectiveness of interventions and are able to convey that belief to their clients achieve more positive responses than healers who remain skeptical about the interventions they are prescribing. An attitude of caring and being in control tends to alleviate clients' anxieties and fears while increasing their hope and positive expectations.

Client–Healer Relationship. A trusting and close relationship between the client and healer has a positive psychological effect on clients and can become the mental catalyst they need for recovery. It is essential for the success of the integrative approach. The ability of healers to communicate in an empathic manner increases client satisfaction with care; increases compliance with mutually set goals; increases feelings of empowerment, self-confidence, and self-worth; and decreases depression and anxiety.

Although conventional health care considers many of these approaches as speculative, incomplete, or insufficient to explain the placebo response, integrative healers see the placebo response as measurable and reproducible evidence that the mind and body are intertwined. The placebo response is viewed as proof that feelings, thoughts, and beliefs can change the physiological and structural functioning of individuals.

Remembered Wellness. The term *remembered wellness* is used to describe the physiological response that occurs after positive therapeutic interventions. Remembered wellness includes the person's prior learning, experiences, environment, beliefs, and perceptions. It can also include biological and genetic factors.

Remembered wellness is triggered by memories of past events or times when good health and feelings of confidence, strength, hope, and peace were part of the person's life. Alternative therapies access these memories by stimulating relaxation, such as the quieting of the body and mind to promote healing. Clinical research has demonstrated relaxation to be effective in treating anxiety, pain, high blood pressure, and tachycardia and in managing stress. Research studies have confirmed a close relationship between the central nervous and immune systems and have shown that interaction occurs between the two mind–body pathways: the autonomic and neuroendocrine systems.

Much more research is required for a full scientific explanation of the how the mind and body interact to produce the placebo response and why remembered wellness produces the positive responses it often does. The placebo response remains an enigma to conventional health care and implies an element of deceitfulness when used deliberately in client treatments. For integrative healing, the placebo response and remembered wellness are forces that can be harnessed to bring about healing.

Energy Systems

It has long been known scientifically that the human body is regulated by its own internal electrical energy system. Human beings cannot survive without the low levels of electricity that sustain and regulate life at the cellular and molecular levels. Electrical–chemical reactions are produced in the nervous system and help regulate other body systems, electrical impulses trigger heartbeats, and minute electrical currents regulate the production of hormones. The blood is composed largely of iron; therefore, magnetic forces exist in all parts of the body.

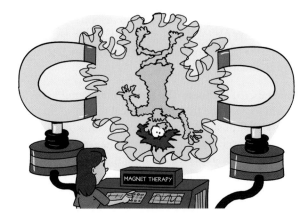

MAGNET THERAPY

Conventional Uses of Energy

Conventional health care has long used various types of energy systems (e.g., electrical, magnetic, microwave, and infrared) for screening, diagnosis, and some types of treatment. Commonly used modalities include electrocardiograms, magnetic resonance imaging, electroencephalograms, electromyograms, x-rays, radiation treatments for cancer,

low-frequency electric current to stimulate growth of bone cells (osteoblasts) to accelerate healing of fractures, types of electric shock therapy for cardiac arrest, cardioversions for cardiac arrhythmia, and pacemakers.

Conventional health care also uses bioenergy (body energy) to determine the degree of injury and estimate recovery times through the study of cells as they decompose, die, reproduce, and respond to pathogens and traumas. The majority of conventional treatments for many diseases are chemical (medications) or surgical or involve immobilizing or manipulating the affected body part. They are used primarily *after* the disease has been diagnosed.

Energy in Alternative Healing

Conventional medicine has long been cynical about integrative practices, and as a result has been slow to recognize how the energy of the body can be used for health promotion and healing. Alternative therapies refer to energy systems as fields, vital essences, balance, and flow that clients can use to prevent illness, promote health, and heal themselves. The basic concept is that external forces are not able to cause harm if the person is in the well state. Alternative healers may be needed to help individuals manipulate the energy system primarily for self-protection or healing. Major alternative and complementary modalities using bioenergy and other energy fields include energy medicine, vital essences and balance, and external energy forces.

Energy Medicine

This therapy includes a number of techniques that use external energy sources to stimulate tissue regeneration or improve the immune system response. Relaxation of muscles through electrical stimulation is thought to promote general body relaxation, increase circulation, enhance waste removal, improve nutrition and oxygenation, and restore energy balance. Examples of energy medicine include biofeedback, magnet therapy, and sound and light therapy.

Vital Essences and Balance

In the integrative models, illness reflects blockage, loss, or imbalance of body energy or vital essence. Disturbance of internal body energy can result from external or internal factors. Treatment may be directed at removing the blockage of energy flow through such measures as acupuncture, acupressure, chiropractic adjustment, craniosacral therapy, or reflexology. It may also be directed at increasing the amount of energy and vital essence to restore balance in the body.

Ways of inducing these changes include diet, herbs, exercises, and spiritual techniques, such as yoga, meditation, and Qi Gong. Therapies related to the creative arts, such as music, drawing, singing, chanting, and dancing, are also used to restore balance and vital essences.

External Energy Forces

It is believed that external energy forces have the capacity for healing. Some of these external forces involve treatments with actual external energy sources, such as whole body vibration (WBV) therapy and electroacupuncture. WBV involves stimulating the client's body with low-frequency vibration in the range of 0.5 to 80 Hz. To be most effective, the vibration should be administered over a wide contact area using a platform to stimulate the feet when standing, or a special chair to stimulate the buttocks when sitting, or the whole back when lying on a vibrating surface. For maximal effect, the client should experience some fatigue or low-level stress. It is believed that the vibration causes the body to learn how to adapt to external stress, which produces increased circulation, improved muscle tone, better joint motion, and activation of osteoblasts that increase bone density. By connecting wires to two acupuncture needles at a time and passing a low-voltage pulsating current of electricity between them, it is believed that electroacupuncture augments the acupuncture experience and is especially effective in the treatment of pain. Several pairs of needles can be electrified at the same time and the procedure should not last more than half an hour.

Other energy force treatments include mobilizing the healing energy of faith, spirituality, prayer, shamanism, crystals, and hand-mediated energetic healing techniques, such as therapeutic touch and healing touch (Box 25.4).

Nutrition

Nutrition and diet have long been recognized by both integrative and conventional healing systems as important in health promotion and illness treatment. They can also be risk factors for or even cause disease.

Box 25.4

Therapeutic Touch

Therapeutic touch (TT) and healing touch (HT) are two forms of hand-mediated energetic healing. TT refers to the Krieger-Kunz method and HT to the techniques taught to health-care professionals and certified by the American Holistic Nurses Association. HT relies on the ability of practitioners to choose appropriate energy healing techniques through their interpretation of the client's energy flow, whereas TT follows a set of rules and protocols based in traditional or ancient healing concepts of energy, such as aura (electromagnetic field), chakras, and prana (life force or vital essence in Ayurvedic medicine).

No physical contact takes place between practitioner and client in either technique. The practitioner's hands are held, palms down, 2 to 6 inches away from the client. Slow, rhythmic motions are made over the client from head to toe to detect blockage in the normal energy flow in the body. When energy blockages or imbalances are detected or sensed, they are rectified by transference of energy from the practitioner's hands to the client's energy field, replenishing the client's energy flow, removing energy obstructions, and releasing energy congestion. The transference of energy stimulates the healing powers of the body through reduction of stress and anxiety, promotion of relaxation, and relief of pain. TT is also believed to relax crying babies, relieve asthmatic breathing, increase wound healing, and reduce fever, inflammation, headache, and postoperative pain.

In conventional health care, nutrition and diet are usually considered as adjuncts to biomedical treatment. In integrative systems, nutrition is commonly seen as a way of life and as a method of preventing illness.

Benefits of Organic Foods

Currently in the United States, there is a trend to use the terms *natural foods, all-natural foods,* and *organic foods* interchangeably; however, there are differences. The definitions for natural and all-natural foods remain vague and have little meaning because of the lack of established quality standards. The implication in labeling a product as natural is that the food is unprocessed or only minimally processed, suggesting that it does not contain "unnatural" or manufactured substances. However, these products may contain natural substances such as salt, and they may be grown with the use of pesticides and chemical fertilizers and may be irradiated after harvesting and still be called *natural.*

In contrast, the term *organic* has been legally defined and has agreed-upon international standards. Foods can be labeled organic only if they are grown using organic farming methods, which eliminate the use of all synthetic products during their growth cycles such as chemical pesticides and synthetic fertilizers. Additionally, organic foods are not irradiated or chemically cleaned and do not contain any synthetic food additives after harvesting. Producers must obtain a special certificate from the U.S. government to market their products as organic.

Conventional health care commonly focuses on the need for food and a well-balanced diet without close regard to food production or processing. The safety of food sources in the contemporary diet has been called into question by both alternative healers and conventional health-care professionals because of increasing evidence of toxins in the food chain. These include:

- Pesticides used in agricultural production, lawn care, and pest control.
- Industrial pollutants discharged into the air and water in which plants and animals live and obtain nutrients.
- Chemicals added to food for preservation, to increase shelf life, or to make food more aesthetically appealing and pleasing in texture and taste.
- Irradiation used to kill organisms, retard sprouting, and preserve shelf life.
- Antibiotics, hormones, and other drugs given to animals to improve their health and increase their size, weight, and speed of growth.
- Alteration of nutrients during food processing.
- Genetic alteration of foods for improved production rates and drought resistance.

Integrative modalities recommend only foods produced in a natural manner and in their natural environment. Emphasis on organic products can be attributed to four primary factors:

1. Concerns about food production and processing
2. The belief that the person-body, as both an energy system and a physical entity, is designed to live in a natural environment

3. The belief that what is eaten directly affects an individual's health
4. Concerns about increased consumption of nutrient-poor and energy-rich foods

Scientific evidence indicates that the more sedentary lifestyle and greater affluence experienced by many have resulted in excessive and unhealthy eating. The end result is a nation that has high rates of obesity, coronary artery disease, micronutrient deficiencies, congenital abnormalities, and cancer. Most alternative systems advocate consumption of plant-based, whole foods and complex carbohydrates. Increasing the amounts of food lower on the food chain helps decrease the amounts of meat, saturated fats, and processed foods that dominate many diets. Examples of natural food diets include the macrobiotic and vegetarian diets.

Dietary Supplements

The FDA defines dietary supplements as "a product intended for ingestion that contains a 'dietary ingredient' intended to add further nutritional value to (supplement) the diet. A 'dietary ingredient' may be one, or any combination, of the following substances:

- A vitamin
- A mineral
- An herb or other botanical
- An amino acid
- A dietary substance for use by people to supplement the diet by increasing the total dietary intake
- A concentrate, metabolite, constituent, or extract

Dietary supplements may be found in many forms such as tablets, capsules, softgels, gelcaps, liquids, or powders. Some dietary supplements can help ensure that you get an adequate dietary intake of essential nutrients; others may help you reduce your risk of disease."[8]

Supplements as Prevention

Conventional health-care professionals typically view nutritional supplements (vitamins and minerals) as replacement or preventive therapy for nutrition-deficient conditions. For example, rickets and osteoporosis can be prevented by adequate vitamin D and calcium intake; adequate ascorbic acid (vitamin C) intake prevents scurvy; and neural tube defects in newborns can be prevented by sufficient maternal intake of folic acid (vitamin B_9) during the prenatal period. Niacin has been shown to lower cholesterol levels. On the basis of research by the National Academy of Sciences, the FDA has established maximum recommended daily allowances (RDAs) for vitamin and mineral intake. These levels are usually well above the amount at which deficiency diseases occur but below the level at which the client would experience toxic side effects.

Rethinking RDA Levels. Studies indicate that approximately two-thirds of adults fail to consume the RDAs of fruits and vegetables. Also, some studies suggest that RDA levels may be too low for certain vitamins, minerals, and micronutrients to prevent the onset of chronic diseases in persons whose diets do not meet the recommended daily nutrient requirements. Especially susceptible are growing children, alcoholics, people with conditions preventing normal nutrient absorption, and pregnant, lactating, and postmenopausal women. Conventional health-care professionals consider general daily supplements, such as vitamin pills, sufficient to prevent deficiency diseases in persons with special dietary needs.

Alternative systems, like conventional health care, regard nutritional supplements as necessary to promote health through assurance of adequate dietary intake and as replacement therapy for conditions caused by nutrition deficiency. Alternative systems also consider orthomolecular therapy or megavitamin therapy (the administration of "megadoses" far in excess of RDAs for vitamins and minerals) as being effective in curing diseases, increasing vitality, and enhancing overall well-being.

Regulation of Supplements

Concern about nutritional supplements also exists because, unlike drugs and most food additives, they are not regulated by the FDA. If manufacturers make no claims that they are effective against a disease, they do not need to be tested for safety and effectiveness before they are sold to the public. However, there has been a gradual increase in the regulation of these products over the past 25 years. The 1994 Dietary Supplement Health and Education Act (DSHEA) created a special category of 20,000 protected substances previously sold as supplements. The DSHEA defined supplements as including vitamins, minerals, amino acids, herbs, botanicals, and other plant-derived products and the extracts, metabolites, constituents, and concentrates of supplements.

What Do You Think?

Should dietary supplements be considered medications? What are the advantages and disadvantages of classifying supplements as medications?

The FDA can remove supplements from the market if it receives reports of their adverse effects and then proves that they are dangerous to consumers' health. The FDA issues public warnings when supplements are linked to safety concerns. The DSHEA also gave the FDA authority to improve and enforce product labeling, package inserts, and accompanying literature. To enhance product comparison, guidelines instituted in 1999 require labels to carry a panel of "supplemental facts" or a "nutrition facts box," which includes ingredients.

The U.S. Postal Service and the Federal Trade Commission (FTC) also regulate nutritional supplements and herbal products. The U.S. Postal Inspection Service monitors products purchased by mail and may intercept supplements shipped through the mail for false claims, such as the statement that they can cure AIDS or cancer. The Office of Criminal Investigation can be contacted at (703) 248-2000.

The FTC has issued guidelines to ensure that advertising claims are substantiated by reliable scientific evidence. Claims of effectiveness and safety based on testimonials and other anecdotal evidence are no longer acceptable. Also outlawed are vague disclaimers, such as "results may vary." The term *traditional use* (e.g., folk remedy), which implies that the product is effective even without scientific evidence, has also been banned. The risks or qualifying information of any product must be prominently displayed and easily understood.

> *Alternative therapies refer to energy systems as fields, vital essences, balance, and flow that clients can use to prevent illness, promote health, and heal themselves. The basic concept is that external forces are not able to cause harm if the person is in the well state.*

Plants as Medicine

Both alternative and conventional health care use plants as medicine. Herbalism, or "botanical medicine," also known as *phytotherapy* or *phytomedicine* in England and other parts of Europe, is the study and use of herbs or crude-based plant products for food, medicine, or prophylaxis. They can also be used to heal, treat, or prevent illness and improve the spiritual and physical quality of life.[9]

Herbs may be angiosperms (flowering plants, trees, or shrubs), algae, moss, fungus, seaweed, lichen, or ferns. Herbs used as medicines come from some part of the plant (leaf, root, flower, fruit, stem, bark, or seed), its syrup-like exudates, or some combination of these. In some herbal traditions, nonplant products are used alone or in combination, with or without plants. They may include animal secretions and parts (e.g., bones, organs, or tissues), stones and gemstones, minerals and metals, shells, and insects and insect products.

Botanical healing in the form of herbal medicines was widely used in the United States until the early 19th century, when it was gradually displaced by the increasing prominence of the scientific method and labeled quackery. Phytomedicine continues to be a prominent branch of conventional health care in Europe. Botanicals are used by 40 percent of German and French physicians in their daily practices.

Integrative systems, like conventional health care, consider nutritional supplements both as necessary to promote health through assurance of adequate dietary intake and as replacement therapy for conditions caused by nutrition deficiency.

Scientists have yet to determine the pharmaceutical qualities of most plants, and little is known about what toxicities they can produce. The world supports an estimated 250,000 to 500,000 flowering plant species, but only 5,000 have been researched for their pharmacological effects.[9]

Herbal Traditions

The use of herbal therapies varies according to culture and tradition. The three major groups of herbal therapies recognized throughout the world are from Western medicine, traditional Chinese medicine, and Ayurvedic medicine.

Western Pharmacology

The Western herbal tradition relies primarily on the pharmacological action of herbs, most of which are derived from the plant kingdom. There are approximately 123 plant-derived pharmaceutical medicines that are in use today. Almost all of the food supplements and herbal over-the-counter products, except for minerals, are plant based. The compounds and chemicals found in plants constitute about 25 percent of prescriptions by conventional health-care professionals. (For information on the specific names of medications that are plant based, go to http://chemistry.about.com/library/weekly/aa061403a.htm.)

Chinese Medicine

Herbology is used in traditional Chinese medicine to enhance the flow and amount of chi, restore the harmonious balance of the complementary forces of yin and yang, and balance the five elements (fire, earth, metal, water, and wood). In the Chinese system, plants are prescribed according to their effects on the five elements and their corresponding body processes, including organs, tissues, emotions, and temperatures (climates).

The Chinese believe that the five elements give rise to the five tastes that produce particular medicinal actions. Bitter-tasting herbs (fire) dry and drain. Sweet-tasting herbs (earth) reduce pain and increase tone. Acrid herbs (metal) rid the body of toxins. Salty herbs (water) nourish the kidney. Sour herbs (wood) clean, helping preserve chi and nourishing yin. Herbs are also symbolically classified according to temperature changes they are thought to produce in the body: cold, cool, neutral, warm, and hot. The temperatures correspond to the symbolic climate qualities of the organs and the five elements.

Ayurvedic Medicine

Ayurvedic medicine is the traditional medical system that has been used in India for thousands of years, and it focuses on producing health by balancing the three key substances of the body. A body out of balance is considered to be in a state of illness, and plant-based substances are used to achieve a balance in the body and restore a state of health. The Ayurvedic system also considers the taste, or "essence," of the herb as an integral element in herbology. Ayurveda recognizes six essences (sweet, sour, salty, pungent, bitter, and astringent) and five elements (ether, water, fire, air, and earth). The elements are manifested as three doshas, or humors (vata, pitta, and kapha), that govern body functioning and that must be kept in balance to maintain or restore a healthy state.

Vata, the principle of air, wind, or movement, is decreased by herbs that are sweet, sour, and salty, which exert a symbolic heating effect on the body. Vata is increased by herbs that are pungent, bitter, astringent, and cooling. Pitta, the principle of fire, is decreased by herbs that are sweet, bitter, astringent, and cooling and is increased by those that are pungent, sour, salty, and heating. Kapha, the principle of water, is decreased by herbs that are pungent, bitter, astringent, and heating and is increased by those that are sweet, sour, salty, and cooling.

Concerns About Herbal Therapies

There is growing concern in the United States about the use of herbal preparations by the general public without consultation with either conventional health-care professionals or alternative healers. Sales of herbal preparations have been growing tremendously, and the safety of the products is a concern. For example, the FDA has found that as many as 20 percent of herbal preparations imported from India and China contain higher than allowed levels of heavy metals such as lead, arsenic, and mercury. Some imported herbs have been banned from entry into the United States. Another concern is the lack of licensing and standards for herbalists. Except for naturopaths, most herbalists have no foundation in phytochemistry or botanical medicine.

Some in the health-care community are increasingly concerned about client safety in the wake of the increasing number of states legalizing the medical use of cannabis. The proponents of medical cannabis cite numerous studies that show the value of the plant in treating ailments such as pain, cancer, multiple sclerosis, rheumatoid arthritis, and inflammatory bowel disease; there is even newer research into neurological disorders such as Alzheimer's disease. They point to the American Medical Association's call to conduct clinical research to develop new cannabinoid-based medicines. (For more information, go to http://norml.org/component/zoo/category/recent-research-on-medical-marijuana.)

The opponents of the legalization of medical cannabis point to the fact that federal statutes still consider it a Schedule I controlled substance, and possession of large quantities is a felony. Although the Obama administration has decided not to enforce this law, future presidents may have a different view of the law and re-criminalize the use of cannabis for any reason. Federal law always supersedes state law. Opponents also point out that testing has shown that "medical-grade" cannabis is the same as cannabis bought off the street and that cannabis plants contain more than 400 potentially dangerous chemical compounds. Medical-grade plants have also tested positive for fungi, bacteria, pesticides, and other dangerous chemicals that are aerosolized and inhaled when smoked. It was originally made illegal because of its high abuse potential. Opponents also highlight the dangerous effects on the lungs of smoking any substance and the demonstrated neurological effects, such as paranoia and psychosis, sometimes seen in longtime cannabis users. Overall, they feel that taking shortcuts to get around the scientific and testing processes used for FDA approval of other medications for the purpose of hastening the use of medical cannabis is a mistake and will have long-term negative consequences on the health of many clients. (For more information, go to http://www.narconon.org/drug-information/dangers-of-marijuana.html.)

Also, in other cultural traditions, herbs are not prescribed for the biological effects of their chemical ingredients. They are commonly prescribed according to the "doctrine of signatures," or their physical and taste characteristics. For example, herbs with heart-shaped leaves may be used to treat heart

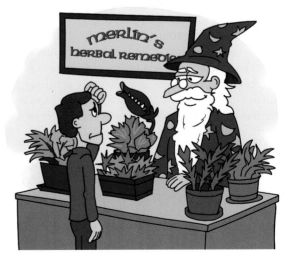

problems, those with red flowers or leaves may be used to control bleeding or blood disorders, and those with a sour taste may be given to decrease swelling or counteract the effects of "sugar" (diabetes mellitus).

Additional problems may arise because the public views most herbal remedies as natural products and therefore considers them to be pure, safe, relatively harmless, and more healthy than manufactured medicines. Recent problems with some natural products indicate that there is no guarantee of safety.

THE PARADOX OF INTEGRATIVE HEALING PRACTICES

Nurses often feel uncomfortable with the use of herbal products and unconventional therapies. This is due to unclear definitions of various integrative practices along with the widespread, yet often unregulated, use of alternative products and healers. This paradox arises because most nursing knowledge comes from the biomedical sciences, but most integrative modalities (1) have not yet been scientifically validated or proven safe by the scientific method and (2) are based in concepts of holism, self-care, and theoretical constructs that emanate from worldviews different from that of biomedicine and the scientific perspective.

A Lack of Validation

Put simply, for most integrative treatment modalities, little is known about whether or how they work, their side effects, or their interactions with conventional or other integrative treatments. Although there is increasing scientific research in this area, claims regarding their effectiveness still come largely from testimonials of users or integrative healers rather than from evidence in scientific studies. Equally limited is valid knowledge about the effectiveness of the various integrative modalities in specific conditions and about their short- and long-term effects.

The nursing profession has worked for many years to build its decision-making skills on knowledge derived from the scientific method and on the use of critical thinking and culture competence. Nurses promote self-care in clients by teaching them to make informed choices about their health-care

options. Many of the integrative health-care practices in use today conflict with the nursing profession's movement toward evidence-based practice.

Few Regulatory Standards

The technical competence and knowledge of integrative healers are of considerable importance to nurses caring for clients who pursue integrative practices. Nurses and the general public are accustomed to determining the qualifications, assumed competency, and scope of practice of conventional health-care practitioners through externally regulated mechanisms. These external regulations include graduation from an accredited school, state-regulated licenses, credentialing, and attainment of specialty certifications from professional organizations or institutions of higher education. No such external processes or criteria exist to validate the competence and knowledge of most integrative practitioners.

The relative lack of regulatory standards makes selection of competent integrative practitioners exceedingly difficult. It is a major concern of conventional health-care practitioners, insurers, and the general public because clients may be subject to financial exploitation, ineffective therapies, and psychological and physical abuse.

A Challenge to Nurses

The challenge presented to nurses by integrative healing modalities relates to professional accountability. Nurses must learn about integrative modalities, their general safety and efficacy, and their use in specific health and illness conditions.

Human caring and cultural competence require that nurses be able to develop therapeutic partnerships with culturally diverse clients and empower them to take charge of their lives and health care. They need to preserve the client's right to self-determination and to practice alternative lifestyles, as well as to pursue a variety of conventional or integrative therapies, with or without consulting alternative healers or conventional health-care professionals. Nurses must keep an open mind while relying on sound evidence for recommendations about alternative practices and practitioners.

Ask Questions

Box 25.5 lists some questions nurses need to ask when determining the quality and validity of information about an integrative modality. It is important

Box 25.5

Questions to Ask About Integrative Modalities

1. What evidence exists that the therapy is effective or harmful?
   - Is there experimental evidence? How effective is the alternative modality when examined experimentally?
   - Is there clinical practice evidence? How effective is the alternative modality when applied clinically?
   - Is there comparative evidence? How effective is the modality when compared with other treatments?
   - Is there summary evidence? Has the modality been evaluated and a consensus reached regarding its use and effectiveness for various health conditions?
   - Is there evidence of demand? Is the modality wanted by clients, practitioners, or both?
   - Is there evidence of satisfaction? Does the alternative modality meet the expectations of clients and practitioners?
   - Is there cost evidence? Is the modality covered by health insurance? Is it cost-effective?
   - Is the meaning evident? Is the modality the best and right one for the client?
2. How strong is the evidence? Is it based on testimonials, clinical observations, or scientific research?
3. Can the results be attributed to the placebo effect? Is the benefit from the placebo effect adequate to the client's needs?
4. Does evidence exist that the benefits of the therapy outweigh the risks?
   - Is the alternative modality potentially useful?
   - Is the modality essentially without value except for the potential placebo effect?
   - Is the modality potentially harmful?
5. Is there another way to obtain the same hoped-for results?
6. Who else has tried this alternative modality, and what was their experience?
7. Are there reputable (licensed and certified) alternative healers available? What has been their experience with this alternative modality?
8. What information do regulatory agencies have about the modality or the alternative healers?
9. What information is available in the popular media about the modality or alternative healers? Has it been or can it be verified by clinical observations or research studies?

Sources: Kurtzweil P. An FDA guide to dietary supplements, 2014. Retrieved September 2014 from http://www.fda.gov/food/guidanceregulation/guidancedocumentsregulatoryinformation/dietarysupplements/default.htm; National Center for Complementary and Alternative Medicine. Considering CAM? 2010. Retrieved November 2010 from http://www.nccam.nih.gov/nccam/fcp/faq/considercam.html; Wiese M, Oster C. "Becoming accepted": The complementary and alternative medicine practitioners' response to the uptake and practice of traditional medicine therapies by the mainstream health sector. *Health: An Interdisciplinary Journal for the Social Study of Health, Illness and Medicine*, 14(4): 415–433, 2010.

to teach clients to ask similar questions so that they can decide about integrative therapy and sort out the often conflicting advice of family, friends, conventional health-care professionals, integrative healers, and the media.

Many clients use integrative healing modalities without ever talking to a conventional health professional about them. They may fear a negative reaction. Others are not aware of the potential harm that may occur, especially when they combine integrative therapies or alternative and conventional therapies. Some may consider the scientific evidence and conclude that most noninvasive and nondrug alternative therapies are harmless. Others may mistakenly assume that integrative therapies are regulated by the government and would not be available if they were dangerous.

Find Information

Lack of scientific information about integrative healing modalities is of concern to integrative healers, conventional health-care professionals, and clients. For nurses and their clients, the need to know where and how to find up-to-date, reliable information on integrative therapies is a must. (Go to any of the sites listed below for more information.)

Information Resources

- Association of Integrative Medicine (AAIM): 877-718-3052 or http://www.aaimedicine.com/contact/

- International College of Integrative Medicine (ICIM): 419-358-0273 or http://www.icimed.com/
- NCCAM offers one of the best general governmental resources for information on alternative modalities at the NCCAM website: http://www.nccam.nih.gov.
- Several authoritative sources on herbal medicines are available for practitioners and clients, such as http://www.nlm.nih.gov/medlineplus/herbalmedicine.html

The FDA maintains a site for reporting and obtaining information about adverse effects and interactions of herbals through MedWatch (800-FDA-1088 or http://www.fda.gov/medwatch).

- F. A. Davis Publishing Company maintains a website on herbal medicines (http://www.DrugGuide.com), as does the U.S. Pharmacopeia (http://www.usp.org/information/index.html).
- The American Botanical Society (800-313-7105) has a website (http://www.herbalgram.org) and publishes the *Herbalgram,* a newsletter on herbal medications.
- MICROMEDEX has an evidence-based series on herbal medicines and dietary supplements, toxicologies, clinical protocols, and client education (800-643-8116 or http://www.micromedex.com). It also links to the electronic database of herbal medicines from the Royal Pharmaceutical Society of Great Britain.
- Tyler's *The Honest Herbal* is one of the most reputable guides for the use of herbs.[6]
- *The Physicians' Desk Reference for Herbal Medicine* contains scientific findings on the efficacy, potential interactions, clinical trials, and case reports of herbs, as well as indexes on Asian, Ayurvedic, and homeopathic herbs.[7]

The Internet has become a primary source of information for both the public and health-care providers about integrative products and local practitioners of integrative therapies. Because information posted to the Internet is not regulated, this avenue of inquiry requires caution. One the earliest and still most useful websites providing reputable information about ACH and specific modalities is http://www.quackwatch.com. There are also several governmental watch sites that can be accessed for information about integrative therapies.

- Quackwatch (http://www.quackwatch.org) offers fact sheets and reviews of specific alternative modalities, as well as those associated with certain illnesses. It also has sections on how to determine whether a website devoted to alternative modalities is trustworthy.

Ask the Client

It is important to ask clients about their use of integrative therapies. Not doing so may place them at risk for adverse health outcomes. When and how to assess for the use of ACH during the client assessment process is a matter of judgment and should be guided by the nurse's knowledge of individual clients. An appropriate time is often after the chief complaint has been documented because this is when questions are asked about the clients' reasons for seeking health care and what they have already done for their problem.

What Do You Think?

Does the facility where you do your clinical practice ask about alternative therapies during the admission assessment? Are you taught to assess for this information in your nursing program?

Discuss the use of integrative therapies tactfully and supportively. Keep complete and accurate documentation of all interactions with clients about integrative therapies and healers. And as much as possible, help direct clients toward the safest therapies and the most qualified practitioners.

Conclusion

Integrative, alternative, and nontraditional health-care practices are a growing part of health care in the United States. It is essential that nurses become aware of what these practices entail and how they may affect or interact with conventional therapies that the client is already receiving. When clients enter the health-care system for whatever reason, admission assessments for these practices should become a routine part of client evaluation. Nurses traditionally have approached health care from a holistic viewpoint that addresses all of the client's needs—mind, body, and spirit. As health care moves more toward integrative practices, nurses are the logical choice to coordinate a comprehensive approach to health care that includes both traditional and alternative practices. Combining these efforts will bind together the fragmented health-care system.

Critical-Thinking Exercises

- Contact three of the websites on alternative practices listed in this chapter. Evaluate them according to their quality, content, and usefulness to your practice.
- Identify a nurse practitioner, physician, or other health-care provider in your area who uses integrative practices. Interview that person and arrange for a presentation to the class about alternative health-care practices.
- Select a client from your clinical experiences who is having pain. How might alternative practices help this client? Develop a care plan using both traditional and alternative methods for pain control.
- Identify and discuss three advantages of and three problems with integrative health-care practices.
- Select three nursing theories from Chapter 3 that use a holistic approach to nursing. Identify how and what alternative practices would work well with each one of these theories.
- Have a class debate about the pros and cons of the use of medical cannabis.

GLOSSARY OF INTEGRATIVE HEALING TERMS

Inclusion of particular ideas or practices in this glossary does not imply endorsement of them. Healthcare practitioners and their clients must carefully evaluate the claims and qualifications of integrative healing practices and practitioners before coming to conclusions about them.

Acupressure Use of fingers or hands to apply pressure over acupuncture points on meridians to restore or enhance the flow of chi. Believed to maintain or restore energy balance. From traditional Chinese medicine.

Acupressure massage Use of massage techniques such as rubbing, kneading, percussion, and vibration over acupuncture points to improve circulation of chi.

Acupuncture Insertion of needles along meridian channels to alleviate blockage of chi and reestablish the balance of energy in the body. The insertion points are believed to be linked to specific internal organs. Originating in traditional Chinese medicine, acupuncture is now commonly considered a complete treatment system on its own.

Alexander technique A technique developed by Frederick Matthias Alexander that realigns body posture through imaging and relaxation. Decreases muscle tension and fatigue, stress, and back and neck pain. Based on the belief that poor posture during daily activities contributes to physical and emotional problems.

Allopathic medicine A synonym for conventional medicine. Practitioner uses medicines to counteract symptoms or heal by producing different effects or a second condition different from the one being treated. From the Greek words *allos* (other) and *pathos* (suffering).

Applied kinesiology Study of muscle activity, strength, and health effects through the muscle-gland-organ link. Muscle dysfunction may be counteracted by nutrition, manual procedures (e.g., massage), pressure over muscle attachment points, and realignment.

Aromatherapy A type of herbal therapy that uses the odors of essential oils extracted from plants to treat various conditions, such as headaches, tension, and anxiety. Chemical composition of the oils produces pharmacological effects that include antibacterial, antiviral, antispasmodic, diuretic, vasodilative, and mood-harmonizing actions. The oils may be applied by massage, inhaled, placed in baths and other forms of hydrotherapy, or taken internally.

Art therapy Use of artistic self-expression through drawing, sculpture, and painting to diagnose and treat behavioral or emotional problems.

Aura Magnetic field thought to surround every person, plant, and animal. Adjustment of the field is believed to affect health, emotions, spirit, and mind.

Auriculotherapy A method developed in France in which points on the external ear are stimulated with acupuncture needles, massage, electronics, or infrared treatment. These points are believed to have neurological connections to other body areas. Also called *ear acupuncture*.

Ayurvedic medicine A personalistic, holistic, and naturalistic approach to health maintenance and treatment of illness, originating in India. Maintains balance of the three doshas (bioenergies) of the body through diet and herbs, meditation, breathing exercises (pranayama), massage with medicated oils, yoga and other forms of vigorous exercise, and exposure to the sun for higher consciousness.

Bach flower essences Homeopathic preparations of oil concentrates extracted from flowers. Originated by Edward Bach, an English physician, this method is aimed at emotional states rather than the signs and symptoms of physical illness. Specific concentrates or combinations of concentrates are associated with various emotional states. Each client is diagnosed individually because there is no corresponding psychological equivalent for every physical state.

Biofeedback Form of training that helps a person to consciously control or change normally unconscious body functions to improve overall health. Also refers to the method of immediately reporting back information to the client about a biological process being measured so the person can consciously alter or influence the process.

Bodywork General term used to describe various forms of massage therapy, energy balancing, deep-tissue manipulation, and movement awareness.

Botanical medicine Use of an entire plant or herb for treating illness or maintaining health.

Chakras Circles found along the midline of the body, in alignment with the spinal cord, that distribute energy throughout the body. If they are blocked, energy flow is inhibited.

Chelation therapy Use of minerals combined with amino acids, given intravenously or orally, to help cleanse the body of unnecessary or toxic minerals that block blood circulation. From the Greek word *chele* (to bind or to claw).

Chi (qi, shi) From traditional Chinese medicine. Chi is the invisible life force that circulates through the body along meridians, or channels. Maintaining or restoring the flow of chi restores and promotes health.

Chiropractic A Western medical system postulating that partial joint dislocations (subluxations) cause the body to be misaligned. Removal or adjustment of subluxations balances the spinal–nervous system and restores and maintains health.

Craniosacral therapy Manipulation of the bones of the skull to treat craniosacral dysfunctions caused by restriction in the flow of cerebrospinal fluid and misalignment of bones. *Cranio* refers to the cranium and *sacral* to the sacrum.

Crystal therapy Use of quartz and other gemstones, believed to emit electromagnetic energy. Frequently used with light and color therapy. Also called *gem therapy*.

Cupping From traditional Chinese and Ayurvedic medicines. Method using a heated cup placed over the skin to draw out impurities, decrease blood pressure, increase circulation, and relieve muscle pain.

Curanderismo Healing tradition, found in Mexican American communities, based in concepts of supernaturalism, balance, and holism. From the Spanish verb *to heal*.

Dance therapy Use of dance movement to enhance wellness and aid healing. Sharpens levels of awareness, enhances self-confidence, helps with motor coordination and physical skills, and assists with communication, especially with severely disturbed psychiatric clients.

Doshas Three basic metabolic types (*vata, pitta,* and *kapha*), life forces, or bioenergies in Ayurvedic medicine. Each has certain characteristics and tendencies that combine to determine a person's constitution. When they are in balance, mind and body are coordinated, resulting in vibrant health and energy. When they are out of balance, the body is susceptible to outside stressors, such as microorganisms, poor nutrition, and work overload.

Energy medicine Measurement of electromagnetic frequencies emitted by the body. The object is to diagnose energy imbalances that may cause or contribute to present or future illnesses and to use electromagnetic forces to counteract imbalances and restore the body's energy balance.

Environmental medicine Method that explores the role of environmental and dietary allergens in health and illness.

Feldenkrais method A type of bodywork or physical movement developed by Moshe Feldenkrais that stresses awareness through movement and helps the body work with gravity. Incorporates imaging, active moving, and forms of directed attention designed to re-educate the nervous system, teach subjects how to learn from their own kinesic feedback, and avoid movements that strain joints and muscles.

Gerson therapy Metabolic therapy developed by Max Gerson, a German physician. It is based on the belief that cancer results from metabolic dysfunctions in cells that can be countered by detoxification, a vegetarian diet, coffee enemas to stimulate excretion of liver bile, the exclusion of sodium, and an abundance of potassium.

Guided imagery A facilitated flow of thoughts that helps a person see, feel, taste, smell, hear, or touch something in the imagination. The power of the mind or imagination is used to stimulate positive physical responses and provide insight into health and an understanding of emotions as a cause of ill health.

Healing touch Healing tradition based on the belief in a universal energy system. Humans are seen as interpenetrating layers of energy systems just above and outside the body that are integrated with energy fields in the environment. Manipulation of such energy fields through touch can help restore a person's energy balance and health.

Hellerwork A type of bodywork developed by Joseph Heller as an outgrowth of Rolfing. It combines dialogue, body movement education, and deep touch to achieve greater mind–body awareness and structural body alignment with gravitational forces. Therapy is individualized to different body types.

Herbal medicine Use of the chemical makeup of herbs in much the same way as conventional medicine uses pharmaceuticals. The most ancient known form of health care, herbal medicine is basic to traditional Chinese, Ayurvedic, and Native American medical systems. Also called *botanical medicine, phytotherapy,* and *phytomedicine.*

Homeopathy A Western medical system based on the principle that "like cures like." Natural substances are prescribed in minute dilutions to cause the symptoms of the disease they are intended to cure, helping the body cure itself.

Humor therapy Deliberate use of laughter to improve quality of life by encouraging relaxation and stress reduction, distracting individuals from awareness of constant pain, and providing symptom relief.

Hydrotherapy Use of hot, cold, or contrasting water temperatures to maintain or restore health. Water, steam, or ice may be used in combination with baths, compresses, hot and cold packs, showers, and enemas or colonic irrigations. Minerals, herbs, and oils may be added to enhance the therapeutic effects. Also known as *water cure.*

Hypnotherapy Use of hypnosis, power of suggestion, and trancelike states to access the deepest levels of the mind. Used to bring about changes in behavior, treat health conditions, and manage medical and psychological problems.

Integrative medicine The practice of conventional health-care professionals who prescribe a combination of therapies from both systems. For more information, contact the American Association of Integrative Medicine (AAIM) at 877-718-3052 or http://www.aaimedicine.com/contact/.

Iridology Iris diagnosis. In this belief system, each area of the body has a corresponding point on the iris of the eye. Thus, the state of health (balance) or disease (imbalance) can be diagnosed from the color, texture, or location of pigments in the eye.

Jin Shin Jyutsu A Japanese form of massage in which combinations of healing points on the body are held for a minute or more with the fingertips. The purpose is to enhance or restore the flow of chi.

Light and color therapy A method by which light is converted into electrical impulses, travels along the optic nerve to the brain, and stimulates the hypothalamus to send neurotransmitters to regulate the autonomic nervous system. Various colors of light are believed to stimulate different parts of the body.

Magnet therapy A type of electromagnetic therapy or energy medicine in which magnets are used to stimulate circulation, increase oxygen to cells, and facilitate healing by correcting disturbed or malfunctioning electromagnetic frequencies that the body emits.

Mantra A type of sound therapy used in Ayurvedic medicine to reach a higher level of spiritual and mental functioning. It changes the "vibratory patterns of the mind" to release unconscious negative thoughts, psychological stress, and emotional distress. Often achieved by uttering a mystical word or phrase and associated with meditation.

Meditation Use of contemplation to exercise the mind. A form of mental cleansing that enhances self-awareness and awareness of one's environment. Also called *mind-cure,* this is an unseen force of healing. Thoughts and deep feelings are considered the primary arbiters of health through relaxation.

Megavitamin therapy A type of orthomolecular medicine in which diseases are prevented and cured by large doses of vitamins and other supplements. Dosages exceed the normal or recommended amounts needed for general good health or prevention of deficiencies. The disease to be treated or prevented determines the type, dosage, and mode of administration of vitamins, minerals, and nutrient supplements.

Meridians Invisible channels by which chi flows through the body. Blockage along a meridian causes illness. From traditional Chinese medicine.

Mind–body medicine Healing based on the interconnectedness of the mind and body, individual responsibility for self-care, and the self-healing capabilities of the body. Uses a wide range of modalities, such as imaging, massage, hypnotherapy, meditation, yoga, concepts of balance, herbs, and diet.

Moxibustion From traditional Chinese medicine, burning of *moxa* (dried or powered herbs) on or close to acupuncture points on the meridians to restore or improve the flow of chi.

Music therapy Use of music to enhance well-being and promote healing. Helps improve physical and mental functioning, alleviate pain, ease the psychological discomfort of illness, and improve quality of life, especially for terminally ill persons. Aids ability of the mentally handicapped, autistic persons, and elderly persons with dementia to interact with others, learn, and relate to their environments.

Naturopathy A Western healing system that uses safe, natural therapies. Promotes holism and use of natural substances, treats cause rather than effect (symptoms), empowers and motivates individuals to take responsibility for their own health, prevents disease through lifestyle and education, and does no harm.

Neurolinguistic programming A system that focuses on how individuals learn, communicate, and change. *Neuro-* refers to the way the brain works and the consistent and observable patterns that emanate from human thinking. *Linguistic* refers to the expression (verbal and nonverbal) of those patterns of thinking. *Programming* refers to the ways such patterns of thinking are interpreted and how they can be changed. Changing the patterns gives people the ability to make better choices for healthy behavior.

Orthodox medicine A synonym for conventional, Western, scientific, biomedicine, or official healthcare system.

Orthomolecular medicine A system that treats physiological and psychological disorders by reestablishing, normalizing, or creating the optimal nutritional balance in the body. Vitamins, minerals, amino acids, and other types of nutritional substances are administered. (*Ortho-* means "normal" or "correct.")

Osteopathy A Western system of medicine that considers the structural integrity of the body the most important factor in maintaining and restoring the person to health. The structural integrity or balance of the musculoskeletal system is maintained through physical therapy, joint manipulation, and postural reeducation.

Oxygen therapy Use of various forms of oxygen to destroy pathogens and promote body healing. Includes hyperbaric, ozone, and hydrogen peroxide therapies.

Pharmacognosy Scientific study of the chemical properties of plants and natural products. A goal is to standardize herbal products to make sure they are free of harmful components and contain the identical amount of active ingredients.

Phytomedicine/phytotherapy A branch of botanical medicine, especially prominent in Europe, that includes the pharmaceutical study and therapeutic use of herbs, herbal derivatives, and herbal synthetics. Merges ancient herbal traditions with contemporary scientific investigation to standardize the active ingredients of herbal products.

Polarity therapy A combination of bodywork and other hands-on techniques to restore the natural flow of energy through the body. Other therapies may include reflexology, hydrotherapy, and breathing techniques.

Prana Vital energy or life force that runs through the body. From Ayurvedic medicine.

Qi Gong (chi kung, chi gong) Technique from traditional Chinese medicine that combines movement, meditation and deep relaxation, and regulation of breathing. Enhanced flow of chi throughout the body nourishes vital organs.

Reflexology Pressure applied to the hands or feet to unblock nerve impulses. In this belief system, every part of the body has a corresponding area on the hands and feet. Thus, body parts can be stimulated by pressure applied to the appropriate sites. Reflexology is used to relieve tension, improve circulation, promote relaxation, and restore energy balance.

Reiki An ancient Buddhist version of healing touch practiced in Tibet and Japan. The word also means *universal life force.* Energy is transferred to the person through the hands of the healer to restore energy balance in the body.

Relaxation response Physiological mechanism described by Herbert Benson in which body stress is reduced through regulation of internal activity, such as reduced metabolism and slowing of other physiological reactions.

Relaxation therapy Use of the relaxation response to reduce stress through release of physical and emotional tension. Various therapies are commonly included in other types of therapeutic programs. Examples are mind–body therapies such as biofeedback, hydrotherapy, imaging and visualization, meditation, Qi Gong, tai chi, and yoga.

Rolfing Technique of deep massage developed by Ida Rolf. Use of the knuckles is meant to counteract the effects of gravity on body balance. Fascia, connective tissue, and muscle are loosened and lengthened to help them return to their correct positions.

Rosen technique A type of bodywork in which muscle tension is seen as repressed emotional conflicts. Deep and gentle pressure is applied as persons are questioned about what they are experiencing.

Shamanism Ancient healing approach found in most cultural systems. Shamans communicate with the spirit world through trances and other altered states of consciousness. They attempt to control spirits and effect change in the physical world. The belief is that the soul of the shaman separates from the body and explores the cosmos in search of cures for ill clients.

Shiatsu Japanese form of massage, literally meaning *finger pressure*. Consists of firm pressure in a sequential and rhythmic manner. Pressure is exerted for 3 to 10 seconds on points along the body that correspond to acupuncture meridians. It is designed to "awaken the meridian."

Sound therapy Use of sound to affect different parts of the brain, regulate corticosteroid hormone levels, and affect the body's own rhythmic patterns.

Spiritual healing Cosmic healing energy transferred or channeled from practitioner to client through laying on of the hands.

Swedish massage The most common form of massage, focusing on superficial muscle layers. Practitioner uses kneading, friction, and long, gliding strokes to relieve muscle tension and promote relaxation.

Tai chi From traditional Chinese medicine. Derived from Qi Gong but practiced at a much slower pace. Also one of the body–mind therapies. Combines contemplation (meditation) with movement or "moving meditation" and coordinated breathing.

Therapeutic massage Manipulation of soft tissues through a variety of techniques to affect the circulatory, lymphatic, and nervous systems.

Therapeutic touch A healing touch modality that does not involve actual touching of the client's body. The therapist's hands are used to sense and interact with the client's energy field to redirect it, alleviate energy blockage, and restore balance.

Traditional Chinese medicine A complete system of healing based on the concept of the uninterrupted flow of chi, or vital essence, and the concept of balance (yin and yang), representing corresponding and interrelated elements in the internal world of the body and the external world. All illness is attributed ultimately to a disturbance of chi.

Trager therapy A method of bodywork, developed by Milton Trager, meant to develop the ability to move more effortlessly. Use of gentle, rhythmic touch and movement exercises to assist in the release of accumulated tensions. Uses sensory-motor feedback or mental gymnastics (mentastics) to learn how the body moves.

Vibration medicine Healing systems that treat the body on an energy level. Cure is effected by ingestion of substances that adjust energy or rate of energy field vibration. Homeopathy is an example.

Visualization Also called *guided imagery, centering, focusing, meditation,* or *distraction.* Use of the imagination or power of the mind to get in touch with one's inner self. Involves all, several, or one of the senses to bridge the mind, body, and spirit.

Yin/yang Complementary but opposing phenomena or correspondents in Taoist philosophical thought that form the underpinning of traditional Chinese medicine. Yin and yang represent the interdependence of all elements of nature and body and mind. Yin represents the female force and passive, still, reflective aspects. Yang represents the male force and active, warm, moving aspects. For health to be maintained and wellness achieved, yin and yang must be in balance.

Yoga Literally meaning *union,* or the integration of mental, physical, and spiritual energies. Part of Ayurvedic medicine. The integration is accomplished through exercise in the form of assuming different body postures, meditating, and breathing.

References

1. Daniel R, Morris D, Jobst KA. Distinguishing between complementary and alternative medicine and integrative medicine delivery: The United Kingdom joins world leaders in professional integrative medicine education. *Journal of Alternative & Complementary Medicine,* 17(6):483–485, 2011.

2. WHO launches the first global strategy on traditional and alternative medicine, 2012. Retrieved April 2013 from http://www.who.int/mediacentre/news/releases/release38/en/

3. What is integrative medicine? Whole Person Health, 2012. Retrieved April 2013 from http://www.wholepersonhealth.com/what-is-integrative-medicine/

4. What is complementary and alternative medicine? NCCAM Publication No. D347 2010. Retrieved April 2013 from http://nccam.nih.gov

5. The use of complementary and alternative medicine in the United States: Cost data, NCCAM. Retrieved April 2013 from http://nccam.nih.gov/news/camstats/costs/costdatafs.htm

6. Acupuncture in the treatment of obesity: A narrative review of the literature. *Acupuncture in Medicine,* 31(1):88-97, 2013.

7. Lemley B. What is integrative medicine? 2013. Retrieved April 2013 from http://www.drweil.com/drw/u/ART02054/Andrew-Weil-Integrative-Medicine.html

8. Foster S, Tyler VM. *Tyler's Honest Herbal: A Sensible Guide to the Use of Herbs and Related Remedies* (5th ed.). Binghamton, NY: Haworth Herbal Press, 2010.

9. Medical Economics Staff. *Physicians' Desk Reference for Herbal Medicines* (4th ed.). New York: Thomson Health Care, 2012. Retrieved from http://www.clinicalkey.com/?campid=2012_10222&utm_campaign=ck_google_adwords_launch&mm=bolandj&reg=na&prod=ck_individual&aud=phy&utm_medium=paid_search&utm_source=google&utm_content=medical_ref_md&utm_term=%2Bphysician%20%2Bdesk%20%2Breference

26 Preparing for Functioning Effectively in a Disaster

Joseph T. Catalano

Learning Objectives

After completing this chapter, the reader will be able to:

- Discuss the nurse's role in preparing for bioterrorism events and disasters
- Distinguish the phases of a disaster
- Identify resources that nurses can use during a disaster
- Identify the main agents used in a bioterrorism attack
- List and discuss the key elements in preparing for a disaster
- Explain the differences in the mechanisms of action of the three types of chemical agents
- Name and explain the three key factors for effective treatment of chemical injuries
- Distinguish between the different classes of protective wear for chemical or biological contamination

DISASTERS ON THE INCREASE

The United States has witnessed an increase in natural and terrorism-related disasters during the past decade. The vast majority of disasters are still considered natural. These range from the catastrophic failure of man-made structures, such as building collapses, to weather-related catastrophes, such as tornadoes, hurricanes, and floods. Most credible scientists believe that because of the significant climate change that is taking place, natural disasters will become more frequent and more destructive for decades to come. They point to hurricanes and superstorms such as Hurricanes Katrina and Sandy that devastated major metropolitan areas and caused billions of dollars in damage.

They also look at tornado events that took place in Joplin, Missouri; Moore, Oklahoma; and El Reno, Oklahoma. Tornadoes in the United States and Canada are rated on a scale from 0 to 5, based on the amount of damage they produce, with 5 causing catastrophic damage. This scale was initially developed by Dr. Tetsuya Fujita in 1971 (the Fujita scale) and then revised in 2007 and is now named the Enhanced Fujita (EF) scale. An EF-5 tornado is the most powerful windstorm on earth with winds in the range of 200 to 300 miles per hour or more with the ability to uproot large trees, vacuum up pavement, completely demolish a well-built house, and remove it from its foundation. A portable Doppler radar truck monitoring the May 5, 2003, Oklahoma City tornado clocked the fastest winds ever recorded on earth at 319 miles per hour. In the past, EF-5 tornadoes were very rare, with one occurring only once a year or about one out of every 1,000 tornadoes that occur every year in the United States. The Moore and El Reno tornadoes were both rated EF-5 and occurred within weeks of each other. The El Reno tornado was the largest tornado on record, measuring almost 3 miles wide. Just 4 months later, an EF-4 tornado struck Washington, Illinois, killing eight people and removing the town from the map.

Disaster Defined

Simply defined, a disaster is a catastrophic event that leads to major property damage, a large number of injuries, displaced individuals, or major loss of life. The American Red Cross defines a disaster as "an occurrence such as a hurricane, tornado, storm, flood, high water, wind-driven water, tidal wave, earthquake, drought, blizzard, pestilence, famine, fire, explosion, building collapse, commercial transportation wreck, or other situations that cause human suffering or create human needs that the victims cannot alleviate without substantial assistance."[1]

Personal and Family Preparation for a Disaster

It is virtually impossible to make preparations to *avoid* disasters caused by acts of terrorism and catastrophic human engineering failures. Most natural disasters, except for earthquakes and volcano eruptions, have a warning period ranging from a few minutes to several hours. However, the aftermath of all disasters is very similar and preparations can be made to deal with those circumstances. Relief and rescue workers generally arrive quickly after a disaster, but they cannot take care of all the injured or trapped at the same time. During the time between the occurrence of the disaster and the rescue, individuals are left to their own devices and resourcefulness for their survival.

Extreme disaster preparedness is seen in those who are known as *doomsday preppers* or just *preppers*. They usually build large, elaborate underground structures costing anywhere from a few hundred thousand dollars to several million dollars. Preppers often make sure to have enough food, water, and other supplies to last up to 6 months without any contact with the outside world. They often have elaborate electrical generators and air-filtration devices to keep out unwanted viruses and toxins. Preppers also are generally armed to the teeth with a variety of powerful military-grade weapons to keep out individuals or groups who are seeking shelter in the preppers'

subterranean enclaves. However, even these strongly built structures can be destroyed by natural events such as earthquakes and floods or man-made devices such as large bombs.

Most U.S. citizens cannot afford or do not even want this type of extreme disaster protection. So what can they do when they are faced with an impending disaster? There are a number of relatively straightforward measures that can be taken when coping with a disaster and its aftermath. These can be modified to some degree to accommodate the most common types of disasters that are likely to be encountered in their areas. For example, an underground storm shelter is great protection from an approaching tornado but would not be appropriate in a coastal area where an approaching hurricane usually causes a great deal of flooding.

As health-care providers, nurses need to make the same basic emergency preparations as the general public to ensure their safety during the emergency so that they can effectively aid those injured during the disaster. An injured health-care provider is just another victim who needs care.

The Federal Emergency Management Agency (FEMA), in conjunction with the Red Cross, recommend the following four steps in preparing for a disaster:

> *Most credible scientists believe that because of the significant climate change that is taking place, natural disasters will become more frequent and more destructive for decades to come.*

1. Get informed
2. Make a plan
3. Assemble a kit
4. Update the plan and the kit[2]

Get Informed

Knowledge is the best preparation for any kind of disaster. Before a plan can be formulated, a sufficient amount of information must be gathered about potential dangers and ways to deal with them. The local emergency management office or local American Red Cross chapter is a good place to start the search for information. Some areas are more likely to experience certain types of disasters than others. Find out what disasters the community has experienced in the past. Is it on a fault line and likely to have earthquakes? Is it located in tornado alley? When was the last time a wildfire broke out? There may be some potential man-made hazards associated with the community. Does it have

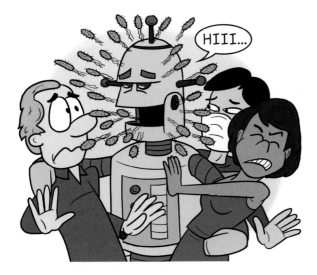

large fertilizer or fireworks plants that may explode? Is there a large oil or natural gas pipeline that runs under the town? How old is the freshwater dam that is located upstream from the community?

All communities should have a written disaster plan that provides information such as how local first responders are to organize rescue efforts, where community emergency shelters are located, and which roads are designated as evacuation routes. These plans will probably be located at the local Red Cross office or at firehouses. Ask for a copy of it. Other information that is valuable includes mass transportation plans. In the event that personal transportation is unavailable or has been destroyed, is public transportation or school buses available to evacuate people? Also find out what types of internal disaster plans schools, businesses, and hospitals have to protect the children, employees, and clients.[2]

All communities should have some type of early warning signals. These are usually sirens or horns, but it is important to learn beforehand what these sound like and know how much time there is between when the signals sound and the disaster hits. Most community disaster plans have some provision for how local authorities and rescuers will provide information to the public before, during, and after the disaster has occurred.

A commonly used method of notification is the National Oceanic and Atmospheric Administration (NOAA) weather radio system and the Emergency Alert System (EAS). Although emergency warnings can be broadcast over the network television system, purchasing an inexpensive NOAA alert radio can

provide warnings 24 hours a day (http://www.noaa.gov). The automatic alert system sends a signal that triggers the radio to turn on. The speakers and audible-visual alert screen automatically turns on to provide instant alerts of conditions that may affect life and property. These radios have Specific Area Message Encoding (SAME) technology, allowing the radio to be programmed to receive only information specific to a particular geographic area. Most TV stations and the Weather Channel have apps that can be downloaded to smartphones or tablets that will also provide instantaneous weather alert information.

Make a Plan

After gathering sufficient information, sit down with all family members and develop a plan for possible looming disasters. Key elements in all emergency disaster plans should include:

An "Out-of-Town" Contact Person. This would most likely be a friend or relative who lives a considerable distance from the community. If they live too close, they may be caught in the disaster too. The contact person's phone number needs to be programmed into all family members' cell phones or memorized by everyone. After a disaster has struck, family members should call this person and tell them where they are and what their condition is. Because of damage to the cell system itself or overload of the system by many callers after a disaster, it is often easier to reach someone on a long-distance call than a family member who may be only a few blocks away.[3] Also, the phone's texting feature uses a different system than the voice phone, and it is often less problematic to get text messages through than a regular call.

A Preselected Meeting Place. Most of the time, disasters do not occur when everyone is together in one place. In the event of a larger disaster where family members are widely dispersed, such as at school and work, and the disaster prevents a return home because of its destruction or debris-blocked streets, select a location for everyone to meet at that is centrally located and likely to survive the disaster.[2]

A Family Communication Plan. All contact information for all family members, at any time, should be easily accessible. This includes work and school phone numbers. Other useful numbers can include National Poison Control Center (1-800-222-1222), local hospitals, and close relatives. These numbers can be programmed into phones or, in case of damage or loss of the phone, listed on a card or a form that should be carried at all times by all family members. A sample of this type of form can be found at http://www.ready.gov or at http://www.redcross.org/contactcard. These websites also provide blank wallet cards on which contact information can be recorded and carried in a wallet, purse, backpack, and so on, for quick reference.[4] It is probably a good idea to get this laminated to make them more durable and able to survive even if they get wet. Children must be taught how to call the emergency phone numbers and in what situation it is appropriate to do so. Also post a copy of the communication plan near each landline house phone, if these are still being used.

Escape Routes and Safe Places. Draw a floor plan of the house that shows all the rooms and the location of stairways, doors, and windows that lead outside. The locations of the utility shut-off points, particularly gas and electricity, should also be shown. There should be at least two ways to exit each room, such as a door and a window or two doors.[2] Everyone in the family should know the best escape routes out of the house and where the safe places are in the house for each possible type of disaster (i.e., if a tornado approaches, go to the storm shelter or basement or the lowest floor of the home or an interior room or closet with no windows). It is recommended that emergency evacuation drills be conducted at least two times a year and whenever any changes are made in the escape plan.

> *Because of damage to the cell system itself or overload of the system by many callers after a disaster, it is often easier to reach someone on a long-distance call than a family member who may be only a few blocks away.*

A Special Plan for Disabled Family Members. Items necessary for mobility such as walkers, crutches, and canes should be kept in the same place all the time so they are easy to get to quickly. For bed-bound individuals who have caregivers, the caregivers need an alternate plan if no one else is at home. Power companies should be notified if the disabled person is dependent on some life-support technology such as a ventilator.[3] Most of these devices have some type of battery backup system for short-term power outages, but there should be a plan for an alternate power source for long-term outages. It may require moving the person to another location. Also have a several-day supply of important medications and other routinely used care items set aside that can be taken with the client.

A Plan for Pets. Pets can create considerable problems for rescue workers. Some people refuse to leave their pets when they are asked to evacuate and other times pets become protective of their injured owners and will not allow rescue workers to approach them, especially large dogs. If forced to evacuate, take the pet along if at all possible. Some individuals have many pets and taking all of them may not be possible. In the past, emergency shelters did not allow any animals other than service animals because of hygiene issues.[2] However, with the many disasters that have occurred in recent years, these rules have been relaxed to some degree. Some shelters are divided into no pets and pets sections. Identify boarding facilities, veterinarians, and "pet-friendly" hotels that would be willing to accept pets when a disaster occurs.

Actions to Take Before a Disaster
Check Key Utilities Locations. Learn how to turn off water, gas, and electricity at the main switches or valves. Show all family members where they are and how to do it. If special wrenches or tools are required, buy a spare one and keep it near the valve or shutoff.[4]

Check Insurance Coverage. Most people tend to automatically renew their homeowners coverage each year when they receive the renewal notification. It is a good idea to sit down with an insurance agent every 1 to 2 years and discuss what is actually covered in the policy. The worst time to find out that a bargain basement online insurance policy does not cover roof or siding damage is after a wind or hailstorm. Homeowners insurance does not cover flood damage. Special flood insurance is available from the U.S. government.[2] Most home insurance does not routinely cover earthquakes either. Special additional coverage must be purchased.

Take a First Aid/CPR and Automated External Defibrillation (AED) Class. Contact the local American Red Cross chapter to find out when they are offering classes. The American Heart Association also provides CPR classes and can be contacted for locations and times of classes. Most hospitals hold classes also, generally for their employees, but they will often allow community members to attend.

Take an Inventory of All Home Possessions. In the past, this type of inventory required several written pages of information.[2] With the advent of phones and other digital devices with built-in cameras, it now is easy to do. Make a movie of the house inside and out, with particular focus on high-dollar items like the 70-inch LED smart-TV and computer equipment. Because the device also records audio, comments such as when it was purchased and particular additional features such as 3-D would be helpful in establishing its value.

Some polices have a "total replacement value" clause that will replace the item with a new one just like it no matter how old it is. These policies are more expensive, obviously. Most homeowner policies prorate the value of the item on its age. For example, if the computer cost $3,000 five years ago, it may be worth only $1,500 today. The $1,500 is all that the insurance company will reimburse the homeowner for this item. Also, make a movie of outbuildings, cars, boats, and recreational vehicles. Obtain professional appraisals of jewelry, collectibles, artwork, or other items that may be difficult to evaluate. Make copies of receipts and canceled checks showing the cost for valuable items. Store this information in a place safe from flood, fire, or other disasters. Paper documents need to be in a safe-deposit box at a local bank. Electronic data can be stored on a flash drive or disk that also can be kept at the bank. In addition, electronic data can be stored at off-site electronic data storage facilities or even in the cloud.

> *The worst time to find out that a bargain basement online insurance policy does not cover roof or siding damage is after a wind or hailstorm.*

Protect Important Records and Documents. These important documents include photocopies of all credit cards, home titles, birth and marriage certificates, Social Security cards, passports, wills, deeds, and financial information such a checking account numbers, insurance policies, and immunizations records. Ideally these should also be in a safe-deposit box, but fire- and water-proof home safes and strongboxes can provide adequate protection and are more convenient to access.

Assemble a Kit

A disaster supplies kit is a collection of basic items a family would probably need to stay safe and be more comfortable during and after a disaster.[3] Store these items in plastic or metal portable containers and keep as close as possible to the exit door or in a secure place such as a storm shelter. At least once a year, the kit should be opened and all items checked. Family members' needs may have changed and certain items will exceed their expiration date. Smaller emergency kits can be kept in each vehicle and at work.

A well-stocked disaster supply kit should include the following:

- Three-day supply of boxed and canned ready-to-eat nonperishable food
- A hand can opener, knives, and other eating utensils (can be plastic)
- Three-day supply of water (1 gallon of water per person, per day)
- Portable, battery-powered radio, citizen band radio, or small television with extra batteries
- Flashlight, portable LED lantern with many extra batteries
- Well-stocked first aid kit with sufficient supplies to stop major bleeding injuries
- Sanitation and hygiene items (hand sanitizer, moist towelettes, and toilet paper)
  - Matches or a lighter in waterproof containers
  - Whistle, horn, or some other type of device that can be used for signaling if trapped
- Extra sturdy clothing and warm blankets
- Photocopies of identification and credit cards
- Cash (several hundred dollars if possible) and coins
- Special needs items such as prescription medications, eyeglasses, contact lens solution, and hearing aid batteries
- If applicable, items for infants, such as formula, diapers, bottles, and pacifiers
- Basic tools (hammer, large pliers, screwdrivers, small pry bar), if applicable, pet supplies
- Jacket or coat
- Long pants and long-sleeve shirt
- Sturdy shoes and socks
- Sleeping bag or warm blanket[2]

Update the Plan and the Kit

Ideally, the plan should be reevaluated every 6 months. Ask family members about it and get their input. Check and replace food supplies that have expired and replace drinking water every 6 months.[4]

Issues in Practice

The 10 Commandments of Disaster Preparedness

Nurses and the general public should take the following preparation steps well before a disaster strikes:

1. Discuss the type of hazards that could affect your family. Know your home's vulnerability to storm surge, flooding, and high wind.
2. Locate a safe room or the safest areas in your home for high wind hazard. In certain circumstances, the safest areas may not be your home but within your community.
3. Determine escape routes from your home and places to meet.
4. Designate an out-of-state friend as a single point of contact for all your family members.
5. Make a plan now for what to do with your pets if you need to evacuate.
6. Post emergency telephone numbers by your phones and make sure your children know how and when to call 911.
7. Check your insurance coverage—flood damage is not usually covered by homeowners' insurance.
8. Stock nonperishable emergency supplies and a disaster supply kit.
9. Purchase and know how to use an NOAA weather radio. Remember to replace its battery every 6 months.
10. Take first aid, cardiopulmonary resuscitation (CPR), and disaster preparedness classes.

Sources: Goodhue CJ, Burke RV, Chambers S, Ferrer RR, Upperman JS. Disaster Olympix: A unique nursing emergency preparedness exercise. *Journal of Trauma Nursing,* 17(1):5–10, 2010; James JJ, Benjamin GC, Burkle FM, Gebbie KM, Kelen G, Subbarao I. Disaster medicine and public health preparedness: A discipline for all health professionals. *Disaster Medicine & Public Health Preparedness,* 4(2):102–107, 2010.

When the Disaster Strikes

Even with all the above listed precautions and preparations in place, when a disaster strikes, it is going to be both physically and emotionally traumatic to the whole family. Keeping a cool head and knowing what to do will allow all involved to survive and make the best of a bad situation.

It is important to follow the instructions of the professional first responders who have trained and planned for a variety of disasters. If a radio or television is available, valuable information can be obtained concerning the location of emergency shelters, the estimated time for rescuers to respond, and the general condition of the surrounding community.

It is important to wear sturdy clothing such as jeans and particularly important to protect feet by wearing sturdy shoes or boots.[2] If attempting to evacuate an area, it is best to use only the travel routes specified by local authorities. Emergency routes are generally the first ones cleared after a disaster where alternate routes and "shortcuts" can be blocked by debris or water and are impassable or dangerous. If at home after a disaster, only use flashlights if it is dark. There may be undetectable gas leaks or other dangerous fumes that can be ignited by matches or candles. Also, keep at least one general purpose fire extinguisher in an easily accessible location.[5]

Downed high-voltage power lines pose a particularly lethal threat to those who are near them. Even if a downed power line is not sparking, it may still be live and stepping on it or driving over it is a potentially deadly mistake. If water is present near the power line, it, too, can become electrified and cause a fatal shock several feet from the actual power line. It's important to check on neighbors, especially those who are elderly or disabled.

Many people have purchased portable generators in recent years as a backup source of power after a disaster. These pose their own set of dangers. The biggest one is carbon monoxide poisoning.[3] Some people think that running the generator in an attached garage is safe because the fumes go out the big open door. This is false! They should only be run outside in a well-ventilated area. In addition, refueling a generator while it is still hot or while it is running can cause a serious fire. Electricity is dangerous and there is always the potential for electrical shock or fire if the wiring is not connected correctly.

There are many resources for dealing with all types of disasters. FEMA's Community and Family Preparedness Program and American Red Cross Community Disaster Education are available online. Almost every agency that deals with disasters has written information that is available.

Health-Care Professional and First Responder Preparation for a Disaster

The information above is general information that all citizens, including health-care providers and first responders, should know in preparing for a variety of disasters. However, by the very nature of their work, health-care providers and first responders require additional knowledge and preparation in dealing with disasters. People look to them for help during their time of need. Although some of the knowledge overlaps, a higher level of preparation is expected of professionals. The information below focuses on this knowledge.

Even if a downed power line is not sparking, it may still be live and stepping on it or driving over it is a potentially deadly mistake.

Disaster Phases

Although there is a considerable amount of overlap, all disasters can be divided into three basic phases: The preimpact phase, the impact phase, and the postimpact phase. Nurses should learn what they need to do to provide care in all of the disaster phases.

The Preimpact Phase

Certain types of natural disasters are preceded by a warning period. For a tornado, this may range from a few minutes to as much as an hour; for hurricanes, it may be as long as several days. During the warning stage, also called the preimpact phase, the focus is on preparation for the aftereffects of the event. This preparation is primarily at the local community level.[6]

Even before a catastrophic event is predicted, first responders and health-care professionals in disaster-prone regions practice with disaster drills. These drills provide valuable training in a low-stress environment and identify the types of resources that may be needed during a disaster. This type of training helps identify unique risk situations for the community and builds the skill and knowledge disaster responders must have to meet the needs of the population.

When the disaster becomes imminent and a warning is issued, preparations such as evacuations are put into operation by the local emergency response unit. Since Hurricane Katrina, FEMA, the Red Cross, and other government agencies have begun the practice of stockpiling essential supplies to be used after the disaster somewhere close to the disaster target area where they can be reached quickly and easily for distribution.

Communication Is Critical

One key element, brought to the forefront by recent disasters, is the ability of the various agencies involved to communicate with each other. The lack of the ability to communicate became painfully evident after the 9/11 disaster. Fire and rescue, first responders, law enforcement, public health, government agencies, and health-care services were using radios that all had different frequencies and were unable to exchange essential information with each other. Large sums of money were spent by the Bush administration to correct this problem so that victims could receive the best possible care. Proficient communication leads to a well-coordinated response. All agencies must have agreements in place and understand the role that each one is to play in the disaster. This preparation will eliminate the turf arguments sometimes seen among agencies.[7] In rural areas, agreements with nearby communities also become important for obtaining mutual aid.

The news media is playing an even larger part in disaster reporting; however, planning for the news media and the flow of information is often overlooked in disaster preparations. Nurses are likely to hear about a disaster from breaking news reports before they learn about it through official channels. One fear that can become real is group panic. Generally, all information released from a health-care facility should go through the public relations representative or the designated spokesperson for the facility. Before any information is released, it should be determined how the news will affect particular populations. Families of victims often cling to every word and may misinterpret what is being said.

> *Often in disaster situations, nurses function outside their usual practice setting and may assume a variety of roles in meeting the needs of the disaster victims. Nurses must be able to perform under stressful and sometimes physically dangerous conditions.*

Persons designated to speak for the health-care facility should have experience with public speaking and be able to convey the information clearly and in terms that the general public can understand. They should also be able to "think on their feet" when responding to questions. However, question-and-answer sessions should be severely limited, especially when national media are involved. Reporters ask the same questions over and over again even when there is no information about the subject.

When people are under stress or have high levels of anxiety, communication must be direct, honest, and to the point. Long technical explanations will only confuse the facts. The public should also be calmed by reassurances that everything possible is being done. Regular updates every 30 to 60 minutes, even if there is little new information, are helpful in reducing anxiety levels.

Who to Contact

The following agencies can help with planning during the preimpact phase:

- *Disaster Medical Assistance Team (DMAT):* A group of frontline medical personnel, including nurses, who provide health care after a disaster. These may include terrorist, natural, or environmental disasters.
- *Medical Reserve Corps:* Part of the USA Freedom Corps, which was developed in 2002 in response to Americans' desire to volunteer and serve their communities in the wake of the 9/11 terrorist attacks.
- *American Red Cross:* Registered nurses (RNs) can join their local Red Cross and receive specialized training in disaster and bioterrorism preparedness.
- *Commission Corps Readiness Force:* Deploys teams to respond to public health emergencies.[6]
- *National Disaster Medical System (NDMS):* Mobilizes comprehensive disaster relief and works closely with local fire, police, and emergency medical services. NDMS also uses volunteer disaster response teams called International Medical and Surgical Response Teams (IMSuRTs), of which nurses are an essential component. The IMSuRTs provide emergency medical services at any place in the world where there is a lack of resources.

The Impact Phase

When the actual disaster strikes, the impact phase begins. The goal during the impact phase is to respond to the disaster, activate the emergency response, and reduce the long-term effects of the disaster as much as possible.[8] Activation of the emergency response plans developed during the preimpact phase mobilizes all agencies involved. Because fire, rescue, and police are usually the first on the scene, they provide and establish the command post from which all other efforts will be coordinated. Their goal is to identify and remove victims from dangerous situations, deal with unstable structures, and provide first aid to those who have been injured.

Because of the recent heightened concern over acts of terrorism, law enforcement may initially take control of the disaster scene until it can be determined that the cause was not a criminal act such as a bombing. Even with natural disasters such as tornadoes or floods, law enforcement is often first on the scene and, by their training, tend to take over control. Nurses working in the early stages of disasters sometimes feel frustrated by law enforcement officers, who may limit their ability to provide care. It is important to remember that law enforcement is concerned with identifying a crime and preserving evidence that may be used later in criminal prosecutions. The whole disaster area is considered a crime scene until released by law enforcement.

The Incident Management System (IMS) is an effective tool in bringing some order to the confusion that always surrounds any disaster event. Based on a military model, IMS is a hierarchy with a well-defined chain of command. At the top is the incident commander or manager, who is responsible for coordinating all rescue efforts. A "job sheet," really a vertical organizational chart, lists all the key people from all the essential agencies involved. It also outlines the responsibilities of each person and agency and must be followed throughout the disaster event for the best coordination of emergency services.[9] Most IMS plans now include hospitals within the service area. Information flows freely from the commander down to paramedics and from the street level back to the top.

Medical assistance is provided in hospitals, local clinics, or the field. Deployable Rapid Assembly Shelters (DRASHs) are mobile shelters that can be used by the IMSuRT team as a small independent hospital. The DRASH is designed with triage emergency care, intensive care units, and surgical rooms.

Protection for First Responders

Nurses and other first responders must always be aware of the potential dangers of any disaster. If the health-care providers become injured during rescue attempts, they can no longer provide care to the victims. As a result, protecting the lives and health of the first responders takes priority over rescue efforts. Because of the wide range of potential hazards, including chemicals such as nerve gas, biological substances, radioactive agents, and explosive devices, care providers must wear appropriate protective equipment.[7] Images of rescue personnel wearing bulky yellow or blue biohazard suits have become ingrained in the public consciousness. The biohazard suits, otherwise known as *personal protective equipment,* actually have a range of protective abilities against many types of substances (Box 26.1).

Most nurses have not received training in donning, wearing, or performing procedures in biohazard suits. If nurses find themselves in situations in which they may be required to wear such protection, it is important to recognize some of the limitations. The heavy gloves significantly reduce manual dexterity, and even routine procedures, such as starting intravenous (IV) lines or dressing wounds, become extremely difficult if not impossible. The hood restricts

---

B o x 2 6 . 1

Protective Levels of Biohazard Suits

Level A: Resistant to all types of chemicals and biological and radioactive substances and is used in situations in which splashing or exposure to unknown agents is possible. Totally encapsulates personnel and has its own internal air supply.

Level B: Has a hood but does not totally encapsulate personnel. Is splash resistant to most chemicals. Has its own internal air supply.

Level C: Has a hood but does not totally encapsulate personnel. Is less resistant to chemical penetration than previous levels. Equipped with a respirator that can filter out most chemical contaminants and biological and radioactive substances.

Level D: Used when there are no chemicals or agents that can affect the respiratory system or penetrate through the skin. Generally consists of a jumpsuit or scrub suit.

Source: http://www.firstrespondernetwork.com.

peripheral vision and the plastic view plate may distort the visual field. Even cursory physical examination, including the ability to use a stethoscope, becomes more difficult. Nurses may also find that the suit itself causes claustrophobia. The unusual taste and smell of the self-contained breathing equipment can sometimes cause nausea.

After exposure to any type of chemical, biological, or radioactive agent, personnel must go through a decontamination procedure. These procedures vary widely, depending on the type of agent. They range from simply removing clothes and showering with water to extensive treatment with various neutralizing agents. Most emergency response teams have a decontamination tent that provides some privacy and contains the equipment necessary for thorough decontamination.

The Postimpact Phase

The postimpact phase may begin as little as 72 hours after the disaster and in some cases may last considerably longer.[8] It may continue for years, as in the aftermath of Hurricane Sandy on the East Coast, Hurricane Katrina in New Orleans, and the attacks on the World Trade Center on 9/11. The activities focus on recovery, rehabilitation, and rebuilding. One vital step during the postimpact phase is the evaluation of the disaster preparations and of how rescue and recovery efforts could be improved.

Many Roles for the Nurse

Every disaster poses its own unique challenges. The role of the nurse in a specific disaster depends on its nature and on the type and numbers of injuries. Although most nurses have some familiarity with the role of nurses when they provide aid in a disaster, they may assume many other roles and function outside their usual practice setting in meeting the needs of the disaster victims.[6] Nurses must be able to perform under stressful and sometimes physically dangerous conditions.

After the hurricanes in Florida in 2005, large numbers of disabled and elderly clients who had been living in nursing homes and extended care facilities were displaced to schools and shelters. Nurses assumed the primary responsibility for caring for these individuals who, because they could not care for themselves and lacked essential medications, needed care at a level above what rescue workers could provide.

Triage Nurse

When the number of injured is very high, more than 1,000, the incident is classified as a mass casualty, and multiple agencies, from the local to federal, become involved. Nurses also can provide direct treatment, which may be brief or may be involved in more complex roles, such as mobile surgical units (Box 26.2).

However, in the early stages of many disasters, nurses may find a lack of essential resources both in the field and in the emergency department. Nurses have a long history of being able to improvise and get by with what is available, and a disaster will certainly challenge their creativity. When there are large numbers of victims in major disasters, nurses are often responsible for triage (from the French word meaning

---

Box 26.2

Responsibilities of the Disaster Nurse

Short-Term

1. Performs triage at the scene or in the emergency department.
2. Provides emergency medical assistance at the scene or in the emergency department. Special attention is given to vulnerable groups, such as handicapped people, children, and the elderly.
3. Provides assistance in the mobilization of necessary resources such as food, shelter, medication, and water.
4. Works in collaboration with existing disaster organizations and uses available resources.

Long-Term

1. Provides assistance with resettlement programs and psychological, economic, and legal needs.
2. Partners with independent, objective media; local and national branches of government; international agencies; and nongovernmental organizations.
3. Warns clients to be aware that many scam artists are present after any disaster and what factors to consider in detecting a scam.

"to sort"), assessing victims and prioritizing care for the best use of resources. Mass casualty situations require a different type of thinking than is usually used in everyday health care. The traditional classification of victims into low risk, intermediate care, and immediate care is reordered. The overriding goal in a disaster is to provide the best care possible for the greatest numbers of victims. Often this involves providing only palliative care to those with critical injuries, allowing more resources to be used for those with a better chance of surviving the disaster.

Triage is performed either in the field or in the emergency department. In the field, usually few medical resources are available, quick evacuation is not possible, and no one knows how soon higher level medical care will arrive. Standard triage systems were developed for fewer numbers of victims who could be moved quickly to a health-care facility; however, they fall short when there are many victims who must remain in the disaster zone for a longer period of time.

The Medical Disaster Response (MDR) system was designed to quickly evaluate and classify victims immediately after a disaster who cannot be evacuated for a substantial period of time. It requires the specialized training of local health-care providers, particularly nurses and first responders. It relies upon a dynamic triage methodology that allows for ongoing triage that may last for hours or even days. The goal is to maximize victim survival and make the best use of existing resources.

Classification Systems

The MDR system is based on the traditional "simple triage and rapid treatment" (START) method but is modified to use palpation of the radial pulse in place of the more difficult capillary refill assessment along with respiratory rate and basic neurological assessment (can the victim respond to commands). It is also combined with the "secondary assessment of victim endpoint" (SAVE) system of triage that was developed to better use limited resources for victims who were most likely to survive and recover. Trauma statistics serve as the basis for the SAVE system, which attempts to determine which victims will best survive with the various types of injuries they have suffered. The formula used is:

Probability of survival (%) = benefit ÷ available recourses.

If it is determined that a victim has a 50 percent or greater chance of surviving, they receive treatment.

Basically, the person conducting the triage makes a cost-benefit analysis in deciding which victims will benefit most for the limited resources on hand. The system places all victims into one of three categories:

Category 1: Those who will die anyway, no matter what resources are used to help them
Category 2: Those who will survive whether or not they are treated
Category 3: Those who can be helped and will gain long-term benefit from intervention and use of resources

The key to the success of the system is to identify and treat those who fall into category 3 as quickly as possible. The first and second category victims will receive only palliative care. Colored tags are also affixed to the victims based on their physical condition and injuries:

Green (category 2): Victims who are able to get up and walk around and require minimal or no treatment to save life or limb.
Red (category 3): Victims who require help breathing or assistance with their airways or whose respiratory rate is greater than 30 breaths per minute. Also included in this group are clients who are breathing but have no pulse at the wrist (radial pulse) and victims who are unable to respond to commands. Some of these victims can be saved and require immediate intervention, but they require the use of a large quantity of already scarce resources.
Yellow (category 3—nonurgent): Those victims who do not meet the criteria for the red category but are not able to walk. These individuals require intervention but usually can tolerate some delay in treatment.
Black (category 1): Those victims who are so severely injured that they have no chance for survival—fatalities.

Other factors that enter into the decision-making process include the victim's age and severity of any preexisting conditions. For example, an elderly victim with a head injury and a Glasgow Coma Scale score of 5 (out of a possible 15—unresponsive to all stimuli) who is wearing a MedicAlert bracelet that says he is on anticoagulant medications would require the use of significant medical resources and would still not likely survive the injury. He would receive a black tag and be placed in the "expectant area." However, a middle-aged adult with 20 percent second-degree burns of the legs would require minimal treatment with dressings and pain medications and has an excellent chance of surviving with full recovery would receive a yellow tag and be moved to a "treatment" area. Victims need to be reassessed frequently because conditions change and they may need to be moved to another area. The MDR-SAVE methodology is a systematic approach to use triage as a tool to maximize victims' survival in the immediate aftermath of a catastrophic disaster.

BIOTERRORISM

Biological weapons include any organism (e.g., bacteria, viruses, or fungi) or toxin found in nature that can be used to kill or injure people. Toxins are poisonous compounds produced by organisms, such as the botulism toxin. Bioterrorism is the use of microorganisms with the deliberate intent of causing infection to achieve military or political goals.[10]

An Acute Health Issue

Biological weapons are one category of weapons of mass destruction because of their ability to disable or kill large numbers of people at one time. Unfortunately, biological weapons are relatively easy and inexpensive to produce. Biological agents can be spread through the air, through water, or in food. It is also possible to use robotic delivery of agents by remote-control devices such as model airplanes. Most frightening of all, biological agents can be spread by "suicide coughers" who have purposely been given the disease and spread it from person to person in a crowded space such as a subway or an airport. After being released, microorganisms can go undetected for an extended period because their effects are not immediate and the initial symptoms are often nonspecific or "flu-like." Person-to-person transmission may continue for days or even weeks before the source is detected and a specific disease-causing organism is identified.

The vulnerability of the United States to a biological attack became painfully apparent with the delivery of anthrax spores through the postal system as an infective agent after the 9/11 attacks. The need to protect a vulnerable American population from

> *"When the number of injured is very high, more than 1,000, the incident is classified as a mass casualty, and multiple agencies, from the local to federal, become involved."*

further terrorist attacks became an acute public health issue.[11] Also, the offensive biological weapons programs of the former Soviet Union produced some deadly weaponized biological agents that cannot be located; this knowledge has increased the national anxiety level concerning bioterrorism in the United States. Since 1998, the American Nurses Association (ANA) has worked in conjunction with the American College of Emergency Physicians (ACEP) to develop strategies for health-care providers to use in responding to nuclear, biological, and chemical incidents.

Early Recognition

For nurses and other clinicians, the key to an effective response is training in the early recognition of a bioterrorist attack. Some biological agents can be detected in the environment using high-tech detection devices (sniffers). Several of the portable sniffer models include the Biological Aerosol Warning System (BAWS), which was used in Iraq, and the Portable Biofluorosensor (PBS).[12] Even newer technology may also play a part in the future of early detection of biological agents. The latest research is focused on developing tiny electronic chips containing living nerve cells that could be worn like a radiation-detection badge. It would warn of the presence of a wide range of bacterial and viral organisms. Another experimental device that would help identify specific pathogens such as botulism and smallpox consists of fiberoptic tubes coated with antibodies. Light-emitting molecules would shine through the antibodies, and the different colors produced would indicate which organism is present.

However, biological agents are most often identified by specific blood tests and cultures or the report of a health-care provider of a particular set of symptoms indicative of a particular disease. Another early warning sign is an unusually large number of ill or dead animals found throughout the community, particularly birds. They are often the first ones to catch lethal illnesses. Health-care providers must be able to identify victims early and recognize the patterns of the disease. If there are a large number of people with the same unusual symptoms, reports of dead animals, or other inconsistent findings, a biological warfare attack should be suspected. Early detection of a biological agent in the environment allows for early and specific treatment and enough time to treat others who were exposed. Currently, the U.S. Department of Defense is evaluating devices to detect clouds of biological warfare agents in the air at higher altitudes.

Are Nurses Ready?

Studies conducted over the past decade provide data indicating that nurses are still not as well prepared as they should be to respond to biological warfare agents.[10] Nurses have been and will remain the frontline first responders to all emergency situations, including a biological attack. Nurse preparedness can only increase through improved education and training in early recognition, detection, and treatment of infected persons. To help achieve this goal, several computerized education programs have been developed to raise the knowledge level of nurses and other first responders.

To educate nurses about bioterrorism, the Centers for Disease Control and Prevention (CDC) have produced online teaching and learning modules. A more comprehensive education program has been developed by the University of California–Los Angeles, in conjunction with content experts. It consists of six interactive case studies that require participants to use their knowledge to identify each biological agent. Pretest and post-test results indicate a marked increase in participant knowledge and ability to detect and distinguish among various biological agents.[10]

Recognizing and treating outbreaks as early as possible is critical for rapid implementation of measures to prevent the spread of disease. Response to bioterrorist attacks is similar to the traditional public health response when communicable disease outbreaks occur naturally, but the focus must be on early detection. However, early recognition is challenging because terrorists may use weaponized biological agents that cause highly variable initial symptoms or symptoms that are ignored until they become debilitating.

Clinical Presentation

Nurses and other clinicians must be familiar with the specific symptoms and clinical syndromes caused by bioterrorism agents (Box 26.3). One of the first indications of a biological attack is an increase in the number of individuals seeking care from public

---

B o x   2 6 . 3

Epidemiological Clues to a Biological Attack

- Many clients with the same disease, indicating the sudden development of a large epidemic
- Multiple clients with unusually severe symptoms or diseases with unusual routes of exposure
- Diseases occurring where they normally do not, or during the wrong season, or at a time when the normal vector is absent (e.g., West Nile virus in the winter—no mosquitoes)
- Multiple simultaneous epidemics of different diseases
- Outbreak of zoonotic disease (diseases transferred from animals to humans)
- Larger than normal numbers of sick, dying, or dead animals in the community
- Unusual strains of contagious organisms or large numbers of antibiotic-resistant organisms
- Higher rates of disease than would normally be seen in persons exposed to the organism
- Reports of a credible threat of a biological attack by official authorities
- Direct evidence of biological attack

---

health agencies, primary care providers, and EDs. Because many of these agents are viruses, the early symptoms often look like a case of the flu. Hospitals, doctors, nurses, and public health professionals will be on the front lines of any attack. A heightened level of suspicion, plus knowledge of the relevant epidemiological clues, should help in the recognition of changes in illness patterns.[6]

Biological Agents

The CDC has developed a list of biological agents that are considered the most likely to be used in a bioterrorist attack (Table 26.1). Infective agents were included for their ability to produce widely disseminated infections, high mortality rates, potential for major public health impact, and ability to cause panic and social disruption. Those that require special action for public health preparedness were also included. Category A agents possess the highest immediate risk for use as biological weapons; category B agents pose the next highest risk. Category C agents have a potential for use but are not considered an immediate risk as biological weapons.

Table 26.1 **Critical Biological Agent Categories for Public Health Preparedness**

Category	Biological Agent	Disease
A: Highest immediate risk	*Variola major*	Smallpox
	Bacillus anthracis	Anthrax
	Yersinia pestis	Plague
	Clostridium botulinum (botulinum toxins)	Botulism
	Francisella tularensis	Tularemia
	Filoviruses and arenaviruses (Ebola and Lassa viruses)	Viral hemorrhagic fevers
B: Next-highest risk	*Coxiella burnetii*	Q fever
	Brucella species	Brucellosis
	Burkholderia mallei	Glanders
	Burkholderia pseudomallei	Melioidosis
	Alphaviruses	Encephalitis (VEE, EEE, WEE)
	Rickettsia prowazekii	Typhus fever
	Toxins (e.g., ricin, staphylococcal enterotoxin B)	Toxic syndromes
	Chlamydia psittaci	Psittacosis
	Food-safety threats (e.g., *Salmonella* species, *Escherichia coli* 0157:H7)	Salmonellosis, diarrheal illness, sepsis, hemolytic uremic syndrome
	Water-safety threats (e.g., *Vibrio cholerae, Cryptosporidium parvum*)	Cholera, cryptosporidiosis
C: Potential, but not an immediate risk	Emerging-threat agents (e.g., Nipah virus, hantavirus)	

EEE = eastern equine encephalitis; VEE = Venezuelan equine encephalitis; WEE = western equine encephalitis.

Effective Response

In the event of a widespread bioterrorism attack, nurses in all levels and types of health-care settings will likely become involved. To develop a prompt and effective response, nurses and other health-care providers must know the modes of transmission, incubation periods, symptoms, and communicable periods of these diseases as outlined by the CDC.[11]

Identification and Management

Once a potential outbreak is detected, it must be brought to the attention of the appropriate health-care agencies or specialist in infective diseases. The CDC is always called in and may "take over" the hospital to prevent the further spread of the biological agent. In cases of suspected bioterrorism, they are given the authority of federal law enforcement personnel.

All nurses should have accurate around-the-clock information on the resources available for their geographic area. Once appropriate notifications have been made, nurses will use their skills of clinical evaluation and history taking to identify the infective organism, mode of transmission, and source of exposure. In addition, nurses play a critical role in managing postexposure prophylaxis and its complications, as well as psychological and mental health problems brought on by the event.

What Do You Think?

Have you received any specialized training in disaster or bioterrorism preparedness? If you have, how does it make you better able to care for victims of disaster or bioterrorism? If you do not eventually receive this training, is it something that you think is important enough to seek out on your own? Do you feel prepared to care for these victims?

Response Training

The American College of Emergency Physicians (ACEP), in alliance with the ANA, submitted a list of recommendations to the Health and Human Services

Office of Emergency Preparedness in April 2001. Included was the recommendation that all basic nurse education programs include information on how to respond to mass casualty events. The task force also recommended that self-study modules and other types of specialty programs be developed for ED nurses that would contain more in-depth information on the detection and management of bioterrorism. (For more information, go to http://www.acep.org for recent updates.)

The ANA is actively involved in developing ways to better prepare nurses to respond to bioterrorist events. In collaboration with the Department of Health and Human Services (DHHS), they established the National Nurses Response Teams (NNRT). This joint effort was unveiled at the ANA's 2002 biennial convention.

Activation and Deployment

In the event that the president declares a bioterrorism state of disaster, the NNRT will be activated to respond by providing mass immunization or chemoprophylaxis to a population at risk. The NNRT, under the auspices of the DHHS, will be quickly deployed in response to a major national event.

> *Since 9/11, the need to protect a vulnerable American population from further terrorist attacks has become an acute public health issue.*

The goal of the ANA and federal officials is to recruit 10 regional teams of 200 nurses. The ANA is working to recruit these nurse teams and will provide ongoing education to the NNRT in disaster response. The DHHS is responsible for the screening and processing of potential nurse team members after they have been recruited by the ANA.

When the NNRT teams are deployed, the members become "federalized," and the federal government will pay their salaries, reimburse them for travel, and cover their housing costs during the duty period. In case of a terrorism disaster, the deployment will be limited to 2 weeks to minimize the impact on the nurses' employers.

The nursing profession faces serious challenges in the response to threats of bioterrorism. The nation is counting on nurses to play a vital role in bioterrorism preparedness and response. The public depends on nurses to be the frontline responders and to protect them from the effects of bioterrorism. Nurses must be able to communicate medical information and educate the public quickly after a crisis. It is imperative that the nursing profession train nurses in appropriate, effective responses to ensure the best outcome in a frightening, unfamiliar event.

MRC

Nurses interested in working with disaster victims might want to consider joining the Medical Reserve Corps (MRC). It is a nationwide network of community-based response units sponsored by the office of the surgeon general of the United States. As a national network of local groups of volunteers committed to improving the health, safety, and resiliency of their communities, anyone can join. The largest single group of volunteers in the MRC is nurses. Each MRC unit is organized and trained to address a wide range of challenges, from public health education to disaster response. The training is specific for the types of disasters that are seen in the units' communities and range from setting up aid stations and administering immunizations to the after care of displaced elderly victims. After a nurse volunteer has been trained and certified, they can respond to a variety of different types of disasters, including those that are out of state. Normally, nurses are not allowed to practice nursing in states in which they are not licensed. Because MRC certification is national, states have agreed to allow certified nurses to practice within their boundaries during disaster events. For more information, please visit http://www.naccho.org/topics/emergency/mrc/ or http://www.medicalreservecorps.gov/.

CHEMICAL WEAPONS

Although the Chemical Weapons Convention of 1993 banned, under the legal threat of punishment, the worldwide production, stockpiling, and use of chemical weapons, a number of countries, including the United States, maintain large aging stockpiles of these horrific weapons. Their storage and use is generally rationalized as a means of defending the country against attack from a hostile aggressor.

Definition

Chemical weapons (CW) are generally defined as devices that use any one of a number of chemicals mixed in such a way as to inflict death or harm to human beings. CWs, along with biological and nuclear devices, generally fall into a class of weapons know as *weapons of mass destruction.* CWs take many forms, including gas, liquids, and solids, that often kill or destroy targets other than the one intended.[13]

There are two general classes of CWs—unitary and binary agents. Unitary chemical agents are effective by themselves and do not require any other substances to be mixed with them to make them lethal. These agents are highly volatile (unstable and return to a gas state quickly) and are the types of agents most commonly stockpiled by nations in their weapons arsenals and preferred by terrorists. Binary CWs only become lethal when two non-dangerous chemicals are mixed together to create a third dangerous chemical.[14] These are more difficult to manufacture and more complicated to activate. However, the reason passengers can no longer take liquids, contained in more than 3-ounce increments, on airplanes is because of a plot by terrorists in Great Britain to use binary agents poured into shampoo bottles and then mixed when they were on the plane with the intention of bringing down international flights.

> *Many CWs kill in a matter of minutes while others can take hours or even days, providing the victims with a chance of survival if quickly decontaminated and treated with the appropriate antidote, if one is available.*

Horrific Results

The first widespread military use of CWs was during World War I. The injuries caused by them were so horrific that, although most major countries now have stockpiles of them, they have been very reluctant to use them. There was some use of CW by Japan against the Chinese at the beginning of World War II, but after seeing the effects, they were not used again. The Aum Shinrikyo cult used sarin, a deadly colorless, odorless nerve gas, on a Tokyo subway in 1995, killing 12 people and injuring more than 5,500.[13] In addition, Saddam Hussein used CWs against the Kurds in the northern part of Iraq. Parts of the country became a desert because CW annihilated all living things and made the area uninhabitable for decades due to contamination of water and food supplies. The half-life of many CWs can last a few years or even decades.

More recently, there were substantiated reports that CWs were used in Syria in 2013 on a limited scale, although it is unclear who actually used them. Experts believed for many years that the Syrian government had a stockpile of CWs, although they consistently denied it. Investigations seemed to point to one of the groups of rebel terrorists fighting against the government had obtained CWs on the black market and used them. Later that year, U.S. vice president Joseph Biden brokered a deal whereby the Syrian government would turn over all the chemical weapons stockpiles that they claimed they never had to Russia for permanent destruction.

Russia reluctantly acknowledged that some of their CWs went missing after the fall of the Soviet Union and may very well have gotten into the hands of terrorists groups. Letters sent to the U.S. president and several high-ranking government officials in the spring of 2013 were laced with ground caster beans, the key ingredient in the deadly poison ricin. If the terrorist bombers at the 2013 Boston Marathon had incorporated chemical agents into their backpack bombs, the death toll and number of injured would have been even more devastating.

Since the September 11, 2001, terrorist attacks on America, the threat of chemical weapons has become an immeasurable concern for both citizens and the government. The government has made preparations to protect the population against CWs and has taken measures to ensure that there is a plan for action in response to a CW attack. The technology to produce CWs is widely available, and key chemicals are available at the tens of thousands of chemical manufacturing plants in the United States and Europe alone.

In 1997, in an attempt to stop the spread and use of CWs, the U.S. Senate ratified a global chemical weapons ban treaty signed by more than 80 other nations. However, terrorists groups do not abide by these treaties and, because of the abysmal effects and fear generated by CWs, seem eager to obtain and use them on Western populations.

Types of Chemical Weapons

The three major groups of chemical weapons are nerve agents, blister agents, and choking agents. They are generally dispensed as aerosols, liquids, or vapors that enter the body through the eyes, lungs, or skin. There are also blood agents, which are inhaled. Their overall effectiveness in killing people can be affected by how old the agent is, its purity, weather conditions such as temperature and humidity, strength and direction of the wind, size of the environment where they are released, and how they are introduced into the environment.[13] Many CWs kill in a matter of minutes; others can take hours or even days, providing the victims with a chance of survival if quickly decontaminated and treated with the appropriate antidote, if one is available. Although symptoms vary based on the class of agent, some general symptoms to look for include immediate failure of the respiratory or nervous system (paralysis), severe skin irritations and blisters, headaches, irregular heartbeat or palpitations, vomiting, and convulsions (Box 26.4).

Nerve Agents

The nerve agents are among the most toxic of all CWs. They are particularly deadly when released in an enclosed area such as a subway train or an airplane. Their initial development was just before World War II for the purpose of controlling insect infestations on farms. Chemically related to the organophosphorus insecticides that are in wide use today, they work by inhibiting the production of acetylcholinesterase throughout the nervous system and causing paralysis of smooth muscles. German scientists of the 1930s soon recognized the lethal potential of these chemicals and began producing concentrated weaponized forms of the substance that could be used on the battlefield and in the gas chambers of the concentration camps.[15]

Causing an excessive accumulation of acetylcholine in the nerve endings of the parasympathetic system, nerve agents inhibit the smooth muscles all along the vagus nerve (cranial nerve X), including the iris of the eye, ciliary bodies in the bronchial tree and gastrointestinal tract, bladder, and blood vessels. They also paralyze the salivary glands and secretory glands of the gastrointestinal tract, the respiratory tract, and eventually the cardiac muscle tissue. Although respiratory symptoms are generally the first to appear after

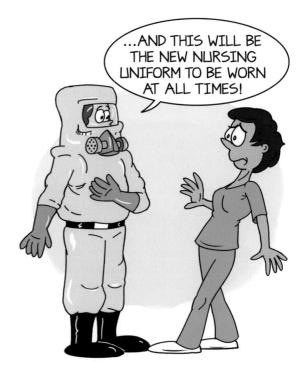

Box 26.4

Classes of Chemical Agents

Nerve Agents	Blister Agents	Respiratory Agents
Tabun (GA)	Sulfur mustard (Yperite) (HD)	Phosgene (CG)
Sarin (GB)	Nitrogen mustard (HN)	Diphosgene (DP)
Soman (GD)	Lewisite (L)	Chlorine (Cl)
Cyclosarin (GF)	Phosgene oxime (CX)	Chloropicrin (PS)
Methylphosphonothioic acid (VX)		

inhalation of nerve agent vapors, if ingested, gastrointestinal symptoms are usually the first to appear. The early symptoms often mimic a heart attack, manifesting with tightness in the chest, shortness of breath, elevated blood pressure, and abnormal heart rhythms. As the effect of the toxin becomes more systemic, the victim will experience increased fatigue and generalized weakness, which increases with activity. Soon after, involuntary muscular twitching, scattered involuntary muscle contractions, and intermittent muscle cramps develop. The skin may be pale due to vasoconstriction. Left untreated or treated too late, nerve agents lead to organ failure, complete shutdown of the nervous system, and death.[13]

The primary treatment is immediate decontamination and the administration of atropine sulfate IV as soon as possible. Atropine blocks the effects of the parasympathetic system and helps breathing by drying secretions and dilating the airways. Atropine also suppresses other symptoms of nerve agents, including nausea, vomiting, abdominal cramping, low heart rate, and sweating. Atropine, however, does not prevent or reverse paralysis. Another medication, pralidoxime chloride, may also be given. It belongs to a family of compounds called *oximes* that bind to organophosphate-inactivated-acetylcholinesterase, thereby "regenerating" or "reactivating" acetylcholinesterase and allowing the synapses to function again.[14] Unfortunately, if it is not given soon after exposure, it may not be able to break the molecular bonds in the synapse and it will be ineffective. If treated early, the serious signs and symptoms of nerve agent toxicity rarely last more than a couple of hours.

Generally, if the victim survives the initial exposure and peak toxic effects, the symptoms usually disappear within 1 day, and the survival rate is excellent. Victims who were exposed but show no symptoms are usually observed for at least 18 hours because some signs and symptoms can show up later.

Blister Agents

Blister agents, sometimes called *vesicants,* burn and blister the exposed skin on any part of the body they contact. With enough exposure or if inhaled in large quantities, they can kill people, but they are more often used to produce large numbers of serious casualties that need extensive care, thus taking away needed resources for fighting. They also force the enemy to wear full protective equipment, making their ability to fight more cumbersome and less effective. When thickened and applied to land, ship decks, or the surfaces of aircraft or vehicles, blister agents become a persistent hazard that makes it challenging to defeat enemies.[15]

Although exposed skin is usually the first area of the body affected, blister agents also can cause major damage to the eyes, mucous membranes, linings of the lungs, and blood-forming organs. In addition, when ingested, they cause vomiting and diarrhea. The most feared and oldest of the blister agents is mustard gas. It is easily made, very stable chemically, remains dangerous on surfaces almost indefinitely, and there is no effective treatment for it even today, making it hard to decontaminate.[13] It was first used in World War I, and the gruesome burns it produced frightened even the people who released it.[15]

Another problem is that exposure to mustard gas is not always evident right away because of the latent and symptom-free period that may occur after skin exposure. This may result in delayed decontamination or failure to decontaminate at all. However, it must be removed from the skin quickly and efficiently. After even as little as a 2-minute exposure, a drop of mustard on the skin can cause serious blisters and burns.

Initial treatment, as with all chemical agents, is immediate decontamination. The chemical chlorination has proven somewhat effective in disabling mustard and several other of the blister agents. There is no practical drug treatment available for preventing the internal effects of mustard. Infection is the most serious complication after exposure to blister agents. Although there is little agreement on the best way to treat exposure to blister agents, most mustard gas victims survive but have protracted and painful recovery periods with the need for multiple skin grafts.

Choking Agents

Choking or respiratory agents work by attacking the tissues of the lungs and produce massive pulmonary

> *Decontamination of the victims as soon as possible is essential to reducing their exposure to the toxins and providing appropriate medical treatment, such as specific antidotes, that will increase their chances for survival.*

edema. The most dangerous of this group of toxins is phosgene and the one that terrorists are most likely to use. Phosgene was used for the first time in 1915, and it accounted for 80 percent of all the deaths attributed to CWs during World War I. Initial symptoms include coughing, choking, a feeling of tightness in the chest, nausea and occasionally vomiting, headache, and excessive tear production.[15]

When delivered in very high concentrations, a painful and agonizing death can occur within several hours. With lower concentrations, death usually occurs in 12 to 24 hours. There is no specific antidote or treatment. Respiratory support by ventilation with positive end expiratory pressure (PEEP) can usually maintain adequate oxygenation of the body. Use of osmotic diuretics can reduce the fluid load in the lungs. Other supportive measures commonly used for persons in pulmonary edema may be helpful. If the victim survives the initial exposure, they usually begin to recover within 48 hours, although there may be permanent lung damage. Respiratory infection is the dreaded major complication. If victims survive longer than 48 hours, they usually make a full recovery.[13]

General Principles of CW Preparation

In reality, many of the measures used by nurses and first responders for preparation and protection for bioterrorism are also effective with CWs. It's imperative that nurses and emergency personnel wear personal protective suits when dealing with chemical contamination due to the persistent nature of some of the agents. Decontamination of the victims as soon as possible is essential to reducing their exposure to the toxins and providing appropriate medical treatment, such as specific antidotes, that will increase their chances for survival.[13]

Personal Protective Equipment

First responders and emergency room personnel are at serious risk for exposure to the chemically contaminated areas (known as *hot zones*). The victims themselves automatically become hot zones and the hot zones can move if the victim is not completely decontaminated. If first responders are unprotected, direct contact to the CW or inhalation of vapors automatically makes them victims as well.

> **It is more likely that any individual would be exposed to a chemical agent from an industrial accident or vehicular mishap.**

If a liquid chemical agent was used, handling the skin and clothing of victims exposes rescue personnel to the same chemical.[13]

Full level D hazardous material (hazmat) suits should be worn until the source of contamination has been completely eliminated. A hazmat suit is an impermeable whole-body garment that is worn as protection against a variety of hazardous materials. To protect against chemical exposures, these suits are made of barrier materials like Teflon, heavy PVC plastic, corrosive-resistant synthetic rubber, or Tyvek (a brand name for cloth made from flash-spun high-density polyethylene fibers).

The high-level suits have self-contained, filtered breathing systems to eliminate any exposure to airborne toxins. These are similar to the suits used for bioterrorism, except they are more resistant to the corrosive effects of some chemical agents. Also, biological protective suits must have fully sealed systems and positive-pressure breathing systems to prevent entry of the biological agent, even if the suit is punctured or torn. Although hazmat suits are mostly used by firefighters, researchers, personnel responding to toxic spills, specialists cleaning up contaminated facilities, and workers in toxic environments, most health-care facilities have them available for personnel who are likely to come into contact with hazardous chemicals.

Decontamination

Decontamination is the physical and chemical removal of toxic agents from people's skin, clothing, equipment, and any environmental surfaces where they were disseminated. Hazardous chemicals remaining on clothing, skin surfaces, and even in the respiratory system can be a source of exposure to others.[13] This is called *secondary exposure* and is the most common type of exposure experienced by first responders and emergency room personnel. Immediate decontamination is a major treatment priority for those with CW exposure. It should include:

• Removing all contaminated clothes and jewelry from the victim and washing the unclothed body thoroughly with warm water and soap.

- Avoiding the use of very hot water and excessively vigorous scrubbing because they may actually force more of the chemical into the skin.
- Decontaminating all victims who have been exposed, even if it is unknown whether it was a vapor or liquid. Vapor exposure alone may not require decontamination; however, some vapors cling to clothing and skin and can be inhaled from these surfaces.
- Decontaminating victims as close as possible to the site of exposure. This minimizes the time of exposure and prevents moving the hot zone to another area. Most hospitals that are certified to treat chemical exposures have policies and procedures about where victims may be decontaminated. Usually it is an area outside the emergency department where a tent is set up to perform initial decontamination before people and equipment are allowed entry. Portable decontamination equipment with showers and runoff water collection systems are commercially available. Some larger facilities have in-house decontamination areas with showers, special ventilation, and various decontamination rooms. All hospitals should have the capacity to safely decontaminate at least one person at a time.[13,14]

Supportive and Specific Therapy

Health-care providers should follow the ABCs of emergency care: airway, breathing, and circulation. Keeping the airway open and making sure victims are able to breathe or are well oxygenated is always the first priority. Intubation and oxygen delivery equipment must be available. Until the specific agent is identified, health-care providers should treat the most serious and life-threatening symptoms first. However, laboratory tests used to identify specific chemical agents are not available in all hospitals. Confirmation of the chemical agent may take several hours or even days. Once the agent has been identified, specific antidotes known to be effective should be used.[13]

The Centers for Disease Control and Prevention is the authority on chemical weapons and their treatments. They have information on treatment options and a decision tree that can be used for deciding what treatments are most likely to be successful. For more information, go to http://www.cdc.gov/nceh/demil/articles/initialtreat.htm.

The Odds Are Good

Realistically, the chances of being exposed to CWs or chemical agents is miniscule. Although some

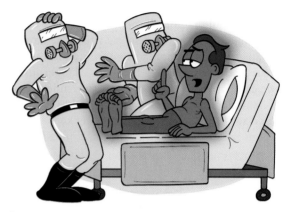

"THIS ISN'T A SIDE EFFECT OF VIAGRA, IS IT?"

terrorist organizations have been successful in obtaining and releasing chemical agents, the reality is that making effective delivery systems is extremely difficult. It is more likely that any individual would be exposed to a chemical agent from an industrial accident or vehicular mishap. There are numerous chemical factories across the nation right now creating chemical toxins that are more deadly than any ever used in weapons. Because of the volatile nature of the chemicals they make, these chemical factories have a disturbing tendency to explode from time to time and spread the toxins over wide areas. Toxic chemicals are regularly shipped by trains and tractor-trailers to all parts of the country. It is not unusual to see a train accident where the large black tank cars lie broken on their sides near a populated area. The chemicals they contain are often highly toxic.

Dangerous Aging Weapons

An even more concerning situation is the aging stockpiles of chemical weapons owned by the U.S. military. Many of these weapons were manufactured over 60 years ago and put into containers that were made to last only a few years. Because of the corrosive nature of these chemicals, many of the containers are developing leaks, exposing personnel to the toxic agents. The only sure way to dispose of these toxins is by burning them at extremely high temperatures, 2,500 to 3,000 degrees, thereby reducing them to their basic elements and rendering them harmless. Unfortunately, there are only a few of these disposal plants for chemical weapons in the country. Disposal of the many aging chemical warheads would require shipping them cross-country by rail or truck to the disposal sites. The dangers of accidents and widespread contamination make this method of eliminating them very dangerous. Some companies have developed large "indestructible" stainless steel tanks located in stable underground salt caves that can theoretically keep these weapons in safe storage for centuries. Unfortunately, the jury is still out on how safe these tanks and salt caves really are.

Nurses must be prepared to deal with all types of disaster. Education for disaster preparedness needs to start in nursing school and continue throughout the nurses' career. It would be highly unlikely that a nurse would not experience some type of disaster during his or her career. Knowledge and skills development are the best preparation.

Issues Now

Disaster Preparedness for . . . Scam?

The sirens were blaring and the emergency radio was shouting "SEEK SHELTER NOW!" The whole family and two dogs scrambled for the storm shelter. We barely got the door closed and bolted down when there was a big crash, a roaring sound (it really does sound like a train), banging and scraping, and the shelter door started to partially lift up. After what seemed like hours (in reality about 5 minutes), there was only dead silence. We carefully pushed up the heavy shelter door, and all we could see was an empty foundation slab, glistening wet from the rain. I guess our house isn't in Kansas anymore!

OMG, what do we do now? We had our disaster plan and supply kit, so at least we had a place to start. I think I went through the five stages of grief in about 10 minutes. It really didn't start to sink in until several days later. I'm going to need to call the insurance company, I thought. I've never even filed a claim for a broken window before. I wonder how you do that. What about the utilities? Do I have to pay for them even though there's no house anymore? Do you still have to pay real estate taxes and fees for garbage pickup? My HD 70-inch flat-screen is sticking out of the side of the neighbor's garage—I don't think we'll get many cable channels there! When are the FEMA guys going to show up?

As I picked through what was left of my belongings, trying to find anything of value, an official-looking, nicely dressed, clean-cut young man walked up to me.

"Hi!" he said.

"Hi!" I answered.

"It looks like that tornado got you real good," he remarked.

"Yeah, me and everyone else on the block," I replied.

"I see you're trying to clean up some. Are you finding anything interesting?" he asked.

"I guess you could say that," I answered. "The real interesting stuff is from my neighbors' houses across the street and next door. I guess it all got mix-mastered into one big pile. I'm trying to keep the piles separated. I have no idea where some of the stuff came from."

"Are you still able to work?" he asked.

"I teach, or used to teach, at the high school you walked past on your way here," I said.

"There's not much left of that either, is there," he observed. "That sure must have affected your income."

"It's not too bad. I usually have the summers off anyway, and my husband is an administrator at a local college who works all year round," I explained.

"That gives you some advantage over some people since you must be used to dealing with paperwork. Are you making any progress with all the paperwork involved after something like this?" he asked.

"I was just thinking about that. I really don't even know where to start with it," I said.

"Maybe I can help. I work with a company associated with the National Relief Agency that specializes in helping disaster victims plow through the mountain of paperwork after tornadoes, floods, and other disasters," he said.

(continued)

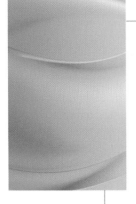

Issues Now continued

He handed me a nice professional-looking red-white-and-blue business card with an official-looking government seal printed on it and National Relief Agency across the top. It had his name, address, phone number, and an e-mail address on it ending in .gov. It even had "BBB Approved" on the bottom of the card.

"How does it work?" I asked, seeing my first glimmer of hope in many days.

"Well, we take care of pretty much everything, from getting your utilities turned off to filing for FEMA assistance. We'll even help file for your building permit when it is time to rebuild. All I need is some basic information, like your name and address," he answered.

"That sounds almost too good to be true. But I think I need some time to think about it," I responded.

"Oh, that may be a problem," he said. "You see, we're a small company and in order to provide the personal service our clients deserve and expect, we only accept a limited number and then cut off enrollment. Actually, I was authorized to accept only one new client today and then we were not going to accept any more for 2 or 3 months until we clear some of our earliest enrollees. You understand, don't you?"

"I think so, but how much does it cost?" I asked suspiciously.

"We ask for $1,000 up front. There may be some additional fees later. However, most of that money is used to pay for costs that you would have spent anyway, such as fees for filing for FEMA assistance, insurance company adjustor fees, any fees charged by utilities for turning off their services, building permit fees, and other stuff like that. We will also work with your insurance company to get you the best settlement possible. We work out of a lawyer's office, and insurance companies don't like dealing with lawyers," he explained.

"So let me get this straight," I said cautiously. "If I don't sign up with you today, it will be several months before I can do so again?"

"Well, it looks like there might be a lot of other people around here that probably would be interested in this type of program," he answered.

"Well, um, I don't know . . . I guess. Okay, let's do it," I said excitedly. I pride myself on always being able to make decisions quickly.

"All you have to do is fill out this one information form and a credit card authorization form," he said.

He removed the forms from his coat pocket and handed them to me. I retrieved the photocopy of the credit cards I had in my emergency kit and filled in the information and signed it. The other form required some basic information, including my Social Security number and bank account number so that, he told me, money from FEMA and the insurance settlement could be direct-deposited into my account. How thoughtful and convenient! He gave me a handwritten receipt and promised he would get started on the paperwork that afternoon. Finally, someone was actually helping me and I felt I could see the light at the end of the tunnel!

No, probably not so much. The light you see at the end of the tunnel is the light on the locomotive of the Scam-line express, roaring down the tracks to flatten your hopes and dreams. It is most likely that you will never see or hear from

Issues Now *continued*

this person again and never see your money again either. And just wait and see what happens when the identity theft starts kicking in. After disasters, scam artists show up like flies at a picnic and there are as many different scams as there are flies. The Better Business Bureau has dubbed these scam artists "storm chasers" because they show up after every major storm or disaster. By the way, although the letters BBB can stand for Better Business Bureau, unless the name is spelled out, the letters probably stand for something else (Big Blue Buttons, Big Best Barbeque, Bob's Best Bikes, etc.).

There were so many scams after Hurricane Katrina that the Department of Justice created a new agency, the National Center for Disaster Fraud, a central information clearinghouse for more than 20 federal agencies where people can report suspected fraudulent activities tied to disasters of all types. Here are some things to keep in mind to keep from being scammed:

- There are *never* fees to apply for FEMA or SBA assistance or to receive property damage inspections. If someone is asking for money, it's a scam.
- Utilities do not charge for turning *off* services. Some charge a small fee for turning them back on, although in disaster situations they often waive the fees.
- If someone claims to be from the government, always ask to see a government-issued photo ID and take a picture of it with your cell phone. In fact, they should volunteer to show you an ID.
- Business cards are not official IDs. With all the online do-it-yourself business card companies these days, it is very easy to make professional-looking business cards that say just about anything, sometimes free for the first 250 cards.
- Government workers or people associated with government agencies will *never* ask for payment to perform their duties or offer to increase your assistance grant for a fee.
- If private insurance adjusters and local building code inspectors visit your property, they, too, should provide identification on demand. They do not charge fees.
- Never hire a laborer or contractor on the spot; good ones don't need to solicit work door to door. Also, check with your neighbors to see if they suffered damage similar to what is being cited at your place.
- For major repairs, get at least three estimates, based on the same specifications and materials. Check their references, licensing, and registration information with the National Association of State Contractors Licensing Agencies (NASCLA), and read reviews posted by the Better Business Bureau.
- Require written contracts that specify work to be done, materials to be used, start and end dates, responsibility for hauling away debris, and costs broken down by labor and materials. Verify that the contractor's name, address, phone number, and license number are included, as well as any verbal promises and warranties.
- Never sign a contract with blank spaces. Unscrupulous contractors sometimes enter unacceptable terms later on.
- Never give out Social Security numbers, credit card numbers, bank account numbers, or personal information about your finances. Employees of legitimate organizations will never ask for them.

(continued)

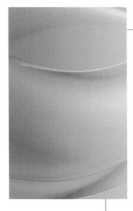

Issues Now _{continued}

- Read the fine print. Some shady contracts include clauses allowing substantial cancellation fees if you choose not to use the contractor after your insurance company has approved the claim. Others require you to pay the full price if you cancel after the cancellation period has expired.
- Ask your contractor to provide proof of his or his company's current insurance that covers workers compensation benefits, property damage, and personal liability. Depending on the size of the job, you may want a performance bond, which protects you if work isn't done according to the contract. Contractors don't like to get these.
- You'll probably be asked to pay an upfront deposit to cover initial materials—one-quarter to one-third is reasonable upon delivery of materials to your home and once work begins. Get a signed receipt for the money you paid.
- Never pay in full in advance, and don't pay cash. Have the contract specify a schedule for releasing payments, and before making the final payment, ask the contractor to provide proof that all subcontractors have been paid—if not, you could be liable for their fees.
- If you suspect anyone—whether an inspector, contractor, disaster survivor, or someone posing as one—of fraudulent activities in relation to a natural or man-made disaster, call FEMA's toll-free Disaster Fraud Hotline at 866-720-5721, or local law enforcement officials.
- If it sounds too good to be true, it probably is.
- If someone uses high-pressure sales tactics, requires full payment up front, asks you to get necessary permits, or offers to shave costs by using leftover materials from another job, it's a scam.

We generally think of the elderly as being most susceptible to scam artists, but these crooks are so slick that anyone can fall for their sales pitches. They know that people who are under stress are much more vulnerable to scams than those who feel secure. Many postdisaster victims have a mild form of post-traumatic stress disorder (PTSD) that may last for many months or even years after the disaster. Making people aware of scams, although not usually thought of as a nursing function, certainly falls into the category of caring.

Sources: Alderman J. Avoiding post-disaster scam artists. Huffington Post, 2013. Retrieved June 2013 from http://www.huffingtonpost.com/jason-alderman/avoiding-post-disaster-sc_b_2916643.html; Kirchheimer S. Avoid post-disaster scams. AARP. Retrieved June 2013 from http://www.aarp.org/money/scams-fraud/info-08-2012/avoiding-post-disaster-scams.html; National Center for Disaster Fraud. Department of Justice, 2013. Retrieved June 2913 from http://www.justice.gov/criminal/oilspill/about/ncdf.html and http://www.justice.gov/opa/pr/2012/November/12-crm-1308.html

Conclusion

The plain and simple truth is that nurses need to be prepared for all types of disasters, including bioterrorism, natural disasters, and chemical weapon exposure. These types of events have unfortunately become a part of post-9/11 life. The tragic events of that day in New York City; Washington, DC; and Pennsylvania revealed how poorly prepared the United States was to deal with disasters. In response, legislation was enacted on federal and state levels that began to address the many issues associated with terrorist acts. Large sums of money were expended to purchase equipment and train health-care workers to be better able to deal with a variety of potential disasters.

Collaboration between groups that often had little to do with each other in the past became an essential component of these plans. The Department of Health and Human Services and the ANA have been working closely to educate nurses in disaster and bioterrorism responses. Although much better preparation was demonstrated in the aftermath of the EF-5 Oklahoma tornadoes in 2013 than in 2005 with the repercussions of Hurricane Katrina, there is still room for improvement. Nurses have dealt with disasters for many years in emergency rooms and working with first responders in the field. Most of their knowledge was accumulated on the job after years of experience. It is essential that the principles involved in disaster preparation and emergency aftercare be taught to the nurse before graduation from nursing school.

Critical-Thinking Exercises

- Obtain the policy and procedure manuals from your nursing school and your primary clinical location. Try to find the procedures for disaster preparedness (note: sometimes these are separate documents). Compare the school's and the facility's policies with each other and the plan in this chapter. How do they compare? Where are the areas that need improvement?
- If you don't have a disaster plan or kit yet for your family, put one together. Show your family and ask for their input.
- Volunteer to work with your local Red Cross chapter. Write a report about what they do and how they are funded.
- Read or reread the Issues Now box "Disaster Preparation for a . . . Scam?" In the conversation, identify the warning signs, if any, that this was likely a scam. What should the person have done?
- Look up the word *acetylcholinesterase*. Prepare a short presentation to the class about how nerve agents affect the sympathetic and parasympathetic nervous systems. Explain why atropine is an effective antidote.

References

1. McCabe OL, Barnett DJ, Taylor HG, Links JM. Ready, willing, and able: A framework for improving the public health emergency preparedness system. *Disaster Medicine & Public Health Preparedness,* 4(2):161–168, 2010.

2. Plan and prepare. Federal Emergency Management Agency, 2013. Retrieved June 2013 from http://www.fema.gov/what-mitigation/plan-prepare

3. Disaster Preparation. General Preparedness Information Flyer, 2013. Retrieved June 2013 from http://nbcert.org/DisasterPreparation.htm

4. Disaster preparedness for healthcare and communities. Response Systems, 2013. Retrieved June 2013 from http://www.disasterpreparation.net/

5. Fire extinguisher types (what type should I use?). Fire Extinguisher 101, 2013. Retrieved June 2013 from http://www.fire-extinguisher101.com/

6. Debisette AT, Martinelli AM, Couig MP, Braun M. US Public Health Service Commissioned Corps Nurses: Responding in times of national need. *Nursing Clinics of North America,* 45(2):123–135, 2010.

7. James JJ, Benjamin GC, Burkle FM, Gebbie KM, Kelen G Subbarao I. Disaster medicine and public health preparedness: A discipline for all health professionals. *Disaster Medicine & Public Health Preparedness,* 4(2):102–107, 2010.

8. Sherly W. Phases of a disaster. Healthy Living. Retrieved June 2013 from http://www.ehow.com/list_6732381_phases-disaster-management.html

9. National Incident Management System. FEMA, 2013. Retrieved June 2013 from http://www.fema.gov/national-incident-management-system

10. Nyamathi AM, Casillas A, King ML, et al. Computerized bioterrorism education and training for nurses on bioterrorism attack agents. *Journal of Continuing Education in Nursing,* 41(8):375–384, 2010.

11. Goodhue CJ, Burke RV, Chambers S, Ferrer RR, Upperman JS. Disaster Olympix: A unique nursing emergency preparedness exercise. *Journal of Trauma Nursing,* 17(1):5–10, 2010.

12. Biological detection systems. National Criminal Justice Reference Service. Retrieved June 2013 from http://www.ncjrs.gov/pdffiles1/nij/190747-b.pdf

13. Federation of American Scientists. Types of chemical weapons. Retrieved May 2013 from http://www.fas.org/programs/bio/chemweapons/cwagents.html

14. Organization for the prohibition of chemical agents. Retrieved May 2013 from http://www.opcw.org/about-chemical-weapons/types-of-chemical-agent/

15. Arnold JL, White S, Talavera F, Roberge RJ. Chemical warfare. eMedicineHealth, 2013. Retrieved May 2013 from http://www.emedicinehealth.com/chemical_warfare/page7_em.htm

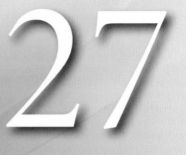

27 Developments in Current Nursing Practice

Joseph T. Catalano

Learning Objectives

After completing this chapter, the reader will be able to:

- Discuss the nurse's role in forensics, entrepreneurship, legal consulting, case management, and nurse navigator, nurse coder, and client safety officer positions
- Discuss ways in which to develop a nurse-run business
- Identify factors that indicate the need for case management
- Give examples of organizations that nurses can become involved in to provide assistance in the event of a disaster

NEW ROLES FOR THE NURSE

The profession of nursing is dynamic and ever-changing. Nursing roles evolve and develop in response to the needs of society. Part of the hope for the Affordable Care Act is that it will open even more doors for professional nurses and provide opportunities for expanded practice. This chapter discusses the new and exciting practice roles in nursing. Included are discussions of forensic nursing, nurse entrepreneurs, nurse case managers, and legal nurse consultants.

FORENSIC NURSING

Forensic nursing is an emerging field that forms an alliance among nursing, law enforcement, and the forensic sciences. The term *forensic* means anything belonging to, or pertaining to, the law.

An Emerging Discipline

Forensic nursing, as defined by the International Association of Forensic Nurses (IAFN), is "the application of nursing science to public or legal proceedings; the application of the forensic aspects of health care combined with the bio-psycho-social education of the registered nurse (RN) in the scientific investigation and treatment of trauma and/or death of victims and perpetrators of abuse, violence, criminal activity and traumatic accidents." [1] Forensic nurses provide a continuum of care to victims and their families, beginning in the emergency room or crime scene and leading to participation in the criminal investigation and the courts of law.[1]

Nurses, particularly emergency department (ED) nurses, have long provided care to victims of domestic violence, rape, and other injuries resulting from criminal acts. They have collected, preserved, and documented legal evidence, often without formal training. It was not until 1992 that the term *forensic nursing* was coined.

What Do You Think?

Do you know any nurses who are involved in forensic nursing? Is this a role that you might be interested in pursuing after graduation?

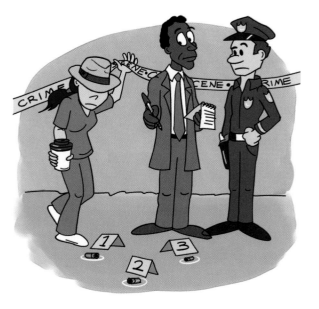

The IAFN was founded in the summer of 1992. Seventy-four nurses, primarily sexual assault nurse examiners, came together in Minneapolis, Minnesota, to develop an organization of nurses who practice within the arena of the law. This very diverse group includes, but is not limited to, legal nurse consultants, forensic nurse death investigators, forensic psychiatric nurses, and forensic correctional nurses.

The organization's membership tripled within its first year. By 1999, the IAFN had more than 1,800 members. The American Nurses Association (ANA) recognized forensic nursing as a subspecialty in 1995, and the Scope and Standards of Forensic Practice was established in 1997. Because this is a relatively new field, the definition of the forensic nurse role is continuing to evolve. With the formation of the IAFN and the designation of the forensic specialty, nurses were given an identity and recognition for a role they have long been performing.

Forensic nurses specialize in several diverse roles and are beginning to find employment in a variety of settings. These roles include the sexual assault nurse examiner (SANE), the forensic nurse death investigator, the forensic psychiatric nurse, the forensic correctional nurse, and the legal nurse consultant.

Sexual Assault Nurse Examiner

A SANE is an RN trained in the forensic examination of sexual assault victims. This person has an advanced education and clinical preparation specialized in this area.

Clients who have been sexually assaulted have unique medical, legal, and psychological needs. As crime victims, they require a competent collection of evidence that assists in both investigation and prosecution of the incident. Their bodies and clothing become a key part of the crime scene and are essential for collection of evidence. The SANE offers the type of compassionate care that is often lacking among law enforcement personnel. The care provided by SANEs has been designed to preserve the victim's dignity and reduce psychological trauma. Research data collected in recent years indicate that the SANE's comprehensive forensic evidence collection leads to more effective investigations and more successful prosecutions.[2]

Usually SANEs work in a hospital or ED with other members of a sexual assault response team (SART). The other team members may include physicians, law enforcement personnel, social workers, child and adult protective service workers, and therapists.

In their training, SANEs learn all aspects of the care of sexually assaulted clients. Their responsibilities include interviewing the victim, completing the physical examination, collecting specimens for forensic evidence, and documenting the findings. They also provide emotional support for victims and family members. When the case goes to court, the SANE testifies as an expert legal witness about how evidence was collected and the physical and psychological condition of the client. The SANE may offer an opinion as to whether a crime occurred.

To become a SANE, an RN must complete an adult/adolescent SANE education program. These programs are available through a traditional university setting and online. The training includes either a minimum of 40 contact hours of instruction or three semester units of classroom instruction by an accredited school of nursing. Trainees also must have clinical supervision until they demonstrate competency in SANE practice. After successful completion of the program, the candidate is able to take the certification examination.

Legal Nurse Consultant

The legal nurse consultant is a licensed RN who critically evaluates and analyzes health-care issues in medically related lawsuits. Because the legal system is involved, nurses acting as consultants are considered to be practicing forensics. Nurses uniquely combine their medical expertise with legal knowledge to assess compliance with accepted standards of health-care practice.

Legal nurse consultants work in collaboration with attorneys and other legal and health-care professionals. They may have independent practices, work in the hospital setting in risk management, or be employed by law firms or health insurance companies.

The following is a list of activities performed by legal nurse consultants that distinguishes their specialty practice:

1. Drafting legal documents under the supervision of an attorney
2. Interviewing witnesses
3. Educating attorneys and other involved parties on health-care issues and standards
4. Researching nursing literature, standards, and guidelines as they relate to issues within a particular case
5. Reviewing, analyzing, and summarizing medical records
6. Identifying and conferring with expert witnesses
7. Assessing causation and issues of damages as they relate to the case
8. Developing a case strategy in collaboration with other members of the legal team
9. Providing support during the legal proceedings
10. Educating and mentoring other RNs in the practice of legal nurse consulting[3]

Forensic Nurse Death Investigator

The role of the nurse death investigator is to advocate for the deceased. In general, a death investigator is a professional with experiential and scientific knowledge who can accurately determine the cause of death. The forensic nurse death investigator is an RN with specialized education who is functioning in the death investigator's role. Nurse death investigators are called upon when law enforcement suspects a death did not result from natural causes. At a natural death scene, there are usually only uniformed officers.

The forensic nurse death investigator may assume several different titles, such as forensic nurse investigator, death investigator, or deputy coroner. In some areas of the country, nurses actually practice as coroners. In the United States, there are currently no standard definitions of "nurse death investigator" or any national credentialing or education requirements. Each region of the country specifies the requirements in its own jurisdictions.

A complete death investigation must have three key elements: (1) history of the victim, including psychological, medical, and social history; (2) a detailed and thorough examination of the victim's body; and (3) a search for evidence in the immediate and extended death area. Nurses who have been trained and certified in forensic investigation and crime techniques are ideal for these types of investigations. To qualify for forensic training, the nurse should have 2 to 5 years of work experience in a critical care setting such as an ED or critical care unit, a high level of critical-thinking ability, and well-developed assessment skills. They must also be able to cope with often violent and gruesome crime scenes. (For more information on forensic education for nurses, go to http://www.nursing-school-degrees.com/Nursing-Careers/nurse-death-investigator.html.)

The basic knowledge and skills in which all nurses are educated, such as physical assessment, pharmacology, anatomy, physiology, growth, and development, are minimum requirements for the death investigation role. This nursing knowledge allows the investigator to sort out factors involved in a death. Nurses also learn advanced communication skills and knowledge of the grief process during their education. These skills are required for notifying next of kin and interviewing witnesses.[4] (For a more complete list of skill requirements for nurse death examiners, see Box 27.1.)

Nurse death investigators can use their skills in a variety of ways and at a number of locations. Work settings range from a coroner's or medical examiner's laboratory, accident sites or sites where a suspicious death has occurred, or at police precincts

B o x   2 7 . 1

Required Skills for a Forensic Nurse Death Investigator

The ability to:
- Collaborate with other disciplines and agencies.
- Use basic nursing knowledge such as anatomy, physiology, pharmacology, and communication techniques during investigations.
- Formulate insightful questions using an evidence-based practice knowledge base.
- Help families and survivors work through the grieving process.
- Know and follow state codes about obtaining evidence and submitting death reports.
- Conduct postmortem sexual assault and child abuse examinations.
- Work with organ and tissue procurement agencies to identify appropriate donors.
- Act as a liaison between medical personnel and police investigative staff.
- Identify subtle signs of abuse and neglect in children and women.

with homicide detectives. Forensic nurse death investigators have many responsibilities. They respond to scenes of deaths or accidents and work in collaboration with law enforcement. At the scene, they examine the body, pronounce death, and take tissue and blood samples. They take pictures of the body and evidence at the scene. Nurse death investigators must be able to recognize and integrate other evidence collected during the investigation, such as patterns of injury, types of wounds, and estimated time of death. They are responsible for record keeping and arranging for the transport of the body to the morgue or to the coroner's office to undergo autopsy for further examination. Nurse death investigators work with the forensic pathologist to collect additional evidence in the lab during the autopsy.

What Do You Think?

Have you ever been involved in a court case or lawsuit? What was your role? How would being a nurse trained in legal issues have changed what you did or said?

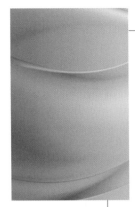

Issues in Practice

If You Were the Nurse on Duty, What Would You Do?

Below are scenarios that exemplify typical situations for the nurse in general practice. Identify your probable response. Critically analyze each situation in terms of what you know and do not know. What types of facts or skills are not part of your current knowledge base?

You are working on a maternity unit when a female inmate from a correctional institution is admitted in an advanced stage of labor. A correctional officer is in attendance; the woman is shackled at the feet and hands. As she is wheeled to the labor room, you note that the client has had 10 previous pregnancies and 4 live births.

Questions for Thought

1. What factors make the care of this woman different from that of other pregnant women?
2. Is she dangerous?
3. How do you maintain confidentiality with this client?
4. As an offender in custody, does she surrender any rights?

You work in a hospital setting that is experiencing an increase in workplace violence. Perpetrators of street, child, and domestic violence often follow their victims to the hospital and continue to pose a significant threat to the whole hospital community. It is important to assess the potential for violence.

Questions for Thought

1. How will you contribute to the reduction of risk in the workplace?
2. Identify risk factors and cues for violence.
3. How would you implement strategies to assist violence management in the acute care setting?

A halfway house for paroled offenders is due to be constructed in your community. Residents are angry and afraid to have ex-convicts living in their neighborhood. A town meeting is scheduled in which the issue will be discussed. Does nursing have anything to contribute to the discussion?

Questions for Thought

1. What do we know about mentally ill offenders, sex offenders, perpetrators of domestic violence, and others?
2. What is the therapeutic outcome for those mentally ill offenders who have completed rehabilitation programs?
3. What is the risk to the community?
4. What stress management strategies are helpful to a community?

Issues in Practice continued

You work at a junior high school, providing sex education and health promotion programs for young teenagers. You notice that more and more young people are wearing gang colors and using gang-related language and hand signals.

Questions for Thought

1. How does this affect your work?
2. Does this change your priorities?
3. Are there referrals or strategies that should be initiated because of the gang affiliations of your students?

Forensic Psychiatric Nurse

Forensic psychiatric nurses work with individuals who have mental health needs and who have entered the legal system. These nurses generally practice in state psychiatric institutions, jails, and prisons.

Nurses in this role perform physical and psychiatric assessments and develop care plans for the clients entrusted to their care. At the most basic level, forensic psychiatric nurses assist clients with self-care, administer medical care and treatment, and monitor the effectiveness of the treatment. Psychiatric interventions are developed to promote coping skills and improve mental health in a therapeutic environment.[5]

Forensic psychiatric nurses may also have advanced practice certification. RNs who have master's degrees in psychiatric–mental health nursing practice work as clinical nurse specialists or nurse practitioners. Nurses in this role are able to diagnose and treat individuals with psychiatric disorders and often are allowed to prescribe medications. They may function as primary care medical and mental health providers, psychotherapists, and consultants. Advanced practice forensic psychiatric nurses may practice independently or in mental health centers, state facilities, and health maintenance organizations (HMOs).

> *Legal nurse consultants work in collaboration with attorneys and other legal and health-care professionals. They may have independent practices, work in the hospital setting in risk management, or be employed by law firms or health insurance companies.*

Forensic Correctional Nurse

Correctional facilities reflect the demographics of the general population, with an increasingly aging incarcerated population who have age-related health-care problems. Forensic correctional nurses provide health care for inmates in correctional facilities such as juvenile centers, jails, and prisons. They manage acute and chronic illness, develop health-care plans, dispense medications, and perform health screenings and health education. Forensic correctional nurses conduct psychiatric assessments and respond to emergency situations. The role of the forensic correctional nurse offers a high level of autonomy compared with other nursing roles.

Evolving Requirements

There is no official certification as a forensic nurse in the United States except for the SANE certification.

Many nurses working in forensic roles believe certification requirements will develop as the specialty of forensic nursing continues to evolve and becomes better defined. In the near future, nursing education will be required to develop classes that teach forensic nursing as a part of their curriculum.

NURSE ENTREPRENEUR

An entrepreneur is someone who establishes and runs his or her own business. A nurse entrepreneur starts a business by combining nursing experience and knowledge with business knowledge.

Should You Be Your Own Boss?

Starting a business can be risky financially and certainly is far different from the nurse's traditional role as an employee in an institution. However, nurses are educated to think independently and are sometimes willing to take risks for the benefit of their clients. As professionals who can translate their expertise and confidence into new arenas, nurses are capable of achieving personal and financial success running their own businesses.[6]

Historically, nurse-run businesses have usually focused on temporary staffing agencies, nursing education, or consultant roles. Nurse entrepreneurs can also include nurse attorneys, nurse case managers, nurse educators, nurse death investigators, nurse midwives, nurse paralegals, psychiatric nurses, legal nurse consultants, and sexual assault nurses. Nurse practitioners in rural areas set up their own primary care clinics and provide care for populations that do not have access to any other type of primary care.

Assess Your Nursing Skills

In making the decision to start a business, nurses need to first assess their nursing experience to determine what type of business would be appropriate for their skill set and knowledge levels. For example, a SANE may contract services to EDs or law enforcement agencies. A critical care nurse may start a home care agency offering high-tech services. Nurses may develop self-defense courses they can market to high-risk professions, such as forensic psychiatric and forensic correctional nurses.

After nurses determine what skills and knowledge they possess, they need to develop a plan on how to establish the business. A basic level of knowledge about finances and the business start-up process is essential for success. The hopeful entrepreneur needs to consider the customer who will be seeking his or her services, what customers need and desire, what start-up costs will be, and who the competition may be. Answering these questions will allow the nurse to assess the potential success of the business.[7]

Any nurse can start a business. Generally, no advanced degrees are required unless the business involves diagnosis and treatment. Key qualities needed for success are a high degree of self-motivation and a passion for the business to succeed. Nurse entrepreneurs are limited only by their creativity and desire to succeed.

CASE MANAGEMENT

Other titles for this position are care coordinator, care manager, transitional care coordinator, nurse care coordinator, and client care coordinator. The Case Management Society of America (CMSA) defines case management as "a collaborative process of assessment, planning, facilitation and advocacy for options and services to meet an individual's health needs through communication and available resources to promote quality, cost-effective outcomes."[8] Effective collaboration among all members of the health-care team is essential to meet the needs of clients in today's complex heath-care system.

A Care Coordinator

In the era of health-care reform, nurse case managers are serving a larger role than previously experienced. The Patient Protection and Affordable Care Act of 2010 includes the Hospital Consumer Assessment of Healthcare Providers and Systems Survey (HCAHPS) among the methods that are being used to calculate value-based incentive payments. The HCAHPS survey asks discharged clients 27 questions that help evaluate their stay in the facility. It is administered randomly between 48 hours and 6 weeks after discharge. Hospitals must submit the results of the HCAHPS survey to receive their full inpatient prospective payment system (IPPS) annual increases in funding. This evaluation system has broad implications for case managers in controlling the resources used in client diagnosis and treatment. They have a key role in ensuring that preadmission tests and results are communicated throughout the health-care system so the unnecessary tests are not replicated.[9]

Nurse case managers act as advocates for clients and their families by coordinating care and linking the client with the physician, other members of the health-care team, resources, and the payer. The goal of the nurse case manager is to help the client obtain high-quality, cost-effective care while preventing the duplication and fragmentation of care. Research data indicate that active participation by a nurse case manager in the care of a client positively affects the client's outcomes.

> *The role of the forensic correctional nurse offers a high level of autonomy compared with other nursing roles.*

What Do You Think?

Do you know any nurses with the title of "case manager"? Interview them and note what duties they perform as part of their roles.

Nurses are uniquely prepared by their education and professional experiences to fulfill the role of case manager. The holistic health-care approach has been an underlying principle of nursing care since the time of Florence Nightingale. Nurses have experience in arranging referrals, providing client education, and acting as a liaison between physicians and specialty care.

Any client who may face challenges regarding care and recovery can benefit from case management. Included are hospitalized clients, those with complex medical conditions, those requiring specialty care, and those who have personal or psychological circumstances that may interfere with recovery.

Factors that indicate the need for a nurse case manager include:

1. A complex treatment plan that requires coordination or a plan that is unclear.
2. An injury or illness that may permanently prevent the client from returning to his or her previous level of health.
3. A preexisting medical condition that may complicate or prolong recovery.
4. A need for assistance in accessing health-care resources.
5. Environmental stressors that may interfere with recovery.

Physicians Catch Up

The CMSA Standards of Practice for Case Management cite the physician and case manager collaboration as essential for successful case management. Although recent research shows that clients benefit from case management, it has been underused by physicians. Case managers and physicians met in 2003 to identify barriers to the use of case management and to explore ways to increase the use of case managers. One result of this meeting was the development of the "Consensus Paper of 2003 Physician and Case Management Summit: Exploring Best Practices in Physician and Case Management Collaboration to Improve Patient Care." This paper identified both barriers and ways to promote effective, collaborative use of case management by physicians (Box 27.2).

The research that attributes improved client outcomes directly to case management is compelling. It appears that nurse case managers will continue to expand their role in the health-care system of the future.

NURSE NAVIGATOR

Although the nurse navigator role is similar to the case manager, it tends to be more focused on only one specialty area, such as cancer clients. The role revolves around clients and families to help them deal with complex care issues. The nurse navigator attempts to eliminate barriers and serves as an advocate for the client to make moving through the treatment maze easier. Some of the obstacles that clients must face include lack of transportation, a myriad of confusing insurance forms, change in financial status,

---

Box 27.2

Collaboration of Case Managers and Physicians

Barriers to the Use of Case Managers by Physicians

1. Lack of resources and financial incentives in medical practice to integrate case management
2. Resistance to change by, and time pressures imposed on, physicians
3. Insufficient awareness of the role of the case manager among physicians and consumers
4. Insufficient promotion of their value by case managers
5. Lack of evidence of the value of case management

Facilitators of the Use of Case Managers by Physicians

1. Recognition, understanding, and use of case management
2. Standardization of the education and definition of case managers
3. Education for physicians and consumers about case management
4. Compensation for physicians who use case manager services
5. Education of clients in accessing case management
6. Validated research on the effectiveness of case management
7. Recognition of the CMSA Standards of Practice for legitimacy and credibility of the nurse case manager role

---

lack of knowledge about the disease and its treatment options, and the side effects of powerful medications. The nurse navigator also works with the client's family, caregivers, and employers to help reduce the client's anxiety and/or depression.[10]

After receiving a referral from a physician, the nurse navigator contacts the client and together they develop an individual plan of care that addresses the client's particular needs. This referral can even be before the client undergoes surgery or first treatments. The nurse navigator takes into consideration the client's perceptions and beliefs about the disease process and the modalities of treatment. It is important that the client maintains a sense of empowerment while undergoing treatment. Regular contact is maintained with the client throughout the treatment regime by personal contact, phone, or e-mail. The client is reassured that the nurse navigator is available to answer any questions or concerns at any time.

Oftentimes, office appointments can trigger anxiety and can be confusing for a client. In those cases, the nurse navigator will accompany the client to the office or clinic to reduce their apprehension and help them understand the treatments or instructions they receive. The nurse navigator also may write up a summary of the interaction with the care provider so they can better remember the instructions given and the date and time for the next appointment.[10] An interprofessional approach to care is used by involving other members of the health-care team such as a social worker, financial counselor, dietician, chaplain, and, if needed, a mental professional. Subsequently, the client is encouraged to participate in rehabilitation programs and other support services.

Nurses who choose this role find it very rewarding. They observe clients go from the depths of treatment and illness to a new state of wellness. Average salaries for nurse navigators depend on the national region but generally range between $57,000 to $74,000 annually.[11] Although there are a number of specialty nurse navigator organizations, general information can be found at http://www.nursenavigator.com.

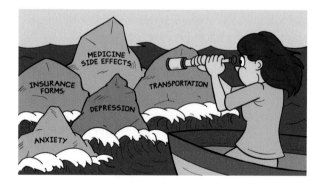

NURSE CODER

Most of the time, nurses do not really think much about the process that allows them to be paid. They get their money direct-deposited into their bank accounts periodically, and as long as it shows up, they do not ask questions. However, the process is much

more complicated. The reimbursement systems used to pay facilities for individual clients from insurance companies and the government are dependent on a coding system for diseases and injuries. Each client is assigned a code or several codes when they are treated. The old coding system (ICD-9) that has been in use for many years was to be replaced October 1, 2013, by a new system, ICD-10, which is much more complicated; however, it was delayed by the Senate for at least 1 year. The number of codes in the ICD-9 system was 14,000. The ICD-10 system has over 70,000 codes. This increase in codes provides for more precise identification of illness, but it also complicates the process immensely.[12] For example, there were about 25 codes used for a knee injury under ICD-9; with ICD-10, that number increases to almost 700.

Although this switch is going to be immeasurably challenging for hospitals and other health-care providers to master, it does open up the door for new nursing roles—certified RN-coders and certified RN-auditors. Because the changes are much more complicated, the knowledge and expertise of nurses will be a remarkable asset.[12]

The origins of the American Association of Clinical Coders and Auditors (AACCA) can be traced back to 2003 when a group of RNs who held MS and PhD degrees, in conjunction with several physicians and a physician's assistant, met to discuss how to improve the quality of coding. Mistakes in coding were costing health-care facilities huge sums of money from third-party payers. The group came up with the idea of certifying individuals who were doing coding by providing a valid test of their coding knowledge and skills. The test would also determine if they were in compliance with the coding rules and documentation, which would help to reduce fraud and abuse of the system. They established a bank of questions and tested them for validity and reliability. Currently, the AACCA has over 4,000 members and has tested/credentialed 3,682 members, 99 percent of whom are RNs. Certification testing is online and results are provided immediately after test completion.

There are training courses for coders online and in person. These courses vary in length from a few weeks full-time to as much as 15 weeks taking classes one day a week.[13] The cost is rather high, ranging from around $1,000 on the low end to $4,000 on the high end. Most of high-end courses include the cost of the certification examination, which is around

$399 for members of the AACCA or $1,200 for non-members. Some colleges and universities offer a BS degree in coding. (For more information, go to http://www.aacca.net/certification.html.)

Nurse coding positions, analyzed by the U.S. Bureau of Labor Statistics (BLS) (http://www.bls.gov), found a faster than average job growth rate, about 20 percent, between 2008 and 2014. Job growth is due in part to an aging population and the transition to the new ICD-10 program. Use of more advanced electronic technology also contributes to the growth in the market for professional coders. The BLS reported that nurse coders' annual wages started at $40,610 a year. The lowest salaries for coders were in the $20,000 a year range, with salaries for experienced coders being $50,000 or higher.[14]

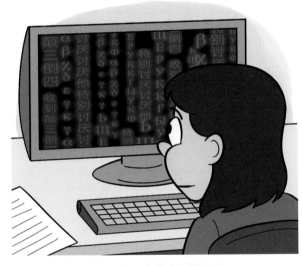

NURSE CODERS DECODE
CONFUSING HEALTH INFORMATION.

CLIENT SAFETY OFFICER

Also known as a client safety nurse, RNs in this position work to lower the risk factors that cause poor or adverse client outcomes. Unlike traditional quality assurance programs that focus primarily on satisfying the Joint Commission and the requirements of other regulatory bodies, client safety officers plan and implement protocols and procedures to eliminate health-care errors. Under the auspices of the National Patient Safety Foundation (NPSF), these nurses provide a more comprehensive approach to safety, including reporting and analyzing adverse events, looking for trends, implementing risk-reduction activities, and developing medication error reduction strategies. They also monitor the effectiveness of the protocols and maintain systems that increase client safety.[15]

One of the most difficult elements of the role is attempting to change the traditional health-care culture that attributes errors in client care to carelessness and incompetence. The client safety officer attempts to establish a new culture of safety in which both individual health-care providers and the organization as a whole see safety in all elements of care. The institution collectively must have an awareness of client safety and make it a part of their mission. An important part of their role is to educate other nurses on the causes of errors and how to eliminate them using evidence-based safety strategies. Although the position can be filled by a relatively new graduate RN, nurses with experience in risk management and quality assurance are frequently recruited for the role.

With the various reports from the Institute of Medicine (IOM) demonstrating an excess of 90,000 deaths per year caused by medical errors, client safety and quality assurance have become a major concern. The client safety officer role evolved from the IOM's goals for high-quality care, including safe, effective, client-centered, timely, efficient, and equitable care.

Traditionally, nursing students were taught the bare minimum about client safety in their classes (see Chapter 14). Although this trend is beginning to wane, most nurses in practice today learned about safety and its application to health care while on the job. In many of the larger health-care facilities, nurse safety officers are required to have an MS in nursing or a higher degree. They also need to take and pass the client safety examination to become certified.

In smaller facilities, the client safety officer often fills one or more roles at the same time, such as infection control or nurse educator. In larger facilities, the client safety officer position may be the only job the nurse has. In extremely large facilities, several client safety officers may be assigned to individual units where there tends to be high error rates with poor outcomes, such as the emergency room, intensive care unit, or the obstetrical unit. Insurance companies and law firms may also hire certified client safety nurses to use their expertise in reducing costly lawsuits and injury settlements.[16]

Most nurses in the safety officer role have a high degree of satisfaction with their position. They get to observe the decrease in errors and the overall increase in safety and quality of care. Because they are usually classified as administration, salaries for client safety officers range from around $50,000 a year to over $80,000 per year. More information can be found at the National Patient Safety Foundation website at http://www.npsf.org.

Conclusion

Florence Nightingale wrote in 1859 that "no man, not even a doctor, ever gives any other definition of what a nurse should be than this 'devoted and obedient.' This definition would do just as well for a porter. It might even do for a horse!"[17] The profession of nursing has come a long way since Nightingale made the first efforts to move it out of its position of servitude to physicians.

Nursing is constantly evolving and defining itself as it strives to include expanded roles of practice. Of the many new and exciting roles for nurses, forensic, legal consultant, entrepreneur, case management, nurse navigator, nurse coder, and nurse safety officer have developed in response to the needs of society.

Although nurses have practiced in these areas for many years, they are only now beginning to be recognized for the unique skills and qualities they bring to these roles. For example, the job description of an emergency department nurse has long included interviews with and assessments of crime victims, collection and proper handling of evidence, and accurate and complete documentation of injuries and information provided by crime victims. In the role of client advocate, nurses have always been case managers through assessment of client needs, coordination of referrals for specialized or long-term care, and coordination of non-nursing services such as diet teaching and social services.

All nurses have the knowledge of anatomy, physiology, growth, and development that is required for the death examiner position. As more nurses seek the specialized training now available for many of these roles and obtain nationally recognized certification as a demonstration of their knowledge, they will gain acceptance as highly qualified and valuable members of these specialized health-care teams.

ASSOCIATIONS AND WEBSITES

American Academy of Forensic Sciences: http://www.aafs.org
American Association of Legal Nurse Consultants: http://www.aalnc.org
American College of Forensic Examiners Institute: http://www.acfei.com
American Forensic Nurses: http://www.amrn.com
American Psychiatric Nurses Association: http://www.apna.org
International Association of Forensic Nurses: http://www.forensicnurse.org or http://www.iafn.org
Journal of Forensic Nursing: http://journals.lww.com/forensicnursing/pages/default.aspx
Legal Nurse Consultant Certificate Program: http://www.aalnc.org/page/ALNCCCertBoard
National Alliance of Sexual Assault Coalitions: http://www.endsexualviolence.org/who-we-are/about-naesv
National Association of Correctional Nursing: http://www.correctionalnursing.org
National Commission on Correctional Health Care: http://www.ncchc.org
National Nurses in Business Association: http://www.nnba.net
Nurse Entrepreneur Network: http://www.Nurse-Entrepreneur-Network.com
Nursing Entrepreneur: http://www.nursingentrepreneurs.com
Office for Victims of Crime: http://www.ojp.usdoj.gov/ovc
Office for Victims of Crime Resource Center: http://www.ncjrs.org
Public Health Functions Projects: http://www.health.gov/phfunctions/public.htm
Rape, Abuse, and Incest National Network (RAINN): http://www.rainn.org
Sexual Assault Resource Service (SARS): http://www.sane-sart.com
Violence Against Women Office: http://www.ovw.usdoj.gov

Critical-Thinking Exercises

APPLICATION OF HUMAN RIGHTS

What information do you need to make a decision? Explore applications of human rights from the point of view of the victim and the perpetrator of the crime. Think about how the issue of human rights would be defined and protected in the following examples. What is the nurse's role?

- A married father of two, an upstanding member of the community, is accused of child molestation and is admitted to the unit for psychiatric evaluation and submission of tissue samples.
- A female inmate becomes pregnant in prison and does not want anyone to know who the father is.
- A young man has a history of substance abuse and mental illness. He refuses medication to control psychotic behavior and is confined in a forensic psychiatric facility because of the claim that he is incompetent to stand trial for car theft.
- A mother of an infant is being interviewed in a suspected child abuse case. She admits that she was sexually and physically abused as a child and throughout her marriage. The priority is to establish her role in the current charges involving injury of her 3-month-old infant.

References

1. Sekula LK, Colbert AM, Zoucha R, Amar AF, Williams J. Strengthening the science of forensic nursing through education and research. *Journal of Forensic Nursing,* 8(1):1–2, 2012.

2. Maier SL. Sexual assault nurse examiners' perceptions of their relationship with doctors, rape victim advocates, police, and prosecutors. *Journal of Interpersonal Violence,* 27(7):1314–1340, 2012.

3. Lukinovich LA, Couvillon J. Evidence-based practice for the legal nurse consultant. *Journal of Legal Nurse Consulting,* 21(3):3–7, 2010.

4. Grinstein-Cohen O, Sarid O. A case report of gunshot terror attack in pregnancy: Implications for forensic nursing. *Journal of Forensic Nursing,* 8(3):138–143, 2012.

5. Rose DN, Peter E, Gallop R, Angus JE, Liaschenko J. Respect in forensic psychiatric nurse-patient relationships: A practical compromise. *Journal of Forensic Nursing,* 7(1):3–16, 2011.

6. Danna D, Porche D. The NP entrepreneur: Nurse entrepreneur as a global executive. *Journal for Nurse Practitioners,* 5(6): 454–455, 2010.

7. Question and Answer with Anthony J. Hall, RN, BSN, nursing entrepreneur and charge nurse in behavioral health. *NEWS-Line for Nurses,* 14(1F):4–7, 2013.

8. Corvol A, Moutel G, Gagnon D, Nugue M, Saint-Jean O, Somme D. Ethical issues in the introduction of case management for elderly people. *Nursing Ethics,* 20(1):83–95, 2013.

9. Cesta Toni. The role of case management in an era of healthcare reform—Part 3. *Hospital Case Management,* 20(9): 135–138, 2012.

10. Horner K, Ludman EJ, McCorkle R, et al. An oncology nurse navigator program designed to eliminate gaps in early cancer care. *Clinical Journal of Oncology Nursing,* 17(1):43–48, 2013.

11. Patient Navigator Salary. CareerBuilder.com. Retrieved April 2013 from http://salary.careerbuilder.com/Patient-Navigator/?bdint=decline

12. Bounos MT. Why ICD10 is the BIGGEST Opportunity for RNs! Retrieved 2013 from http://www.aacca.net/icd10opportunityforrns.html

13. Wexler JM. Code green or why every RN should know how to code. Nurse Entrepreneur Network, 2013. Retrieved April 2013 from http://www.nurse-entrepreneur-network.com/public/403.cfm

14. U.S. Bureau of Labor Statistics. Retrieved April 2013 from http://www.bls.gov

15. Shulkin DJ. Interview with a quality leader: John J. Kelly, MD, on quality and patient safety. *Journal for Healthcare Quality: Promoting Excellence in Healthcare,* 35(2):47–49, 2013.

16. Nedved P, Chaudhry R, Pilipczuk D, Shah S. Impact of the unit-based patient safety officer. *Journal of Nursing Administration,* 42(9):431–434, 2012.

17. Nightingale F. *Notes on Nursing.* Oxford, UK: Dover, 1860.

abandonment Leaving a client without the client's permission; terminating the professional relationship without providing for appropriate continued or follow-up care by another equally qualified professional.

accountability Concept that each individual is responsible for his or her own actions and the consequence of those actions; professional accountability implies a responsibility to perform the activities and duties of the profession according to established standards.

accreditation Approval of a program or institution by a voluntary professional organization to provide specific education or service programs.

act Legislation that has become law.

active euthanasia Acts performed to help end a sick person's life.

acute-severe condition Health problem of sudden onset; a serious illness or condition.

adaptation Process of exchange between a person and the environment to maintain or regain personal integrity; the key principle in the Roy Model of Nursing.

administrative A governmental agency that implements legislation.

administrative rule or regulation An operating procedure that describes how a government agency implements the intent of a statute; state boards of nursing implement the nurse practice act.

advanced nursing education Master's- or doctoral-level education that provides knowledge and skills in areas such as research, education, administration, or clinical specialties.

advanced placement A process by which a student is given credit for a required course through transfer or examination rather than by enrolling in and completing the course.

advanced practice Extended role; increased responsibilities and actions undertaken by an individual because of additional education and experience; nurse practitioners are advanced practice nurses.

advocate One who pleads for a cause or proposal; one who acts on behalf of another.

affective domain objectives Goals established in conjunction with the client that are directed toward changing feelings, values, and attitudes necessary for a positive effect on the client's health.

affidavit Written, sworn statement.

affiliation agreement A formal agreement between an educational institution and another agency that agrees to provide clinical areas for student practice.

aggressiveness Harsh behavior that may result in physical or emotional harm to others.

ambulatory care center Type of primary care facility that provides treatment on an outpatient basis.

answer Document filed in the court by the defendant in response to the complaint.

anxiety Uneasiness or apprehension caused by an impending threat or fear of the unknown.

apathy Lack of interest.

appeal Request to a higher court to review a decision in the hopes of changing the ruling of a lower court.

appellant Person who seeks an appeal.

arbitrator Neutral third party who assesses facts independently of the judicial system.

articulation Type of education program that allows easy entry from one level to another; for example, many BSN programs have articulation for nurses with associate degrees.

artificial insemination Insertion of sperm into the uterus with a syringe.

assault An overt threat to violate the a person's right to self determination or an overt threat of bodily harm coupled with an apparent, present ability to cause the harm. The actual production of harm is *battery*.

assertiveness Ability to express thoughts, feelings, and ideas openly and directly without fear.

assessment Process of collecting information about a client to help plan care.

assignment Designating tasks for ancillary personnel that fall under their *own level of practice* according to facility policies, position descriptions, and, if applicable, state practice act.

associate degree nursing program Type of nursing education program that leads to an associate degree with a major in nursing; usually located in a community or junior college, these programs normally last 2 years.

asymmetrical information The use of multiple data sources in economics and business that produces a better understanding of day-to-day economic activity.

audit Close review of records or documents to detect the presence or absence of specific information.

auscultation Assessment technique that requires listening with a stethoscope to various parts of the body to detect sounds produced by organs.

authoritarian Type of leadership style in which the leader gives orders, makes decisions for the group as a whole, and bears most of the responsibility for the outcomes. Also called autocratic, directive, or controlling.

autonomy State of being self-directed or independent; the ability to make decisions about one's future.

autopsy Examination of a body after passing to determine the cause of death.

baccalaureate degree nursing program Type of nursing education program that leads to the bachelor's degree with a major in nursing; usually located in a college or university, the length of the program is 4 years.

bargaining agent Organization certified by a governmental agency to represent a group of employees for the purpose of collective bargaining.

baseline data Initial information obtained about a client that establishes the norms for comparison as the client's condition changes.

basic human rights Those considerations society deems reasonably expected for all people: right to self-determination, protection from discomfort and harm, dignity, fair treatment, and privacy.

battery Nonconsensual touching of another person that does not necessarily cause harm or injury.

behavior modification Method to change behavior through rewards for positive behavior.

behaviorism Psychological theory based on the belief that all behavior is learned over time through conditioning.

belief Expectations or judgments based on attitude verified by experiences.

benchmarking Written outcome standards used to classify acceptable levels of performance to maintain high quality care.

beneficence Ethical principle based on the beliefs that the health-care provider should do no harm, prevent harm, remove existing harm, and promote the good and well-being of the client.

bereavement State of sadness brought on by the loss or death of a loved one.

bill Proposed law that is moving through the legislative process.

bill of rights List of statements that outline the claims and privileges of a particular group, such as the Client's Bill of Rights.

bioethical issues Issues that deal with the health, safety, life, and death of human beings, often arising from advances in medical science and technology.

biofeedback Ability to control autonomic responses in the body through conscious effort.

Biological Aerosol Warning System (BAWS) A high-tech biological agent detection device that is capable of detecting biological agents in the environment.

bioterrorism The use of microorganisms with the deliberate intent of causing infection to achieve military or political goals.

Black belts Individuals certified as Six Sigma Consultants through the Institute of Industrial Engineers or the American Society for Quality who are trained employees of Six Sigma working as well-paid consultants for hospitals and other institutions.

body substance isolation (BSI) Universal precautions; guidelines established by the Centers for Disease Control and Prevention (CDC) and the Occupational Safety and Health Administration (OSHA) to protect health-care professionals and the client from diseases carried in the blood and body fluids, such as HIV and hepatitis B; involves the use of gloves whenever one is in contact with blood or body fluids and the use of masks, gowns, and eye covers if a chance of aerosol contact with fluids exists.

brain death Irreversible destruction of the cerebral cortex and brain stem manifested by absence of all reflexes; absence of brain waves on an electroencephalogram.

breach of contract Failure by one of the parties in a contract to fulfill all the terms of the agreement.

bullying A type of uncivil behavior that could reasonably be considered humiliating, intimidating, threatening or demeaning to an individual or group of individuals. It can occur anywhere and at times becomes habitual, being repeated over and over.

burden of proof Requirement that the plaintiff submit sufficient evidence to prove a defendant's guilt.

burnout syndrome A state of emotional exhaustion that results from the accumulative stress of an individual's life, including work, personal, and family responsibilities.

cadaver donor Clinically or brain-dead individual who previously agreed to allow organs to be taken for transplantation.

capitated payment system System of reimbursement in which a flat fee is paid for health-care services for a prescribed period of time. Expenses incurred in excess of this fee are provider losses.

capricious Unpredictable; arbitrary.

career ladder Articulation of educational programs that permit advancement from a lower level to a higher level without loss of credit or repetition of coursework.

career mobility Opportunity for individuals in one occupational area to move to another without restrictions.

case management Health-care delivery in which a client advocate or health-care coordinator helps the client through the hospitalization to obtain the most appropriate care.

case manager Health-care provider who coordinates cost-effective quality care for individuals who are generally at high risk and require long-term complex services.

certification Official recognition of a degree of education and skills in a profession by a national specialty organization; recognition that an institution has met standards that allow it to deliver certain services.

challenge examination Examination that assesses levels of knowledge or skill to grant credit for previous learning and experience; passing a challenge examination gives the individual credit for a course not actually taken.

chart Legal document that contains all the pertinent information about a client who is in a hospital or clinic; usually includes medical and nursing history, medical and nursing diagnosis, laboratory test results, notes about the client's progress, physician's orders, and personal data.

charting Process of recording (written or computer-generated) specific information about the client in the chart or medical record.

civil law Law concerned with the violation of the rights of one individual by another; it includes contract law, treaty law, tax law, and tort law.

claims-made policy Type of malpractice insurance that protects only against claims made during the time the policy is in effect.

client More modern term for patient; an individual seeking or receiving health-related services.

client goal Statement about a desired change, outcome, or activity that a client should achieve by a specific time.

clinical education Hands-on part of a nursing program that allows the student to practice skills on actual clients under the supervision of a nursing instructor.

clinical forensic nurse Professional nurse who specializes in management of crime victims from trauma to trial through collection of evidence, assessment of victims, or making judgments related to client treatment associated with court-related issues.

clinical ladder Type of performance evaluation and career advancement in which nursing positions for direct client care have two or more progressive levels of required skill leading to advancement in salary and responsibility; it allows nurses to remain in direct client care while making career advancements rather than having to move into administration.

clinical pathways Case-management protocols used to enhance quality of care, encourage cost-effectiveness, and promote efficiency.

closed system System that does not exchange energy, matter, or information with the environment or with other systems.

code of ethics Written values of a profession that act as guidelines for professional behavior.

cognitive domain objectives Most basic type of objectives for client learning that merely outline the knowledge that will be taught to the client.

collective bargaining Negotiations for wages, hours, benefits, and working conditions for a group of employees.

collective bargaining unit Group of employees recognized as representatives of the majority, with the right to bargain collectively with their employer and to reach an agreement on the terms of a contract.

committee Group of legislators, in the House or Senate, assigned to analyze bills on a particular subject.

common law Law based on past judicial judgments made in similar cases.

community rating A method of calculating health insurance premium costs that is based on the risk factors attributed to all people in a particular region or the nation as a whole. It requires the health insurance company to charge everyone in the group the same rates and prevents them from changing rates based on the history of claims or the health status of any one or small group of individuals. It is rarely used in the private insurance market but widely used by the government.

comparable worth Method for determining employees' salaries within an organization so that the same salary is paid for all jobs that have equivalent educational requirements, responsibilities, and complexity regardless of external market factors.

compensatory damages Awards that cover the actual cost of injuries and economic losses caused by the injury in a law suit including all medical expenses related to the injury and any lost wages or income that resulted from extended hospitalization or recovery period. Also called actual damages.

competencies Behaviors, skills, attitudes, and knowledge that an individual or professional has or is expected to have.

competency-based education Courses or programs based on anticipated student outcomes.

Competency Outcomes Performance Assessment (COPA) model An assessment tool used by medical schools and some schools of nursing to validate the skills and knowledge of their graduates and promote competency for clinical practice at all levels.

complaint Legal document filed by a plaintiff to initiate a lawsuit, claiming that the plaintiff's legal rights have been violated.

compliance Voluntary following of a prescribed plan of care or treatment regimen.

computer technology Use of highly advanced technological equipment to store, process, and access a vast amount of information.

concept Abstract idea or image.

conceptual framework Concept, theory, or basic idea around which an educational program is organized and developed.

conceptual model Group of concepts, ideas, or theories that are interrelated but in which the relationship is not clearly defined.

confidentiality Right of the client to expect the communication with a professional to remain unshared with any other person unless a medical reason exists or unless the safety of the public is threatened.

conflict management The use of interpersonal communication skills and reason to reduce the tension and disagreement between employees who hold strong opinions and views about a particular project or idea with the goal of achieving conflict resolution.

conflict resolution Using conflict management skills to bring together individuals or groups who disagree so that conflicts are resolved fairly and closure is achieved on the disagreement, moving the group towards achievement of the ultimate goal.

consensus General agreement between two or more individuals or groups regarding beliefs or positions on an issue or finding.

consent Voluntary permission given by a competent person.

consortium Two or more agencies that share sponsorship of a program or an institution.

constitutional law Law contained within a federal or state constitution.

continuing care Nursing care generally provided in geriatric day-care centers or in the homes of elderly clients.

continuing education Formal education programs and informal learning experiences that maintain and increase the nurse's knowledge and skills in specific areas.

continuing education unit (CEU) Specific unit of credit earned by participating in an approved continuing education program.

continuous quality improvement (CQI) Type of total quality management whose primary goal is the improvement of the quality of health care.

contract Legally binding agreement between two or more parties.

contractual obligation Duty to perform a service identified by a contract.

copayment Percentage of the cost of a medical expense that is not covered by insurance and must be paid by the client.

core curriculum Curriculum design that enables a student to leave a career program at various levels, with a career attained and with the option to continue at another higher level or career; it is organized around a central or core body of knowledge common to the profession.

coroner Elected public official, usually a physician, who investigates deaths from unnatural causes, including homicide, violence, suicide, and other suspicious circumstances.

correctional/institutional nurse Registered nurse who specializes in the health care of those in custody in secure settings such as jails or prisons.

credentialing Process whereby individuals, programs, or institutions are designated as having met minimal standards for the safety and welfare of the public.

crime Violation of criminal law.

criminal action Process by which a person charged with a crime is accused, tried, and punished.

criminal law Law concerned with violation of criminal statutes or laws.

criterion-referenced examination Test that compares an individual's knowledge to a predetermined standard rather than to the performance of others who take the same test.

critical discernment The ability to sift through and carefully assess all available and credible research findings by analysis and judgment so that recommendations for using the best practice techniques can be made on the basis of best evidence.

critical incident stress debriefing (CISD) A process to help health-care providers deal with major acts of violence and trauma. The process is performed by teams of mental health professionals specially trained in crisis intervention, stress management, and treating post-traumatic stress disorder with the goal of encouraging the participants to verbalize their feelings and thoughts, identify and develop their coping skills, and generally lower overall grief and anxiety levels.

critical thinking The intellectual process of rationally examining ideas, inferences, assumptions, principles, arguments, conclusions, issues, statements, beliefs, and actions for which all the relevant information may not be available. This process involves the ability to use the five types of reasoning (scientific, deductive, inductive, informal, practical) in application of the nursing process, decision-making, and resolution of ambiguous issues.

cultural competence The provision of effective care for clients who belong to diverse cultures, based on the nurse's knowledge and understanding of the values, customs, beliefs, and practices of the culture.

cultural synergy The commitment that health-care providers make not only to learn about other cultures but also to immerse themselves in those cultures. Nurses achieve cultural synergy when they begin to

selectively include values, customs, and beliefs of other cultures in their own world views.

curriculum Group of courses that prepare an individual for a specific degree or profession.

customary, prevailing, and reasonable charges The typical rate in a specific locale that payers traditionally reimburse physicians.

damages Money awarded to a plaintiff by a court in a lawsuit that covers the actual costs incurred by the plaintiff.

dashboards Electronic tools that act as a scorecard providing retrospective or real-time data to assess the quality of client care and assisting the process of quality improvement.

database Information collected by a computer program on a specific topic in a specified format.

death panels The false belief that the Affordable Care Act had groups of individuals who would decide which persons should live and which should die as a cost-saving measure.

defamation of character Communication of information that is false or detrimental to a person's reputation.

defendant Person accused of criminal or civil wrongdoing. A party to a lawsuit against whom the complaint is served.

delegation Assignment of specific duties by one individual to another individual.

democratic Type of leadership style in which the leader shares the planning, decision-making, and responsibilities for outcomes with the other members of the group. Also called participative leadership.

deontology Ethical system based on the principle that the right action is guided by a set of unchanging rules.

dependent practitioner Provider of care who delivers health care under the supervision of another health-care practitioner; for example, a physician's assistant is supervised by a physician, or an LPN is supervised by an RN.

deposition Sworn statement by a witness that is made outside the courtroom; sworn depositions may be admitted as evidence in court when the individual is unable to be present.

diagnosis Statement that describes or identifies a client problem and is based on a thorough assessment.

diagnosis-related groups (DRGs) Prospective payment method used by the U.S. government and many insurance companies that pay a flat fee for treatment of a person with a particular diagnosis.

differentiated practice Organizational process of defining nursing roles based on education, experience, and training.

dilemma Predicament in which a choice must be made between two or more equally balanced alternatives; it often occurs when attempting to make ethical decisions.

directed services Health-care activities that require contact between a health-care professional and a client.

discharge planning Assessment of anticipated client needs after discharge from the hospital and development of a plan to meet those needs before the client is discharged.

disease Illness; a functional disturbance resulting from an individual organism's inability to adapt to certain stressors; an abnormal physiologic state caused by microorganisms, cancer, or other conditions.

distributive justice Ethical principle based on the belief that the right action is determined by that which will provide an outcome equal for all persons and will also benefit the least fortunate.

due process Right to have specific procedures or processes followed before the deprivation of life, liberty, or property; the guarantee of privileges under the 5th and 14th Amendments to the U.S. Constitution.

duty Obligation to act created by a statute, contract, or voluntary agreement.

emerging health occupations Health-care occupations that are not yet officially recognized by government or professional organizations.

employee Individual hired for pay by another.

Employee Retirement Income Security Act (ERISA) Federal law that grants incentives to employers to offer self-funded health insurance plans to their employees.

employer Individual or organization that hires other individuals for pay to carry out specific duties during certain hours of employment.

empowerment Process in which the individual assumes more autonomy and responsibility for his or her actions.

end product Output of a system not reusable as input.

endorsement Reciprocity; a state's acceptance of a license issued by another state.

energy Capacity to do work.

entry into practice Minimal educational requirements to obtain a license for a profession.

environment Internal and external physical and social boundaries of humans; all those things that are outside a system.

essentials for accreditation Minimal standards that a program must meet to be accredited.

ethical dilemma Ethical situation that requires an individual to make a choice between two equally unfavorable alternatives.

ethical rights (moral rights) Rights that are based on moral or ethical principles but have no legal mechanism of enforcement.

ethical system System of moral judgments based on the beliefs and values of a profession.

ethics Principles or standards of conduct that govern an individual or group.

ethnic group Individuals who share similar physical characteristics, religion, language, or customs.

euthanasia Mercy killing; the act or practice of killing, for reasons of mercy, individuals who have little or no chance of recovery by withholding or discontinuing life support or by administering a lethal agent.

evaluation Fifth step in the nursing process; used to determine whether goals set for a client have been attained.

evaluation criteria Outcome criteria; desired behaviors or standards.

evidence reports Provide a scientific basis for a disease or a nursing practice and then integrate research data into actions used in practice. They synthesize previous and current knowledge related to the topic, review the information for quality and documentation, explain how evidence-based practice (EBP) is currently being used, and discuss how useful the EBP is to the clinical practice.

expanded role Extended role; increased responsibilities and actions undertaken by an individual because of additional education and experience.

experience rating Similar in concept to risk rating, experience rating establishes insurance premiums based on the history of the individual. Often used in calculating lost work days due to illness or injury in workman's compensation cases, it compares the lost days of the individual to what would normally be expected for individuals in the same class.

expert witness Individual with knowledge beyond the ordinary person, resulting from special education or training, who testifies during a trial.

external degree Academic degree granted when all the requirements have been met by the student; a type of outcomes-based education in which credit is given when the individual demonstrates a certain level of knowledge and skill, regardless of how or when these skills are attained; challenge examinations are often used.

false imprisonment Intentional tort committed by illegally confining or restricting a client against his or her will.

family Two or more related individuals living together.

Federal Tort Claims Act Statute that allows the government to be sued for negligence of its employees in the performance of their duties; many states have similar laws.

fee for service Payment is expected each time a service is rendered. Includes physicians' office visits, diagnostic procedures (laboratory tests, x-rays), and minor surgical procedures.

feedback Reentry of output into a system as input that helps maintain the internal balance of the system.

feedback loop As used in Systems Theory or Nursing Care Models, it is the continuous provision of information about the effectiveness of treatments back to the health care provider that allows him or her to adjust the treatments for optimal effectiveness.

fellowship Scholarship or grant that provides money to individuals who are highly qualified or highly intelligent.

felony Serious crime that may be punished by a fine of more than $1000, more than 1 year in jail or prison, death, or a combination thereof.

fidelity The obligation of an individual to be faithful to commitments made to self and others.

for-profit Health-care agencies in which profits can be used to raise capital to pay stockholders dividends on their investments. Also called proprietary agencies.

foreign graduate nurse Individual graduated from a school of nursing outside the United States. This individual is required to pass the U.S. NCLEX-RN CAT to become a registered nurse in the United States.

forensic nurse Registered nurse who specializes in the integration of forensic science and nursing science to apply the nursing process to individual clients, their families, and the community, bridging the gap between the health-care system and the criminal justice system.

forensic psychiatric nurse Registered nurse who specializes in application of psychosocial nursing knowledge linking offending behavior to client characteristics; nurse specializing in forensic psychological evaluation and care of offender populations with mental disorders.

forensic science Body of empirical knowledge used for legal investigation and evidence-based judgment in police or criminal cases.

fraud Deliberate deception in provision of goods or services; lying.

functional nursing Nursing care in which each nurse provides a different aspect of care; nurses are assigned a set of specific tasks to perform for all clients, such as passing medications.

general damages Monetary awards in a lawsuit for injuries for which an exact dollar amount cannot be calculated including pain and suffering, loss of companionship, shortened life span, loss of reputation, and wrongful death.

general systems theory Set of interrelated concepts, definitions, and propositions that describe a system.

genetics Scientific study of heredity and related variations.

gerontology Study of the process of aging and of the effects of aging on individuals.

goal Desired outcome.

Good Samaritan Act Law that protects health-care providers from being charged with contributory negligence when they provide emergency care to persons in need of immediate treatment.

grievance Complaint or dispute about the terms or conditions of employment.

group practice Three or more physicians or nurse practitioners in business together to provide health care.

health Complete physical, mental, and social well-being; a relative state along a continuum ranging from severe illness to ideal state of being; the ability to adapt to illness and to reach the highest level of functioning.

health-care consumer Client or patient; an individual who uses health-care services or products.

health-care team Group of individuals of different levels of education who work together to provide help to clients.

health insurance purchasing cooperative (HIPC) Large groups of people or employers who band together to buy insurance at reduced costs. HIPCs may be organized by private groups or the government.

health literacy A client's ability to read, comprehend, and act on health-care instructions provided by a nurse or other health-care worker.

health maintenance organization (HMO) Prototype of the managed health-care system; method of payment for a full range of primary, secondary, and tertiary health-care services; members pay a fixed annual fee for services and a small deductible when care is given.

health policy Goals and directions that guide activities to safeguard and promote the health of citizens.

health practitioner Individual, usually licensed, who provides health-care services to individuals with health-care needs.

health promotion Interventions and behaviors that increase and maintain the level of well-being of persons, families, groups, communities, and society.

health systems agency (HSA) Local voluntary organization of providers and consumers that plans for the health-care services of its geographic region.

hearsay Evidence not based on personal knowledge of the witness and usually not allowed in courts.

holistic Treatment of the total individual, including physical, psychological, sociological, and spiritual elements, with emphasis on the interrelatedness of parts and wholes.

home health care Health-care services provided in the client's home.

honesty, integrity, respect, responsibility, and ethics (HIRRE) Type of honor code in which students and faculty sign a pledge not to cheat or plagiarize.

horizontal violence Type of peer-to-peer incivility or negative interaction.

hospice care Alternative way of providing care to terminally ill clients in which palliative care is used; the major goals of hospice care are control of pain, provision of emotional support, promotion of social interaction, and preparation for death; family support measures and anticipatory grief counseling are also used if appropriate.

hospital privileges Authority granted by a hospital, usually through its medical board, for a health-care practitioner to admit and supervise the treatment of clients within that hospital.

humor me approach A communication method used with clients in the denial stage of grief to help them comply with the treatment regimen.

hypothesis Prediction or proposition related to a problem, usually found in research.

ideal role image Projection of society's expectations for nurses that clearly delineates the obligations and responsibilities, as well as the rights and privileges those in the role can lay claim to. Is often unrealistic.

illness Disease; a functional disturbance resulting from an individual organism's inability to adapt to certain stressors; an abnormal physiologic state caused by microorganisms, cancer, or other conditions.

implementation Fourth step in the nursing process, in which the plan of care is carried out.

incidence Number of occurrences of a specific condition or event.

incident report Document that describes an accident or error involving a client or family member that may or may not have resulted in injury; the purpose of the incident report is to track incidents and to make changes in the situations that caused them; the incident report is not part of the chart.

incivility Failure to be civil; any speech or behavior that disrupts the harmony of the work or educational environment.

incompetency Inability of an individual to manage personal affairs because of mental or physical conditions; the inability of a professional to carry out professional activities at the expected level of functioning because of lack of knowledge or skill or because of drug or alcohol abuse.

indemnity insurance Health insurance in which the contractual agreement is between the consumer and the insurance company. Providers are not involved in these arrangements, and rates are not pre-established.

independent nurse practitioner Nurse who has a private practice in one of the expanded roles of nursing.

independent practice association (IPA) Type of HMO usually organized by physicians that requires fee-for-service payment.

independent practice organization (IPO) Type of IPA in which a group of providers deals with more than one insurer at a time.

independent practitioner Health-care provider who delivers health care independently with or without supervision by another health-care practitioner.

indirect services Health-care actions that do not require direct client contact but that still facilitate care, such as the supply and distribution department of a hospital.

individual mandate The requirement that all US citizens must purchase some type of health insurance with the goal of spreading the costs across a large population and lowering premiums.

informed consent Permission granted by a person based on full knowledge of the risks and benefits of participation in a procedure or surgery for which the consent has been given.

injunction Court order specifying actions that must or must not be taken.

input Matter, energy, or information entering a system from the environment.

inquest Formal inquiry about the course or manner of death.

institutional licensure Authority for an individual health-care provider to practice that is granted by the individual's employing institution; the institution determines the educational preparation, training, and functions of each category of provider it employs; no longer legally permitted, unlicensed assistive personnel (UAPs) act under a form of de facto institutional licensure.

intentional tort A willful act that violates another person's rights or property and may or may not cause physical injury.

interprofessional education Two or more students from different professions learning about, from and with each other to enable effective collaboration and improve health outcomes.

interrogatories Written questions directed to a party in a lawsuit by the opposing side as part of the discovery process.

intervention Nursing action taken to meet specific client goals.

invasion of privacy Type of quasi-intentional tort that involves (1) an act that intrudes into the seclusion of the client, (2) intrusion that is objectionable to a reasonable person, (3) an act that intrudes into private facts or published as facts or pictures of a private nature, and (4) public disclosure of private information.

Joint Commission Formerly Joint Commission on Accreditation of Healthcare Organizations (JCAHO), an organization that performs accreditation reviews for health-care agencies.

judgment Decision of the court regarding a case.

junk policies Low-cost health insurance policies that sound good when advertised but include riders that severely limit what is covered. They are marketed to people who tend not to read the fine print such as young adults and the elderly.

jurisdiction Authority of a court to hear and decide lawsuits.

justice Fairness; giving people their due.

just culture The establishment of a positive work environment that has a commitment to safety and quality, transparency, and using errors as learning opportunities and allowing employees to report errors and near misses voluntarily and anonymously. Also called a blame-free culture.

Kardex Portable card file that contains important client information and a care plan.

laissez-faire Type of leadership style in which the leader does little planning, sets few goals, avoids decision-making, and fails to encourage group members to participate. Also called permissive or nondirective leadership.

lateral violence Is also known as horizontal violence is found in the workplace and can include name calling, threatening body language, physical hazing, bickering, fault finding, negative criticism, intimidation, gossip, shouting, blaming, put-downs, raised eye brows, rolling of the eyes, verbally abusive sarcasm with rude tones, or physical acts such as pounding on a table, throwing objects or shoving a chair against a wall, unfair assignments, marginalizing a person, refusing to help someone, ignoring, making faces behind someone's back, refusing to work with certain people, whining, sabotage, exclusion, and fabrication.

law Formal statement of a society's beliefs about interactions among and between its citizens; a formal rule enforced by society.

Leapfrog Group Launched in 2000 by The Robert Wood Johnson Foundation, the Leapfrog groups' mission is to promote giant leaps forward in the safety, quality, and affordability of health care by using incentives and rewards.

legal complaint Document filed by a plaintiff against a defendant claiming infringement of the plaintiff's legal rights.

legal obligations Obligations that have become formal statements of law and are enforceable under the law.

legal rights (welfare rights) Rights that are based on a legal entitlement to some good or benefits and are enforceable under the legal system with punishment for violations.

legislator Elected member of either the House of Representatives or the Senate.

legislature Body of elected individuals invested with constitutional power to make, alter, or repeal laws.

liable Obligated or held accountable by law.

libel Written defamation of character.

license Permission to practice granted to an individual by the state after he or she has met the requirements for that particular position; licensing protects the safety of the public.

licensed practical nurse (LPN) Licensed vocational nurse; technical nurse licensed by any state, after completing a practical nursing program, to provide technical bedside care to clients.

licensing board Government agency that implements the statutes of a particular profession in accordance with the Professions Practice Act.

licensure Process by which an agency or government grants an individual permission to practice; it establishes a minimal level of competency for practice.

Licensure, Accreditation, Certification and Education (LACE) A report issued in 2008 by the APRN Consensus Work Group and the National Council of State Boards of Nursing (NCSBN) APRN Advisory Committee addressing the lack of common definitions regarding APRN practice, the ever increasing numbers of specializations, the inconsistency in credentials and scope of practice and the wide variations in education for ARNPs.

licensure by endorsement Method of obtaining a license to practice by having a state acknowledge the individual's existing comparable license in another state.

licensure by examination Method of obtaining a license to practice by successfully passing a state-board examination.

living will Signed legal document in which individuals make known their wishes about the care they are to receive if they should become incompetent at a future date; it usually specifies what types of treatments are permitted and what types are to be withheld.

lobbyist Person who attempts to influence political decisions as an official representative of an organization, group, or institution.

locality rule standard of care Legal process that holds an individual nurse accountable both to what is an acceptable standard within his or her local community and to national standards as developed by nurses throughout the nation through the American Nurses Association (ANA), national practice groups, and health-care agencies.

malfeasance Performance of an illegal act.

malpractice Negligent acts by a licensed professional based on either omission of an expected action or commission of an inappropriate action resulting in damages to another party; not doing what a reasonable and prudent professional of the same rank would have done in the same situation.

managed care System of organized health-care delivery systems linked by provider networks; health maintenance organizations are the primary example of managed care.

mandatory licensure Law that requires all who practice a particular profession to have and to maintain a license in that profession.

manslaughter Killing of an individual without premeditated intent; different degrees of manslaughter exist, and most are felonies.

mediation Legal process that allows each party to present their case to a mediator, who is an independent third party trained in dispute resolution.

Medicaid State health-care insurance program, supported in part by federal funds, for health-care services for certain groups unable to pay for their own health care; amount and type of coverage vary from state to state.

medical examiner Coroner; a physician who investigates deaths that appear to be from other than natural causes.

medically indigent Individuals who cannot personally pay for health-care services without incurring financial hardship.

Medicare Federally run program that is financed primarily through employee payroll taxes and covers any individual who is 65 years of age or older as well as blind and disabled individuals of any age.

Medicare Utilization and Quality Peer Review Organization (PRO) Organization that reviews the quality and cost of Medicare services.

Medigap policies Health insurance policies that are purchased to cover expenses not paid by Medicare.

middle range theory A set of relatively concrete concepts or propositions that lie between a minor working hypothesis found in every-day nursing research and a well developed major nursing theory. They are less comprehensive and more focused than the major nursing theories but not as specific or concrete as situation-specific practice theories and they generally contain only a few basic ideas or concepts that the researcher is attempting to prove or illustrate.

midwife Individual experienced in assisting women during labor and delivery; they may be lay midwives, who have no official education, or certified nurse midwives, who are RNs in an expanded role, having received additional education and passed a national certification examination.

misdemeanor Less serious crime than a felony; punishable by a fine of less than $1000 or a jail term of less than 1 year.

model Hypothetical representation of something that exists in reality. The purpose of a model is to attempt to explain a complex reality in a systematic and organized manner.

Modular Synthetic Research Evaluation and Extrapolation Tool (mSTREET) A learning game developed by the Community Health Nursing Serious Game designed to deliver computerized virtual training. In the game, students can investigate and respond to a variety of settings as they "walk" through the streets of a virtual city.

moral obligations Obligations based on moral or ethical principles but *not* enforceable under the law.

morality Concept of right and wrong.

morals Fundamental standards of right and wrong that an individual learns and internalizes during the early stages of childhood development, based primarily on religious beliefs and societal norms.

mores Values and customs of a society.

mortality Property or capacity to die; death.

motivation Internal drive that causes individuals to seek achievement of higher goals; desire.

multicompetency technician Allied health-care provider who has skills in two or more areas of practice through the process of cross-training.

multiskilled practitioner Health-care professional who has skills in more than one area of health care, such as an RN who has training in physical therapy.

national health insurance Proposed system of payment for health-care services whereby the government pays for the costs of the health care.

National Nurses Response Teams (NNRT) Teams of nurses under the auspices of the Department of Health and Human Services, who will be quickly deployed in response to major national bioterrorism events to provide mass immunization or chemoprophylaxis to high risk populations.

negative entropy Tendency toward increased order in a system.

negligence Failure to perform at an expected level of functioning or the performance of an inappropriate function resulting in damages to another party; not doing what a reasonable and prudent person would do in a similar situation.

never events A list of reasonably preventable medical errors that occur in hospitals that will no longer be paid for by Medicare in an attempt to control costs.

no-code order Do not resuscitate (DNR) order; an order by a physician to withhold cardiopulmonary resuscitation and other resuscitative efforts from a client.

nonfeasance Failure to perform a legally required duty.

nonmaleficence Ethical principle that requires the professional to do no harm to the client.

nontraditional education Methods of education that do not follow the traditional lecture and clinical practice methods of learning; may include computer-simulated learning, self-education techniques, or other creative methods.

nonverbal A type of communication that uses any methods except written and spoken messages and constitutes 93 percent of the communication between individuals. It includes body language, gestures, facial expression, tone, pace, personal space, etc.

normal damages Money awarded when the law requires a judge and jury to find a defendant guilty but no real harm happened to the plaintiff. The award is usually very small, generally in the sum of $10.00.

normative ethics Questions and dilemmas requiring a choice of actions whereby there is a conflict of rights or obligations between the nurse and the client, the nurse and the client's family, or the nurse and the physician.

norm-referenced examination Examination scored by comparison with standards established on the performance of all others who took the same examination during a specific time; the NLN achievement examinations are norm referenced.

not-for-profit (nonprofit) agencies Agencies in which all profits must be used in the operation of the organization.

nurse clinician Registered nurse with advanced skills in a particular area of nursing practice; if certified by a professional organization, a nurse clinician may also be a nurse practitioner, but more often this designation refers to nurses in advanced practice roles such as nurse specialists.

nurse practice act Part of state law that establishes the scope of practice for professional nurses, as well as educational levels and standards, professional conduct, and reasons for revocation of licensure.

nurse practitioner Nurse specialist with advanced education in a primary care specialty, such as community health, pediatrics, or mental health, who is prepared independently to manage health promotion and maintenance and illness prevention of a specific group of clients.

nurse specialist (clinical nurse specialist) Nurse who is an expert in providing care focused on a specialized field drawn from the range of general practice, such as cardiac nurse specialist.

nurse theorist Nurse who analyzes and attempts to describe what the profession of nursing is and what nurses do through nursing models or nursing theories.

nursing assessment Systematic collection and recording of client data, both objective and subjective, from primary and secondary sources using the nursing history, physical examination, and laboratory data, for example.

nursing diagnosis Statements of a client's actual or potential health-care problems or deficits.

nursing order Statement of a nursing action selected by a nurse to achieve a client's goal; may be stated as either the nurse's or the client's expected behavior.

nursing process Systematic, comprehensive decision-making process used by nurses to identify and treat actual and potential health problems.

nursing research Formal study of problems of nursing practice, the role of the nurse in health care, and the value of nursing.

nursing standards Desired nursing behaviors established by the profession and used to evaluate nurses' performances.

obligations Demands made on individuals, professions, society, or government to fulfill and honor the rights of others. Obligations are often divided into two categories—moral and legal (welfare).

occurrence policy A type of malpractice insurance that protects against all claims that occurred during the policy period regardless of when the claim is made.

omission Failure to fulfill a duty or carry out a procedure recognized as a standard of care; often forms the basis for claims of malpractice.

oncology Area of health care that deals with the treatment of cancer.

open curriculum Educational system that allows a student to enter and leave the system freely; often uses past education and experiences.

open system System that can exchange energy, matter, and information with the environment and with other systems.

option rights Rights that are based on a fundamental belief in the dignity and freedom of humans.

ordinance Local or municipal law.

out-of-pocket expenses Amount the client is responsible for paying for a health-care service.

outcome criteria Standards that measure changes or improvements in clients' conditions.

output Matter, energy, or information released from a system into the environment or transmitted to another system.

palliative Type of treatment directed toward minimizing the severity of a disease or illness rather than curing it; for example, for a client with terminal cancer, relief of pain is the main goal (palliative), rather than cure.

panel of approved providers A list of physicians, nurse practitioners, pharmacies, and other health-care providers that are approved by an insurance plan and to whom reimbursement will be made by the insurer.

paraverbal The tone, pitch, volume, and diction used when delivering a verbal message that comprises approximately 38 percent of the total message and is often considered part of nonverbal communication.

passive learning A type of client education in which the material is merely presented to the client without his or her involvement. Least effective type of learning because it usually does not change attitudes or behaviors.

patient Client; an individual seeking or receiving health-care services.

patient day Client day; the 24-hour period during which hospital services are provided that forms the basis for charging the patient, usually from midnight to midnight.

pediatrics Study and care of problems and diseases of children younger than the age of 18.

peer review Evaluation against professional standards of the performance of individuals with the same basic education and qualifications; formal process of review or evaluation by coworkers of an equal rank.

perceived role image The individual's own definition of the role, which is usually more realistic than the ideal role, involving rejection or modification of some of the norms and expectations of society.

percussion Physical examination involving the tapping of various parts of the body to determine density by eliciting different sounds.

performed role image The duties performed by the practitioner of a role. Often produces reality shock in new graduate nurses.

perjury Crime committed by giving false testimony while under oath.

permissive licensure Law that allows individuals to practice a profession as long as they do not use the title of the profession; no states now have permissive licensure.

personal space The distance from others that individuals maintain around themselves in most casual social situations. Is often culturally based.

phenomenology Philosophical approach that holds that consciousness determines reality in space and time.

plaintiff Individual who charges another individual in a court of law with a violation of the individual's rights; the party who files the complaint in a lawsuit.

point-of-service plans Insurance plans in which consumers can select providers outside of a prescribed provider panel if they are willing to pay an additional fee.

political action Activities on the part of individuals that influence the actions of government officials in establishing policy.

political capital The goodwill or favorable sentiment that a politician gains after winning an election, initiating a successful program, passing other politicians' bills or making a public appearance after a natural disaster that accentuates their leadership abilities. It is sometimes called the "Honeymoon" period of a presidency and like money, must be spent soon or it will evaporate.

political involvement Group of activities that, individually or collectively, increase the voice of nursing in the political or health-care policy process.

politics Process of influencing the decisions of others and exerting control over situations or events; includes influencing the allocation of scarce resources.

practical nursing program Vocational nursing program; a program of study leading to a certificate in practical nursing, usually 12 to 18 months in length; these programs are located in a vocational or technical school or in a community or junior college; after passing the NCLEX-LPN CAT examination, students become licensed practical nurses (LPNs).

precedent Decision previously issued by a court that is used as the basis for a decision in another case with similar circumstances.

preceptor Educated or skilled practitioner who agrees to work with a less-educated or less-trained individual to increase the individual's knowledge and skills; often staff nurses who work with student nurses during their senior year.

precertification Approval for reimbursement of services before their being rendered.

preferred provider organization (PPO) Method of payment for employee health-care benefits in which employers contract with a specific group of health-care providers for a lower cost for their employees' health-care services but require the employee to use the providers listed.

premium Amount paid on a periodic basis for health insurance or HMO membership.

prescriptive authority Legal right to write prescriptions for medications, granted to physicians, veterinarians, dentists, and advanced practice nurses.

presumed consent law A law that presumes that all reasonable and prudent persons would normally wish to donate their organs upon their death. It is often associated with the issuance of a new driver's license; however, those not wishing to be organ donors are able to "opt-out" of the process, which is a reversal of the current asking for consent to donate process.

preventive care Well care; nursing care provided for the purpose of maintaining health and preventing disease or injury, often through community health clinics, school nursing services, and storefront clinics.

primary care Type of health care for individuals and families in which maintenance of health is emphasized; first-line health care in hospitals, physicians' offices, or community health clinics that deal with acute conditions.

primary care nurse Hospital staff RN assigned to a primary care unit to provide nursing care to a limited number of clients who are followed by the same nurse from admission to discharge.

primary intervention Health promotion, illness prevention, early diagnosis, and treatment of common health problems.

private-duty nurse Nurse in private practice; nurse self-employed for providing direct client care services either in the home or the hospital setting.

privileged communication Information imparted by a client to a physician, lawyer, or clergyman that is protected from disclosure in a court of law. Communication between a client and a nurse is not legally protected, but nurses can participate in privileged communication when they overhear information imparted by the client to the physician.

process consent A requirement that the researcher renegotiate the consent if any unanticipated events occur during the process of gathering data.

profession Nursing; an occupation that meets the criteria for a profession, including education, altruism, code of ethics, public service, and dedication.

professional review organization Multilevel program to oversee the quality and cost of federally funded medical care programs.

professionalism Behaviors and attitudes exhibited by an individual that are recognized by others as the traits of a professional.

prospective payment system (PPS) System of reimbursement for health-care services that establishes the payment rates before hospitalization based on certain criteria, such as diagnosis-related groups (DRGs).

protocol Written plan of action based on previously identified situations; standing orders are a type of protocol often used in specialty units that have clients with similar problems.

provider Person or organization who delivers health care, including health promotion and maintenance and illness prevention and treatment.

provider panel Health-care providers selected to render services to a group of consumers within a managed-care plan.

proximate cause Nearest cause; the element in a direct cause-and-effect relationship between what is done by the professional and what happens to the client. For example, when a nurse fails to raise the side rails on the bed of a client who has received a narcotic medication, and the client falls out of bed and breaks a hip as a result.

psychomotor domain objectives Goals established with input from the client that deal with changes in behavior or learned skills.

public policy Decision made by a society or its elected representatives that has a material effect on citizens other than the decision-makers.

punitive damages Money awarded in a law suit in addition to compensatory and general damages when the actions that caused the injury to the client were judged to be willful, malicious, or demonstrated an extreme measure of incompetence and gross negligence. The primary purpose of punitive damages is to "punish" the plaintiff and deter him or her from ever acting in the same way again. Also called exemplary damages.

qualitative research design Investigates the why and how of decision making and not just what, where, when it happened with the goal of gathering an in-depth understanding of human behavior and the reasons that govern such behavior.

quality Level of excellence based on pre-established criteria.

Quality and Safety Education for Nurses (QSEN) Nursing education curriculum designed to prepare future nurses with the knowledge, skills, and attitudes (KSAs) necessary to continuously improve the quality and safety of the health-care system in which they work.

quality assurance Activity conducted in health-care facilities that evaluates the quality of care provided to ensure that it meets pre-established quality standards.

quality indicators Measures of health-care quality from easily accessible inpatient hospital administrative data that includes prevention, inpatient, patient, and pediatric safety and are used to focus efforts on potential quality concerns so they may be addressed by further investigation as well as tracking changes over time.

quantitative experimental research designs Are guided by a somewhat rigid set of rules that gives the most importance to the *process* of inquiry and are highly respected by researchers.

quasi-intentional tort A violation of a person's reputation or personal privacy.

Rapid Response Teams (RRT) Teams of individuals from various disciplines who can rescue clients whose conditions are deteriorating to prevent codes and in-hospital deaths using specific communication models to make interdisciplinary communication clearer, a workspace that promotes efficiency and waste reduction, professional support programs, and liberalized diet plans and meal times.

reality shock (transition shock) A sudden and sometimes traumatic realization on the part of the new graduate that the ideal or perceived roles do not match the actual performed role.

recertification Periodic renewal of certification by examination, continuing education, or other criteria established by the accrediting agency.

reciprocity Endorsement; a state's acceptance of a license issued by another state.

recision The practice of health insurance companies to cut or cancel health care plans already in place usually because of the high costs associated with the client's illness.

registration Listing of a license with a state for a fee.

registry Published list of those who are registered; the agency that publishes the list of individuals who are registered.

regulations Rules or orders issued by various regulatory agencies, such as a state board of nursing, which have the force of law.

rehabilitation Restoration to the highest possible level of performance or health of an individual who has suffered an injury or illness.

relative intensity measures (RIMs) Method for calculating nursing resources needed to provide nursing care for various types of clients; helps determine the number and type of staff required based on client acuity and needs.

respondeat superior Legal doctrine that holds the employer or supervisor responsible for the actions of the employees or of those supervised; for example, under this doctrine, RNs are held responsible for the actions of unlicensed assistive personnel under their supervision.

responsibility Accountability; the concept that all individuals are accountable for their own actions and for the consequences of those actions.

restorative care Curative care; nursing care that has as its goal cure and recovery from disease.

resume Curriculum vitae; a summary of an individual's education, work experience, and qualifications.

retrospective payment system Payment system for health care in which reimbursement is based on the actual care rendered rather than on preset rates.

right Just claim or expectation that may or may not be protected by law; legal rights are protected by law, whereas moral rights are not.

risk management Evaluating the risk of clients and staff for injuries and for potential liabilities and implementing corrective and preventive measures.

risk rating A method of calculating the rate for health insurance premiums based on various characteristics of an individual or small group of individuals, such as previous history of claims filed, characteristics of the individual's or group's health practices, or changes in the individual's or group's overall health status that might increase the risk for claims. It is the most commonly used method of calculating health insurance premiums and allows companies to change their rates at will.

root cause analysis A type of assessment that tracks events leading to error, identifies faulty systems, and processes and develops a plan to prevent further errors.

secondary care Nursing care usually provided in short-term and long-term care facilities to clients with commonly occurring conditions.

secondary intervention Acute care designed to prevent complications or resolve health problems.

secured settings Any institutional setting imposing restriction of movement, confinement, and limitations to activity and access; jails, locked units or locked mental institutions, prisons.

sentinel event Unexpected occurrence involving death or serious physical or psychological injury, or the risk thereof including loss of limb or function. Relatively infrequent, occurring independently of a client's condition, that commonly reflect hospital system and process deficiencies and result in negative outcomes for clients. Sentinel events are not the same as medical errors.

service insurance Health insurance in which services are provided for a prescribed fee that is established between the providers and the insurance company.

sexual assault nurse examiner (SANE) A registered nurse specializing in care of victims of sexual assault, performing physical and psychosocial examination, collection of physical evidence, and therapeutic interventions to minimize trauma.

significant other Individual who is not a family member but is emotionally or symbolically important to an individual.

situation–background–assessment–recommendation (SBAR) Communication technique used between members of the health-care team when a client's condition requires immediate attention and action; an easy-to-remember, concrete mechanism frames the conversation efficiently.

Six Sigma Business management strategy that has been adapted to the health-care industry to identify wasteful practices and lower costs while improving the overall quality of care.

slander Oral defamation of character.

sliding-scale fees Fees for services that are based on the client's ability to pay.

slow-code order Physician's order that the efforts for resuscitation of a client who is terminally ill should be initiated and conducted at a leisurely pace; the goal of a slow-code order is to allow the client to die during an apparent resuscitation. Slow-code orders are not acceptable practice and do not meet standards of care.

special damages Money awarded to the plaintiff for out-of-pocket expenses related to the trial. It would cover the expenses of taking a taxi back and forth to the courthouse, use of special assistive equipment, and special home health-care providers and other expenses that are not covered under actual damages.

staff nurse Nurse generalist who works as an employee of a hospital, nursing home, community health agency, or some other organization providing primary and direct nursing care to clients.

standard of best interest A type of decision made about an individual's health care when he or she is unable to make the informed decision for his or her own care; based on what the health-care providers and/or the family decide is best for that individual.

standards Norms; criteria for expected behaviors or conduct.

standards of care Written or established criteria for nursing care that all nurses are expected to meet.

standards of practice Written or established criteria for nursing practice that all professional nurses are expected to meet.

standing order Written order by physician for certain actions or medication administration to be initiated or given in certain expected circumstances; similar to protocols.

statute Law passed by a government's legislature and signed by its chief executive.

statute of limitations Specific time period in which a lawsuit must be filed or a crime must be prosecuted; most nursing or medical lawsuits have a 2-year statute of limitations from the time of discovery of the incident.

statutory law Law passed by a legislature.

stereotype Fixed or predetermined image of or attitude toward an individual or group.

stress Crisis situation that causes increased anxiety and initiation of the flight-or-fight mechanism.

stressor Internal or external force to which a person responds.

structure criteria Physical environmental framework for client care.

subpoena Court document that requires an individual to appear in court and provide testimony; individuals who do not honor the subpoena can be held in contempt of court and jailed or fined.

subsystem Smaller system within a large system.

summary judgment Decision by a judge in cases in which no facts are in dispute.

sunset law Law that automatically terminates a program after a pre-established period of time unless that program can justify its need for existence.

support system Environmental factors and individuals who can help an individual in a crisis cope with the situation.

systems theory Theory that stresses the interrelatedness of parts in any system in which a change in one part affects all other parts; often, the system is greater than the sum of its parts.

taxonomy Classification system.

team nursing Method of organizing nursing care in which each client is assigned a team consisting of RNs, LPNs, and nursing assistants to deliver nursing care.

technician Individual who carries out technical tasks.

technology Use of science and the application of scientific principles to any situation; often involves the use of complicated machines and computers.

telehealth The use of electronic information and communications technologies to provide and support health care when distance separates the health care provider and the client including "plain old telephone service" (POTS), highly sophisticated digitized cameras, telemetry, voice systems, and even interactive robots that can be controlled by the practitioner to assess clients and administer treatments.

telemedicine One of the services provided by the overall telehealth system that primarily involve consultation with a physician.

teleology Utilitarianism; an ethical system that identifies the right action by determining what will provide the greatest good for the greatest number of persons. This system has no set, unchanging rules; rather, it varies as the situation changes.

tertiary care Nursing care usually provided in long-term care and rehabilitation facilities for chronic diseases or injuries requiring long recovery.

tertiary intervention Provision of advanced and long-term health-care services to acutely ill clients, including the use of advanced technology, complicated surgical procedures, rehabilitation services, and care of the terminally ill.

testimony Oral statement of a witness under oath.

theory Set of interrelated constructs (concepts, definitions, or propositions) that presents a systematic view of phenomena by specifying relations among variables with the purpose of explaining and predicting phenomena.

third-party payment Payment for health-care services by an insurance company or a government agency rather than directly by the client.

third-party reimburser Organization other than the client, such as an employer, insurance company, or governmental agency, that assumes responsibility for payment of health-care charges for services rendered to the client.

throughput Matter, energy, or information as it passes through a system.

tort Violation of the civil law that violates a person's rights and causes injury or harm to the individual. Civil wrong independent of an action in contract that results from a breach of a legal duty; a tort can be classified as unintentional, intentional, or quasi-intentional.

tort-feasor Person who commits a tort.

total quality management (TQM) Method for monitoring and maintaining the quality of health care being delivered by a particular institution or health-care industry.

treble damages A provision in the laws of some states that allows the judge, in certain instances, to triple the actual damage award amount as an additional form of punitive damages in a law suit.

trial Legal proceedings during which all relevant facts are presented to a jury or judge for legal decision.

Tri-Council Nursing group composed of the American Nurses Association (ANA), National League for Nursing (NLN), American Association of Colleges of Nursing (AACN), and American Organization of Nurse Executives (AONE).

two plus two (2 + 2) program Nursing education program that starts with an associate (2-year) degree and then moves the individual to a baccalaureate degree with an additional 2 years of education.

Uniform Anatomical Gift Act Legislation providing for a legal document signed by an individual indicating the desire to donate specific body organs or the entire body after death.

unintentional tort A wrong occurring to a person or that person's property even though it was not intended; negligence.

universal health-care coverage Health-care reimbursement benefits for all U.S. citizens and legal residents.

universal precautions Body substance isolation; guidelines established by the Centers for Disease Control and Prevention (CDC) and the Occupational Safety and Health Administration (OSHA) to protect health-care professionals and clients from diseases carried in the blood and body fluids, such as HIV and hepatitis B; involves the use of gloves whenever in contact with blood or body fluids and masks, gowns, and eye covers if a chance exists of contact with aerosol fluids.

upward mobility Movement toward increased status and power in an organization through promotion.

utilitarianism Teleology; an ethical system that identifies the right action by determining what will provide the greatest good for the greatest number of persons. This system has no set, unchanging rules; rather, it varies as the situation changes.

utilization guidelines Guidelines that stipulate the amount of services that can be delivered by a health-care provider.

value Judgment of worth, quality, or desirability based on attitude formed from need or experience; a strong belief held by individuals about something important to them.

values clarification Process by which individuals list and prioritize the values they hold most important.

veracity The principle of truthfulness. It requires the health-care provider to tell the truth and not intentionally deceive or mislead clients.

verbal A type of communication based on written or spoken messages that constitute approximately 7 percent of the total communication between individuals.

vertical violence The use of inappropriate coercive power by a superior to harass and bully subordinates.

veto Signed refusal by the president or a governor to enact a bill into law. If the president vetoes a bill, the veto may be overridden by a two-thirds vote of the membership of both the House and Senate.

vicarious liability Imputation of blame on a person for the actions of the other.

victimization Experience of physical, emotional, or psychological trauma in which the individual suffers injury, fear, self-blame, and/or other dysfunction.

vocational nursing program Licensed practical nursing program in Texas and California; a program of study leading to a certificate in vocational nursing, usually 12 to 18 months in length; these programs are located in vocational and technical schools and community and junior colleges; after passing the NCLEX-LPN CAT examination, students become licensed vocational nurses (LVNs).

Note: *b* indicates box; *f*, figure; *n*, footnote, and *t*, table.

2 + 2 program, 88
3-D printing, 159–160

A

abandonment, 187
abortion, 146–147, 355
accountability
    professionalism and, 16
    responsibility and, 5–6
accreditation
    of health-care institutions, 104
    of nursing schools, 83–84, 85–86, 110
Accreditation Commission for Education in Nursing (ACEN), 110
acculturation, 542–543
active euthanasia. *See* euthanasia
act utilitarianism, 134
acupressure, 623, 640
acupressure massage, 640
acupuncture, 619, 631, 640
acute (secondary) care, 363
Adams, Isabel. *See* Hampton, Isabel Adams Robb
additive manufacturing (3-D printing), 159–160
advance directive, 163–165, 167, 194
    common questions about, 194*b*
    nurse's role in, 195
    sample, 168*f*
    See also do-not-resuscitate (DNR) order
advanced practice registered nurse(s) (APRNs), 91–93
    certification of, 104
    conflict between American Medical Association and, 105–106
    definition of, 107–108
    education for, 108
    growing role of, 107
    licensing model for, 107–109
    types of, 10–12
advocacy group, 464
AED (automated external defibrillation) class, 649
Affordable Care Act (ACA) of 2010
    advanced practice registered nurses and, 107
    arguments against, 500–504
    arguments for, 498–500
    concerns about, 355
    elderly population and, 567–568, 570
    evaluation of, 505, 508
    full implementation of, 508–510
    funding for nursing research from, 584
    future challenges of, 512–513
    impact of repeal of, 510

increased coverage due to, 356
integrative health care and, 613–614, 616
lack of public knowledge about, 511–512
nursing and, 355–356
provisions in, 354–355
standards of care and, 196
summary of, 504–505, 505–507*t*
waivers to, 510–511, 511*b*
    See also health-care reform
agencies
    legislation and government, 464
    volunteer health, 370
Agency for Healthcare Research and Quality (AHRQ), 381, 389, 582, 591*b*, 601
aggressive communication, 290–291
aging population. *See* elderly population
AIDS and HIV, 169–170
Alexander, Frederick Matthias, 640
Alexander technique, 640
Alliance for the Mentally Ill, 370
allopathic medicine, 640
alternative medicine. *See* complementary and alternative medicine (CAM); integrative health care
altruism, 6, 9
American Academy of Nursing (AAN), 391–392
American Association of Clinical Coders and Auditors (AACCA), 683
American Association of Colleges of Nursing (AACN), 110
    competencies of, 94
    Essentials of Baccalaureate Education by, 76, 77*b*
    on incivility, 421–422
    position paper on education by, 82–83
    position statement on nursing shortage by, 453
American Botanical Society, 638
American Cancer Society, 370
American College of Emergency Physicians (ACEP), 659–660
American Holistic Nurses Association (AHNA), 530*b*
American Hospital Association
    Blue Cross insurance plans and, 490
    on staffing ratios, 372
American Journal of Nursing (AJN), 32, 137, 472
American Medical Association (AMA)
    on cannabis research, 635
    conflict between nursing profession and, 105–106
American Nurse, 472
American Nurses Association (ANA), 9, 110–111
    culturally competent care standards of, 562
    definition of nursing by, 20
    on delegation, 396, 406

on do-not-resuscitate (DNR) order, 195–196
on health-care reform, 504
on informatics, 433
nursing research and, 586, 588, 590*b*, 601
position paper on education by, 82–83
position papers on lateral violence by, 415
as potential source of power, 16
recommendations for mass-casualty events, 659–660
sexual-harassment approach by, 338–339
on staffing, 273
on staffing ratios, 372
workplace violence task force of, 421
See also American Nurses Credentialing Center (ANCC)
American Nurses Association (ANA) Code of Ethics, 9, 137, 138, 603
2001 and 2015 versions of, 139*b*
on delegation, 406
on incivility, 421
American Nurses Association (ANA) Council of State Boards of Nursing, 101
American Nurses Association (ANA) Political Action Committee (ANA-PAC), 111, 453
American Nurses Credentialing Center (ANCC), 103, 434
American Pain Society, 601
American Recovery and Reinvestment Act of 2009
computerized medical records and, 431
funding for nursing research by, 584
American Red Cross, 32, 652, 653
Amos, 521
ANA Basic Guide to Safe Delegation, 406
ANA Principles of Staffing, 273
ancient Egypt, 21
ancient Greeks, 21–22
ancient Hebrews, 21
ancient Rome, 22
anger as communication blocker, 299–300
answer (in lawsuit), 189
antidepressants, 336
applied ethics, 122
applied kinesiology, 640
Applied Nursing Research, 588
APRN Consensus Model (Model of Regulation), 107–109
arbitration, 193, 306
Aristotle, 521
Army Nurse Corps, 24, 25
aromatherapy, 640
articulation. *See* ladder programs
art therapy, 640
assault and battery, 186
assertive communication, 286–289, 290*b*
assertiveness, 287, 289*b*
assignment *versus* delegation, 397
assisted living center, 367
assisted suicide, 167–169. *See also* right to die
associate degree nurse (ADN), 26
associate degree nursing (ADN) program, 84–85
Association of Integrative Medicine (AAIM), 637
associations. *See* organizations; professional organizations
assumption of risk, 192
asymmetrical information, 431
atropine, 663
aura, 640
auriculotherapy, 640
authoritarian leadership, 258*t*, 259–260
automated health record. *See* electronic health record (EHR)
autonomy (self-determination)
assisted suicide and, 168–169
of client, 124–125, 166

genetic screening and, 148–149
of incompetent client, 195
of nursing practice, 9–10
Ayurvedic medicine, 634–635, 640

B
Babylonian Empire, 21
baccalaureate degree nursing programs, 85–86, 96
baccalaureate ladder program, 87–88
Bach, Edward, 640
Bach flower essences, 640
backstabber. *See* sneak (difficult coworker)
bargaining, 305
battery, 186
Bellevue Training School nursing cap, 28–29
beneficence, 125–126
Berners-Lee, Tim, 8
Bertalanffy, Ludwig von, 53
best interest, standard of, 129–130
best practice, 593–594, 607. *See also* evidence-based practice
Best Practices Network, 601
bias, 607
Biden, Joseph, 661
bioethics, 134
abortion and, 146–147
assisted suicide and, 167–169
child-related issues and, 171–175
cord blood banking and, 150–151
fetal tissue research and, 149–150
genetic research and, 147–149
HIV and AIDS and, 169–170
organ donation and transplantation and, 151–156, 154*b*, 159–160
prolonging life and, 160–162
right to die and, 162–167
See also ethics
biofeedback, 640
biohazard suit, 654–655, 654*b*
biological interventions, 622*b*, 623
biologically based therapies, 621*b*, 623
biological weapons/agents, 657
categories of, 658, 659*t*
early detection of, 657–658
epidemiological clues to attack with, 658*b*
response to attack with, 659–660
biopsychosocial relationship, 41
Bismarck, Otto von, 490
Bixler, Elizabeth, 5
black humor, 337
Blackman, Lewis, 390–391
blister agents, 663
blogger.com, 235
Blue Cross/Blue Shield, 490
bodywork therapies, 618, 619*b*, 622*b*, 623, 640
Bolton Act, 25
botanical medicine, 641. *See also* herbalism
Bowman, James, 156
brain death, 152–153
breach of confidentiality, 188
"BSN in Ten" proposal, 82. *See also* baccalaureate degree nursing programs
Buddha, 521
Buddhism, 21
budget preparation, 271–272
bullying, 414–416. *See also* incivility
Burke, Edmund, 468

burnout, 244–245
  spiritual perspective of, 535
  symptoms of, 244*b*
  techniques for countering, 245, 248–249
Bush, George W., 195, 491

C

Cadet Nurse Corps, 25
California Nurses Association, 113
Canada Health Act (CHA), 359–360
cannabis, medical, 635
cap, nursing, 28–29, 29*f*
capitated payment system, 361
Capitol Update, 472
cardiopulmonary resuscitation and right to die, 162–163
care coordinator, 681–682
care delivery (client-care) models, 279–281, 280*t*
career ladder program. *See* ladder programs
career *versus* job, 10
care management, 81
Carter, Jimmy, 489
case law. *See* common law
case management/manager, 12, 681–682
  collaboration between physicians and, 682*b*
  in nursing curriculum, 81
  protocols for, 381
case study, 607
categorical imperative, 136
Catholic Church, 23
causal relationship, 607
Center for Quality Improvement and Patient Safety, 389
Center for Research for Nursing, 588
Centers for Disease Control (CDC)
  classification of biological agents by, 658, 659*t*
  information on chemical weapons/treatments
    from, 665
Centers for Medicare and Medicaid Services (CMS),
    107, 389
Centre for Health Evidence, 599
certification, 103–104, 107
certified nursing assistant (CNA), 102–103
certified transcultural nurse (CTN), 562
chakras (energy centers), 527, 641
change agent, 277*b*, 280*t*
charge nurse, 279
Charleston Area Medical Center, Tabata v., 441
charting by exception, 199. *See also* medical records
chelation therapy, 641
chemical weapons (CW), 660
  aging stockpiles of, 665–666
  definition of, 661
  odds of exposure to, 665
  preparation for, 664–665
  types of, 662–664, 662*t*
  use of, 661
Chemical Weapons Convention, 660
chi, 641
chi gong (Qi Gong), 643
chi kung (Qi Gong), 643
child abuse, 171, 172–173
children
  ethical issues involving, 171–175, 174*b*
  as organ donors, 152
  spirituality in, 528
Children's Health Insurance Program, 490
Chinese medicine, traditional, 634, 644. *See also* acupuncture;
    Oriental medicine
chiropractic care, 623, 641

choking agent, 663–664
Christianity, 22
chronic disease, 566, 571
church nurse. *See* parish nurse
CINAHL, 591*b*
civility
  in classroom and clinical setting, 418*b*
  communication and, 412
  definition of, 411–412
  job satisfaction and, 426
  model for, 420, 420*f*
  in nursing, 412
  See also incivility
civil law, 180
Civil Rights Act of 1964, 412
Civil War (U.S.), 24
claims-made insurance policy, 201
client-care (care delivery) models, 279–281, 280*t*
client data. *See* electronic health record (EHR);
    medical records
client education
  for elderly population, 572–573
  quality of care and, 387
client-focused care (modular nursing), 280*t*, 281
client outcomes. *See* health outcomes
client(s)
  abandonment of, 187
  autonomy of, 124–125, 166, 195
  concepts of, 41, 51
  as consumer, 82
  in Johnson Behavioral System Model, 64
  in King Model of Goal Attainment, 60
  in Neuman Health-Care Systems Model, 66
  in Orem Self-Care Model, 58
  as partner, 52
  in Roy Adaptation Model, 55, 57
  satisfaction of, 378
  in Watson Model of Human Caring, 61
  See also difficult clients
client safety officer, 684–685
clinical nurse leader (CNL), 92
clinical nurse specialist (CNS), 12, 92
clinical pathways (case management protocols), 381
clinical psychologist, 11*t*
clinics, 366. *See also* nurse-run health center
Clinton, Bill, 489
Clinton, Hillary Rodham, 489
closed system, 54
Cochrane Collaboration, 593, 599
code of ethics, 123, 137–138. *See also* American Nurses Association
    (ANA) Code of Ethics
coder, nurse, 683–684
codes of conduct, 422
coercive power, 14
cognitive dissonance, 228
cognitive science, 432, 437
collaboration, 607. *See* team nursing; teamwork and health-care
    quality
collective bargaining, 305
collective power, 14
Commission Corps Readiness Force, 653
Commission on Education of Health Care Professionals in the
    21st Century, 94–95
Commission on Nursing Research, 601
common law, 179
communication, 285–286
  barriers to and benefits of clear, 286, 287*b*
  civility and, 412

during disasters, 653
effective, 197–199
nonverbal, 291
paraverbal, 291
privileged, 188
scenario on, 307
styles of, 286–291
technology and, 431
transcultural, 553, 554b, 555, 557–558
verbal, 291
communication blocker(s), 291, 293–297
communication builder(s), 291–293
community health center, 366
Community Health Nursing Serious Game, 79, 80
community rating system, 490
comparative effectiveness research (CER), 598–599, 607
comparative (descriptive) ethics, 122
comparative negligence, 191–192
compassion, 522
compassion fatigue, 233
competence, 41
competencies, 41, 42–51t
    American Association of Colleges of Nursing (AACN), 94
    assessment of, 76
    Institute of Medicine (IOM), 75, 77b
    in nursing research, 601–602
    Pew Commission report on, 62, 74
    Quality and Safety Education for Nurses (QSEN), 75–76, 77b, 386, 388
competency-based education, 87
Competency Outcomes Performance Assessment (COPA), 75, 386, 388
competition, 278–279
complaining and whining, 339
    approaches to, 342–343, 349–350
    case study on, 344–348
    causes of, 339–340
    effects of, 340–341
    types of, 341–342
    unsuccessful approaches to, 350
complaint (legal), 189
complementary and alternative medicine (CAM) 615-616
    See also integrative health care
computerized health record. See electronic health record (EHR)
computer systems. See informatics
conceptual framework, 607
conceptual model, 607
confidentiality
    breach of, 188
    electronic health record and, 441
    establishing trust with, 320–321
    genetic screening and, 148
    Health Insurance Portability and Accountability Act and, 442
conflict
    contributing factors to, 301–302
    focusing on strengths in, 304
    in home health care, 365
    role, 226–227
    strategies for resolving, 303–304
    successful handling of, 304
conflict resolution tips, 290b
Confucius, 521
congregational nursing, 370, 531b
consent. See informed consent
consequentialism. See utilitarianism
conservative, 457

consistency, 320
constituency group, 464, 476
consultant, legal nurse, 676
contextual informed consent, 531
continuous quality improvement (CQI), 377–378, 381
contract negotiation, 305
contributory negligence, 191
controlling leadership. See authoritarian leadership
conventional medicine, 623–625, 643
cord blood banking, 150–151
correctional nurse, 680
correlation, 607
Corso, Thomas v., 203
cost containment, 360–361, 486, 512
cover letter, 236, 236b
coworkers. See difficult behaviors; difficult coworkers
craniosacral therapy, 641
credentials. See certification; licensure
criminal law, 179–180
criterion-referenced examination, 205–206
critical incident stress debriefing (CISD), 249–250
critical thinking
    in health-care reform debate, 488
    in nursing curriculum, 77–78
Crossing the Quality Chasm, 377, 412
Cruzan, Nancy, 160, 195
crystal therapy, 641
Culp, Connie, 157–158
cultural assessment, 549–550, 549b, 553
cultural-awareness development, 545
cultural beliefs, purposes of, 545–546
cultural belief system, 545
cultural competency, 365, 544, 553
cultural conflict, 559, 560–561
cultural diversity, 542
culturally competent care, 553
cultural relativism, 543
cultural synergy, 559
cultural values, 546, 548
culture(s)
    assessment of, 549–550, 549b, 553
    as barrier to care, 541–542
    concepts of, 542
    definition of, 540
    organ donation and, 551–552
    similarities among, 559
    See also transcultural nursing
cupping, 641
curanderismo, 641

D

Dalai Lama, 529
damages (in lawsuit), 190–191
D'Amour and Oandasan model of interprofessional nursing, 94
dance therapy, 641
Danforth, John, 194
dashboard, 378
data, 432
day-care center, 369
deaconess, 28
death
    organ donation and determination of, 152–153
    and right to die, 162–167
    See also near-death experience
death investigator, nurse, 676–677, 677b
decision-making process, ethical, 138–142, 140f

decompression routine, 252
decontamination, 664–665
defamation of character, 187–188
defendant, 179, 180
defense of the fact, 192–193
delegation, 396, 407*f*
    advantages of, 405
    versus assignment, 397
    barriers to effective, 404*b*
    decision tree for, 405*b*
    definitions of, 187*b*, 397
    developing skills in, 404–405
    direct and indirect, 406
    five "rights" of, 401*b*
    inappropriate tasks for, 404–405
    legal issues in, 405–406
    National Council Licensure Examination (NCLEX) and, 406
    responsibility and accountability in, 397–399
    of uncomplicated tasks, 401
democratic (transformational) leadership, 258–259, 258*t*, 425, 425*b*
deontology, 135–136
Deployable Rapid Assembly Shelter (DRASH), 654
deposition (in lawsuit), 189, 190*b*
descriptive ethics, 122
developmental crisis, 520
diagnosis-related group (DRG), 361
diet. *See* diet therapies; nutrition and diet
Dietary Supplement Health and Education Act (DSHEA), 633
dietary supplements, 632–633
diet therapies, 621*b*, 623
difficult behaviors, 311
    basic principles in dealing with, 312–313
    complaining and whining as, 339–350
    identifying people with, 311–312
    sexual harassment as, 336–339
    understanding needs while dealing with, 312
    See also difficult clients; difficult coworkers
difficult clients
    establishing trust of, 320–321
    sexual harassment from, 337–339
    stages of grief and, 319–320
        acceptance, 336
        anger, 323–328
        bargaining, 328–332
        denial, 321–323
        depression, 332–336
difficult coworker(s), 314
    persecutor as, 314–316
    sexual harassment from, 336–337
    sneak as, 316–319
dilemma, 123–124, 131, 133
diploma schools, 83–84
directed (organ) donation, 155
directive leadership. *See* authoritarian leadership
Disaster Medical Assistance Team (DMAT), 653
disaster(s)
    10 commandments of preparedness for, 651
    biological weapons and, 657–660
    chemical weapons and, 660–666
    communication during, 653
    definition of, 647
    elderly population and, 573
    impact phase of, 654–655
    postimpact phase of, 655
    preimpact phase of, 652–653
    preparation for, 647–650

protection for first responders in, 654–655
    roles of nurse in, 655–656, 655*b*
    scam artists and, 667–670
    triage during, 656–657
    what to do during, 652–655
disciplinary hearing, 202
discovery (in lawsuit), 189
disease, chronic, 566, 571
distributive justice, 125, 128
diversity and workplace conflict, 302–303. *See also* cultural diversity;
        culture(s)
Dock, Lavinia Lloyd, 33
doctoral programs, 90
doctor of nursing education (DNEd), 90
doctor of nursing practice (DNP), 90, 92–93, 108
doctors. *See* physicians
documentation. *See* medical records
donation after cardiac death (DCD), 153
donor registry, 159
do-not-resuscitate (DNR) order, 195–196. *See also* advance directive
doomsday prepper, 647
doshas, 641
double-crosser. *See* sneak (difficult coworker)
downed power lines, 652
durable power of attorney for health care (DPOAHC), 130, 194.
        See also advance directive
duty-based ethics. *See* deontology

E
EBSCOhost, 591*b*
education
    1940s studies on, 587
    for advanced practice, 91–93
    American Nurses Association (ANA) position paper on, 82–83
    associate degree nursing (ADN) program, 84–85
    baccalaureate, 85–86, 96
    changes in health-care system and, 72–73
    competencies and, 74–76
    diploma schools and, 83–84
    doctoral programs, 90
    electronic, 79–80
    faculty shortage in, 455
    future curricular revisions in, 76–78, 81–82
    grants for, 73*b*
    incivility in, 416–421, 417*b*
    interprofessional, 93–95
    ladder programs in, 87–89
    master's program in, 89–90
    nursing shortage and, 17, 228
    Pew Commission's key areas for, 62–63
    practical/vocational nursing programs in, 86–87
    quality care and, 386, 388, 391
    spirituality in, 576
    tuition debt and, 453–454
    See also client education
educational (mobility) ladder. *See* ladder programs
e-health, 370
Eisenhower, Dwight, 490
elderly population
    chronic conditions of, 566, 571
    disaster preparation for, 573
    economic impact of, 571–572
    Gerontological Nursing Interventions Research Center and, 601
    growth of, 571
    health-care coverage for, 566–567
    mobile acute care (MACE) for, 569

nursing and effects of, 572–573
self-care of, 566
spirituality of, 574–577
elections, 462–463, 468–470
electroacupunture, 631
electronic health care (e-health), 370
electronic health record (EHR), 438–441
ethics, security, and confidentiality of, 441–444
implementation of, 431
Emergency Alert System (EAS), 648
emergency (secondary) care, 363
emotional distress, intentional infliction of, 186
emotional intelligence, 412
emotions and conflict, 301
empirical evidence, 607
employment. *See* job search
employment settings, 73
empowerment, 12–14
endorphins, 629
energy centers (chakras), 527
energy fields/systems, 525, 532, 630
energy therapies, 618, 619*b*, 623, 630–631, 641
Enhanced Fujita (EF) scale, 646
entrepreneur, nurse, 680–681
environment
concept of, 51–52
in Johnson Behavioral System Model, 65
in King Model of Goal Attainment, 60
in Neuman Health-Care Systems Model, 66
in Orem Self-Care Model, 58–59
quality care and, 391–392
in Roy Adaptation Model, 57
in Watson Model of Human Caring, 61
environmental communication blockers, 295–297
environmental communication builders, 293
environmental medicine, 641
epidemiologist, 607
errors. *See* medical errors
Essentials of Baccalaureate Education for Professional Nursing Practice, 76, 77*b*
ethical decision-making process, 138–142, 140*f*
ethical dilemma, 123–124, 131, 133
ethical rights, 132
ethical standards, 607
ethics
categories of, 122
committees on, 132
definition of, 123
delegation and, 405–406
of health insurance practices, 494–497
in home health care, 365
incivility and, 421–422
key concepts in, 124–127, 129–130, 132
in nursing research, 602–604
systems of, 134–136
terminology in study of, 122–124
See also American Nurses Association (ANA) Code of Ethics; bioethics; code of ethics
ethnic minority(ies)
growth of population of, 544
insurance coverage for, 545
See also culture(s)
ethnography, 607
euthanasia, 167–169. *See also* right to die
evidence-based medicine (EBM), 581
Evidence-Based Nursing, 593

evidence-based practice (EBP), 6, 38–39, 581–582, 589, 607
versus best practice, 593–594
goals and features of, 601
incorporation of, 582, 598, 604–606, 606*b*
informatics and, 435
on-the-job research in, 436
organizations for, 601
quality care and, 390
relation of nursing to, 597*b*
systematic reviews *versus* primary research in, 598–599
usefulness of information in, 599
See also evidence reports; nursing research
evidenced-based health care (EBHC), 581
evidence reports, 589
evaluation of, 593
sources of, 590–592*b*, 593
types of evidence in, 589, 593
executive branch, 458, 459*b*
executive order, 467
exercise, 246–247, 251–252
expanded practice. *See* advanced practice registered nurse (APRN)
experience rating system, 490
experiential learning (trial and error), 582
experimental research design, 607
expert power, 13
exploratory study, 607
externship, 230
extraordinary treatments, 162
eye contact, 291–292, 558
eye donation, 155

F
face transplant, 156, 157–158
false imprisonment, 186
fast-track education programs, 88
Federal Emergency Management Agency (FEMA), 652
Federal Trade Commission (FTC), 633
feedback loop, 54–55
Feldenkrais, Moshe, 641
Feldenkrais method, 641
felony, 179
fetal tissue research, 149–150
fidelity, 125
First-Aid/CPR class, 649
fiscal note, 466
Fletcher, Joseph, 134
Flexner, Abraham, 5
followers, 265–267, 266*t*
food, organic, 631–632
Food and Drug Administration (FDA), 632, 633, 638
Ford, Loretta C., 33–34, 468
foreign graduate nurse, 103
forensic nursing, 674–677, 680
formalistic system of ethics. *See* deontology
Franklin, Benjamin, 24
Fry, Elizabeth, 24
Fujita, Tetsuya, 646
functional nursing, 279–280, 280*t*

G
gallows humor, 337
gem (crystal) therapy, 641
general systems theory, 52–55
generator, portable, 652
Genetic Information Nondiscrimination Act (GINA), 147–148
genetic research, 147–149

genetic screening, 148–149
Gerontological Nursing Interventions Research Center, 601
Gerontological Society of America (GSA), 570
Gerson, Max, 641
Gerson therapy, 641
goal setting, 248
Goodrich, Annie W., 33, 101
Good Samaritan Act, 192
governance, 270–271, 270*f*. *See also* leadership; management
government
    local, 459*b*
    organizational structure of, 460*b*
    state, 459*b*
    three branches of federal, 458, 459*f*, 460–461
governors, state, 470
grassroots organizations, 113
grassroots politics, 455, 470
Great Depression, 25
Gretter, Lystra E., 137
grief, stages of. *See under* difficult clients
grounded theory, 607
group dynamics, 277–279
guided imagery (visualization), 532, 641, 644. *See also* meditation

H

Hampton, Isabel Adams Robb, 32, 33
Hanberry, Pat, 159
hazmat suit, 664
Healing Matrix, 618–620, 619*b*
healing touch, 641
health
    concept of, 51
    in Johnson Behavioral System Model, 65
    in King Model of Goal Attainment, 60
    in Neuman Health-Care Systems Model, 66
    in Orem Self-Care Model, 58
    in Roy Adaptation Model, 57
    U.S. *versus* world indicators of, 360
    in Watson Model of Human Caring, 61
    World Health Organization definition of, 615
health care
    ethics of child, 174–175
    as industry, 357
    restriction of expensive treatments in, 162
    expenditures on, 492, 566, 570, 571
health-care plans
    how to identify quality, 379*b*
    types of, 362*b*
health-care proxy. *See* durable power of attorney for health care
    (DPOAHC)
health-care reform
    adapting other countries' approaches to, 513
    American Nurses Association (ANA) position on, 504
    critical thinking in debate on, 488
    debate on, 497–504
    history of, 487, 489–491
    nature of, 521–524
    need for, 491–497
    nurses as partners in, 485–486, 513–514
    See also Affordable Care Act (ACA) of 2010
health-care system(s)
    in Canada, 359–360
    changes in, 72–73
    cost-containment measures in, 360–361, 486, 512
    effects of aging population on, 357
    levels of service in, 363

settings in, 363–371
    in third-world nations, 358
    types of, 357–358, 358*t*
    See also health care; health-care plans
health-care team members, 10, 11*t*
health deviation self-care, 58
Healthfinder (website), 444
health informatics, 432. *See also* informatics
health insurance
    private, 362*b*
    unethical practices of, 494–497, 498*t*
    See also health-care system(s), types of
Health Insurance Portability and Accountability Act (HIPAA)
    of 1996, 188, 442, 496
health insurance purchasing cooperative (HIPC), 369
health literacy, 512
health outcomes
    baccalaureate degrees and improved, 96
    in U.S., 494
Health Promotion Model, 68
Healthy People 2020, 383, 571
Heller, Joseph, 641
Hellerwork, 641
Henderson, Virginia, 588
herbalism, 621*b*, 623, 634–636, 638, 641–642
heritage consistency, 543
Heritage Foundation, 509
heroic measures, 162
Herzberg, Frederick, 274–275
Hinduism, 21
Hippocrates, 22, 122
Hippocratic Oath, 22
HIRRE honor code, 422
historical study, 607
HIV and AIDS, 169–170
Ho, Sinwan, 556
holism, 616, 626. *See also* integrative health care
holistic nursing, 529. *See also* spiritualism
home health care, 363–365, 449
homeopathy, 642
homeowners insurance, 649, 650
homologous recombination, 147
Honest Herbal, The, 638
horizontal (lateral) violence, 315, 414, 415, 423–425
Hosea, 521
hospice, 369
Hospital Care Quality Information from the Consumer Perspective
    (HCAHPS), 378
Hospital Consumer Assessment of Healthcare Providers and Systems
    Survey (HCAHPS), 681
hospitals, 366–367
    early military, 23
    how to identify quality, 379*b*
    magnet, 73, 392, 454–455
hospital skills, 77
hot zones, 664
housekeeping bill, 466
Human Genome Project, 149
human interaction theory of management, 267, 269
human (option) rights, 132
humor, gallows, 337
humor therapy, 642
Hussein, Saddam, 661
hydrotherapy, 642
hypnotherapy, 642
hypothesis, 38, 607

I

ICD-10, 683
ideology(ies), 457–458
illness, conventional *versus* holistic view of, 626–627
imagery, 530
"I" message, 293
immigrants, 542–543, 544. *See also* culture(s)
impeaching the witness, 189
Incident Management System (IMS), 654
incivility, 413–416
    continuum of, 413*f*
    ethical prohibitions to, 421–422
    in media, 411
    in nursing education, 416–421, 417*b*
    spiral of, 423, 423*f*
    in workplace, 422–425
    See also civility
independence of practice, 9–10
Independent Payment Advisory Board (IPAB), 500
indigenous medical systems, 620*b*
individual certification, 103–104
induced abortion, 146
Industrial Revolution, 24
informatics, 391
    definitions of, 431–432, 433, 434
    evidence-based practice and importance of, 435
    health-care cost cutting and, 431
    human factors in, 436–438
    models of, 432–433
    as specialty, 433–434
    technology, nursing theory, function, and, 433
information, 432
    explosion of, 436
    principles for access to, 437*b*
information science, 432
informed consent
    children and, 173–174
    contextual, 531
    definition of, 607
    exceptions to, 194
    genetic screening and, 148
    key elements of, 605*b*
    litigation and, 193–194
    non-English-speaking clients and, 556
    in nursing research, 603–604
    sharing of client data and, 442
ingested or applied substances, 618, 619*b*
initiation rite, 419
inpatient, 363
input, 54, 55
insecurity and conflict, 301–302
Institute for Healthcare Improvement (IHI), 390, 591*b*
Institute of Medicine (IOM)
    competencies of, 75, 77*b*
    Crossing the Quality Chasm report by, 412
    health-care quality recommendations by, 376–377
    priorities for research by, 584, 585*b*
    report on future of nursing by, 74–75
institutional licensure, 103
institutional review board (IRB), 602–603, 607
instrumental interventions, 622*b*, 623
insurance
    homeowners, 649, 650
    liability, 200–202, 201b
    See also health insurance
integrative healer, 626*b*

integrative health care, 611–612
    classification of
        Healing Matrix, 618–620, 619*b*
        NCCAM, 620, 620–622*b*, 623
    complementary and alternative medicine and, 615–616
    definition of, 615, 642
    difference between conventional medicine and, 623–625, 624*b*, 626–627
    discussion with client about, 638
    federal support for, 613–614, 616
    glossary of terms related to, 640–644
    holistic approach of, 625–626
    lack of validation and regulation of, 636
    nutrition and diet in, 631–632
    placebo response and, 628–630
    principles of, 626*b*
    questions nurses should ask about, 636–637, 637*b*
    reasons for use of, 616–618, 617*b*
    self-care in, 628
    sources of information about, 637–638
    See also individual types of alternative practices
intentional infliction of emotional distress, 186
Interactive Community Simulation Environment for Community Health Nursing. *See* Community Health Nursing Serious Game
interdisciplinary (interprofessional) education, 93–95
International Association of Forensic Nurses (IAFN), 674, 675
International Center for the Integration of Health and Spirituality (ICIHS), 532*b*
International College of Integrative Medicine (ICIM), 638
International Council of Nurses (ICN), 101, 112, 588
International Medical and Surgical Response Team (IMSuRT), 653
International Parish Nurse Resource Center, 531*b*
Internet
    code of conduct for, 422
    evaluating sources on, 7–8
    personal reputation on, 242–243
    personal Web page on, 235
    politics and, 461–462
    as resource for consumers, 444
    as resource for nursing research information, 590–592*b*
    as resource for professionals, 444
    as resource on herbalism, 638
internship, 230
interprofessional education, 93–95
interventions. *See* Iowa Interventions Project
interview, job. *See* job interview
invasion of privacy, 188
in vitro fertilization, 150
Iowa Interventions Project, 39–41, 40*b*
iridology, 642
Isaiah, 521
Issues in Practice
    10 commandments of disaster preparedness, 651
    caring for relatives at work site, 15
    client autonomy, 166
    communication, 307
    compassion fatigue, 233
    complaining behavior, 344–348
    conflict of interest in funding storefront clinic, 115
    cultural aspects of organ donation, 551–552
    cultural conflict, 560–561
    distributive justice, 128
    ethical dilemmas, 131, 133
    health-care reform debate and critical thinking, 488

leadership/management case studies
  poor staff performance, 402–403
  revolving staff, 268
lobbying, 474–475
malpractice, 35, 182, 184–185
managing change in workplace, 282, 298
politics, 479
refusal of treatment for religious reasons, 534
reporting of child abuse, 171
scenarios in legal/criminal issues, 678–679
short staffing in an emergency, 600
spirituality of the elderly, 574–575
tube feedings, heroic measures, and death with dignity, 161
Issues Now
  civility and job satisfaction, 426
  client education, 387
  disaster victims and scam artists, 667–670
  evaluating Internet sources, 7–8
  exercise myths, 246–247
  federal support for integrative medicine, 613–614
  five "rights" of medication administration, 447–448
  handling anxiety about NCLEX, 207
  Healthy People 2020, 383
  informed consent and non-English-speaking clients, 556
  minority nurses, 547
  Mobile Acute Care for the Elderly (MACE), 569
  nursing home falls, 368
  nursing research, 584–585
  professional nurse coach, 400
  travel nursing, 31

J

Jefferson, Thomas, 468
Jin Shin Jyutsu, 642
Joanna Briggs Institute, 590*b*
job
  versus career, 10
  definition of, 4
job interview, 239–242
  fashion do's and don'ts of, 239–240*b*
  questions interviewees should ask during, 241*b*
  worst mistakes in, 241*b*
job search
  cover letter and, 236, 236*b*
  employer requirements and, 231
  employer's response to application, 237
  interview and, 239–240*b*, 239–242, 241*b*
  interview follow-up and, 243–244
  personal reputation on Internet and, 242–243
  personal Web page and, 235
  portfolio and, 237, 238*b*, 239
  résumé and, 231–232, 231*b*, 234–235
  sample follow-up letter and, 243*b*
Johnson, Dorothy E., 64
Johnson, Lyndon Baines, 489
Johnson Behavioral System Model, 56*t*, 64–65
Johnson v. Women's Hospital, 186
Joint Commission (JC), 104
  guidelines for incivility by, 421
  National Patient Safety Goals of, 382
  sentinel events and, 384
  on teamwork, 93–94
Joint Committee on Nursing, 25
Joint Statement on Academic Progression for Nursing Students and Graduates, 391
Journal of Transcultural Nursing, 562

journals, peer-reviewed, 7
judicial branch, 458, 459*b*, 460
junk insurance policy, 495
just culture organization, 391
justice, 125, 128

K

Kaiser Family Foundation (KFF), 491, 511
Kasper, Anna, 157–158
Keck, Schessler v., 187
Kennedy, John F., 489
Kevorkian, Jack, 167
kinesiology, applied, 640
King, Martin Luther Jr., 468
King Model of Goal Attainment, 56*t*, 60–61
Kluger, Lawrence, 556
Knight Hospitallers, 27
knowledge, 432
knowledge, skills, and attitudes (KSAs), 75, 76
Kübler-Ross's stages of grief, 319
Kyslinger v. United States, 387

L

ladder programs, 87–89
"Lady of Light," 26
laissez-faire leadership, 258, 258*t*
lamp (nursing symbol), 26–27
language, nursing. *See* nursing, language of
Lao-tzu, 521
lateral (horizontal) violence, 315, 414, 415, 423–425
law(s), 123
  civil, 180
  common, 179
  criminal, 179–180
  sources of, 178–179, 179*b*
  statutory, 178–179
  See also legislation
leadership
  case studies in
    poor staff performance, 402–403
    revolving staff, 268
  key behaviors of, 261–263, 270*f*
  key qualities of, 263–265, 263*b*
  versus management, 269–270
  theories of, 257–261
  transformational, 425, 425*b*
  See also governance; management
leadership-style theory, 258–260, 258*t*
Lean Six Sigma quality-improvement program, 385–386
Leapfrog Group, 378, 380–381
legal nurse consultant, 676
legal obligation, 130
legal (welfare) rights, 132
legislation
  enactment process of, 465–466
  non-passage of, 477
  sources of, 463–465
legislative branch, 459*b*, 460–461
legislator, 14
legitimate power, 14
liability insurance, 200–202, 201*b*
libel, 187
liberal (progressive), 457
libertarian, 458
library, principles for access to, 437*b*
licensed practical nurse (LPN), 10, 86–87, 407*f*

licensed vocational nurse (LVN), 86–86
licensure, 9
    examinations for, 101. *See also* National Council Licensure Examination (NCLEX)
    history of, 100–101
    for practical/vocation nurses, 86
    purpose of, 187*b*
    revocation of, 100*b*, 202
    types of, 102–103
    universal, 101–102
Licensure, Accreditation, Certification, and Education (LACE), 107, 109
life assistance services, 364
life expectancy, 494
life-prolonging measures, 160–162
light and color therapy, 642
lines of defense (client-system boundary), 66
linkedin.com, 235
litigation. *See* lawsuit, malpractice
living will, 163–165, 167, 194
    checklist for evaluation of, 163*b*
    common questions about, 194*b*
    See also advance directive
Lloyd, Lavinia. *See* Dock, Lavinia Lloyd
lobbyist/lobbying, 455–456, 464, 473–475
long-term care facility, 367
loyalty, 321

M
magnet hospitals, 73, 392, 454–455
magnet therapy, 642
malpractice, 180–186
    considerations for nursing, 181*b*
    types of, 186–188
malpractice lawsuits
    alternatives to, 193
    common issues in, 193–197
    examples of, 184–185, 203
    possible defenses against, 191–193
    prevention of, 197–200
    process of, 188–191
Maltese cross, 27
managed care organization (MCO), 361, 362*b*
management
    care delivery models and, 279–281, 280*t*
    case studies in
        poor staff performance, 402–403
        revolving staff, 268
    competition and, 278–279
    group dynamics and, 277–278
    leadership *versus*, 269–270
    motivational theory and, 274–275
    theories of, 267, 269
    workplace changes and, 275–277, 282, 298
    See also case management/manager; governance; leadership
manager
    budgeting by, 271–272
    key behaviors of, 269, 270*f*
    unit staffing by, 273–274
mandatory licensure, 102
manipulation (bodywork therapy), 618, 619*b*, 622*b*, 623
Man-Living-Health Model, 67
mantra, 642
mantra meditation. *See* transcendental meditation (TM)
marijuana, medical. *See* cannabis, medical
Maslow, Abraham, 274
Maslow's hierarchy of needs, 313, 313*f*

massage, 644. *See also* bodywork therapies
master's ladder, 88
master's programs, 89–90
McCain, John, 491
media and politics, 461–463
mediation, 193, 306
Medicaid, 362*b*, 566–567, 568, 570
Medical Disaster Response (MDR), 656
medical doctors. *See* physicians
medical errors, 129
    categories of, 438
    incivility and, 414
medical home, 94
medical informatics, 431. *See also* informatics
medical records
    advantages and disadvantages of paper, 439*b*
    documentation guidelines for, 200*b*
    lawsuit prevention and, 199
    lawsuits and electronic, 188
    Nursing Minimum Data Set (NMDS) and, 435
    purposes of, 438
    unified nursing language for, 434, 434*b*
    See also electronic health record (EHR)
Medical Reserve Corps, 653, 660
Medicare, 566, 567
    definition of, 362*b*
    "never events" and, 390
    Part D program of, 491
Medicare and Medicaid Act of 1965, 489
medication
    errors with, 438
    five "rights" of administration of, 447–448
    nocebo effect and, 531
    remembered wellness (placebo effect) and, 530–531, 628–630
    Western, 634
medicine, conventional (orthodox), 623–625, 643
Medieval Ages, 23
meditation, 530, 531–532, 642. *See also* guided imagery (visualization)
MEDLINE, 435–436
Megan's Law, 464
megavitamin therapy, 642
mental (psychic) therapy, 619, 619*b*
mercy killing, 167
meridians, 642
meta-ethics, 122
metaparadigm, 608
MICROMEDEX, 638
middle-range theory(ies), 67–68
midwife. *See* nurse midwife
military hospitals, early, 23
mind-body medicine, 621*b*, 623, 642
mind-cure. *See* meditation
minority nurses, 544, 547
miscarriage, 146
misdemeanor, 179
Mobile Acute Care for the Elderly (MACE), 569
model, 39
modular nursing, 280*t*, 281
Montague, Mildred, 84
Moore, Thomas, 526
moral obligation, 132
moral philosophy, 123
moral (ethical) rights, 132
morals, 123
Mosaic Code of Laws, 21
motivational theory, 274–275

motivation-hygiene theory, 274–275
moveabletype.com, 235
moxibustion, 642
multicultural health care. *See* transcultural nursing
multiculturalism, 542–543
multitasking, 536
music therapy, 642
mustard gas, 663
Mutual Recognition Model for Nursing Licensure, 101
mystics, 528–529

N
Napoleon, 476
National Center for Complementary and Alternative Medicine
       (NCCAM), 638
    classification of CAM by, 620, 620–622*b*, 623
    definition of CAM by, 615
National Center for Disaster Fraud, 669
National Center for Nursing Research (NCNR), 588
National Council Licensure Examination (NCLEX), 101, 205–206
    background information on, 218–219
    changes in, 206
    cognitive-ability levels component in, 208–210
    difficulty level of questions in, 217
    grading of, 216–217
    handling anxiety about taking, 207
    number of questions in, 215–216
    nursing-process questions in, 210–211
    preparing for day of, 222–223
    questions about client health needs in, 206, 208
    questions about delegation in, 406
    study strategies for, 220–222
    time limit of, 216
    types of questions in, 212–215, 212–215*f*
    zone of knowledge in, 217–218
National Council Licensure Examination Computerized Adaptive
       Testing, for Registered Nurses (NCLEX-RN, CAT),
       101, 206
National Disaster Medical System (NDMS), 653
National Guideline Clearinghouse, 591*b*, 593, 601
National Healthcare Workforce Commission, 510
National Institute of Nursing Research (NINR), 588
National Institutes of Health (NIH), 592*b*
National League for Nursing (NLN), 9, 32, 109–110
    accreditation of schools by, 84, 85–86, 110
    program on incivility by, 417
National League for Nursing Accrediting Commission (NLNAC),
       84. *See also* Accreditation Commission for Education in
       Nursing (ACEN)
National League for Nursing Testing Division, 101
National Library of Medicine, 591*b*
National Nurses Response Team (NNRT), 660
National Nursing Accrediting Service, 84
National Oceanic and Atmospheric Administration (NOAA)
       weather radio, 648
National Organ Transplant Act, 153
National Patient Safety Foundation (NPSF), 512
National Research Act, 602–603
National Security Administration (NSA), 443
National Student Nurses' Association (NSNA), 111–112
natural foods, 631–632
naturopathy, 642–643
navigator, nurse, 682–683
NCLEX. *See* National Council Licensure Examination (NCLEX)
near-death experience, 527–528
negative feedback, 55

negligence, 180, 191–192. *See also* malpractice; malpractice lawsuits
negotiation, 304–305
nerve agent, 662–663
networking, 16–17
Neuman, Betty, 65, 525
Neuman Health-Care Systems Model, 56*t*, 65–67
neurolinguistic programming, 643
"never events," 390
New York Nurses Association licensure bill, 101, 101*b*
Nightingale, Florence, 5, 26–27, 28, 30, 100–101
    on delegation, 396
    nursing pin designed by, 27, 28*f*
    research by, 587
    spirituality and, 524–525
Nightingale Pledge, 137
Nightingale School of Nursing, 83
Nixon, Richard, 489
nocebo effect, 531
nonassertive communication, 289–290
non-English-speaking clients, communication with, 553, 554*b*, 555,
       557–558
nonfeasance, 180
nonmaleficence, 126, 169
nonprobability sampling, 608
nonsummativity, 60*n*
nonverbal communication, 291
nonverbal communication blockers, 293–294
nonverbal communication builders, 291–292
normative ethics, 122, 134
norm-referenced examination, 205–206
Notes on Nursing, 587
Nuremberg Code, 602, 603*b*, 608
nurse coach, 400
nurse midwife, 104
nurse practice acts, 100, 197
nurse practitioner (NP), 11–12, 91
    founding of practice of, 33–34
    increased health-care demand and, 486
    proposed blended roles of clinical nurse specialist and, 12
    state limitations on advanced practice of, 454
nurse residency (NR) program, 230
nurse-run health center, 370–371
nurse(s)
    employment settings of, 73
    high demand for. *See* nursing shortage
    minority, 544, 547
    new roles for, 674–685
    origin of term, 22
    types of, 10–12
Nurses Associated Alumnae of the United States and Canada, 32,
       101
Nurses Network (website), 444
Nurses of Pennsylvania, 113
nursing
    autonomy and independence of, 9–10
    concept of, 52
    definitions of
        American Nurses Association, 20
        International Council of Nurses, 588
    forensic, 674–680
    functional, 279–280, 280*t*
    future trends of, 17
    hierarchy in, 23–24
    historical leaders of, 29–30, 32–34. *See also* Nightingale, Florence
    history of U.S., 24–26
    in Johnson Behavioral System Model, 65

in King Model of Goal Attainment, 61
language of, 434, 434*b*
modular, 280*t*, 281
in Neuman Health-Care Systems Model, 66–67
in Orem Self-Care Model, 59
origins of, 20–24
primary care, 280–281, 280*t*
in Roy Adaptation Model, 57
as spiritual calling, 535
symbols of, 26–29
team, 25, 280, 280*t*
traits of, 5–6, 9
travel, 31
in Watson Model of Human Caring, 64
Nursing and Health Care, 472
nursing cap, 28–29, 29*f*
nursing diagnosis, 57
nursing home (retirement center), 367, 368
nursing intervention classifications systems (Iowa Project), 39–41, 40*b*
Nursing Minimum Data Set (NMDS), 435
nursing models and theories
    challenges to, 68–69
    key concepts of, 41, 51–52
    major, 55, 56*t*, 57–61, 64–67
    middle-range, 67–68
    nursing activities and, 39
    trends for future in, 67
nursing orders, 23–24, 28
Nursing Organizations Alliance, 424
nursing pin, 27–28, 28*f*
nursing research
    centers for, 587, 588
    competencies in, 601–602
    critical discernment of findings of, 588–589, 593–594
    definitions of, 583, 608
    ethical issues in, 602–604
    evidence reports and, 589, 590–592*b*, 593
    federal funding for, 584
    gap between practice and, 595–598
    glossary of terms in, 607–608
    goals and purposes of, 583
    informed consent in, 603–604
    Institute of Medicine's priorities for, 584, 585*b*
    origins and development of, 587–588
    priorities for, 586
    process of, 594–595
    research problem and, 586
    See also evidence-based practice (EBP)
nursing science, 6, 432
nursing shortage
    education and, 17, 228
    elderly population and, 572
    origins of current, 371
    political activism and, 453
    projected estimates of, 17, 62, 79, 229
    reasons for, 229
    state licensing of foreign nurses and, 454
    stress caused by, 371
nutrition and diet, 631–632. *See also* diet therapies

O

Obama, Barack, 73*b*, 164, 489, 490, 491, 508, 513, 566
obesity rates, 494
obligations, 130, 132
occupation, 4

occupational health clinic, 366
Occupational Safety and Health Administration workplace violence guidelines, 422
occurrence insurance policy, 201
Office of Human Research Protections, U.S. (OHPR), 592*b*
Office of Research Integrity, U.S., 592*b*
"old boy" system, 16
Omnibus Budget Reconciliation Act (OBRA) of 1990
    advance directives and, 164
    durable power of attorney and, 130
Oncology Nursing Society, 601
Online Journal for Knowledge Synthesis in Nursing, 593
Online Journal of Clinical Innovations, 593
open curriculum, 88
open system, 54
operational budget, 271–272
option rights, 132
Orem, Dorothea E., 58
Orem Self-Care Model, 56*t*, 58–60
organ donation. *See* transplantation and organ donation
organic foods, 631–632
Organisation for Economic Co-operation and Development (OECD), 492
organizational certification (accreditation), 104
organizations
    grassroots, 113
    specialty, 113–114
    See also professional organizations
organizer, political, 476, 476*b*
organ transplantation. *See* transplantation and organ donation
Oriental medicine, 620, 620*b*
orthodox (conventional) medicine, 623–625, 643
orthomolecular medicine, 621*b*, 623, 643
osteopath, 625
osteopathy, 643
outcomes. *See* health outcomes
outpatient, 363
output, 54, 55, 57
oxygen therapy, 643

P

paraphrasing, 293
paraverbal communication, 291
paraverbal communication builders, 292–293
parish nurse, 370, 531*b*
Parse, Rosemary Rizzo, 67
participative leadership. *See* democratic (transformational) leadership
partisanship, 456
passive euthanasia, 167
passive obedience, 558–559
paternalism, 130
patient. *See* client(s)
Patient Self-Determination Act of 1990, 194
Patriot Act, 443
Pavalko, Eliza, 5
peer abuse, 414
peer evaluation, 279
peer-reviewed journal, 7
Pender, Nola, 68
permissive licensure, 102
persecutor (difficult coworker), 314–316
personal directive. *See* living will
personality, 310–311
personality disorder, 314
personal matters, 557

personal protective equipment, 654–655, 664
personal space, 558
PES (problem-etiology-signs and symptoms) statement, 57, 58*f*
Pew Commission
    report on competencies and professional education, 62–63, 74
    report on health professions, 74
pharmacist, 11*t*
pharmacognosy, 643
pharmacological interventions, 622*b*, 623
phenomenology, 521, 608
phosgene, 664
physical therapist, 11*t*
physician assistant, 11*t*
physicians
    collaboration between case managers and, 682, 682*b*
    conflict between nursing profession and, 105–106
    how to identify quality, 379*b*
    nursing in office of, 366
    per capita, 494
    types of, 11*t*
Physician's Desk Reference for Herbal Medicine, 638
phytotherapy/phytomedicine (herbalism), 621*b*, 623, 634–636, 638,
        641–642, 643
PICO question, 586, 608
pin, nursing (symbol), 27–28, 28*f*
Pio, Padre, 528
placebo effect (remembered wellness), 530–531, 628–630
plaintiff, 180
Plato, 521
pocket veto, 466
polarity therapy, 643
policy limit cap, 495
political action, 16
    alliances and, 471–472, 476
    constituent groups' levels of involvement in, 467–468
    definition and examples of, 455
    elections and, 468–470
    grassroots, 113, 455, 470–471
    issue awareness and, 472
    lobbying and, 455–456, 464, 473–475
    organizing nurses and, 476
    questions to ask while engaging in, 477
    reasons for engaging in, 467
    tactics and, 472–473
politics
    definition of, 455
    media and, 461–463
    nursing-related issues in, 453–454
    partisanship, self-interest, and ideology in, 456–457
    personal effects of, 479
    See also legislation
Pomahac, Bohdan, 156
Population, Intervention, Comparison and Outcome (PICO)
        question, 586, 608
population trends
    of the elderly, 571
    of ethnic minorities, 543–544
populist, 457–458
portable generator, 652
portfolio, 237, 238*b*, 239
position, 4
positive feedback, 54–55
post-traumatic stress disorder (PTSD), 249–250
power, 12–14, 16–17
power of attorney. *See* durable power of attorney for health care
        (DPOAHC)

practical nursing programs, 86–87
pralidoxime chloride, 663
prana, 643
prayer, 530
preceptorship, 230
preferred provider organization (PPO), 362*b*
prepper, 647
preventive care, 356. *See also* primary care
primary care, 363, 369
primary care nursing, 280–281, 280*t*
primary research, 598–599
primary research source, 608
principle system of ethics. *See* deontology
privacy
    HIV and AIDS and, 169
    invasion of, 188
private insurance, 362*b*
privileged communication, 188
problem solving, 300–301
process approach for defining a profession, 4
process consent, 604, 608. *See also* informed consent
procrastination, 250–251
profession, 4
professional, 4
professional development continuum, 4
professional education. *See* education
professional identity, 10
professionalism, 4, 16
professional misconduct, 183
professional nurse coach, 400
professional organizations, 9, 109–14
    collective power of, 14, 16, 109
        grassroots, 113
        special-interest, 113–114
    See also individual organizations
professional portfolio, 237, 238*b*, 239
professional standards review organization (PSRO), 360
progressives, 457
prospective payment system (PPS), 361
psychiatric nurse, 680
psychologist, clinical, 11*t*
public health department, 363
public service function of nursing, 6
Purnell's Model for Cultural Competence, 549*b*

Q

qi (chi), 641
Qi Gong, 643
Quackwatch (website), 638
qualitative research design, 594–595, 595*b*, 608
Quality and Safety Education for Nurses (QSEN) competencies,
        75–76, 77*b*, 386, 388
    opposing opinions about, 388
    workplace incivility and, 423–424
quality assurance (QA), 377
quality care
    client education and, 387
    definition of, 376
    federal initiatives for, 389
    how to identify, 379*b*
    key factors to, 390–392
    methods to measure and improve, 377–378, 380–382, 384–386
    nursing education and, 386, 388, 391
Quality Improvement Organization (QIO), 389
quality indicators (QIs), 381
quantitative research design, 583*f*, 594–595, 596*b*, 608

quasi-experimental design, 608
Quinlan, Karen, 160

R
radical, 458
random sample, 608
reactive change, 276
Reagan, Ronald, 457
reciprocity in licensing, 103
recommended daily allowances (RDAs), 633
Red Cross. *See* American Red Cross
referent power, 13
reflexology, 643
registered nurse (RN), 10, 102. *See also* advanced practice registered
    nurses (APRNs)
Registered Nurse Safe Staffing Act, 273
registration of nurses, 102
rehabilitation center, 367
reiki, 643
reincarnation, 527
relationship-task orientation theory of leadership, 260
relaxation response, 643
relaxation therapy, 643
reliability, 608
religion, 522–523. *See also* spirituality
religious orders, 23–24, 28
remembered wellness, 530–531, 629–630
Renaissance, 23
replication study, 608
rescission (cancellation of insurance), 495–496, 498*t*
research. *See* nursing research
research design(s), 594–595, 608
research-practice gap, 595–598
research process, 608
research randomizers, 592*b*
residency program. *See* nurse residency (NR) program
resistance (client-system boundary), 66
respect, 320
respiratory (choking) agents, 663–664
respiratory therapist, 11*t*
responsibility. *See* accountability and responsibility
restating, 293
résumé, 231–232, 231*b*, 234–235
retirement center (nursing home), 367, 368
review of literature, 608
Revolutionary War (U.S.), 24
reward source of power, 13–14
Richtman, Max, 568
rights, 132
rights-in-trust, 175
right to die, 162–167
right to know, 126–127
risk management, 381–382
RN-coder/auditor, 683–684
Robb, Isabel. *See* Hampton, Isabel Adams Robb
Robert Wood Johnson Foundation Transforming Care at the
    Bedside, 390
Roe v. Wade, 146
Rogers, Martha, 525, 532
role conflict, 226–227
Rolf, Ida, 643
rolfing, 643
Romney, Mitt, 489
Roosevelt, Franklin Delano, 489
Roosevelt, Theodore, 489, 490
Rosen technique, 643

Roy, Callista, 55
Roy Adaptation Model, 55, 56*t*, 57, 58*f*
rule utilitarianism, 134
rural primary care, 369. *See also* telehealth

S
Safe Nursing and Patient Care Act of 2007, 73*b*
safety officer, client, 684–685
Sai Baba, 528
sample, 608
sampling
    Internet sources for information on, 592*b*
    nonprobability, 608
SAVE (secondary assessment of victim endpoint), 656
SBAR system, 198–199
Schessler v. Keck, 187
Schiavo, Terri, 160, 195, 526
school-based health care, 365–366
schools of nursing, 83–84. *See also* education
Science of Unitary Human Beings, 525, 532
scientific inquiry, 583*f*, 608
secondary care, 363
secondary exposure, 664
secularism, 523
selective serotonin reuptake inhibitors (SSRIs), 336
self, components of, 519, 520*f*
self-care
    in integrative health care, 628
    for nurses, 251
    in Orem Self-Care Model, 58
self-determination. *See* autonomy (self-determination)
self-healing, 625, 628
self-interest, 456–457
senior citizens. *See* elderly population
sentinel event, 384
sexual assault nurse examiner (SANE), 675–676
sexual harassment
    by client, 337–339
    by coworker, 336–338
Shamanism, 643–644
shi (chi), 641
shiatsu, 644
short staffing during emergency, 600
Sigma Theta Tau, 112, 424, 590*b*
Silver, Henry K., 33
simple triage and rapid treatment (START), 656
situation, background, assessment, recommendation (SBAR)
    system, 198–199
situational theory of leadership, 261
situation ethics. *See* utilitarianism
Six Sigma quality-improvement program, 384–386
slander, 187
sneak (difficult coworker), 316–319
social worker, 11*t*
Socrates, 456
soul, the, 526–527
sound therapy, 644
special interest group, 464
specialty organizations, 113–114
speech patterns, 555, 557
spiritual distress, 525–526
spiritual healing, 644
spirituality
    in children, 528
    definitions of, 521, 522
    developmental stages of, 524

differences between religion and, 522–523
of the elderly, 574–577
elements involved in, 537, 537*f*
Florence Nightingale and, 524–525
health effects of, 577
maintaining and restoring balance through, 535–536
manifestations of, 523–524
in nursing education, 576
in nursing theories, 525
practices incorporating, 530–533
questions for assessing, 529
questions of, 522*b*
refusal of treatment and, 534
from religious perspective, 522
secular, 523
sense of oneness and, 520–521
the soul and, 526–527
themes of, 522
spiritual therapy, 619, 619*b*
staffing, 273–274. *See also* short staffing during emergency
staff-to-client ratios, 273, 371–373
standard of best interest, 129–130
standards of care, 196–197
START (simple triage and rapid treatment), 656
state boards of nursing (SBNs), 100
State University of New York (SUNY), 593
statute of limitations, 189
statutory law, 178–179
St. Augustine, 521
stem cell research, 149–150
stimuli. *See* environment, in Roy Adaptation Model; input
stress
    communication blockers and, 296–297
    eliminating source of, 299
    major, 249–250
    problem-solving techniques for, 250–252
    See also burnout
stressors, 66
subcultures, 542
submissive (nonassertive) communication, 289–290
supervision skills, 404
supplements, dietary, 632–633
supportive leadership. *See* democratic (transformational) leadership
Swanson, Kristen M., 68
Swedish massage, 644
symbols, nursing, 26–29
Synthetic Training Research Evaluation and Extrapolation Tool (mSTREET), 79
system, 53
systematic reviews, 598
systems theory, general, 52–55

T

Tabata v. Charleston Area Medical Center, 441
tactics, 472–473
tai chi, 644
Tavenner, Marilyn, 452
team nursing, 25, 280, 280*t*
teamwork and health-care quality, 390–391
technology
    communication and, 431
    well-designed, 438, 439*b*
    See also informatics
telehealth, 369, 445, 449
teleology (utilitarianism), 134
tertiary care, 363

theoretical framework, 608
theory, 38
Theory of Caring, 68
therapeutic communication techniques. *See* communication builders
therapeutic massage, 644
therapeutic relationship, 81
therapeutic touch (TT), 532, 623, 631*b*, 644
therapists, physical and respiratory, 11*t*
Thomas v. Corso, 203
throughput, 54
time management, 250
time-motion theory of management, 267
tissue and eye donation, 155
To Err Is Human: Building a Safer Health System, 376
tornadoes, 646–647
tort, 180
    intentional, 186–187
    quasi-intentional, 187–188
    unintentional, 180–186
tortfeasor, 180
total quality management (TCM). *See* continuous quality improvement (CQI)
touching, 557–558
Trager, Milton, 644
Trager therapy, 644
trait approach for defining a profession, 5
trait theory of leadership, 257–258, 258*b*
transcendental meditation (TM), 530, 531–532
transcultural nursing
    information sources for, 562
    recognition of traditional health practices in, 548–549
Transcultural Nursing Society, 562
transformational (democratic) leadership, 258–259, 258*t*, 425, 425*b*
transformational theory of leadership, 261
transplantation and organ donation, 151–155, 154*b*
    child donors, 152
    cultural aspects, 551–552
    determination of death, 152–153
    donor registries, 159
    faces and hands, 156, 157–158
    tissue and eye, 155
transprofessional education. *See* interprofessional education
travel nursing, 31
triage, 656–657
triage nurse, 655–656
trial (in lawsuit), 189–190
trial and error, 582
Tri-Council for Nursing Issues, 391
Truman, Harry, 489
truthfulness. *See* veracity
tube feeding, 160, 161
tuition debt, 453–454
two plus two (2 + 2) program, 88

U

unavoidable accident, 192
unfunded mandate, 466
Unified Nursing Language System (UNLS), 434
Uniform Anatomical Gift Act (UAGA) of 1968, 153
uninsured, 493
United Network for Organ Sharing (UNOS), 153
United States, Kyslinger v., 387
unit service assistant. *See* unlicensed assistive personnel (UAP)
universal self-care, 58

University of Minnesota, Evidence-Based Health Care Project, 591*b*
unlicensed assistive personnel (UAP), 10, 102–103, 281, 398*b*. *See also* delegation
U.S. Department of Health and Human Services (HHS)
    Culturally and Linguistically Appropriate Services (CLAS) Standards, 554–555*b*
    Healthy People 2020, 383
U.S. Postal Service and dietary supplements, 633
utilitarianism, 134–135

V
validity, 608
validity, internal, 592*b*
value-based purchasing (VBP), 486
values, 122–123. *See also* cultural values
variable, 608
ventilation and right to die, 162
veracity, 126, 129
verbal communication, 291
verbal communication blockers, 294–295
verbal communication builders, 293
vertical violence, 315, 415
vesicants (blister agents), 663
veto, 466
vibration medicine, 644
Vietnam War, 26
violence
    lateral (horizontal), 315, 414, 415, 423–425
    vertical, 315, 415
    workplace, 422–424. *See also* incivility
virtual learning, 79–80
visualization (guided imagery), 532, 641, 644. *See also* meditation
vocational nursing programs, 86–87
volunteer health agency, 370
Voting Rights Act, 469

W
Wade, Roe v., 146
Wald, Lillian, 32, 33, 101
water cure (hydrotherapy), 642
Watson, Jean, 61, 68, 525
Watson Model of Human Caring, 56*t*, 61, 64, 412, 412*b*
weapons of mass destruction. *See* biological weapons/agents; chemical weapons (CW)
weather radio, 648
websites. *See* Internet
welfare rights, 132
wellness and holism, 626–627
whiner *versus* winner, 265*t*. *See also* complaining and whining
whole body vibration (WBV), 631
Women's Hospital, Johnson v., 186
wordpress.com, 236
Work Complexity Assessment (WCA), 40–41
workplace issues
    burnout, 244–245, 244*b*, 248–249, 535
    instituting change in workplace, 275–277, 282
    major stressful events, 249–250
    problem-solving techniques for stress, 250–252
    reality shock, 226–227
    transition from student to professional, 230
    workplace incivility, 422–425. *See also* incivility
World Health Organization (WHO), 94
    on alternative health care, 611–612
    definition of health by, 615
    informed consent template by, 592*b*
World War I, 25
World War II, 25

Y
yin/yang, 644
yoga, 644
"you" messages, 294
Young, Ron, 159